T

D0305705

HEART FUNCTION AND METABOLISM

Proceedings of the Eighth International Meeting of the
International Study Group for Research
in Cardiac Metabolism
[now the International Society for Heart Research]
26—29 May, 1976
Tokyo, Japan

Organized by the
Japanese Study Group for Research in Cardiac Metabolism,
the Japanese Circulation Society, and
the Japan Heart Foundation

Recent Advances in Studies on Cardiac Structure and Metabolism

Series Editor: G. Rona (*formerly with the late E. Bajusz*)

Volume   1: **MYOCARDIOLOGY** (edited by E. Bajusz and G. Rona)
Volume   2: **CARDIOMYOPATHIES** (edited by E. Bajusz and G. Rona, with A. J. Brink and A. Lochner)
Volume   3: **MYOCARDIAL METABOLISM** (edited by N. S. Dhalla)
Volume   4: **MYOCARDIAL BIOLOGY** (edited by N. S. Dhalla)
Volume   5: **MYOCARDIAL CELL DAMAGE** (edited by A. Fleckenstein and N. S. Dhalla)
Volume   6: **PATHOPHYSIOLOGY AND MORPHOLOGY OF MYOCARDIAL CELL ALTERATIONS** (edited by A. Fleckenstein and G. Rona)
Volume   7: **BIOCHEMISTRY AND PHARMACOLOGY OF MYOCARDIAL HYPERTROPHY, HYPOXIA, AND INFARCTION** (edited by P. Harris, R. I. Bing, and A. Fleckenstein)
Volume   8: **THE CARDIAC SARCOPLASM** (edited by P.-E. Roy and P. Harris)
Volume   9: **THE SARCOLEMMA** (edited by P.-E. Roy and N. S. Dhalla)
Volume 10: **THE METABOLISM OF CONTRACTION** (edited by P.-E. Roy and G. Rona)
Volume 11: **HEART FUNCTION AND METABOLISM** (edited by T. Kobayashi, T. Sano, and N. S. Dhalla)
Volume 12: **CARDIAC ADAPTATION** (edited by T. Kobayashi, Y. Ito, and G. Rona)

Recent Advances in Studies on
Cardiac Structure and Metabolism, Volume 11

HEART FUNCTION AND METABOLISM

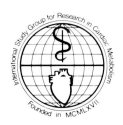

Edited by

Tachio Kobayashi, M.D., F.A.C.C.
Professor and Chairman, Showa University Fujigaoka Hospital,
Honorary Professor
of the University of Tokyo
Tokyo, Japan

Toyomi Sano, M.D., F.A.C.C.
Professor and Head
Institute for Cardiovascular Diseases
Tokyo Medical and Dental University
Tokyo, Japan

and

Naranjan S. Dhalla, Ph.D., F.A.C.C.
Professor of Physiology
Faculty of Medicine
University of Manitoba
Winnipeg, Canada

UNIVERSITY PARK PRESS
Baltimore · London · Tokyo

UNIVERSITY PARK PRESS
International Publishers in Science and Medicine
233 East Redwood Street
Baltimore, Maryland 21202

Copyright © 1978 by University Park Press

Typeset by The Composing Room of Michigan, Inc.
Manufactured in the United States of America by
Universal Lithographers, Inc., and
The Optic Bindery Incorporated

Library of Congress Cataloging in Publication Data

International Society for Heart Research.
   Heart function and metabolism.

   (Recent advances in studies on cardiac structure and metabolism; v.11)
   "Proceedings of the eighth international meeting of the International Study
Group for Research in Cardiac Metabolism (presently, the International Society
for Heart Research) 26–29 May 1976, Tokyo, Japan."
   Includes bibliographies and indexes.
   1. Heart – Congresses.   2. Metabolism – Congresses.
I. Kobayashi, Tachio, 1912–   II. Sano, Toyomi, 1918–   III. Dhalla,
Naranjan S.   IV. Title.   V. Series.

RC667.R4   Vol. 11 [QP111.2]   616.1'2'008s   [599'.01'16]
ISBN 0-8391-0671-8   77-25145

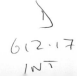

6 12·17
INT

Contents

Contributing Authors xi
Editorial Foreword xv

Electrophysiological Aspect

Fozzard, H. A., and Gibbons, W. R.: Electrical Aspects of Excitation-
    Contraction Coupling 3
Coraboeuf, E.: Ionic Basis of Excitation Mechanism in Cardiac Muscle . 11
Jongsma, H. J., Lieberman, M., de Bruijne, J., and van Ginneken, A. C.
    G.: Electrophysiological Properties of Rat Heart Cells *in vitro* and in
    Tissue Culture 19
Noma, A., and Irisawa, H.: Voltage-clamp Experiments by Double
    Micorelectrode Technique in Rabbit Sinoatrial Node Cell 25
Hiraoka, M., and Sano, T.: Role of Slow Inward Current on Premature
    Excitation in Ventricular Muscle 31
Goto, M., Yatani, A., and Tsuda, Y.: Membrane Calcium Current in
    Cardiac Excitation: Effects of ATP and Related Substances and
    Sodium Pump on Bullfrog Atrium 37
Saikawa, T., Arita, M., and Nagamoto, Y.: Electrically Induced
    Automaticity in Canine Ventricular Myocardium 45
MacKaay, A. J. C., Bleeker, W. K., and Bouman, L. N.: Chronotropic
    Effects of Calcium and Magnesium Ions at Different Temperatures . . 51
Ikemoto, Y., and Goto, M.: Effects of Acetylcholine and Cyclic
    Nucleotides on the Bullfrog Atrial Muscle 57
Nishi, K., Yoshikawa, Y., and Takenaka, F.: Contribution of an
    Electrogenic Sodium Pump to the Response of Sinoatrial Node
    Cells to Acetylcholine 63
Ruiz-Ceretti, E., Ponce Zumino, A., and Schanne, O. F.: Selective
    Effects of TTX and Verapamil on the Upstroke Components of the
    Action Potential from the Atrioventricular Node 69
Abe, Y., Aomine, M., and Goto, M.: Dual Effects of Fluoride on the
    Action Potential, Contraction, and Membrane Currents in Frog
    Atrial Muscle 73
Sano, T., Hiraoka, M., and Sawanobori, T.: Effects of Anoxia and
    Metabolic Inhibitors on Reaction of the Fast Sodium System 79
Arita, M., Nagamoto, Y., and Saikawa, T.: Intraventricular Conduction
    Disturbance due to Delayed Recovery from Ventricular Inactivation
    in Chlorpromazine-Treated Dogs 85

Biophysical Aspect

Ebashi, S., Kitazawa, T., Kohama, K., and van Eerd, P.-C.: Calcium
    Ion in Cardiac Contractility 93
Wikman-Coffelt, J., and Mason, D. T.: Binding of Divalent Cations by
    Canine Cardiac Myosin: Differences in Normal Right and Left
    Ventricles Dependent upon Number of Light Chains 103

Cole, H. A., Frearson, N., Moir, A. J. G., Perry, S. V., and Solaro, R. J.:
Phosphorylation of Cardiac Myofibrillar Proteins   111

Prasad, K., Singal, P. K., and Khatter, J. C.: Frequency-Dependent
Changes in the Electromechanical and (Na^+, K^+)-ATPase Activity of
Cardiac Muscle   121

Saeki, Y., and Kamiyama, A.: Possible Mechanism of Rate-Dependent
Change of Contraction in Dog Ventricular Muscle: Relation to
Calcium Movements   131

Horackova, M., and Vassort, G.: Sodium-Calcium Exchange in
Regulation of Cardiac Contraction   137

Vassort, G., Roulet, M. J., Mongo, K., and Clapier-Ventura, R.:
Relaxation of Frog Myocardium   143

Mashima, H.: Dynamics of Contraction with Special Reference to
Calcium   149

Toll, M. O.: Isometric Dynamic Response of Mammalian Heart Muscle
due to Step Changes in the Calcium Concentration of the Perfusing
Medium   159

Templeton, G. H., Willerson, J. T., Platt, M. R., and Weisfeldt, M.:
Contraction Duration and Diastolic Stiffness in Aged Canine Left
Ventricle   169

Reichel, H., and Baumann, K.: Delay in Diastolic Restitution of Full
Myocardial Contractility in Guinea Pig Atrium   175

Kurihara, S., and Sakai, T.: Effect of Rapid Cooling on Toad and
Guinea Pig Cardiac Muscles   181

Koizumi, T., Ito, Y., and Ebashi, S.: Regulatory Mechanism in
Arterial Smooth Muscle Contraction   185

Biochemical Aspect

Schwartz, A., Levey, G. S., Entman, M. L., Ezrailson, E. G., Van
Winkle, W. B., Bornet, E. P., and Pitts, B. J. R.: Modulation of
Calcium in the Heart   195

Will, H., Blanck, J., Smettan, G., and Wollenberger, A.: Quench-Flow
Measurements of Initial Rates of Ca^{2+} Accumulation by Isolated
Cardiac Sarcoplasmic Reticulum   199

Katz, A. M., Shigekawa, M., Repke, D. I., and Hasselbach, W.: Calcium
Transport and Release by the Sarcoplasmic Reticulum   205

Dunnett, J., and Nayler, W. G.: Substitution of Phosphate for Oxalate
in the Study of Calcium Accumulation and Release by Cardiac
Microsomal Fractions   213

Besch, H. R., Jr., Jones, L. R., and Watanabe, A. M.: Intact Vesicles
of Membranes in Cardiac Microsomes: Evidence from Vectorial
Properties of Integral Enzymes   219

Jones, L. R., Besch, H. R., Jr., and Watanabe, A. M.: Subcellular
Localization of Cardiac Adenylate Cyclase: Sarcolemma or
Sarcoplasmic Reticulum?   227

St. Louis, P. J., and Sulakhe, P. V.: Isolation and Enzymatic
Characterization of Guinea Pig Cardiac Sarcolemma   235

Sulkahe, P. V., and St. Louis, P. J.: Characteristics of Heart
Sarcolemmal Calcium Transport System and Effect of Protein Kinase
on Sarcolemmal Calcium Accumulation   241

Ma, S. K., Sulakhe, P. V., and Leung, N. L.-K.: Binding of [^{3}H] Atropine
by Cardiac Plasma Membrane-Enriched Fractions   249

Sulakhe, S. J., and Sulakhe, P. V.: Properties of Membrane-Bound and
Soluble Guanylate Cyclase of Cardiac and Skeletal Muscle   257

Tada, M., and Kirchberger, M. A.: Significance of the Membrane
Protein Phospholamban in Cyclic AMP-Mediated Regulation of
Calcium Transport by Sarcoplasmic Reticulum   265

Matsushita, S., Sakai, M., Kaku, T., Nakano, T., Kuramoto, K., and
Murakami, M.: An Adenosine 3':5'-Monophosphate-Dependent
Protein Kinase from Human Heart   273

Ohmori, F., Tada, M., Kinoshita, N., Matsuo, H., Sakakibara, H.,
Nimura, Y., and Abe, H.: Effect of Protein Kinase Modulator on
cAMP-Dependent Protein Kinase-Catalyzed Phosphorylation of
Phospholamban and Stimulation of Calcium Transport in Cardiac
Sarcoplasmic Reticulum   279

Kirchberger, M. A., and Raffo, A.: Phosphoprotein Phosphatase-
Catalyzed Dephosphorylation of the 22,000-dalton Phosphoprotein
of Cardiac Sarcoplasmic Reticulum   285

Ito, Y., Matsuura, H., and Ueba, Y.: Effect of Increased cAMP Content
on Intracellular Distribution of Calcium and Contractility in Rabbit
Heart   293

Krasnow, N.: Interaction of Lanthanides with Muscle Microsomes   297

Metabolic Aspect

Tamura, M., Oshino, N., and Chance, B.: A New Spectroscopic
Approach to Cardiac Energy Metabolism   307

Aoyagi, R., Aizawa, K., Aizawa, Y., Murooka, H., Tamura, K., and
Matsuoka, M.: Significance of Heat Loss in Energetics of Left
Ventricle   313

Isselhard, W., Eitenmüller, J., Mäurer, W., Welter, H., and Reinecke, H.:
Myocardial Adenine Nucleotides after Infusion of Adenosine   319

Anazawa, S., Saito, N., and Nagano, M.: Metabolic Effect of pH on
Myocardium of Heart-Lung Preparation   325

Imai, S., Otorii, T., Takeda, K., Katano, Y., and Nakagawa, Y.: Effects
of Catecholamines on Myocardial Energy Metabolism as Studied by an
Organ Redoximeter   335

Tsuyuguchi, N., Matsumura, K., Mikawa, K., Niki, T., Mori, H., and
Aki, K.: Characteristics of Energy Metabolism in Specialized Heart
Muscle of Bovine Heart   343

Whitty, A. J., Dimino, M. J., Elfont, E. A., Hughes, G. W., and Repeck,
M. W.: Transmural Mitochondrial Differences in Myocardium   349

Wahlqvist, M. L., Carlson, L. A., Kaijser, L., Löw, H., Peak, H. J.,
Wide, L., and Wilmshurst, E. G.: Uptake and Release of Immuno-
reactive Insulin in Coronary Circulation in Man: Studies at Rest, During
Exercise, and During Glucose and Insulin Infusions.   355

Schraven, E.: Influence of Carbocromene on Free Fatty Acid
Metabolism of the Heart 363
Kako, K. J., Vasdev, S. C., and Zaror-Behrens, G.: Metabolism of
Individual Fatty Acids in Heart Muscle 369
Takenaka, F., and Takeo, S.: Myocardial Fatty Acid and Cardiac
Performance 379
Julien, P., Dagenais, G. R., Gailis, L., and Roy, P.-E.: Free Fatty Acid
Content of Myocardial Interstitial Spaces of Dog 385

Pharmacological Aspect

Klaus, W., and Fricke, U.: Electrolyte-Dependence of Cardiac Glycoside
Actions at the Cellular and Subcellular Level 393
Akera, T., Olgaard, M. K., and Brody, T. M.: Effect of Ouabain on
Sodium Movement in Cardiac Cells 401
Taubert, K., Willerson, J. T., Shapiro, W., and Templeton, G. H.:
Effects of Hypoxia and Digitalis Glycosides on Myocardial Stiffness . 407
McNeill, J. H.: Thyroid Hormone-Induced Supersensitivity to the
Cardiac Phosphorylase-Activating Effect of Adrenergic Amines 413
Nawrath, H.: Evidence for Opposing Influences of Cyclic GMP and
Cyclic AMP on Force of Contraction in Mammalian Myocardium ... 419
Watanabe, A. M., Hathaway, D. R., and Besch, H. R., Jr.: Mechanism of
Cholinergic Antagonism of the Effects of Isoproterenol on Hearts
from Hyperthyroid Rats 423
Watanabe, A. M., Besch, H. R., Jr., Hathaway, D. R., Harris, R. A., and
Farmer, B. B.: Alpha-Adrenergic Reduction of Cyclic Adenosine
Monophosphate Levels in Rat Ventricular Myocardial Cells 431
Nagao, T., Ikeo, T., Sato, M., Nakajima, H., and Kiyomoto, A.: Effect
of Diltiazem on Calcium- and Noradrenaline-Induced Contractions in
Isolated Rabbit Aorta 437
Imanaga, I.: Effects of Insulin on Mammalian Cardiac Muscle 441
Hashimoto, K., Tsukada, T., and Matsuda, H.: Inotropic and
Chronotropic Effects of Antiarrhythmic Agents on Isolated Blood-
Perfused Canine Ventricular Tissue 451
Harrow, J. A. C., and Dhalla, N. S.: Influence of Quinidine on ATP-
Linked Calcium Binding by Heart Mitochondria and Microsomes ... 457
Saito, T., Okazaki, K., Ohta, N., Sakata, S., Tanaka, Y., Tonogai, R.,
Tomino, T., and Tomino, Y.: Effects of Halothane Anesthesia on
Myocardial Contractility, Coronary as well as Systemic
Hemodynamics, and Myocardial Metabolism in Dogs 467
Merin, R. G., Kumazawa, T., and Luka, N. L.: Dose-Dependent
Depression of Cardiac Function and Metabolism by Inhalation
Anesthetics in Chronically Instrumented Dogs 473
Kumazawa, T., Nakagawa, M., Ikezono, E., Sunamori, M., Hatano, R.,
Yamamoto, N., and Suzuki, T.: Effects of Morphine and Halothane
on Canine Cardiac Function Before and After Cardiopulmonary
Bypass 481
Nayler, W. G., and Fassold, E.: Effect of Acetaldehyde on Functioning
of Cardiac Muscle at the Ultrastructural Level 489

Szelkeres, L., Vághy, P., Bor, P., and Csete, K.: Possible Mode of
  Action of Nitroglycerin on Heart Mitochondria   495
Rudolph, W., Fleck, E., Dirschinger, J., Loracher, C., Brandt, R., Redl,
  A., and Hall, D.: Alterations of Left Ventricular Function and
  Regional Myocardial Blood Flow Induced by Nitrates in Patients with
  Coronary Artery Disease   501

Pathophysiological Aspect

Bricknell, O. L., and Opie, L. H.: Glycolytic ATP and Its Production
  During Ischemia in Isolated Langendorff-Perfused Rat Hearts   509
Williamson, J. R., Steenbergen, C., Deleeuw, G., and Barlow, C.:
  Control of Energy Production in Cardiac Muscle: Effects of Ischemia
  in Acidosis   521
Peng, C. F., Murphy, M. L., Kane, J. J., and Straub, K. D.: Alteration
  in Calcium Metabolism in Mitochondria Isolated from Ischemic and
  Reperfused Myocardium   533
Yamagami, T., Shibata, N., Akagami, H., and Toyama, S.: Relationship
  between Energy Liberation and Utilization in Ischemic Cardiac
  Muscle   539
Ueno, T., Ishiyama, T., Morita, Y., Hatanaka, Y., Azuma, J., Tanimoto,
  T., Ogura, K., Hasegawa, H., Shin, K. S., Tsukamoto, N., and
  Yamamura, Y.: An Experimental Study of the Effect of Glucose-
  Insulin-Potassium Solution on Energy Metabolism of Infarcted
  Cardiac Muscle   549
Minaga, T., Takeda, K., Nakamura, T., Kizu, A., and Ijichi, H.: Effect
  of Xanthine Oxidase Inhibitor on Myocardial Ischemia   555
Boink, A. B. T. J., Ruigrok, T. J. C., Maas, A. H. J., and Zimmerman,
  A. N. E.: Calcium Paradox: Changes in High-Energy Phosphate
  Compounds of Isolated Perfused Rat Hearts   559
Ruigrok, T. J. C., Boink, A. B. T. J., and Zimmerman, A. N. E.:
  Influence of ATP or Oxygen plus Substrate on Occurrence of the
  Calcium Paradox   565
Gudbjarnason, S., Oskarsdottir, G., Hallgrimsson, J., and Doell, B.:
  Role of Myocardial Lipids in Development of Cardiac Necrosis   571
Ishiyama, T., and Morita, Y.: Energy Liberation in Abnormal Cardiac
  Muscle   583
Seki, I., Akioka, H., Goto, N., Kamide, H., Higashihara, Y., Mori, K.,
  Fujiwara, K., Higuchi, H., Terauchi, A., Sano, I., Imaoka, A.,
  Kishima, N., Kondo, K., and Miyagi, T.: Myocardial Energy and
  Electrolyte Metabolism during Exercise in Patients with Circulatory
  Disease   589
Suzuki, Y., Yamazaki, N., Ogawa, K., Mizutani, K., Kakizawa, N.,
  Yamamoto, M., Okubo, M., and Yoshida, M.: Studies on Myocardial
  Mitochondria in Failing Dog Hearts: Studies by Electron Spin
  Resonance (ESR) Spectrometry   599
Tanimoto, T., Ishiyama, T., Morita, Y., Hatanaka, Y., Ueno, T., Azuma,
  J., Ogura, K., Hasegawa, H., Yamamura, Y., and Tsukamoto, N.:
  Disturbance of Myocardial Energy Liberation in Experimental
  Charcoal Embolism of Canine Pulmonary Artery   605

Honda, T., Goshima, K., Takeda, Y., and Miwatani, T.: A Bacterial
Cardiotoxin: Thermostable Direct Hemolysin Produced by *Vibrio
parahaemolyticus* 609
Goshima, K., Honda, T., Takeda, Y., and Miwatani, T.: Stopping of
Spontaneous Beating of Cultured Mouse and Rat Myocardial Cells
by a Toxin (Thermostable Direct Hemolysin) from *Vibrio
parahaemolyticus* 615
Seyama, I., Irisawa, H., Takeda, T., and Miwatani, T.: Increase in
Membrane Conductance and Positive Inotropic Action of Hemolysin
Produced by *Vibrio parahaemolyticus* on Rabbit Myocardium 621

Author Index 627
Subject Index 631

Contributing Authors

Abe, H., *Osaka* (Japan)
Abe, Y., *Fukuoka* (Japan)
Aizawa, K., *Niigata* (Japan)
Aizawa, Y., *Niigata* (Japan)
Akagami, H., *Osaka* (Japan)
Akera, T., *East Lansing, Mich.* (U.S.A.)
Aki, K., *Tokushima* (Japan)
Akioka, H., *Takatsuki* (Japan)
Anazawa, S., *Tokyo* (Japan)
Aomine, M., *Fukuoka* (Japan)
Aoyagi, R., *Niigata* (Japan)
Arita, M., *Fukuoka* (Japan)
Azuma, J., *Osaka* (Japan)
Barlow, C., *Philadelphia, Pa.* (U.S.A.)
Baumann, Kl., *Hamburg* (Federal Republic of Germany)
Besch, H. R., Jr., *Indianapolis, Ind.* (U.S.A.)
Blanck, J., *Berlin-Buch* (German Democratic Republic)
Bleeker, W. K., *Amsterdam* (The Netherlands)
Boink, A. B. T. J., *Utrecht* (The Netherlands)
Bor, P., *Szeged* (Hungary)
Bornet, E. P., *Houston, Tex.* (U.S.A.)
Bouman, L. N., *Amsterdam* (The Netherlands)
Brandt, R., *Munich* (Federal Republic of Germany)
Bricknell, O. L., *Cape Town* (South Africa)
Brody, T. M., *East Lansing, Mich.* (U.S.A.)
Carlson, L. A., *Canberra* (Australia)
Chance, B., *Philadelphia, Pa.* (U.S.A.)
Clapier-Ventura, R., *Orsay* (France)
Cole, H. A., *Birmingham* (England)
Coraboeuf, E., *Orsay* (France)
Csete, K., *Szeged* (Hungary)
Dagenais, G. R., *Ste-Foy, Que.* (Canada)
de Bruijne, J., *Amsterdam* (The Netherlands)
Deleeuw, G., *Philadelphia, Pa.* (U.S.A.)
Dhalla, N. S., *Winnipeg, Man.* (Canada)
Dimino, M. J., *Detroit, Mich.* (U.S.A.)
Dirschinger, J., *Munich* (Federal Republic of Germany)
Doell, B., *Reykjavik* (Iceland)
Dunnett, J., *London* (England)
Ebashi, S., *Tokyo* (Japan)
Eitenmüller, J., *Koln* (Federal Republic of Germany)
Elfont, E. A., *Detroit, Mich.* (U.S.A.)
Entman, M. L., *Houston, Tex.* (U.S.A.)
Ezrailson, E. G., *Houston, Tex.* (U.S.A.)

Farmer, B. B., *Indianapolis, Ind.* (U.S.A.)
Fassold, E., *London* (England)
Fleck, E., *Munich* (Federal Republic of Germany)
Fozzard, H. A. *Chicago, Ill.* (U.S.A.)
Frearson, N., *Birmingham* (England)
Fricke, U., *Koln* (Federal Republic of Germany)
Fujiwara, K., *Takatsuki* (Japan)
Gailis, L., *Ste-Foy, Que.* (Canada)
Gibbons, W. R., *Burlington, Vt.* (U.S.A.)
Goshima, K., *Osaka* (Japan)
Goto, M., *Fukuoka* (Japan)
Goto, N., *Takatsuki* (Japan)
Gudbjarnason, S., *Reykjavik* (Iceland)
Hall, D., *Munich* (Federal Republic of Germany)
Hallgrimsson, J., *Reykjavik* (Iceland)
Harris, R. A., *Indianapolis, Ind.* (U.S.A.)
Harrow, J. A. C., *Winnipeg, Man.* (Canada)
Hasegawa, H., *Osaka* (Japan)
Hashimoto, K., *Niigata* (Japan)
Hasselbach, W., *Heidelberg* (Federal Republic of Germany)
Hatanaka, Y., *Osaka* (Japan)
Hatano, R., *Tokyo* (Japan)
Hathaway, D. R., *Indianapolis, Ind.* (U.S.A.)
Higashihara, Y., *Takatsuki* (Japan)
Higuchi, H., *Takatsuki* (Japan)
Hiraoka, M., *Tokyo* (Japan)
Honda, T., *Osaka* (Japan)
Horackova, M., *Halifax, N.S.* (Canada)
Hughes, G. W., *Detroit, Mich.* (U.S.A.)
Ijichi, H., *Kyoto* (Japan)
Ikemoto, Y., *Fukuoka* (Japan)
Ikeo, T., *Saitama* (Japan)
Ikezono, E., *Tokyo* (Japan)
Imai, S., *Niigata* (Japan)
Imanaga, I., *Ishikawaken* (Japan)
Imaoka, A., *Takatsuki* (Japan)
Irisawa, H., *Hiroshima* (Japan)
Ishiyama, T., *Osaka* (Japan)
Isselhard, W., *Koln* (Federal Republic of Germany)
Ito, Y., *Kobe* (Japan)
Ito, Y., *Tokyo* (Japan)
Jones, L. R., *Indianapolis, Ind.* (U.S.A.)
Jongsma, H. J., *Amsterdam* (The Netherlands)
Julien, P., *Ste-Foy, Que.* (Canada)
Kaijser, L., *Uppsala* (Sweden)
Kakizawa, N., *Nagoya* (Japan)
Kako, K. J., *Ottawa, Ont.* (Canada)

Kaku, T., *Tokyo* (Japan)
Kamide, H., *Takatsuki* (Japan)
Kamiyama, A., *Yokohama* (Japan)
Kane, J. J., *Little Rock, Ark.* (U.S.A.)
Katano, Y., *Niigata* (Japan)
Katz, A. M., *New York, N.Y.* (U.S.A.)
Khatter, J. C., *Saskatoon, Sask.* (Canada)
Kinoshita, N., *Osaka* (Japan)
Kirchberger, M. A., *New York, N.Y.*
(U.S.A.)
Kishima, N., *Takatsuki* (Japan)
Kitazawa, T., *Sendai* (Tokyo)
Kiyomoto, A., *Saitama* (Japan)
Kizu, A., *Kyoto* (Japan)
Klaus, W., *Koln* (Federal Republic of
Germany)
Kohama, K., *Tokyo* (Japan)
Koizumi, T., *Tokyo* (Japan)
Kondo, K., *Takatsuki* (Japan)
Krasnow, N., *Brooklyn, N.Y.* (U.S.A.)
Kumazawa, T., *Rochester, N.Y.* (U.S.A.)
Kumazawa, T., *Tokyo* (Japan)
Kuramoto, K., *Tokyo* (Japan)
Kurihara, S., *Tokyo* (Japan)
Leung, L.-K., *Saskatoon, Sask.* (Canada)
Levey, G. S., *Miami, Fl.* (U.S.A.)
Lieberman, M., *Amsterdam* (The
Netherlands)
Loracher, C., *Munich* (Federal Republic of
Germany)
Löw, H., *Uppsala* (Sweden)
Luka, N. L., *Rochester, N.Y.* (U.S.A.)
Ma, S. K., *Saskatoon, Sask.* (Canada)
Maas, A. H. J., *Utrecht* (The
Netherlands)
Mackaay, A. J. C., *Amsterdam* (The
Netherlands)
Mashima, H., *Tokyo* (Japan)
Mason, D. T., *Davis, Calif.* (U.S.A.)
Matsuda, H., *Niigata* (Japan)
Matsumura, K., *Tokushima* (Japan)
Matsuo, H., *Osaka* (Japan)
Matsuoka, M., *Niigata* (Japan)
Matsushita, S., *Tokyo* (Japan)
Matsuura, H., *Kobe* (Japan)
Mäurer, W., *Koln* (Federal Republic of
Germany)
McNeill, J. H., *Vancouver, B. C.* (Canada)
Merin, R. G., *Rochester, N.Y.* (U.S.A.)
Mikawa, K., *Tokushima* (Japan)
Minaga, T., *Kyoto* (Japan)
Miwatani, T., *Hiroshima* (Japan)
Miyagi, T., *Takatsuki* (Japan)
Mizutani, K., *Nagoya* (Japan)
Moir, A. J. G., *Birmingham* (England)
Mongo, K., *Orsay* (France)

Mori, H., *Tokushima* (Japan)
Mori, K., *Takatsuki* (Japan)
Morita, Y., *Osaka* (Japan)
Murakami, M., *Tokyo* (Japan)
Murooka, H., *Niigata* (Japan)
Murphy, M. L., *Little Rock, Ark.* (U.S.A.)
Nagamoto, Y., *Fukuoka* (Japan)
Nagano, M., *Tokyo* (Japan)
Nagao, T., *Saitama* (Japan)
Nakagawa, M., *Tokyo* (Japan)
Nakagawa, Y., *Niigata* (Japan)
Nakajima, H., *Saitama* (Japan)
Nakamura, T., *Kyoto* (Japan)
Nakano, T., *Tokyo* (Japan)
Nawrath, H., *Mainz* (Federal Republic of
Germany)
Nayler, W. G., *London* (England)
Niki, T., *Tokushima* (Japan)
Nimura, Y., *Osaka* (Japan)
Nishi, K., *Kumamoto* (Japan)
Noma, A., *Hiroshima* (Japan)
Ogawa, K., *Nagoya* (Japan)
Ogura, K., *Osaka* (Japan)
Ohmori, F., *Osaka* (Japan)
Ohta, N., *Tokushima* (Japan)
Okazaki, K., *Tokushima* (Japan)
Okubo, M., *Nagoya* (Japan)
Olgaard, M. K., *East Lansing, Mich.* (U.S.A.)
Opie, L. H., *Cape Town* (South Africa)
Oshino, N., *Philadelphia, Pa.* (U.S.A.)
Oskarsdottir, G., *Reykjavik* (Iceland)
Otorii, T., *Niigata* (Japan)
Peak, H. J., *Canberra* (Australia)
Peng, C. F., *Little Rock, Ark.* (U.S.A.)
Perry, S. V., *Birmingham* (England)
Pitts, B. J. R., *Miami, Fl.* (U.S.A.)
Platt, M. R., *Dallas, Tex.* (U.S.A.)
Ponce Zumino, A., *Sherbrooke, Que.*
(Canada)
Prasad, K., *Saskatoon, Sask.* (Canada)
Raffo, A., *New York, N.Y.* (U.S.A.)
Redl, A., *Munich* (Federal Republic of
Germany)
Reichel, H., *Hamburg* (Federal Republic
of Germany)
Reinecke, H., *Koln* (Federal Republic of
Germany)
Repeck, M. W., *Detroit, Mich.* (U.S.A.)
Repke, D. I., *New York, N.Y.* (U.S.A.)
Roulet, M. J., *Orsay* (France)
Roy, P.-E., *Ste-Foy, Que.* (Canada)
Rudolph, W., *Munich* (Federal Republic
of Germany)
Ruigrok, T. J. C., *Utrecht* (The
Netherlands)
Ruiz-Ceretti, E., *Sherbrooke, Que.* (Canada)

Saeki, Y., *Yokohama* (Japan)
Saikawa, T., *Fukuoka* (Japan)
Saito, N., *Tokyo* (Japan)
Saito, T., *Tokushima* (Japan)
Sakai, M., *Tokyo* (Japan)
Sakai, T., *Tokyo* (Japan)
Sakakibara, H., *Osaka* (Japan)
Sakata, S., *Tokushima* (Japan)
Sano, I., *Takatsuki* (Japan)
Sano, T., *Tokyo* (Japan)
Sato, M., *Saitama* (Japan)
Sawanobori, T., *Tokyo* (Japan)
Schanne, O. F., *Sherbrooke, Que.* (Canada)
Schraven, E., *Frankfurt* (Federal Republic of Germany)
Schwartz, A., *Cincinnati, Ohio* (U.S.A.)
Seki, I., *Takatsuki* (Japan)
Seyama, I., *Hiroshima* (Japan)
Shapiro, W., *Dallas, Tex.* (U.S.A.)
Shibata, N., *Osaka* (Japan)
Shigekawa, M., *New York, N.Y.* (U.S.A.)
Shin, K. S., *Osaka* (Japan)
Singal, P. K., *Saskatoon, Sask.* (Canada)
Smettan, G., *Berlin-Buch* (German Democratic Republic)
Solaro, R. J., *Birmingham* (England)
Steenbergen, C., *Philadelphia, Pa.* (U.S.A.)
St. Louis, P. J., *Saskatoon, Sask.* (Canada)
Straub, K. D., *Little Rock, Ark.* (U.S.A.)
Sulakhe, P. V., *Saskatoon, Sask.* (Canada)
Sulakhe, S. J., *Saskatoon, Sask.* (Canada)
Sunamori, M., *Tokyo* (Japan)
Suzuki, T., *Tokyo* (Japan)
Suzuki, Y., *Nagoya* (Japan)
Szekeres, L., *Szeged* (Hungary)
Tada, M., *Osaka* (Japan)
Takeda, K., *Kyoto* (Japan)
Takeda, K., *Niigata* (Japan)
Takeda, T., *Osaka* (Japan)
Takeda, Y., *Osaka* (Japan)
Takenaka, F., *Kumamoto* (Japan)
Takeo, S., *Kumamoto* (Japan)
Tamura, K., *Niigata* (Japan)
Tamura, M., *Osaka* (Japan)
Tanaka, Y., *Tokushima* (Japan)
Tanimoto, T., *Osaka* (Japan)
Taubert, K., *Dallas, Tex.* (U.S.A.)

Templeton, G. H., *Dallas, Tex.* (U.S.A.)
Terauchi, A., *Takatsuki* (Japan)
Toll, M. O., *London* (England)
Tomino, T., *Tokushima* (Japan)
Tomino, Y., *Tokushima* (Japan)
Tonogai, R., *Tokushima* (Japan)
Toyama, S., *Osaka* (Japan)
Tsuda, Y., *Fukuoka* (Japan)
Tsukada, T., *Niigata* (Japan)
Tsukamoto, N., *Osaka* (Japan)
Tsuyuguchi, N., *Tokushima* (Japan)
Ueba, Y., *Kobe* (Japan)
Ueno, T., *Osaka* (Japan)
Vághy, P., *Szeged* (Hungary)
Van Eerd, P.-C., *Zurich* (Switzerland)
Van Ginneken, A. C. G., *Amsterdam* (The Netherlands)
Van Winkle, W. B., *Houston, Tex.* (U.S.A.)
Vasdev, S. C., *Ottawa, Ont.* (Canada)
Vassort, G., *Orsay* (France)
Wahlqvist, M. L., *Canberra* (Australia)
Watanabe, A. M., *Indianapolis, Ind.* (U.S.A.)
Weisfeldt, M., *Baltimore, Md.* (U.S.A.)
Welter, H., *Koln* (Federal Republic of Germany)
Whitty, A. J., *Detroit, Mich.* (U.S.A.)
Wide, L., *Canberra* (Australia)
Wikman-Coffelt, J., *Davis, Calif.* (U.S.A.)
Will, H., *Berlin-Buch* (German Democratic Republic)
Willerson, J. T., *Dallas, Tex.* (U.S.A.)
Williamson, J. R., *Philadelphia, Pa.* (U.S.A.)
Wilmshurst, E. G., *Canberra* (Australia)
Wollenberger, A., *Berlin-Buch* (German Democratic Republic)
Yamagami, T., *Osaka* (Japan)
Yamamoto, M., *Nagoya* (Japan)
Yamamoto, N., *Tokyo* (Japan)
Yamamura, Y., *Osaka* (Japan)
Yamazaki, N., *Nagoya* (Japan)
Yatani, A., *Fukuoka* (Japan)
Yoshida, M., *Nagoya* (Japan)
Yoshikawa, Y., *Kumamoto* (Japan)
Zaror-Behrens, G., *Ottawa, Ont.* (Canada)
Zimmerman, A. N. E., *Utrecht* (The Netherlands)

Editorial Foreword

This volume of the series *Recent Advances in Studies on Cardiac Structure and Metabolism* represents a part of the proceedings of the Eighth International Meeting of the International Study Group for Research in Cardiac Metabolism held in Tokyo from May 26–29th, 1976. Selected papers dealing with diverse problems in the area of heart function and metabolism have been arranged in different sections for the convenience of our readers. These sections, which reflect the broad-based interests of the participants in the meeting, deal with electrophysiological, biophysical, biochemical, metabolic, pharmacological, and pathophysiological aspects of heart function and metabolism. In fact, the Tokyo meeting will be considered a landmark in the history of our Society because it was at this meeting that the International Study Group for Research in Cardiac Metabolism was renamed the International Society for Heart Research. This step was essential in view of the ever expanding and varied backgrounds of the members of our Society. As will be apparent from the contents of this book, it is our contention that further insight into cardiac function and metabolism under normal, pharmacological, and pathological situations can only be gained from multidisciplinary approaches.

The link between heart function and heart metabolism has always intrigued investigators in the field of experimental cardiology. It is now well established that ATP derived from oxidative metabolism of different substrates, as well as from the process of glycolysis to some extent, is utilized directly by the contractile machinery and various transmembrane pump operations. Likewise, the participation of calcium in the process of excitation-contraction coupling has also been recognized, and an analogous hypothesis implicating calcium in excitation-metabolic stimulation is emerging rapidly. On the other hand, cAMP has been shown to be a unique substance that is capable of stimulating myocardial function and metabolism markedly; these effects of cAMP appear to be mediated through the phosphorylation of different membrane systems, contractile apparatus, and several enzymes involved in the metabolic processes. It may well be that heart function and metabolism are linked by calcium and ATP, while cAMP plays a regulatory role in these events. It is hoped that the material presented in this book will provide some supportive evidence within the framework of this general concept. If this volume poses more questions than answers to students and investigators engaged in heart research, we will regard it as a success for the nature of scientific enquiry.

We wish to thank the Japanese Study Group for Research in Cardiac Metabolism, Japanese Circulation Society, Japan Heart Foundation, Science Council of Japan, and several pharmaceutical and other companies in Japan for their financial and organizational support. The advice and cooperation of the members of the International Executive and Coordination Committee for planning the program of this meeting are gratefully acknowledged. We also express our sincere gratitude to the editorial staff of University Park Press for their assistance in preparing this book.

HEART FUNCTION AND METABOLISM

Electrophysiological Aspect

Recent Advances in Studies on
Cardiac Structure and Metabolism, Volume 11
Heart Function and Metabolism
Edited by T. Kobayashi, T. Sano, and N. S. Dhalla
Copyright 1978   University Park Press   Baltimore

ELECTRICAL ASPECTS OF
EXCITATION-CONTRACTION COUPLING

H. A. FOZZARD[1]
and W. R. GIBBONS[2]

[1] Departments of Medicine and The Pharmacological and Physiological Sciences,
The University of Chicago, Chicago, Illinois, USA:
[2] Department of Physiology and Biophysics, University of Vermont,
Burlington, Vermont, USA

SUMMARY

Control of contraction in heart muscle is an interesting question partly because it is so complex. Contraction can vary by as much as an order of magnitude under the influence of drugs, or by different patterns of stimulation. Membrane depolarization is the initial determinant of contraction. It appears to be initiated by a membrane Ca current that causes graded release of Ca from a cellular store. This cellular store is quite labile; it is increased by entry of Ca by the transmembrane current and is decreased by a membrane Ca pump. Recovery of contraction requires recovery of the store into a releasable form and recovery of the membrane "trigger" current. A plausible scheme for contraction can be proposed without a direct role of membrane depolarization in Ca release, but a direct effect cannot yet be dismissed. Key future studies will require direct monitoring of the sarcoplasmic reticulum transmembrane potential and cytoplasmic Ca, and definition of the factors controlling the size of the Ca store.

INTRODUCTION

The simple temporal relationship between the cardiac action potential (AP) and contraction suggested that the AP in some way caused the contraction. The AP is a complex ionic event, and it is not immediately obvious which aspect is the one responsible for producing tension. The potassium contracture used by Kuffler and Niedergerke, in its simplist interpretation, demonstrated that membrane depolarization itself was an important link in excitation-contraction coupling (Kuffler, 1946; Niedergerke, 1956). Niedergerke further demonstrated a graded dependence of contracture on voltage and external Ca in the frog ventricle. In the decade subsequent to Niedergerke's work it became apparent that the sarcoplasmic reticulum in fast skeletal muscle was the origin of contractile Ca (for review, see Ebashi and Endo, 1968). Cardiac physiologists assumed

Supported in part by USPHS 11665 (Harry A. Fozzard) and USPHS 14614 (W. Ray Gibbons).

the same mechanism in heart muscle, but this was never compatible with the striking dependence of heart muscle on outside Ca. Certainly cardiac muscle lost its contraction rapidly in a Ca-free medium, so that either the Ca in the cardiac SR was quite labile, or the Ca involved in contraction came from outside the cell.

In the years that followed, we have learned that the cardiac cell has a transmembrane Ca current that is closely linked to contraction (Reuter, 1967). In part, the voltage-dependency of contraction is secondary to the voltage-dependency of this Ca current (Beeler and Reuter, 1970b). However, efforts to correlate this current directly to contraction have been only partially successful (Gibbons and Fozzard, 1975b). One of the most commonly suggested explanations for these properties of heart muscle is that the Ca current acts to fill or replenish a store of Ca in the sarcoplasmic reticulum (SR), which normally contains less Ca than is needed for full activation of contraction. According to this scheme the cell can lower its Ca store to a basal level by a pump. This store could be depleted by repetitive stimulation, unless replenished by the Ca current. Contraction during any individual excitation is heavily dependent on the previous history of the fiber, which determines if the store is full or empty.

Missing from this scheme is a mechanism by which depolarization triggers Ca release. At least two mechanisms have been proposed in skeletal muscle. One suggested mechanism is that a small Ca current causes a regenerative release of Ca from the SR (Ford and Podolsky, 1969; Endo, Tanaka, and Ogawa, 1970). The second suggestion is that the membrane depolarization is somehow transferred to the SR, which has a depolarization-induced Ca permeability change. How these SR, which has a depolarization-induced Ca permeability change. How these mechanisms may function in heart muscle will be reconsidered after we discuss the voltage-dependency of contraction.

VOLTAGE-CLAMP STUDIES

Systematic studies of voltage-tension relations using a double micropipette method of voltage clamping were begun by Fozzard and Hellam (1968) and Morad and Trautwein (1968). They found that contraction in response to a voltage step followed a time course similar to that produced by an AP. The contraction was reduced in amplitude if the size of the voltage step was reduced, producing a voltage-tension relationship very much like that seen by Niedergerke with potassium contractures. Partial contractions could also be produced by short depolarizations. Recovery of contraction was a function of both time and voltage, much in the fashion of contracture recovery of skeletal muscle (Hodgkin and Horowicz, 1960).

These characteristics of contraction are consistent with the concept introduced before, that the voltage-dependency of contraction is through a voltage-

and time-dependent Ca current. This current was first related to contraction by Beeler and Reuter (1970b). They and many others have shown the presence of a transmembrane inward current that is largely dependent on calcium ions for its charge source. For convenience we will refer to this current as calcium current, although there are still important questions regarding its nature. If this putative calcium current is important to the voltage control of contraction, several points can be examined.

Point #1. Voltage Threshold for
Force Development and for Calcium Current Should Be the Same

This finding, reported by Gibbons and Fozzard (1971), occurred when threshold was changed by varying the holding potential prior to the test depolarization. New and Trautwein (1972) examined threshold for calcium current and tension development with variable external Ca and Na concentrations. They state that they were never able to see tension development in the absence of the current. Beeler and Reuter (1970b) found small tension development between threshold for Na current and threshold for Ca current (a "foot" on the voltage-tension relation), which they ascribed to loss of good voltage control because of the large Na current. The experimental evidence seems in favor of this hypothesis, with one exception. Morad and Orkand (1971) failed to find Ca current in their studies of frog ventricle.

The finding of this similar voltage value of threshold is consistent with the idea that the Ca current causes tension, but does not prove it. The relationship could be coincidental; both events could be independent and caused by the same prior event, such as depolarization; or the depolarization could cause intracellular Ca release, which in turn causes a change of sarcolemmal conductance.

If the transmembrane current is an early step in a sequence of events that leads to contractions, then it might be possible to separate the two events temporally. As the fiber recovers its ability to contract, Gibbons and Fozzard (1975b) found that the current indeed recovered faster than the contraction, suggesting that there was at least one intermediate step between the events, which had a slower time course of recovery. Reuter (1973) and Trautwein, McDonald, and Tripathi (1975) found time courses of recovery of Ca current and tension that were coincidental. Their results do not disprove a sequence of events in the contraction process, since the recovery of the secondary process would simply be faster under their experimental conditions than recovery of the primary process.

Gibbons and Fozzard (1975a) reported the puzzling observation that recovery of tension after a depolarizing step was partly a function of the duration of that depolarizing step. Recovery was faster after a long step. While a variety of ideas can be suggested to explain this result, one that is consistent with the two-part process for recovery is that one begins with relaxation of the fiber and the other begins only with repolarization. If the one that is not voltage-dependent is slower than the other, then it has additional time to recover before the voltage-dependent recovery begins. While in no way proved by those experiments, the result is in line with recovery of a step in addition to the calcium current stage that is independent of voltage.

Point #2. If the Membrane Calcium Current is Causative, Then the Tension Should Vary as Some Function of the Current

The early experiments of Beeler and Reuter (1970b) and of New and Trautwein (1972) suggest that a relation exists between the calcium current and the size of the contraction produced by a train of voltage steps after a steady tension response was established (after the staircase). This relation can be seen in a simultaneous plot of current and tension versus voltage, such as that shown by Trautwein (1973) and Vassort (1973). A direct plot of maximal Ca current versus tension on the first beat after a rest was made by Gibbons and Fozzard (1975b), showing a linear relation between tension and the magnitude of small currents near threshold. In their experiments, other currents interfered with measurements over the entire voltage range.

This apparent correlation is reassuring in some respects; however, it does not necessarily imply that the Ca entering through the membrane is the same Ca that activates the contractile proteins. Efforts to calculate the amount of Ca entering via the current give confusing results because of the large number of assumptions that must be made. Certainly there is no reason to expect that tension is a linear function of free cytoplasmic Ca. Direct measurements show a sigmoid relation of tension to the logarithm of Ca (Fabiato and Fabiato, 1975). If the Ca current were directly responsible for contraction, one would expect a threshold amount of current to be required before tension would develop, and an exponential relation between current and tension thereafter. A more plausible suggestion is that the current is an important step in the production of tension, but only one of a sequence.

Support for a close relation between the current and tension is provided indirectly by the observation that the steady-state activation and inactivation properties of the current are almost identical to those of tension (Beeler and Reuter, 1970b; New and Trautwein, 1972; Gibbons and Fozzard, 1971, 1975a,b).

A puzzle that has not been resolved is what happens to contractions as one changes the inside potential to markedly positive values. If the contraction is some simple function of calcium current, then as the inside voltage approaches the Ca equilibrium potential (E_{Ca}) the current should decline and cease. No direct measure of inside Ca for calculation of E_{Ca} is available. Indeed, we expect that Ca_i changes during activation. The activity coefficient of Ca is not necessarily the same inside and outside. Consequently only approximate calculations of E_{Ca} can be made. Further, it has been difficult to accept the experimental values of reversal potential of the Ca current as valid estimates of E_{Ca} because they are so low (Beeler and Reuter, 1970; Ochi, 1970; New and Trautwein, 1972). A plausible explanation of the low values of reversal potential for Ca is that Na can also enter through the same membrane channel, so that the current is a mixed one. While this seems likely, sufficient experimental studies of this have not yet been reported.

Even in the absence of accurate measurements of Ca current at inside-positive voltages, it is appropriate to predict that contraction should be less. The original voltage-tension studies probably did not depolarize enough to test this implication (Fozzard and Hellam, 1968; Beeler and Reuter, 1970b; Gibbons and Fozzard, 1971). Subsequently, Trautwein (1973) showed a decline in calcium current with maintenance of a plateau of tension response. However, Reuter (1973) clearly showed a decline in contraction with depolarization beyond +40 mV. This was also seen under some circumstances by New and Trautwein (1972), Morad and Goldman (1973), and Gibbons and Fozzard (1975a).

A valuable observation was made by Vassort (1973) that would clarify part of this problem. He showed that the contraction of frog atrial muscle was clearly made up of two components—a phasic contraction and a tonic one. When he exposed the tissue to solutions containing Li instead of Na, only the phasic contraction could be seen. Under these conditions the correlation between current and contraction persisted to markedly positive internal potentials. This result may have two origins. In Li-Ringer solution the Ca current may be undistorted by movement of Na ions through that channel. In addition, the internal store of Ca may be altered. In conclusion, it seems apparent that at least one component of tension declines as E_{Ca} is approached, as one would predict if the calcium current is a determining factor in causing contraction.

Point #3. The Ca Current Causes Release of Ca from an Internal Store

In addition to the evidence offered above that the Ca current is a necessary step, but does not supply the Ca directly for contraction, a number of other observations suggest that it somehow releases an intracellular Ca store. During a staircase the tension can be seen to increase or decrease with no change in the Ca current. This is well demonstrated in the studies of Beeler and Reuter (1970b) and New and Trautwein (1972). A complete picture of the events in staircase is difficult to illustrate, because of the influence of resting potential, clamp magnitude, duration, interval, and the composition of the solution bathing the muscle. One conclusion that is generally accepted is that after a change in these factors about 8–10 contractions must occur before a steady state is reached. Because neither the depolarization itself nor the Ca current is changing during this time, both candidates for the trigger are in a steady state. The most plausible explanation is that the amount of Ca that is releasable is changing. It could be increased by the calcium current itself. The mechanism of loss of Ca is not so clear.

Cardiac cells have been shown to have a Na:Ca exchange mechanism (Reuter and Seitz, 1968). This is one possible method of removing Ca from the cell. Its role in the staircase phenomenon is not known, but it is likely to be a key factor in determining the size of contraction with steady stimulation. No matter what the mechanism, the cells must have some means for controlling Ca content. Until we understand this mechanism and develop methods to keep the intracellular store constant under experimental conditions, it will be difficult to determine the role of voltage in causing contraction.

An experiment that illustrates this problem is that of determining the voltage-tension relationship. If one allows the fiber to rest for a long time, it presumably comes to a steady level of Ca in the intracellular store. A simple step of voltage can be given to test the effect of variable trigger for release. If, however, the fiber is stimulated regularly, it would exhibit a sequential change in trigger, in Ca influx, in Ca efflux, and in recovery of the store. After a steady state of a train is established, an individual contraction results from both the size of the trigger event and the amount of Ca in the cell, as well as from the extent to which it has recovered to a releasable form.

NATURE OF THE Ca RELEASE

The studies of voltage, tension, and Ca current have shown important aspects of excitation-contraction coupling. The Ca current appears to be an important step in causing intracellular release, although the mechanism of this release is far from clear. By analogy with skeletal muscle studies using the Natori preparation, a Ca-triggered release of Ca from the sarcoplasmic reticulum has been suggested. The existence of this mechanism has been established for heart muscle and carefully studied by Fabiato and Fabiato (1975). They also showed that the effect is a graded one—a larger amount of Ca used as a trigger causes a larger release from the SR. While in skeletal muscle this mechanism is in doubt for several reasons (Endo, 1975), the studies of Fabiato and Fabiato support the suggestion quite strongly for heart muscle.

A direct effect of sarcolemmal depolarization in Ca release cannot be discounted. This mechanism has been shown in the skinned skeletal muscle by change in anions in the solutions to which a skinned fiber is exposed. This change in anion appears to result in a depolarization of the sarcoplasmic reticulum. Kerrick and Best (1974) have demonstrated this phenomenon in heart muscle, but it requires much more study.

PROBLEMS FOR THE FUTURE

Application of the voltage-clamp technique has been very helpful in providing insignts into excitation-contraction coupling. It is possible to conclude from voltage-clamp studies that:

1. Sarcolemmal depolarization is the initial step in causing contraction in heart muscle.

2. Contraction is graded as a function of membrane voltage.

3. A transmembrane Ca current is the likely mediator of the depolarization signal.

4. This current causes a graded release of Ca from the SR by an unknown mechanism.

5. The amount of Ca in the SR is variable, being increased by Ca current and decreased by a Ca pump, probably the Na:Ca exchange system.

6. Recovery of contraction requires recovery of the Ca current system and recovery of Ca into a releasable form in the SR.

The voltage-clamp technique limits us to measurement of membrane voltage, membrane current, and contraction. This is insufficient to provide direct information about the intermediate steps involved in Ca release. Key questions that remain before us include:

1. What are the factors controlling Ca loss from the cell, when in the cycle does it occur, etc.?

2. What are the value and origin of potential difference across the SR membrane?

3. How is Ca stored in the SR? Is the membrane a barrier, so that its depolarization alters Ca permeability?

4. If depolarization of the SR occurs, is it mediated by an ionic change, or is it coupled more directly to the sarcolemma?

5. Is the contraction a simple function of cytoplasmic Ca activity?

To approach these questions, we need tools to permit dynamic monitoring of the SR potential. We need to have the capability to examine the SR membrane permeabilities and factors controlling them. In addition to recording contraction, we must monitor cytoplasmic Ca directly. These questions can be asked with isolated SR, with "skinned" cardiac cells, and with intact cells, if we take proper advantage of the optical techniques now emerging.

REFERENCES

BEELER, G. W., JR., and REUTER, H. 1970a. Membrane calcium current in ventricular myocardial fibres. J. Physiol. 207:191–209.

BEELER, G. W., JR., and REUTER, H. 1970b. The relation between membrane potential, membrane currents, and activation of contraction in ventricular myocardial fibers. J. Physiol. 207:211–229.

EBASHI, S., and ENDO, M. 1968. Calcium ion and muscle contraction. Prog. Biophys. Mol. Biol. 18:123–183.

ENDO, M. 1975. Conditions required for calcium-induced release of calcium from the sarcoplasmic reticulum. Proc. Jpn. Acad. 51:467–72.

ENDO, M., TANAKA, M., and OGAWA, Y. 1970. Calcium-induced release of calcium from the sarcoplasmic reticulum of skinned skeletal muscle fibres. Nature 228:34–36.

FABIATO, A., and FABIATO, F. 1975. Contractions induced by a calcium-triggered release of calcium from the sarcoplasmic reticulum of single skinned cardiac cells. J. Physiol. 249:469–495.

FORD, L. E., and PODOLSKY, R. 1969. Regenerative calcium release within muscle cells. Science 167:58–59.

FOZZARD, H. A., and HELLAM, D. C. 1968. Relationship between membrane voltage and tension in voltage clamped Purkinje fibres. Nature 218:588–589.

GIBBONS, W. R., and FOZZARD, H. A. 1971. Voltage-dependence and time-dependence of contraction in sheep cardiac Purkinje fibers. Circ. Res. 28:446–460.

GIBBONS, W. R., and FOZZARD, H. A. 1975a. Relationships between voltage and tension in sheep cardiac Purkinje fibers. J. Gen. Physiol. 65:345–365.

GIBBONS, W. R., and FOZZARD, H. A. 1975b. Slow inward current and contraction of sheep cardiac Purkinje fibers. J. Gen. Physiol. 65:367–384.

HODGKIN, A. L., and HOROWICZ, P. 1960. Potassium contractures in single muscle fibres. J. Physiol. 153:386–403.

KERRICK, W. G. L., and BEST, P. M. 1974. Calcium ion release in mechanically disrupted heart cells. Science 183:435–437.

KUFFLER, S. W. 1946. The relation of electric potential changes to contracture in skeletal muscle. J. Neurophysiol. 9:367–377.

MORAD, M., and GOLDMAN, Y. 1973. Excitation-contraction coupling in heart muscle: membrane control of development of tension. Prog. Biophys. Mol. Biol. 27:257–313.

MORAD, M., and ORKAND, R. K. 1971. Excitation-contraction coupling in frog ventricle: evidence from voltage clamp studied. J. Physiol. 219:167–189.

MORAD, M., and TRAUTWEIN, W. 1968. The effect of the duration of the action potential on contraction in mammalian heart tissue. Pfluegers Arch. 299:66–82.

NEW, W., and TRAUTWEIN, W. 1972. The ionic nature of slow inward current and its relation to contraction. Pfluegers Arch. 334:24–38.

NIEDERGERKE, R. 1956. The potassium chloride contracture of the heart and its modification by calcium. J. Physiol. 134:584–599.

OCHI, R. 1970. The slow inward current and the action of manganese ions of guinea-pig's myocardium. Pfluegers Arch. 316:81–94.

REUTER, H. 1967. The dependence of slow inward current in Purkinje fibers on the extracellular calcium concentration. J. Physiol. 192:479–492.

REUTER, H. 1973. Time- and voltage-dependent contractile responses in mammalian cardiac muscle. Eur. J. Cardiol. 1/2:177–181.

REUTER, H., and SEITZ, N. 1968. Dependence of calcium efflux from cardiac muscle on temperature and external ion composition. J. Physiol. 209:25–43.

TRAUTWEIN, W. 1973. The slow inward current in mammalian myocardium. Eur. J. Cardiol. 1/2:169–175.

TRAUTWEIN, W., McDONALD, J. F., and TRIPATHI, O. 1975. Calcium conductance and tension in mammalian ventricular muscle. Pfluegers Arch. 354:55–74.

VASSORT, B. 1973. Influence of sodium ions on the regulation of frog myocardial contractility. Pfluegers Arch. 339:225–244.

Mailing address:
Harry A. Fozzard,
Department of Medicine,
The University of Chicago,
Chicago, Illinois 60637 (USA).

Recent Advances in Studies on
Cardiac Structure and Metabolism, Volume 11
Heart Function and Metabolism
Edited by T. Kobayashi, T. Sano, and N. S. Dhalla
Copyright 1978   University Park Press   Baltimore

IONIC BASIS OF
EXCITATION MECHANISM IN CARDIAC MUSCLE

E. CORABOEUF

Laboratory of Comparative Physiology,
University of Paris XI, Orsay, France

SUMMARY

Cardiac electrical activity is due to passive ionic permeabilities and, partially, to nonneutral (electrogenic) active transport, but extracellular accumulation or depletion of potassium is also of importance. The rapid sodium current responsible for the spike of the action potential and the slow calcium or calcium and sodium inward current responsible for the plateau are governed by activation and inactivation variables, but the range of potential in which the corresponding conductances "open" or "close" differs markedly. For that reason, partially depolarized fibers exhibit slow action potentials deprived of a rapid ascending phase. The normal sinoatrial and atrioventricular node action potentials are of this type. Several components of outward (repolarizing) currents, mainly carried by potassium ions (although anions may also carry repolarizing currents), exist, some of them being controlled by intracellular calcium. Repolarization is a much more labile process in Purkinje fibers than in myocardium. Recovery from inactivation of rapid and slow inward currents is important in controlling the shape of the action potential as a function of the previous diastole.

POSSIBLE ELECTROGENIC TRANSPORT MECHANISMS

Electrical activity may be due to passive ionic permeability, electrogenic active transport, or ionic exchange. According to present knowledge, the first mechanism is responsible for the greatest part of cardiac electrical phenomena, but there is growing evidence that the second may also participate. As to the third, its electrogenicity is not yet established.

Passive ionic permeabilities or conductances give rise to passive transmembrane ionic currents as a consequence of electrochemical gradients. In the resting state, inward positive currents (for example, sodium current) and outward positive currents (for example, potassium current) are equal, so that no net current crosses the membrane. The changes in intracellular concentrations of sodium and potassium that result from these currents are corrected by active transport, essentially the sodium pump [(Na,K)-ATPase], much of the internal sodium being probably compartmentalized or sequestered (Lee and Fozzard, 1975). During activity, changes in transmembrane ionic currents develop that are governed by changes in ionic conductances that are voltage- and

11

time-dependent (Hodgkin and Huxley, 1952), although in cardiac tissues some of them may be considered to be totally or partially controlled by quasi-instantaneous (time-independent) inward-going rectifiers (Noble and Tsien, 1968). When the sum of inward currents becomes greater than the sum of outward currents, a net flux of positive charges enters the cell and the membrane depolarizes. It repolarizes when inward current becomes smaller than outward current. Complete reconstruction of the electrical activity of cardiac Purkinje fibers has been performed by McAllister, Noble, and Tsien (1975).

Among possible electrogenic active transport mechanisms, the sodium pump has been extensively studied (for review, see Thomas, 1972). If equal numbers of sodium and potassium ions are transported, the pump will be electrically neutral, but if the carrying system extrudes more sodium ions than potasssium ions taken up, as is generally accepted, an excess of positive charges is ejected from the cell, giving rise to an outward repolarizing current. As a consequence, activation of the sodium pump should hyperpolarize the cell, whereas its inhibition should depolarize the cell or possibly prevent it from repolarizing. Since the early paper by Page and Storm (1965) several authors have presented evidence for the existence of an electrogenic sodium pump in cardiac fibers (for references see Sano, Hiraoka, and Sawanobori, 1975). Such a pump contributes to the membrane potential of beating guinea pig auricle (Glitsch, 1973). The electrogenic sodium pump has also been demonstrated in Purkinje fibers (Vassalle, 1970) and in rabbit sinoatrial node cells (Noma and Irisawa, 1974). It is questioned whether the electrogenic sodium pump generates outward current large enough to significantly participate in the repolarization of the normal cardiac action potential. Evidence in favor of such a possibility has been provided in Purkinje fibers (Isenberg and Trautwein, 1974), whereas in ventricular muscle no such large contribution of an electrogenic sodium pump has been observed (McDonald, Nawrath, and Trautwein, 1975). However, the possibility exists that in Purkinje fibers large changes in the equilibrium potential for potassium ions occur as a consequence of their accumulation in the narrow intercellular clefts after inhibition of the sodium pump (Cohen, Daut, and Noble, 1976). Extracellular potassium accumulation of about 1 mM has also been measured in frog ventricular muscle with potassium-sensitive microelectrodes in the course of each action potential (Kline and Morad, 1976). But greater accumulations seem to be possible, depending on the tissue and the experimental conditions.

Another possible electrogenic system contributing to electrical phenomena in cardiac tissues is the Na-Ca exchange mechanism described in nerve and cardiac muscle (see Baker, 1972; Reuter, 1974). In giant axons the system might be electrogenic (Baker, 1972), whereas in cardiac muscle it has been described as an electro-neutral system (Reuter, 1974). This system is certainly responsible for a large portion of the calcium efflux, the energy for calcium extrusion being provided by the transmembrane sodium gradient maintained by the sodium pump.

SODIUM AND CALCIUM CURRENTS

In the course of the last decade, voltage- and time-dependent conductances have been extensively studied in cardiac tissues, using voltage-clamp techniques (see reviews by Reuter, 1973; Trautwein, 1973; Weidmann, 1974). In spite of criticisms resulting from limitations of the technique (see Tarr and Trank, 1974), transmembrane microelectrode recordings during voltage-clamp experiments, using the vaseline-sealing double sucrose-gap method, have recently indicated satisfactory voltage control, even during the flow of the peak inward current (de Hemptinne, 1976). Results obtained in several laboratories have confirmed the existence of a rapid sodium inward current responsible for the development of the spike of the action potential and a slow calcium (or calcium-sodium) inward current responsible for the development of the plateau.

Rapid conductance for sodium ions and slow conductance for calcium ions are both governed by activation and inactivation processes (see Rougier et al., 1969), but the range of potential in which the corresponding conductances "open" or "close" differs markedly (Reuter, 1973), as is shown schematically in Figure 1. For that reason, in partially depolarized fibers the rapid sodium system may be partially or even completely inactivated (by closure of the "h" gate) while the slow calcium system is still fully available, giving rise to slow action potentials deprived of ascending phase. Such slowly developing, and consequently slowly conducting, action potentials may be the source of cardiac arrhythmias (Cranefield, 1975). It must be remembered that the normal sino-atrial and atrioventricular node action potentials are also slow action potentials. It may be questioned whether the membrane of the weakly polarized, tetrodo-toxin-insensitive, nodal cells possess a rapid sodium channel or not. In the atrioventricular node, increasing the resting potential by applying hyperpolarizing current strongly increases the maximum rate of rise of the action potential (Shigeto and Irisawa, 1972). In sinoatrial true pacemaker cells, carbamylcholine-induced hyperpolarization (Kreitner, 1975) produces an increase in the maximum rate of rise that is suppressed by tetrodotoxin. It may be concluded that these cells possess a rapid channel that is normally inactivated as a consequence of the low take-off potential.

The participation of sodium ions in the slow inward current, described by Rougier et al. (1969) in frog atrial fibers, seems very limited in normal cat ventricular myocardium (Weiss, Tritthart, and Walter, 1974). However, it becomes very large in calcium-free magnesium-free media (Garnier et al., 1969) and is also important in embryonic chick hearts (Shigenobu and Sperelakis,

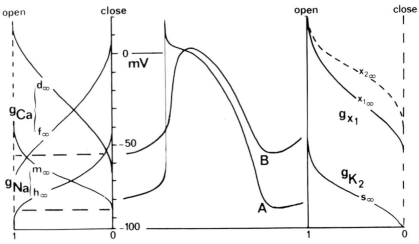

Figure 1. Diagrammatic representation of steady-state activation and inactivation variables controlling ionic membrane conductances in cardiac tissues as a function of membrane potential (*ordinate,* mV). *Left:* conductances responsible for inward depolarizing currents. *Right:* conductances responsible for outward repolarizing currents. When a fiber is suddenly depolarized, activation gates, m and d (which control, respectively, sodium and calcium conductances, g_{Na} and g_{Ca}), "open" rapidly (m is however more rapid than d), while corresponding inactivation gates, h and f, "close" more slowly. Each inward current flows when its activation gate is already open and its inactivation gate not yet closed. When a fiber is partially depolarized, h may be permanently closed (h_∞ = 0), the sodium current is therefore inactivated, and only the calcium current remains available, giving rise to action potentials deprived of a rapid ascending phase (slow action potentials, *B*). The diastolic depolarization is due to the deactivation of g_{K_2} in normally polarized fibers (*A*) and to the deactivation of g_{x_1} in partially depolarized fibers (*B*).

1971). The participation of sodium in the slow inward current has been studied by Verdonck and Carmeliet as a function of external calcium concentration (see Carmeliet, 1975). In frog atrial fibers, addition of magnesium readily suppresses slow inward sodium current, which is also more strongly inhibited by acid media than is calcium current (Chesnais *et al.,* 1975).

For a given slow inward current, the amplitude of the plateau will be increased if the simultaneous outward current is decreased. This is achieved through anomalous rectification, which consists of a quasi-instantaneous decrease in potassium conductance when the membrane depolarizes. Progressive decrease in slow inward current as well as progressive increase in outward current must lead to termination of the cardiac action potential. The decrease in slow inward current is due to its inactivation. As a consequence of the f_∞-Em relationship (Figure 1) the inactivation of the calcium current remains incomplete for depolarizations more negative than zero or +10 mV, but it seems also that in Purkinje fibers a certain proportion of slow channels do not possess inactivation mechanism (see McAllister *et al.,* 1975). Decrease in slow inward current may also, in hearts possessing a sarcotubular system, be caused by an increase in calcium concentration in the very small space between the sarcolemma and the terminal cisternae as a result of the previous entry of calcium (Bassingthwaighte and Reuter, 1972).

The increase in outward current during the plateau may be attributable to: 1) an entry of anions into the cell—a transient increase in chloride conductance has been described in Purkinje fibers (see Fozzard and Hiraoka, 1973) but not in myocardium; and 2) a release of cations—Noble and Tsien (1969) have analyzed several components of outward current carried mainly by potassium ions and showing no detectable inactivation (Figure 1). Among those components, g_{K_2} participates little in the repolarization process, except in its late phase, since it is inhibited by an intrinsic anomalous rectification mechanism in the plateau range of membrane potential, the inhibition being greater for a given potential (say −50 mV) when the external potassium concentration is low (Noble and Tsien, 1968). By contrast, g_{x_1} develops in the plateau range. It is responsible for the delayed rectification observed in Purkinje fibers as well as in other cardiac tissues and plays a role in the termination of the action potential of these tissues. However, it has been shown that increase in outward current does not contribute much to repolarization in sheep or calf ventricular muscle (McGuigan, 1974). Several authors have suggested that the relationship between increasing intracellular calcium and increase in potassium conductance, initially observed in neurons (Meech and Strumwasser, 1970), may also be valid in cardiac tissues. Such a mechanism could play a role in several conditions when a shortening of the action potential is observed (calcium-rich media, increase in frequency, action of certain metabolic inhibitors). Demonstration of a shortening of the action potential duration after iontophoretic intracellular injection of calcium has been given in Purkinje fibers (Isenberg, 1975). Which component of outward current is controlled by internal calcium is still unclear.

An important point is that in Purkinje fibers repolarization is obviously a very labile process as compared to that in myocardium. Situations in which inward current is increased, e.g., with veratrine (Arbel, Lazzari, and Glick, 1975), or in which outward currents are apparently decreased, e.g., in respiratory acidosis, may lead to alterations of repolarization and to the development of humps. Such humps can trigger reactivation and therefore act as ectopic pacemakers (Coraboeuf, Deroubaix, and Hoerter, 1976). They are limited to the Purkinje fibers and are absent in His and myocardial action potentials.

Another important feature of cardiac electrical activity is the change in the shape of the action potential that accompanies modifications of the interval between beats. Such a change is obviously very complex but is primarily controlled by recovery from inactivation of rapid and slow inward currents ("reactivation" or repriming). The first process controls the redevelopment of the rapid ascending phase (spike), the second the redevelopment of the plateau.

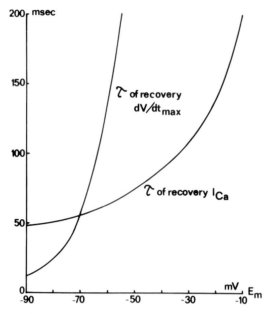

Figure 2. Time constants of recovery from inactivation of dV/dt_{max} and of inward calcium current (after a conditioning action potential or depolarizing pulse), as a function of diastolic potential. Schematically redrawn from Gettes and Reuter (1974).

According to Gettes and Reuter (1974), the relationship of the time constant of repriming as a function of membrane potential is very different for dV/dt_{max} and I_{Ca} (Figure 2). It may be deduced from their data that, in fibers with a high resting potential, the spike will recover earlier than the plateau, while the reverse is true in fibers with a lower resting potential. Several other mechanisms must also play a role in determining changes in the shape of an action potential occurring as a function of the duration of the previous diastole. The amplitude of the plateau increases markedly when rabbit atrial fibers are submitted to repetitive stimulation after a long period of rest. This effect, which seems not to depend on the presence of chloride ions, has been attributed to a progressive increase in anomalous rectification (Saito, 1972). Very little is actually known about this possible mechanism. In cat and dog ventricular muscle, the plateau of interpolated extrasystolic action potentials is also markedly enhanced as compared to the plateau of action potentials triggered at a constant frequency (Bass, 1975; Hiraoka and Sano, 1976), a phenomenon paralleled by transient increase in slow inward current. It is obvious that further work will be necessary to clarify this kind of very complex, but functionally very important, behavior.

REFERENCES

ARBEL, E. R., LAZZARI, J., and GLICK, G. 1975. Effect of veratrine on repolarization in the canine right bundle branch. Amer. J. Physiol. 229:1254–1260.

BAKER, P. F. 1972. Transport and metabolism of calcium ions in nerve. Prog. Biophys. Mol. Biol. 24:117–123.

BASS, B. G. 1975. Restitution of the action potential in cat papillary muscle. Amer. J. Physiol. 228:1717–1724.

BASSINGTHWAIGHTE, J. B., and REUTER, H. 1972. Calcium movements and excitation contraction coupling in cardiac cells. In W. C. DeMello (ed.), Electrical Phenomena in the Heart, pp. 353–393. Academic Press, New York.

CARMELIET, E. 1975. The ionic basis of membrane excitation in ordinary myocardial fibers: some aspects of the sodium and calcium conductance. In A. Fleckenstein and N. S. Dhalla (eds.), Basic Functions of Cations in Myocardial Activity, pp. 3–11. University Park Press, Baltimore.

CHESNAIS, J. M., CORABOEUF, E., SAUVIAT, M. P., and VASSAS, J. M. 1975. Sensitivity to H, Li and Mg ions of the slow inward sodium current in frog atrial fibers. J. Mol. Cell. Cardiol. 7:627–642.

COHEN, I., DAUT, J., and NOBLE, D. 1976. An analysis of the actions of low concentrations of ouabain on membrane currents in Purkinje fibers. J. Physiol. (Lond.) 260: 75–104.

CORABOEUF, E., DEROUBAIX, E., and HOERTER, J. 1976. Control of ionic permeabilities in normal and ischemic heart. Circ. Res. 38 (suppl. 1):92–98.

CRANEFIELD, P. F. 1975. The conduction of the cardiac impulse. Futura Publishing Company, New York. 404 pp.

de HEMPTINNE, A. 1976. Voltage clamp analysis in isolated cardiac fibres as performed with two different perfusion chambers for double sucrose gap. Pfluegers Arch. 363: 87–95.

FOZZARD, H. A., and HIRAOKA, M. 1973. The positive dynamic current and its inactivation properties in cardiac Purkinje fibres. J. Physiol. (Lond.) 234:569–586.

GARNIER, D., ROUGIER, O., GARGOUIL, Y. M., and CORABOEUF, E. 1969. Analyse électrophysiologique du plateau des réponses myocardiques; mise en évidence d'un courant lent entrant en absence d'ions bivalents. Pfluegers Arch. 313:321–342.

GETTES, L. S., and REUTER, H. 1974. Slow recovery from inactivation of inward currents in mammalian myocardial fibres. J. Physiol. (Lond.) 240:703–724.

GLITSCH, H. G. 1973. An effect of the electrogenic sodium pump on the membrane potential in beating guinea pig atria. Pfluegers Arch. 344:169–180.

HIRAOKA, M., and SANO, T. 1976. Role of slow inward current on premature excitation in ventricular muscle. Abstracts of the Eighth International Meeting of the International Study Group for Research in Cardiac Metabolism, Toyko. p. 125.

HODGKIN, A. L., and HUXLEY, A. F. 1952. Currents carried by sodium and potassium ions through the membrane of the giant axon of Loligo. J. Physiol. (Lond.) 116: 449–472.

ISENBERG, G. 1975. Is potassium conductance of cardiac Purkinje fibres controlled by $[Ca^{2+}]_i$? Nature 253:273–274.

ISENBERG, G., and TRAUTWEIN, W. 1974. Effect of dihydro-ouabain and lithium ions on the outward current in cardiac Purkinje fibers. Pfluegers Arch. 350:41–54.

KLINE, R., and MORAD, M. 1976. Potassium efflux and accumulation in heart muscle. Biophys. J. 16:367–372.

KREITNER, D. 1975. Evidence for the existence of a rapid sodium channel in the membrane of rabbit sinoatrial cells. J. Mol. Cell. Cardiol. 7:655–662.

LEE, C. O., and FOZZARD, H. A. 1975. Activities of potassium and sodium ions in rabbit heart muscle. J. Gen. Physiol. 65:695–708.

McALLISTER, R. E., NOBLE, D., and TSIEN, R. W. 1975. Reconstruction of the electrical activity of cardiac Purkinje fibres. J. Physiol. (Lond.)251:1–59.

McDONALD, T. F., NAWRATH, H., and TRAUTWEIN, W. 1975. Membrane currents and tension in cat ventricular muscle treated with cardiac glycosides. Circ. Res. 37:674–682.

McGUIGAN, J. A. S. 1974. Some limitations of the double sucrose gap and its use in a study of the slow outward current in mammalian ventricular muscle. J. Physiol. (Lond.) 240:775–806.

MEECH, R. W., and STRUMWASSER, F. 1970. Intracellular calcium injection activates potassium conductance in Aplysia nerve cells. Fed. Proc. 29:834.

NOBLE, D., and TSIEN, R. W. 1968. The kinetics and rectifier properties of the slow potassium current in cardiac Purkinje fibres. J. Physiol. (Lond.) 195:185–214.

NOBLE, D., and TSIEN, R. W. 1969. Reconstruction of the repolarization process in cardiac Purkinje fibers based on voltage clamp measurements of membrane current. J. Physiol. (Lond.) 200:233–254.

NOMA, A., and IRISAWA, H. 1974. Electrogenic sodium pump in rabbit sinoatrial node cell. Pfluegers Arch. 351:177–182.

PAGE, E., and STORM, S. R. 1965. Cat heart muscle in vitro. VIII. Active transport of sodium in papillary muscles. J. Gen. Physiol. 48:957–972.

REUTER, H. 1973. Divalent cations as charge carriers in excitable membranes. Prog. Biophys. Mol. Biol. 26:3–43.

REUTER, H. 1974. Exchange of calcium ions in the mammalian myocardium. Circ. Res. 34:599–605.

ROUGIER, O., VASSORT, G., GARNIER, D., GARGOUIL, Y. M., and CORABOEUF, E. 1969. Existence and role of a slow inward current during the frog atrial action potential. Pfluegers Arch. 308:91–110.

SAITO, T. 1972. Changes in a train of actions potentials in a rabbit atrium after a rest period. Effects of polarizing currents. Jpn. J. Physiol. 22:239–251.

SANO, T., HIRAOKA, M., and SAWANOBORI, T. 1975. Electrogenic contribution to resting potential in different cardiac tissues. In M. Lieberman and T. Sano (eds.), Developmental and Physiological Correlates of Cardiac Muscle, pp. 299–310. Raven Press, New York.

SHIGENOBU, K., and SPERELAKIS, N. 1971. Development of sensitivity to tetrodotoxin of chick embryonic hearts with age. J. Mol. Cell. Cardiol. 3:271–286.

SHIGETO, N., and IRISAWA, H. 1972. Slow conduction in the atrioventricular node of the cat: A possible explanation. Experientia 28:1442–1443.

TARR, R., and TRANK, J. W. 1974. An assessment of the double sucrose gap voltage clamp technique as applied to frog atrial muscle. Biophys. J. 14:627–643.

THOMAS, R. C. 1972. Electrogenic sodium pump in nerve and muscle cells. Physiol. Rev. 52:563–594.

TRAUTWEIN, W. 1973. Membrane currents in cardiac muscle fibers. Physiol. Rev. 53: 793–835.

VASSALLE, M. 1970. Electrogenic suppression of automaticity in sheep and dog Purkinje fibers. Circ. Res. 27:361–377.

WEIDMANN, S. 1974. Heart: Electrophysiology. Annu. Rev. Physiol. 36:155–169.

WEISS, R., TRITTHART, H., and WALTER, B. 1974. Correlation of Na-withdrawal effects on Ca-mediated action potentials and contractile activity in cat ventricular myocardium. Pfluegers Arch. 350:299–307.

Mailing address:
Prof. E. Coraboeuf,
Laboratoire de Physiologie Comparée,
Batiment 443, Université Paris XI,
91405-Orsay Cedex (France).

Recent Advances in Studies on
Cardiac Structure and Metabolism, Volume 11
Heart Function and Metabolism
Edited by T. Kobayashi, T. Sano, and N. S. Dhalla
Copyright 1978 University Park Press Baltimore

ELECTROPHYSIOLOGICAL PROPERTIES OF RAT HEART CELLS *IN VITRO* AND IN TISSUE CULTURE

H. J. JONGSMA, M. LIEBERMAN, J. DE BRUIJNE, and
A. C. G. VAN GINNEKEN

Department of Physiology, University of Amsterdam,
Amsterdam, The Netherlands

SUMMARY

Some electrical properties of right ventricles of neonatal rats and of aggregates from collagenase-dissociated cells from the same tissue are compared. The duration of the action potential does not change upon changing the stimulation frequency both in ventricles and aggregates; a decrease in temperature increases duration in both preparations to the same extent. The take-off potential and the maximal rate of rise of the action potential decrease in the same way in both preparations, while the time course of these changes is also comparable. It is concluded that the dissociation and aggregation procedure does not interfere with the membrane properties upon which the measured parameters are based; thus, aggregates are well suited for a realistic voltage-clamp analysis.

INTRODUCTION

It is well known that pieces of intact heart are difficult to investigate using voltage-clamp techniques, because of their complex geometry and the inaccessibility of their intercellular space (Johnson and Lieberman, 1971; Tarr and Trank, 1974). For that reason an increasing use is being made of preparations of tissue-cultured heart cells, which have a defined geometry and presumably an easily accessible intercellular space. In order to extrapolate voltage clamp data from tissue-cultured preparations to the intact heart, it is necessary to establish that the process of tissue culturing does not change the membrane properties. For this reason we compared some action potential parameters of right ventricles of neonatal rats with those of a tissue-cultured preparation made from the same tissue.

METHODS

Right ventricles of two-day-old rats were excised from the anesthetized animals, mounted in a tissue bath, and superfused with gassed McEwen solution (pH 7.35 ± 0.05).

Aggregates of collagenase-dissociated heart cells of two-day-old rats were prepared by rotatory shaking of cell suspensions (5×10^5 cells/3 ml) for 48–72 hr at 70 rpm at 37° C. After the aggregates were plated in dishes, they were incubated for 2–4 hr in a pH- and humidity-controlled incubator at 37° C. At the time of experimentation the dishes were placed on the heated stage of an inverted microscope and superfused with a gassed McEwen solution (pH 7.35 ± 0.05). For both preparations temperature was kept constant, within 0.2° C at any value between 31 and 36° C. The aggregates used were spherical, with a diameter ranging between 100 and 400 μm. From electron micrographs we know that there are virtually no fibroblasts present in the aggregates. Both preparations were stimulated with extracellular electrodes. Action potentials were recorded with the conventional glass microelectrode technique. The desired parameters were obtained from the tape recorded signals, using both analog and digital data processing techniques.

RESULTS AND DISCUSSION

Figure 1 shows action potentials from ventricles and aggregates at different driving frequencies and two temperatures. The action potentials shown were

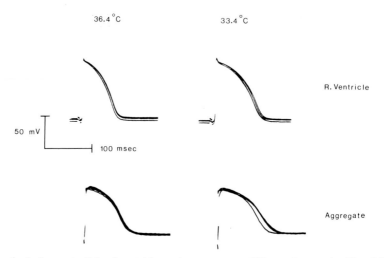

Figure 1. Action potentials of ventricles and aggregates at different frequencies. Ventricle: 1,2,3, and 4 Hz. Aggregate: 1,2,4, and 6 Hz.

recorded at the end of each stimulation period of 30–60 sec. It may be seen that the influence of frequency on action potential duration is very slight. Temperature decrease, on the other hand, increases action potential duration, as is known.

Figure 2 quantifies this. Here, action potential area (measured according to Anderson and Johnson, 1976) is plotted against the stimulation frequency. As expected, there is only a small effect of frequency increase on the area of the action potentials.

The temperature effect is much larger: a $3°$ C decrease in temperature increases the area of the ventricular action potentials about 30% at all frequencies, while a $5°$ C decrease in temperature increases the action potentials area of aggregates 15–20%.

Figure 3 shows the relation between maximal rate of rise of the action potential and driving frequency in the upper half of the figure, and the take-off potential against frequency plot in the lower half. It may be seen that the maximal rate of rise decreases as frequency increases. The take-off potential in ventricles also decreases steadily, while in aggregates we see first a small rise in take-off potential. $\dot{V}_{max}$ is determined by the number of available sodium carriers, which in its turn is strongly voltage-dependent (see Weidmann, 1955); thus, the relations shown in Figure 3 are as expected—only the take-off potential in aggregates rises slightly at the lower frequencies. This might be due to increased action of the Na-K pump. This is seen better from Figure 4, which shows the change in $\dot{V}_{max}$ and take-off potential during stimulation at a fixed frequency, both for ventricle and aggregates. It is clear that in both cases $\dot{V}_{max}$

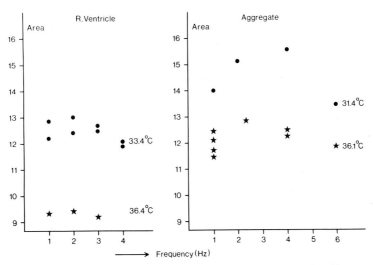

Figure 2. Action potential area at different stimulation frequencies. Area in arbitrary units.

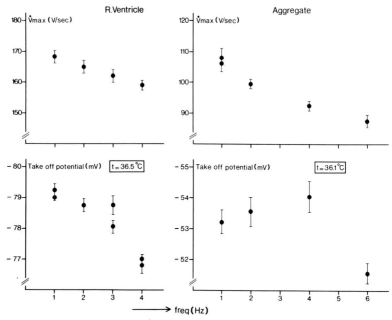

Figure 3. Maximal rate of rise ($\dot{V}_{max}$) and take-off potential at different stimulation frequencies. Each point is the mean of ten consecutive values. *Vertical bars:* ± 1 times standard deviation.

decreases concomitantly with the decrease in take-off potential, as expected. After the initial fast depolarization, the membrane potential stabilizes and later on starts repolarizing again. This repolarization is stronger in aggregates than in ventricle and might be due to electrogenic action of the sodium-potassium pump. During the repolarization $\dot{V}_{max}$ does not increase to the value that would be expected if the availability of the sodium carriers were the only governing factor. It seems that there is an accumulation of intracellular sodium, which decreases the driving force for this ion and stimulates the action of the sodium-potassium pump. This holds true both for ventricle and aggregate and also for rabbit atrium, as shown by Pasmooij *et al.* (1976).

Finally, it may be seen from Figure 4 that the initial depolarization is larger in ventricle than in aggregates. In our opinion this is caused by accumulation of potassium in the intercellular space of the ventricle. Due to this accumulation, membrane permeability for potassium increases and a larger outflow of potassium ensues than is the case in aggregates, where there seems to be a much smaller intercellular space.

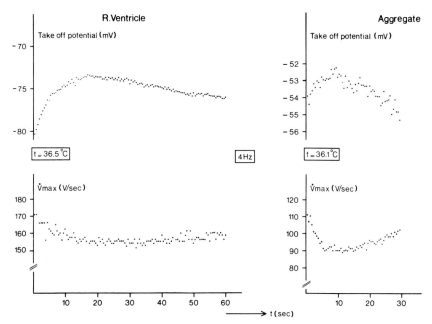

Figure 4. Time course of change in $\dot{V}_{max}$ and take-off potential at 4 Hz. The value measured from every other action potential is plotted.

CONCLUSION

From the foregoing results we conclude that, with respect to action potential duration, take-off potential and $\dot{V}_{max}$, aggregates and ventricles show qualitatively the same changes upon increasing the stimulation frequency. Quantitatively there are some differences, presumably due to differences in geometry between the two preparations. The membrane properties upon which the parameters measured are based are not changed by the dissociation procedure. This fact, together with the indications we have that there is much less intercellular space in aggregates than in ventricle and the ideal passive electrical properties of aggregates, as measured by De Haan and Fozzard (1975), makes them, in our opinion, very well suited for a realisic voltage-clamp analysis.

REFERENCES

ANDERSON, T. W., and JOHNSON, E. A. 1976. The repolarization phase of the cardiac action potential: A comparative study of rate induced changes in its waveform. J. Mol. Cell. Cardiol. 8:103–121.

De HAAN, R. L., and FOZZARD, H. A. 1975. Membrane response to current pulses in spheroidal aggregates of embryonic heart cells. J. Gen. Physiol. 65:207–222.

JOHNSON, E. A., and LIEBERMAN, M. 1971. Heart: excitation and contraction. *In* V. E. Hall, A. C. Giese, and R. Sonnenschein (eds.), Annual Reviews of Physiology, Vol. 33, pp. 479–532. Annual Reviews Inc., Palo Alto, California.

PASMOOIJ, J. H., VAN ENST, B. C., BOUMAN, L. N., ALLESSIE, M. A., and BONKE, F. I. M. 1976. The effect of heart rate on membrane responsiveness of rabbit atrial muscle. Pfluegers Arch. 366:223–231.

TARR, M., and TRANK, J. W. 1974. An assessment of the double sucrose-gap voltage clamp technique as applied to frog atrial muscle. Biophys. J. 14:627–643.

WEIDMANN, S. 1955. The effect of the cardiac membrane potential on the rapid availability of the sodium carrying system. J. Physiol. 127:213–224.

Mailing address:
Dr. H. J. Jongsma
Department of Physiology,
University of Amsterdam,
le C. Huygensstraat 20, Amsterdam (The Netherlands).

Recent Advances in Studies on
Cardiac Structure and Metabolism, Volume 11
Heart Function and Metabolism
Edited by T. Kobayashi, T. Sano, and N. S. Dhalla
Copyright 1978   University Park Press   Baltimore

VOLTAGE-CLAMP EXPERIMENTS BY DOUBLE MICROELECTRODE TECHNIQUE IN RABBIT SINOATRIAL NODE CELL

A. NOMA and H. IRISAWA

Department of Physiology, School of Medicine, Hiroshima University,
Kasumi-cho, Hiroshima, Japan

SUMMARY

When a man-made strand of the rabbit sinoatrial node (S-A node) was shortened by ligation, the spatial decay of the electrotonic potential decreased and the input impedance increased. A satisfactory voltage clamp was achieved in the small S-A node specimen using the double microelectrode technique (Deck, Kern, and Trautwein, 1964).

INTRODUCTION

Information concerning the automaticity of the myocardium has been obtained from voltage-clamp experiments in Purkinje fibers (Trautwein, 1973; McAllister, Noble, and Tsien, 1975). It is still necessary to analyze the ionic mechanisms of S-A node cell activity, since it is the primary pacemaker of the heart. The cable properties of the S-A node tissue (Bonke, 1973; Seyama, 1976) suggest that voltage-clamp experiments are possible in the S-A node.

METHODS

The S-A node tissue was dissected out of the rabbit. The details of the method are described elsewhere (Noma and Irisawa, 1976). In addition to the routine two microelectrodes, one for applying current (current electrode) and the other for recording the membrane potential (control electrode), a third one (monitor electrode) was used to record the membrane potential at a point not included in the feedback circuit.

RESULTS

Specimen

A strand of the S-A node tissue, 0.3 mm in both width and thickness, was shortened by ligation consecutively from 1.5 to 0.6 and 0.3 mm. After each ligation, electronic potentials in response to anodal current pulses were recorded simultaneously at two different distances from the current electrode. The initial peak amplitude of the electrotonic potential was plotted against the applied current (Figure 1). In accordance with the cable properties of the strand, the difference in amplitude between the two electrotonic potentials decreased and the input impedance increased as the strand was shortened. Spatial homogeneity was achieved in the 0.3-mm specimen which was the smallest size to maintain the spontaneous activity.

Voltage-Clamp Experiment

When depolarizing clamp pulses were applied to the specimen slightly longer than 0.3 mm, the potential at the monitor electrode gradually deviated from the controlled value associated with the increase in the membrane current due to the delayed rectification (Figure 2A). Upon repolarization, the potential profile reversed between the two points; the membrane potential at the monitoring electrode was more negative than that at the control electrode. This result indicates considerably large decay of the applied current in a relatively large specimen.

Figure 2, *B* and *C,* demonstrate spatial nonhomogeneity caused by transient inward current. Removal of the inactivation for the inward current system

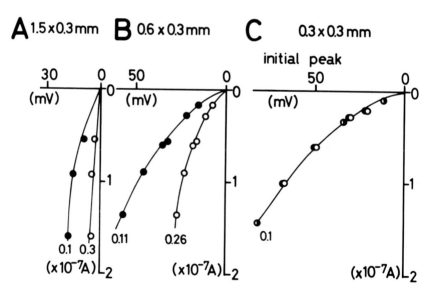

Figure 1. Relation between the amplitude of the electrotonic potential (*abscissa*) and the applied current (*ordinate*) obtained from a specimen of three different lengths. Numerals in the graph indicate the distance in mm between the recording electrode and the current electrode.

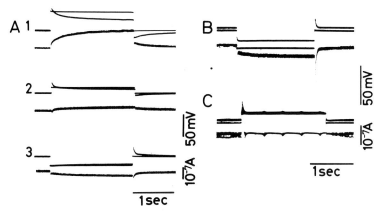

Figure 2. Three types of nonhomogeneity under the voltage-clamp conditions. The *upper* two traces are the potential records, and the *lower* trace is the current record. The difference in the pulse amplitude between the two voltage traces in *B* and *C* was mainly due to incomplete impalement of the monitoring electrode.

during hyperpolarization resulted in both a large inward current and an over-shoot of the potential from the monitor electrode at the break of the pulse (Figure 2*B*). Figure 2*C* shows a repetitive notch in both the current and monitoring voltage traces. This notch might be due to the action potential occurring in incompletely controlled cells within the specimen.

A successful voltage clamp was achieved in several specimens smaller than 0.3 mm in diameter. In these examples the potential from the monitor electrode was similar to that from the voltage electrode (Figure 3). At the beginning of the record the membrane potential was clamped at a potential equivalent to the resting potential (Noma and Irisawa, 1975). After the current activated during the preceding action potential subsided, test pulses were applied. Upon depolarization, the capacitive surge was followed by a transient inward current. Slowly increasing outward current followed the transient inward current, and upon repolarization the outward current slowly declined. Upon hyperpolarization, inward current flowed and its magnitude slowly increased with time during the pulse.

DISCUSSION

With the reported space constant of 0.8 mm (Seyama, 1976), the cable equation (Weidmann, 1952) gives a decay by less than 5% of the electrotonic potential along the 0.3-mm−long specimen. In agreement with this notion, the magnitude of the electrotonic potential was almost identical between two different points within the small specimen (Figure 1). Furthermore, a satisfactory voltage clamp was achieved in the small S-A node specimen (Figure 3). The incompleteness of

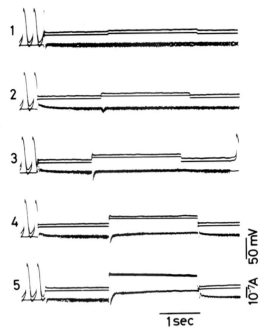

Figure 3. Spatial homogeneity under the voltage-clamp conditions. *Top* trace was recorded by the monitor electrode. The true membrane potential at the monitor electrode was calculated by the ratio of the action potential amplitude recorded by the monitor electrode to that recorded by the control electrode. The two recorded step potentials differed only by 0.8 mV on depolarization of 36.5 mV. The slight decrease with time of the depolarizing pulse amplitude in trace 5 might be caused by high resistivity of the current electrode.

the voltage clamp in several specimens might have occurred because of the complex construction of the S-A node (Irisawa, 1976). It was concluded that the double microelectrode technique, first applied to Purkinje fibers (Deck *et al.,* 1964), may also be useful in the S-A node by using a specimen less than 0.3 mm in diameter.

REFERENCES

BONKE, F. I. M. 1973. Electrotonic spread in the sinoatrial node of the rabbit heart. Pfluegers Arch. 339:17–23.
DECK, K. A., KERN, R., and TRAUTWEIN, W. 1964. Voltage clamp technique in mammalian cardiac fibres. Pfluegers Arch. 280:50–62.
IRISAWA, A. 1976. Fine structure of the sino-atrial node of the rabbit heart. The Eighth International Meeting of the International Study Group for Research in Cardiac Metabolism. 151, Tokyo.

McALLISTER, R. E., NOBLE, D., and TSIEN, R. W. 1975. Reconstruction of the electrical activity of cardiac Purkinje fibres. J. Physiol. 251:1–59.

NOMA, A., and IRISAWA, H. 1975. Effects of Na^+ and K^+ on the resting membrane potential of the rabbit sinoatrial node cell. Jpn. J. Physiol. 25:287–302.

NOMA, A., and IRISAWA, H. 1976. Membrane currents in the rabbit sinoatrial node cell as studied by the double microelectrode method. Pfluegers Arch. 364:45–52.

SEYAMA, I. 1976. Characteristics of the rectifying properties of the sino-atrial node cell of the rabbit. J. Physiol. 255:379–397.

TRAUTWEIN, W. 1973. Membrane currents in cardiac muscle fibers. Physiol. Rev. 53: 793–835.

WEIDMANN, S. 1952. The electrical constants of Purkinje fibres. J. Physiol. 129:568–582.

Mailing address:
Dr. H. Irisawa
Department of Physiology,
School of Medicine,
Hiroshima University,
Kasumi 1-2-3, Hiroshima 734 (Japan).

Recent Advances in Studies on
Cardiac Structure and Metabolism, Volume 11
Heart Function and Metabolism
Edited by T. Kobayashi, T. Sano, and N. S. Dhalla
Copyright 1978   University Park Press   Baltimore

ROLE OF SLOW INWARD CURRENT
ON PREMATURE EXCITATION
IN VENTRICULAR MUSCLE

M. HIRAOKA and T. SANO

Institute for Cardiovascular Diseases,
Tokyo Medical and Dental University, Tokyo, Japan

SUMMARY

Action potential durations in premature excitations showed paradoxical prolongation at the shorter coupling intervals; this was abolished by manganous ions. Voltage-clamp experiments also disclosed a transient increase of slow inward current in premature excitations. These results indicate that prolongation of action potential durations was mainly brought about by changes in slow inward current, especially in its characteristics of recovery from inactivation.

INTRODUCTION

The durations of action potentials in cardiac muscle are dependent on preceding diastolic intervals (PDI) and heart rate (Hoffman and Cranefield, 1960). However, premature excitations (PE) in ventricular muscles show paradoxical prolongation of action potential durations (APD) at short PDI (Gettes, Morehouse, and Surawicz, 1972; Bass, 1975; see also references listed in them). The present experiments were carried out to study the mechanism of this phenomenon.

METHODS

All the experiments were carried out with right ventricular papillary and trabecular muscles of dogs. The preparations were driven by externally applied pulses with various basic cycle lengths (BCL). Premature stimuli were applied at every eighth stimulus after seven basic ones. Membrane current was measured by a single sucrose-gap voltage-clamp technique similar to the method described by Giebisch and Weidmann (1971). The normal Tyrode solution was aerated by $95\% \, O_2 + 5\% \, CO_2$. Temperature of the bath was maintained at $33-35°$ C.

RESULTS

When PE were elicited with progressively shorter coupling intervals, APD became shorter at first, but then increased transiently at coupling intervals of 60–350 msec (Figure 1). At the same coupling intervals, second depolarization of action potentials also showed transient increase; however, the maximum dV/dt of action potentials changed independent of these two parameters (Figure 1). These changes in PE were always observed at different BCL (500–3000 msec) in the six preparations studied.

Voltage-clamp experiments were done with the same program, and results are shown in Figures 2 and 3. Seven basic pulses of 500 msec duration were applied with BCL of 1600 msec, and PE were given at various diastolic intervals. Slow inward current (SIC) in PE was larger than the basic one at shorter diastolic intervals of 65–400 msec. On the other hand, outward current changed litt,e or slightly increased at shorter diastolic intervals. The transient increase of SIC in PE was always observed in six preparations and the phenomenon was also seen with three preparations treated with 2×10^{-5}M tetrodotoxin. To examine the mechanism underlying the transient increase in SIC, the recovery from inactivation of SIC was examined (Figure 4). The recovery of SIC took place very rapidly at first, with a time constant of less than 100 msec, and then was

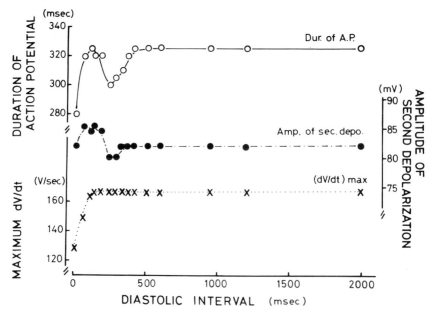

Figure 1. Changes in action potential parameters in PE. *Abscissa* indicates preceding diastolic intervals of PE. Symbols are APD (○), amplitude of second depolarization (●), and maximum dV/dt of action potentials (X).

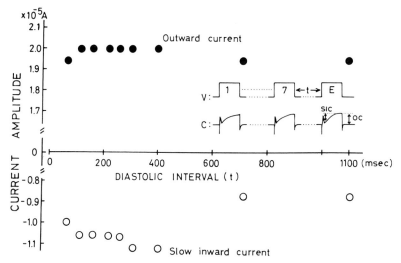

Figure 2. Membrane current changes in PE. *Abscissa* indicates PDI of PE. *Ordinate* is current amplitude of SIC (*lower portion*) and of outward current (*upper portion*). Experimental program is schematically shown in the inset.

followed by slower recovery with a time constant of 500–700 msec. Thus, the recovery of SIC seems to take place by two phases. The same type of results was obtained in three preparations. Finally, the effects of manganous ions, which were shown to block SIC (Ochi, 1970), were tested on PE. In Mn^{2+} solution, transient prolongation of APD in PE was never observed in four fibers examined.

DISCUSSION

PE of ventricular muscles show prolonged APD at the shorter coupling intervals. These results confirm the results of others (Gettes *et al.,* 1972; Bass, 1975). Voltage-clamp experiments disclosed a transient increase of SIC in PE, the time course of which was very similar to changes in APD. Since repolarization of ventricular muscles is mainly determined by development of SIC (Giebisch and Weidmann, 1971), the behavior of SIC can be predicted by its contribution to premature action potentials. This suggestion was further supported by abolition of APD prolongation in Mn^{2+} solution.

The mechanism for increased SIC in PE is partially explained by two phases of recovery from inactivation, but it is still hard to explain why SIC after full recovery, e.g., after 2000-msec rest, was smaller than that of PE with diastolic intervals of 100–300 msec. Therefore, some other mechanism may be involved in this phenomenon; for example, the ionic currents generated during the

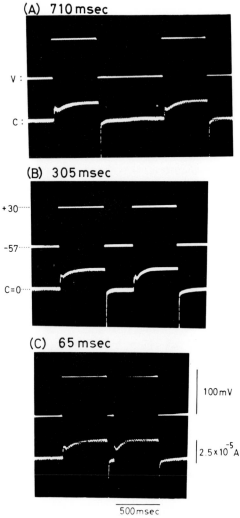

Figure 3. Actual experimental records taken from the same experiments shown in Figure 2. In each picture the *upper record* indicates membrane voltage and the *lower record* is membrane current. Only the seventh basic pulse and premature one are shown, and PDI is indicated at the top of each picture.

preceding response may affect the duration of the subsequent response. Recovery from inactivation of SIC was studied by several authors (Gettes and Reuter, 1974; Trautwein, McDonald, and Tripathi, 1975; Kohlhardt *et al.*, 1975). These authors reported a single exponential recovery, and their results are different from ours. The reason for this discrepancy was not known, but we used much

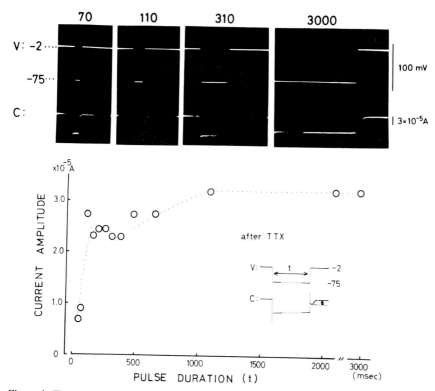

Figure 4. Time course of recovery from inactivation of SIC (*lower half*) and actual experimental records (*upper half*). The experimental program is schematically shown in the inset. The preparation was treated with 2×10^{-5} M tetrodotoxin.

longer duration for full recovery of SIC. This may explain a part of the difference.

REFERENCES

BASS, B. E. 1975. Restitution of the action potential in cat papillary muscle. Amer. J. Physiol. 228:1717–1724.

GETTES, L. S., MOREHOUSE, N., and SURAWICZ, B. 1972. Effect of premature depolarization on the duration of action potentials in Purkinje and ventricular fibers of the moderator band of the pig heart. Circ. Res. 30:55–66.

GETTES, L. S., and REUTER, H. 1974. Slow recovery from inactivation of inward currents in mammalian myocardial fibres. J. Physiol. 240:703–724.

GIEBISCH, G., and WEIDMANN, S. 1971. Membrane currents in mammalian ventricular heart muscle fibers using a voltage-clamp technique. J. Gen. Physiol. 57:290–296.

HOFFMAN, B. F., and CRANEFIELD, P. F. 1960. Electrophysiology of the heart. McGraw-Hill, New York.

KOHLHARDT, M., KRAUSE, M., KÜBLER, M., and HERDEY, A. 1975. Kinetics of inactivation and recovery of the slow inward current in the mammalian ventricular myocardium. Pfluegers Arch. 355:1–17.

OCHI, R. 1970. The slow inward current and the action of manganese ions in guinea-pig's myocardium. Pfluegers Arch. 316:81–94.

TRAUTWEIN, W., McDONALD, T. F., and TRIPATHI, O. 1975. Calcium conductance and tension in mammalian ventricular muscle. Pfluegers Arch. 354:55–74.

Mailing address:
Dr. M. Hiraoka
Institute for Cardiovascular Diseases,
Tokyo Medical and Dental University, Tokyo (Japan).

Recent Advances in Studies on
Cardiac Structure and Metabolism, Volume 11
Heart Function and Metabolism
Edited by T. Kobayashi, T. Sano, and N. S. Dhalla
Copyright 1978   University Park Press   Baltimore

MEMBRANE CALCIUM CURRENT IN CARDIAC EXCITATION: EFFECTS OF ATP AND RELATED SUBSTANCES AND SODIUM PUMP ON BULLFROG ATRIUM

M. GOTO, A. YATANI, and Y. TSUDA

Department of Physiology, Faculty of Medicine,
Kyushu University, Fukuoka, Japan

SUMMARY

In association with the modes of action of catecholamine and acetylcholine (ACh), the effects of ATP, GTP, and related substances on the membrane potential, current, and tension components of the bullfrog atrium were studied. Exogenously applied ATP (0.05–1.0 mM) produced an immediate increase in overshoot and duration of action potential and an augmentation of contraction that were followed by secondary inhibitions. Under voltage clamp, I_{Ca}, I_{Ca}-dependent tension, and, later, delayed outward current (I_x) were enhanced, while slow sodium inward current (I_{Nas}) and I_{Ca}-independent tension diminished. GTP (0.05–1.0 mM) unexpectedly produced almost the same effects. These catecholamine-like actions of ATP and GTP were not eliminated by β-blockers, propranolol (10^{-6} M), and pindolol (10^{-7} M). Adenine and guanine nucleotides, which lack energy-rich phosphate bond ($\sim$P), merely showed a negative inotropic effect under voltage clamp and depressed I_x.

K-depleted Ringer solution produced biphasic positive inotropic effects. Voltage-clamp studies during the initial inotropic phase disclosed an enhancement of I_{Ca} and I_{Ca}-dependent tension, indicating some K-Ca antagonism at the slow channel. During the late inotropic phase, contrarily, I_{Ca}-dependent phasic tension diminished while I_{Ca}-independent tonic tension markedly augmented. The fast (I_{Naf}) and slow inward currents (I_{Nas}, I_{Ca}), the leaky membrane current (I_l), as well as the current of anomalous rectification (I_{Kl}) were gradually depressed. Since ouabain (10^{-6} M) produced comparable effects, an inhibition of Na-pump was estimated responsible for the late inotropic and related effects.

INTRODUCTION

The vertebrate cardiac action potential can be divided into two components, the spike and the plateau. Voltage-clamp studies have clarified that a fast Na inward current (I_{Naf}) is responsible for electrogenesis of the early spike component and a slow Ca and/or Na current (I_{Ca}, I_{Nas}) for the plateau component (cf. Reuter, 1973; Trautwein, 1973). This slow inward current now attracts a keen interest because of its essential roles not only in coupling the membrane excitation to activation of contraction (cf. Langer, 1973; Coraboeuf, 1974) but also in coupling the cardiac metabolism to the electrogenesis of myocardium. Actually,

37

the plateau duration of action potential was elucidated to relate with the amount of ATP derived mainly from glycolytic processes (Girardier, 1971; McDonald and MacLeod, 1973). Moreover, Na pump of the membrane, which depends on a hydrolysis of ATP, is known to become electrogenic in some conditions and to modify the resting potential as well as the configuration of action potential (Senberg and Trautwein, 1974).

In connection with these findings, the present study is concerned with the effects of exogenously applied ATP and related substances and of Na pump on membrane currents and contractile tension components of the bullfrog atrium under voltage-clamped and unclamped conditions.

METHODS

The preparations used were thin muscle bundles (diameter 0.4–0.6 mm) isolated from the right atrium of the bullfrog *Rana catesbiana*. The membrane potential, current, and tension were measured simultaneously by means of the conventional double-gap method (described in Goto, Wada, and Saito, 1974), in which the width of central test chamber was 0.3–0.5 mm. With this apparatus a gap action potential of more than 100 mV was commonly obtained, and its short-circuiting factor exceeded 0.8. Compositions of normal Ringer solution and test solutions used for the purpose of isolation of specific membrane currents are shown in Table 1. All experiments were performed at a constant temperature between $16-17°C$.

RESULTS

Effects of ATP, GTP, and
Related Nucleotides on Membrane Currents and Tension Components

ATP in low concentrations (0.05–0.2 mM) produced an immediate increase of overshoot and duration of action potential and an augmentation of twitch contraction enhancing the rate of rise and fall of tension, as first observed on frog ventricle in Ca-deficient condition (Antoni, Engstfeld, and Fleckenstein, 1960). Higher concentrations of ATP (0.2–1.0 mM), however, elicited a gradual

Table 1. Composition of solutions (mM/liter)

Solution	NaCl	Sucrose	KCl	CaCl$_2$ 2H$_2$O	Tris-Cl	EDTA	MnCl$_2$ 4H$_2$O	Glucose
A	109.84	—	2.56	1.80	10.0	—	—	5.80
B	—	219.67	2.56	1.80	10.0	—	—	5.80
C	109.84	—	2.56	—	10.0	5×10^{-2}	—	5.80
D	109.84	—	2.56	1.80	10.0	—	3.00	5.80

inhibition of contractility after the initial inotropic effect, reducing the enhanced overshoot and duration of action potential concomitantly. All these effects were reversible and eliminated neither by propranolol (10^{-6} M), pindolol (10^{-7} M), nor atropine (10^{-7} M).

Under voltage-clamped conditions also, a marked positive inotropic effect of ATP was observed (Figure 1A), although a long application or higher concentration of ATP elicited similar late inhibitions. The inotropic effects under a constant clamp pulse indicate that ATP definitely affects the excitation-contrac-

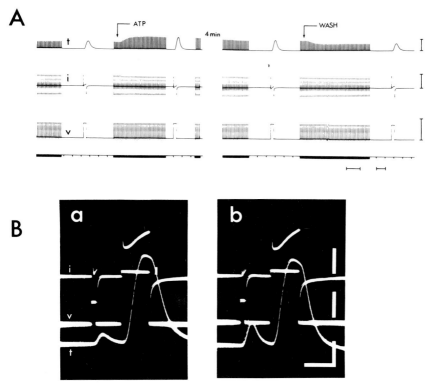

Figure 1. A, Effects of ATP (0.05 mM) on the tension (t) and membrane current (i) of bullfrog atrial muscle under voltage clamp (v). I_{Ca}-dependent responses to small short depolarizing pulses (75 mV, 0.2 sec) are recorded under the presence of TTX (5×10^{-7} g/ml). Note an augmentation of the tension and slow inward current. *B,* Effects of ATP (0.1 mM) on I_{Ca}-dependent and independent tensions in response to small (70 mV, 0.15 sec) n and large pulses (150 mV, 1.0 sec), respectively. *a:* control. *b:* 5 min after ATP. Again, I_{Ca}-dependent tension increased. Note also an inhibition of tonic terminal tension, which represents I_{Ca}-independent tension. Holding potentials were −70 mV (resting potential level) in both figures, *A* and *B,* and TTX (5×10^{-7} g/ml) was present throughout. Vertical calibrations are 0.05 g, 10 μA, and 100 mV in *A,* and 20 μA, 50 mV, and 0.02 g in *B.* Horizontal calibrations in *A* are 1.0 sec and 1.0 min for slow and fast records, respectively, and in *B,* 1.0 sec.

tion coupling process of the myocardium. Examination of the relationship among the amplitude of depolarizing pulse, membrane current, and tension in absence or presence of TTX (5×10^{-7} g/ml) disclosed that ATP produced a marked enhancement of slow inward current and I_{Ca}-dependent tension and an inhibition of I_{Ca}-independent tonic tension (Figure 1B). The delayed outward current (I_X) tended to increase with time. The increase of slow inward current was prominent at lower voltages, and that of I_X at higher voltages (Figure 2A). The I_{Naf}, anomalous rectification (I_{KI}), and leaky current (I_l) did not show any appreciable change. These characteristics could account for the specific configuration change of action potential after ATP. Furthermore, voltage-current relationships in Na-free or Ca-free (+EDTA 5×10^{-5} M, TTX 5×10^{-7} g/ml) Ringer solution have elucidated that I_{Ca} markedly increased while slow Na inward current (I_{Nas}) decreased (the figure is not shown). Correspondingly, in the voltage-tension relationships ATP enhanced I_{Ca}-dependent phasic tension selectively, while I_{Ca}-independent tonic tension was inhibited (Figure 2B).

GTP (0.05–1.0 mM) produced, unexpectedly, almost the same effects as ATP, and induced two sites of action: first, an enhancement of I_{Ca} and I_{Ca}-dependent phasic tension, and, second, an inhibition of I_{Ca}-independent

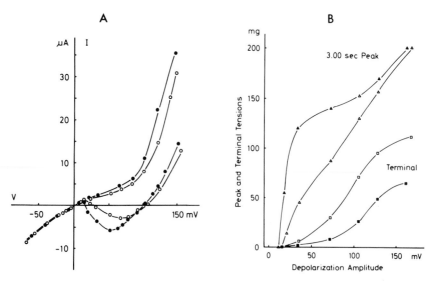

Figure 2. A, Voltage-current relationships before (○) and after (●) ATP application (0.05 mM) in the presence of TTX (5×10^{-7} g/ml). Note an increase of slow inward and delayed outward currents. *B,* Voltage-tension relationships. Long depolarizing pulses of 3.0 sec were used, and peak (△,▲) and terminal tension (□,■) before and after ATP (0.2 mM) were plotted. A marked augmentation of peak tension at low voltages and an inhibition of terminal tension at higher voltages are seen. The former relates mainly to I_{Ca}-dependent phasic tension, and the latter to I_{Ca}-independent tonic tension.

tonic tension and a gradual increase of I_X. Meanwhile, adenine and guanine nucleotides, which lack energy-rich phosphate bond ($\sim$P), merely showed a negative inotropic effect under voltage clamp and depressed I_X. These observations suggest that $\sim$P, together with Ca, is indispensable for the enhancement of I_{Ca} and I_{Ca}-dependent tension, and also that exogenous GTP does not simply counteract with ATP.

Genesis of these actions is uncertain at present. What is apparent is only that the modes of action are quite similar to those of adrenaline. Adrenaline is known to cause a positive inotropic effect by enhancing I_{Ca}, which is thought to act via cyclic adenosine $3':5'$-monophosphate (Reuter, 1974). An increase of I_x component (Tsien, 1973) and an inhibition of tonic tension are also known (Morad and Rolett, 1972). Moreover, ATP derived from glycolysis relates closely with the generation of the plateau potential, as noted (Girardier, 1971; McDonald and MacLeod, 1973). These facts, when considered together, strongly suggest that in the frog atrium ATP attaches or penetrates the membrane more easily at low temperatures and contributes directly to the enhancement of I_{Ca} and I_{Ca}-dependent tension or indirectly to increased cyclic AMP (Rasmussen and Tenenhouse, 1968), so that adrenaline-like actions are produced. The rapid action of exogenously applied ATP and its complete recovery after washing strongly support a physiological action of ATP on the cell membrane.

Na Pump Inhibition and Late Potentiating Effect of Low-K Ringer Solution

It is generally known that when muscle is soaked in K-depleted fluid the membrane (Na, K)-ATPase and the activity of the Na pump are inhibited (Bonting, 1970) and Na ions progressively accumulate within the cells (Desmedt, 1953). In myocardium the accumulation or a rise of $[Na]_i$ produces a secondary increase of $[Ca]_i$ due to Na-Ca exchange diffusion and further a positive inotropic effect (Reuter and Seitz, 1968; Poole-Wilson and Langer, 1975). Thus, Ehara (1974) has demonstrated a delayed potentiating effect of K-deficiency probably due to Na-Ca exchange mechanism in addition to its well-known immediate inotropic effect. Present study aims to clarify further the nature of these inotropic actions, analyzing the membrane currents, potentials, and tension components in the frog myocardium under voltage-clamped and unclamped conditions.

In most atrial preparations, K-depleted Ringer solution produced biphasic positive inotropic effects and immediate and delayed potentiations (Figure 3A), as in the ventricle, but the effects appeared 3–5 times faster in the former than in the latter, probably because of thinness of the atrial fibers and preparations. The initial inotropic effect was accompanied by a hyperpolarization of membrane, a rise in threshold, and an increase in amplitude and duration of action potential, while during the delayed inotropic effect a gradual depolarization and a lowering and prolongation of plateau were produced, together with increase of

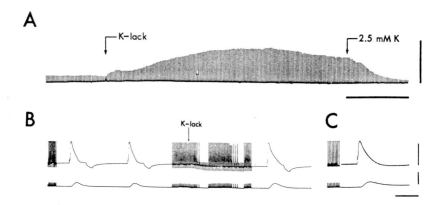

Figure 3. *A,* Immediate and delayed inotropic effects of K-lack Ringer solution. *B,* Effects of K depletion on the membrane potential and contractility. A hyperpolarizing pulse was added after each action potential. *C,* The same as *B,* but the record was obtained 15 min after K depletion. Note an increase in membrane cord resistance and a hyperpolarization followed by a gradual depolarization. Vertical calibrations, 0.1 g in *A,* and 100 mV and 0.1 g in *B* and *C.* Horizontal calibration, 1 sec and 1 min for fast and slow records, respectively.

membrane resistance (Figure 3*B*). The augmented twitch contraction showed a special pattern of fast tension development and slow relaxation.

Voltage-clamp studies during the initial inotropic phase disclosed that I_{Ca} and I_{Ca}-dependent tension were augmented, probably due to some K-Ca antagonism at the slow channel (the figure is not shown). During the late inotropic phase, contrarily, the fast and slow inward currents, especially the latter, were depressed. On the tension components, I_{Ca}-dependent phasic tension diminished, whereas I_{Ca}-independent tension was markedly augmented (Figure 4*A*). Voltage-current relationships (Figure 4*B*) also showed a decrease of the slow inward currents in all voltages, and an increase of anomalous rectification (I_{K1}), which was accompanied by a reduction of leaky current (I_l). These characteristics again account for the typical configuration change of AP in K-lack media—depressed plateau and long tail. A marked reduction of electrogenic outward current by inhibition of Na pump, as demonstrated in sheep Purkinje fibers (Isenberg and Trautwein, 1974) was not seen in the frog atrium, although a presence of electrogenic potential was noticed in the final depressive stage after a few hours of soaking (Figure 3*C*).

Thus, the principal cause of the delayed inotropic effect of K-depleted solution was an augmentation of I_{Ca}-independent tension component and prolongation of action potential. Notable facts were that, except for the initial specific actions of low-K solution, many late effects on the membrane potentials, currents, and tensions appeared quite similar to those of ouabain (unpub-

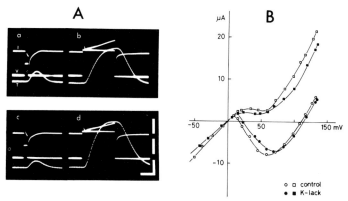

Figure 4. A, Effects of K depletion on I_{Ca}-dependent and independent tension responses for small (70 mV, 0.1 sec) and large (150 mV, 1.0 sec) depolarizing pulses in the presence of TTX (5×10^{-7} g/ml), respectively. I, membrane current; V, voltage; and T, tension. *a, b:* control records. *c, d:* records 15 min after K-depletion. Note a depression of slow inward current and I_{Ca}-dependent tension in *c,* and a marked augmentation of I_{Ca}-independent tension in *d.* B, Voltage-current relationships before ($\circ,\square$) and after ($\bullet,\blacksquare$) k-depletion in the presence of TTX (55×10^{-7} g/ml). The slow inward current and the leaky membrane current were depressed.

lished observations; see also Greenspan and Morad, 1975; McDonald, Nawrath, and Trautwein, 1975). Moreover, ouabain was elucidated to increase solely the I_{Ca}-independent tonic tension (Vassort, 1973). Thus the delayed effect of low-K solution observed can safely be ascribed to an inhibition of the Na pump.

I_{Ca}-independent tension is known to relate closely with Na-Ca exchange mechanism (Goto *et al.,* 1972; Vassort, 1973) and, actually, Ca-influx occurs during sustained depolarization (Kavaler, 1974), while in mechanically and chemically skinned myocardial fibers active doses of ouabain have no effect on the contractility (Fabiato and Fabiato, 1973; Nayler, 1973). Thus, an increase in $[Na]_i$ after inhibition of Na-pump and a following increase of $[Ca]_i$ due to Na-Ca exchange across or with the cell membrane are considered as the most possible genesis of the inotropic affect.

REFERENCES

ANTONI, H., ENGSTFELD, G., and FLECKENSTEIN, A. 1960. Inotrope Effekte von ATP und Adrenalin am hypodynamen Froschmyocard nach elektro-mechanischer Entkoppelung durch Ca^{++}-Entzug. Pfluegers Arch. 272:91–106.

BONTING, S. L. 1970. Sodium-potassium activated adenosinetriphosphatases and cation transport. *In* E. E. Bittar (ed.), Membrane and Ion Transport, Vol. 1, pp. 257–363. John Wiley and Sons, London.

CORABOEUF, E. 1974. Membrane electrical activity and double component contraction in cardiac tissue. J. Mol. Cell. Cardiol. 6:215–225.

DESMEDT, J. E. 1953. Electrical activity and intracellular sodium concentration in frog muscle. J. Physiol. 121:191–205.

EHARA, T. 1974. Late potentiating effect of low-K Ringer solution on the contractility of the bullfrog ventricle. Jpn. J. Physiol. 24:329–342.

FABIATO, A., and FABIATO, F. 1973. Activation of skinned cardiac cells: Subcellular effects of cardioactive drugs. Eur. J. Cardiol. 1–2:143–155.

GIRARDIER, L. 1971. Dynamic energy partition in cultured heart cells. Cardiology. 56:88–92.

GOTO, M., KIMOTO, Y., SAITO, M., and WADA, Y. 1972. Tension fall after contraction of bullfrog atrial muscle examined with voltage clamp technique. Jpn. J. Physiol. 22:637–650.

GOTO, M., WADA, Y., and SAITO, M. 1974. Tension components and tension fall of the bullfrog atrial muscle during depolarization. Jpn. J. Physiol. 24:359–375.

GREENSPAN, A. M., and MORAD, M. 1975. Electromechanical studies on the inotropic effects of acetylstrophanthidin in ventricular muscle. J. Physiol. 253:357–384.

ISENBERG, G., and TRAUTWEIN, W. 1974. Effects of dihydro-ouabain and lithium-ions on the outward current in cardiac Purkinje fibers: Evidence for electrogenicity of active transport. Pfluegers Arch. 350:41–54.

KAVALER, F. 1974. Electromechanical time course in frog ventricle: Manipulation of calcium level during voltage clamp. J. Mol. Cell. Cardiol. 6:575–580.

LANGER, G. A. 1973. Heart: Excitation-contraction coupling. Annu. Rev. Physiol. 35:55–86.

McDONALD, T. F., and MacLEOD, D. P. 1973. Metabolism and electrical activity of anoxic ventricular muscle. J. Physiol. 229:559–582.

McDONALD, T. F., NAWRATH, H., and TRAUTWEIN, W. 1975. Membrane currents and tension in cat ventricular muscle treated with cardiac glycosides. Circ. Res. 37:674–682.

MORAD, M., and ROLETT, E. L. 1972. Relaxing effects of catecholamines on mammalian heart. J. Physiol. 224:537–558.

NAYLER, W. G. 1973. Effect of inotropic agents on cardiac trabecular muscle rendered highly permeable to calcium. Amer. J. Physiol. 225:918–924.

POOLE-WILSON, P. A., and LANGER, G. A. 1975. Glycoside inotropy in the absence of an increase in potassium efflux in the rabbit heart. Circ. Res. 37:390–395.

RASMUSSEN, H., and TENENHOUSE, A. 1968. Cyclic adenosine monophosphate, Ca^{++} and membranes. Proc. Natl. Acad. Sci., USA 59:1364–1370.

REUTER, H. 1973. Divalent cations as charge carriers in excitable membranes. Prog. Biophys. Mol. Biol. 26:1–43.

REUTER, H. 1974. Localization of beta adrenergic receptors, and effects of noradrenaline and cyclic nucleotides on action potentials, ionic currents and tension in mammalian cardiac muscle. J. Physiol. 242:429–451.

REUTER, H., and SEITZ, N. 1968. The dependence of calcium efflux from cardiac muscle on temperature and external ion composition. J. Physiol. 195:451–470.

TRAUTWEIN, W. 1973. Membrane currents in cardiac muscle fibers. Physiol. Rev. 53:793–835.

TSIEN, R. W. 1973. Adrenaline-like effects of intracellular ionophoresis of cyclic AMP in cardiac Purkinje fibres. Nature (New Biol.) 245:120–122.

VASSORT, G. 1973. Influence of sodium ions on the regulation of frog myocardial contractility. Pfluegers Arch. 339:225–240.

Mailing address:
Masayosi Goto,
Department of Physiology,
Faculty of Medicine,
Kyushu University, Fukuoka (Japan).

Recent Advances in Studies on
Cardiac Structure and Metabolism, Volume 11
Heart Function and Metabolism
Edited by T. Kobayashi, T. Sano, and N. S. Dhalla
Copyright 1978   University Park Press   Baltimore

ELECTRICALLY INDUCED AUTOMATICITY IN CANINE VENTRICULAR MYOCARDIUM

T. SAIKAWA, M. ARITA, and Y. NAGAMOTO

Department of Physiology, Faculty of Medicine,
Kyushu University, Fukuoka, Japan

SUMMARY

Repetitive spontaneous action potentials (SAP) could be induced in canine ventricular and atrial muscle, although this inhibitory action was antagonized by the pretreatment with voltage range between about -60 mV and 0 mV. The SAP seemed dependent on both slow inward Ca^{2+} and Na^+ currents and was suppressed by verapamil, Mn^{2+}, and diltiazem, but not by tetrodotoxin. The increase of extracellular potassium concentration also suppressed the SAP. Acetylcholine could not block the SAP in ventricular muscle, but inhibited that in atrial muscle, although this inhibitory action was antagonized by the pretreatment with atropine. The automatic activity was attributed to slow inward Ca^{2+} and Na^+ currents modified by decreasing time-dependent K^+ outward current and K^+ anomalous rectification.

INTRODUCTION

Recently the development of pacemaker activity has been reported in electrically depolarized guinea pig ventricular papillary muscle (Katzung, 1974; Surawicz and Imanishi, 1974). It has been also reported that an abnormal automaticity did occur in ventricular muscle excised from infarcted canine hearts (Solberg, TenEick, and Singer, 1972). The development of such automaticity is interesting and may be important because it implies a possible role of common cardiac muscle in initiation of arrhythmias. Thus, using canine ventricular and atrial myocardium, we studied the nature of the spontaneous action potentials induced by depolarizing currents.

METHOD

Small ventricular papillary muscles and atrial trabeculae were excised from adult mongrel dogs anesthetized with sodium pentobarbital (30 mg/kg, I. P.). The preparations were mounted in a single sucrose-gap chamber. Driving stimuli and depolarizing currents were delivered through a sucrose gap. For control records, the preparations were perfused with Tyrode solution (NaCl, 137; NaHCO₃,

11.9; KCl, 2.7; $CaCl_2$, 1.8; $MgCl_2$, 0.52; NaH_2PO_4, 0.42; and glucose, 5.0 mM).
Verapamil, $MnCl_2$ diltiazem hydrochloride, and acetylcholine were diluted with
Tyrode solution to appropriate concentrations. In some experiments a part of
NaCl was substituted for choline chloride. $CaCl_2$ and KCl were added or
subtracted to change Ca^{2+} and K^+ concentrations, respectively. The intracellular
potential recorded with conventional microelectrodes, the intensity of depolarizing currents, and the first derivative of membrane potential were displayed on an
oscilloscope and recorded with an ink-writing recticorder. Each solution was
bubbled with a mixture of 95% O_2–5% CO_2 and pH was adjusted to 7.3.
Temperature was kept at 36.5° C throughout the experiments.

RESULTS

Spontaneous action potentials (SAP) could be induced in 70% of canine ventricular muscles and 40% of atrial muscles tested in the potential range between –60
mV and 0 mV (Figure 1). The overshoot and maximum rate of rise $(dV/dt)_{max}$
of SAP decreased while the firing rate increased with decreasing membrane
potentials. The fact that the SAP was produced in such a low membrane
potential range suggested that slow inward currents may contribute to the
development of SAP. This assumption was ascertained by the finding that
verapamil (2–6 μg/ml) effectively suppressed the activity. On the other hand,
tetrodotoxin produced little change on the SAP. We also investigated the effect
of extracellular concentrations of Ca and Na ions, $(Ca^{2+})_o$ and $(Na^+)_o$. When
$(Ca^{2+})_o$ was increased, $(dV/dt)_{max}$ and firing rate were increased, whereas
overshoot was not affected. On the other hand, reduction of $(Na^+)_o$ to one-
fourth of Tyrode solution decreased the overshoot, $(dV/dt)_{max}$, and firing rate
altogether. Diltiazem hydrochloride, a new slow channel antagonist (Arita,
Saikawa, and Nagamoto, 1975), inhibited the SAP completely at a concentration
of 5μg/ml, but lidocaine (4–16 μg/ml) was ineffective. Adrenaline (5 μg/ml),
which was known to increase slow inward current, accelerated the SAP. It has
been well known that the pacemaker potential of normal Purkinje fiber is
sensitive to the extracellular potassium concentrations. Thus we tested the effect
of change in $(K^+)_o$. The activity was accelerated by a decrease of $(K^+)_o$ from 2.7
to 0.75 mM, while an increase to 10.8 mM suppressed it. Unfortunately,
however, the resting membrane potential was decreased with increasing $(K^+)_o$.
Therefore, two possibilities must be considered to explain the results, i.e., "Was
the automaticity suppressed by increased permeability to K ions, or by reduced
membrane potential per se?" To clarify this, we set off the high $(K^+)_o$-induced
depolarization by passing hyperpolarizing currents; however, the depressant
action of high $(K^+)_o$ on the automaticity still remained unchanged. The result
meant that the depressant effect of K ions was due to increase in K^+ permeabil-

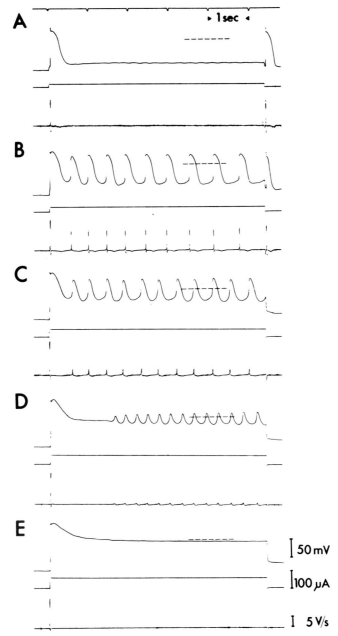

Figure 1. Automaticity of canine ventricular myocardium induced during a passage of depolarizing currents. In each panel, *top trace* is membrane potential; *middle trace,* the currents applied; *bottom trace,* the rate of rise. *Dotted line* is zero potential. The current intensity was increased stepwise through *A* to *E*. Note that the automaticity appeared when the membrane was depolarized to −58 mV (*B*) and disappeared at −5 mV (*E*).

ity. Finally, we measured slope resistance change during pacemaker potential, because it appeared that deactivation of potassium conductance might be a factor in the development of the pacemaker depolarization. As was expected, the slope resistance increased with time during phase 4, suggesting participation of time-dependent decrease of outward K^+ current. The current may be comparable with i_{x1} current in Purkinje fibers (Noble and Tsien, 1969), which is activated and deactivated in the potential range where the SAP was elicited (see Figure 1). However, similar decrease in slope conductance was observed also when the membrane was depolarized electrically by passing a gradually increasing ramp current. It suggests that anomalous rectification may also participate in the increase of slope resistance during pacemaker depolarization. Thus the voltage range where anomalous rectification becomes marked is always coincident with the range of appearance of the SAP. Accordingly, anomalous rectification may be another important factor in triggering and sustaining the automatic activity. In atrial muscle, SAP could be induced by the same method. The SAP was suppressed by verapamil. Acetylcholine ($1-5$ μg/ml), which was known to block slow inward current (TenEick et al., 1976), inhibited the SAP completely while it failed to suppress the ventricular automaticity. This suppressive effect of acetylcholine on atrial automaticity was antagonized by the pretreatment with atropine (1 μg/ml).

DISCUSSION

Spontaneous automatic activity could be induced by an application of small depolarizing currents in canine ventricular and atrial muscles. The activity was blocked by verapamil, Mn^{2+}, and diltiazem, but not by tetrodotoxin. It was concluded that the activity was triggered and sustained by slow inward currents in combination with the anomalous rectification and i_{x_1}-like current. Similar automaticity was reported to be induced in the ventricular muscle of guinea pig (Katzung, 1974; Surawicz and Imanishi, 1974), cat (Sakson, Kukushkin, and Zintsadze, 1975), and dog (Arita, Saikawa, and Nagamoto, 1976), in which significant i_{x_1}-like current was identified (Beeler and Reuter, 1970; Ochi, 1970; Trautwein, McDonald, and Tripathi, 1975). On the contrary, in the sheep ventricular muscle, with no significant i_{x_1}-like current (McGuigan, 1974), no automaticity could be induced by depolarizing currents (Trautwein and Kassebaum, 1961). These findings lend support to the contribution of i_{x_1}-like currents to the development of the automaticity. The clinical implication of the automaticity seems important, because it suggests a possible role of common cardiac muscle in initiation of arrhythmias. Such a situation may be encountered when the muscle is depolarized by an injury current from the infarcted myocardium.

REFERENCES

ARITA, M., SAIKAWA, T., and NAGAMOTO, Y. 1975. Effect of diltiazem hydrochloride(CRD-401) on canine cardiac fibers. Jpn. J. Clin. Exper. Med. 52:2156–2161. (In Japanese.)

ARITA, M., SAIKAWA, T., and NAGAMOTO, Y. 1976. Spontaneous electrical activity induced by depolarizing currents in canine ventricular myocardium. Jpn. Heart J. 17:248–262.

BEELER, G. W., and REUTER, H. 1970. Voltage clamp experiments on ventricular myocardial fibers. J. Physiol. 207:165–190.

KATZUNG, B. G. 1974. Electrically induced automaticity in ventricular myocardium. Life Sci. 14:1133–1140.

McGUIGAN, J. A. S. 1974. Some limitations of the double sucrose gap, and its use in a study of slow outward current in mammalian ventricular muscle. J. Physiol. 240: 775–806.

NOBLE, D., and TSIEN, R. W. 1969. Outward membrane currents activated in the plateau range of potentials in cardiac Purkinje fibers. J. Physiol. 200:205–231.

OCHI, R. 1970. The slow inward current and the action of manganese ions in guinea pig's myocardium. Pfluegers Arch. 316:81–94.

SAKSON, M. E., KUKUSHKIN, N. I., and ZINTSADZE, M. A. 1975. Induced automatics (repeated responses) of ventricular fibers of cat heart. Biofizika 20:101–106.

SOLBERG, L., TenEICK, R., and SINGER, D. 1972. Electrophysiological basis of arrhythmia in infarcted ventricle. Circulation 45 and 46 (suppl. II)–116.

SURAWICZ, B., and IMANISHI, S. 1974. Mechanism of automaticity in depolarized guinea pig ventricular myocardium. Circulation 45 and 46 (suppl. II)–84.

TenEICK, R., NAWRATH, H., McDONALD, T. F., and TRAUTWEIN, W. 1976. On the mechanism of the negative inotropic effect of acetylcholine. Pfluegers Arch. 360: 207–213.

TRAUTWEIN, W., and KASSEBAUM, D. G. 1961. On the mechanism of spontaneous impulse generation in the pacemaker of the heart. J. Gen. Physiol. 45:317–330.

TRAUTWEIN, W., McDONALD, T. F., and O. TRIPATHI. 1975. Calcium conductance and tension in mammalian ventricular muscle. Pfluegers Arch. 354:55–74.

Mailing address:
M. Arita, M.D.,
Associate Professor, Department of Physiology,
Faculty of Medicine,
Kyushu University, Fukuoka 812 (Japan).

Recent Advances in Studies on
Cardiac Structure and Metabolism, Volume 11
Heart Function and Metabolism
Edited by T. Kobayashi, T. Sano, and N. S. Dhalla
Copyright 1978   University Park Press   Baltimore

CHRONOTROPIC EFFECTS OF CALCIUM AND MAGNESIUM IONS AT DIFFERENT TEMPERATURES

A. J. C. MACKAAY, W. K. BLEEKER, and L. N. BOUMAN

Department of Physiology, University of Amsterdam,
Amsterdam, The Netherlands

SUMMARY

In the isolated right atrium of rabbit hearts, excess calcium causes an increase of heart rate at 38° C; this effect is absent or even reversed at a temperature of 30° C. From microelectrode studies it seems that when the calcium concentration is increased the pacemaker shifts within the sinoatrial node to cells in which excess calcium causes an acceleration of diastolic depolarization (type A). In fibers where the impulse originates at low calcium (type B), excess calcium causes a deceleration of diastolic depolarization. At low temperature, the effects on type A fibers are completely absent. Excess magnesium has a negative chronotropic effect at both temperatures, mainly by a deceleration of diastolic depolarization in type B fibers.

INTRODUCTION

The chronotropic action of calcium ions on the mammalian heart is still a matter of controversy. From experiments on rabbit hearts, Seifen *et al.* (1964) described a positive chronotropic effect when the external calcium concentration was increased. Toda (1969) observed no effect at all, whereas Lenfant (1972) found a small fall in heart rate. Close examination of the methods used by these authors revealed that the positive chronotropic response was obtained only at normal temperature; either a negative chronotropic response or the absence of any response was found at low temperatures.

METHOD

The aim of our investigation was to elucidate a possible interference of a low temperature with the positive chronotropic action of calcium ions on the rabbit heart. The right atrium, including the sinoatrial node, was isolated from 35 adult rabbits and kept in a tissue bath. Calcium chloride was added to the perfusion fluid in concentrations between 1.1 and 6.6 mmol/liter. A cardiotachogram was derived from the right atrial electrogram. In addition, the electrical activity of single fibers in the sinoatrial node was conventionally recorded by means of glass microelectrodes in 25 preparations.

RESULTS

In all preparations a positive chronotropic response occurred when the calcium concentration was raised at a temperature of 38° C. An increase from 1.1 to 2.2 mmol/liter shortened the interbeat interval 6.7% ± 1.39 ($n = 10$), while an increase from 1.1 to 3.3 mmol/liter caused a shortening of 12.9% ± 1.0 ($n = 25$). An increase up to 6.6 mmol/liter reduced the interval 17.2% ± 0.85 ($n = 4$). The chronotropic response was not affected by the addition of propranolol in a concentration of 8.10^{-6} mol/liter. The effects of the increase of the external calcium concentration on the electrical activity of a fiber in the sinoatrial node are shown in Figure 1. An increase from 1.1 to 2.2 mmol/liter caused mainly an acceleration of the diastolic depolarization. When more calcium was added, the maximal diastolic potential was also reduced, while the duration of the action potential increased. Furthermore, the sequence of discharge of the nodal fiber and the atrium was reversed. At the lowest calcium concentration the impaled fiber discharged later than the atrium, whereas the reverse was observed at higher calcium concentrations.

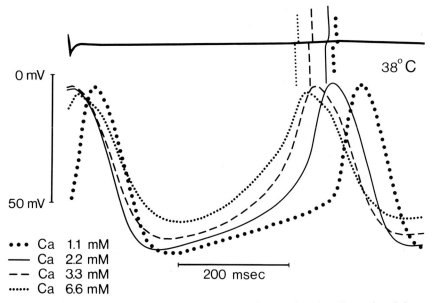

Figure 1. Effect of four different calcium concentrations on heartbeat interval and sino-atrial nodal pacemaker potential. *Upper tracing:* atrium electrogram. *Lower tracing:* trans-membrane potential of a single fiber in the sinoatrial node.

This reversal of the order of activation might be caused by a pacemaker shift within the sinoatrial node. In order to exclude possible side effects of this shift on the shape of the recorded electrical activity, the effect of calcium was also studied during pacing of the right atrium with a constant frequency; the acceleration of diastolic depolarization was still present and in the same order of magnitude (Figure 2, *upper record*). When the temperature of the perfusion fluid was lowered to 30° C, the shortening of the interbeat interval as well as most of the effects on the electrical activity of the fibers disappeared completely. In most preparations even a slight negative chronotropic effect could be observed.

The disappearance of the effects of calcium on the electrical activity of the nodal fibers can also be observed when the preparation is driven. Figure 2 (*lower record*) shows the effects of 1.1 and 3.3 mmol calcium at a temperature of 30° C on the same fiber that provided the upper registration.

CONCLUSIONS

From this series of experiments we conclude that a calcium-dependent process, probably a calcium influx, is involved in the diastolic depolarization; this process is highly temperature-sensitive.

From the previously mentioned reversal of the order of sinoatrial activation we assumed that at different concentrations of external calcium the impulse will originate in different nodal fibers. This assumption could be affirmed experimentally by the localization of the impulse origin by means of multiple impalements. At a low calcium concentration (1.1 mmol/liter) the impulse arose in fibers in the vicinity of the crista terminalis (type B fibers). When the calcium concentration was raised, the site of origin of the impulse was shifted toward the center of the node (type A fibers).

The response of a nodal fiber to an increase of the external calcium concentration, as shown in Figure 1, is typical for the latter group of fibers. The type B fibers behaved completely differently. When the external calcium concentration was raised, in those fibers the diastolic depolarization was slowed down; the order of activation was also reversed, i.e., in high calcium these fibers discharged after the atrium.

There is some evidence that at low temperatures the type B fibers regain their leading role in the origination of the heart impulse. They still showed a deceleration of the diastolic depolarization when the external calcium concentration was raised. This observation is in agreement with the observation of Lenfant (1972) that at 30° C in many preparations a negative chronotropic effect can be observed.

In five experiments the action of excess magnesium was tested by increasing the extracellular concentration from 0.6 to 2.8 mmol/liter at different calcium concentrations and different temperatures. In agreement with earlier observa-

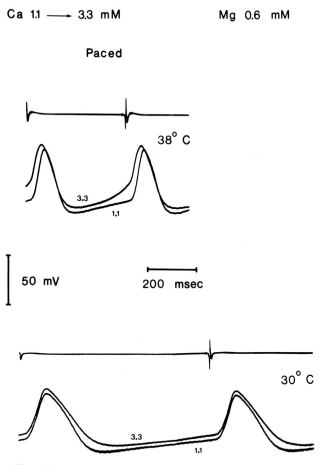

Ca 1.1 ⟶ 3.3 mM   **Mg 0.6 mM**

Paced

38° C

50 mV   200 msec

30° C

Figure 2. Effect of temperature on the response to calcium.

tions on the guinea pig heart (Schaer, 1968; Seifen, 1968) a negative chrono-tropic effect of magnesium was found that is more pronounced at a low calcium concentration; this effect was not abolished by a lowering of the temperature. From these observations we infer that magnesium inhibits diastolic depolarization mainly in the B type fibers.

From voltage-clamp experiments on frog atrial fibers (Chesnais *et al.*, 1975) it has been suggested that magnesium inhibits a slow inward current of sodium ions. In Figure 3 the observed effects on diastolic depolarization are sum-marized; the hypothesis is put forward that type A and B fibers differ with respect to the slow inward current of cations during diastole. These influxes, together with the well-established fall in K efflux, can be held responsible for the diastolic depolarization.

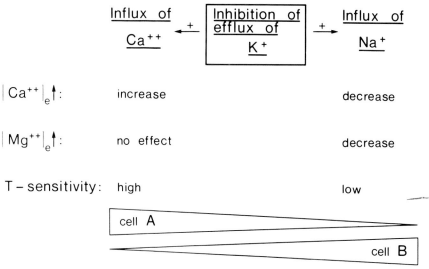

Figure 3. Hypothetical mechanisms of diastolic depolarization. In cell A a relatively strong calcium influx is assumed.

REFERENCES

CHESNAIS, J. M., CORABOEUF, E., SAUVIAT, M. P., and VASSAS, J. M. 1975. Sensitivity to H, Li and Mg ions of the slow inward current in frog atrial fibers. J. Mol. Cell. Cardiol. 7:627–642.

LENFANT, J. 1972. Analyse des propriétés de la membrane myocardique sino-auriculaire: genèse de l'activité spontanée. Thesis. Poitiers.

SCHAER, H. 1968. Antagonistische Wirkungen von Magnesium-, Calcium- und Natrium-ionen auf die Impulsbildung im Sinusknoten des Meerschweinchenherzens. Pfluegers Arch. 298:359–371.

SEIFEN, E. 1968. Dependency on Mg⁻ and Ca⁻ concentration on cyclic length in spontaneously beating guinea-pig atria. Pfluegers Arch. 304:46–56.

SEIFEN, E., SHAER, H., and MARSHALL, J. M. 1964. Effect of calcium on the membrane potential of single pacemaker fibers and atrial fibers in isolated rabbit atria. Nature 202: 1223–1224.

TODA, N. 1969. Electrophysiological effects of potassium and calcium ions in the sino-atrial node in response to sympathetic nerve stimulation. Pfluegers Arch. 310:45–63.

Mailing address:
Dr. L. N. Bouman,
Professor of Physiology, Department of Physiology,
University of Amsterdam,
le C. Huygenstraat 20, Amsterdam (The Netherlands).

Recent Advances in Studies on
Cardiac Structure and Metabolism, Volume 11
Heart Function and Metabolism
Edited by T. Kobayashi, T. Sano, and N. S. Dhalla
Copyright 1978   University Park Press   Baltimore

EFFECTS OF ACETYLCHOLINE AND CYCLIC NUCLEOTIDES ON THE BULLFROG ATRIAL MUSCLE

Y. IKEMOTO and M. GOTO

Department of Physiology, Faculty of Medicine,
Kyushu University, Fukuoka, Japan

SUMMARY

Effects of ACh on the slow inward current and tension components of bullfrog atrial muscle were examined with voltage-clamp technique. ACh decreased the phasic component of contractile tension and the slow inward current with a reduction of $\bar{g}_{Ca}$. Contracture tensions were augmented by ACh and decreased by adrenaline. Intracellularly injected cGMP through microelectrode decreased the overshoot and the plateau level of action potential without affecting the resting membrane potential, indicating a decrease in the slow inward current. cAMP enhanced the overshoot and the plateau. ACh seems to reduce the slow inward current through an elevation of intracellular cGMP concentration.

INTRODUCTION

Acetylcholine (ACh) has long been known to produce a negative inotropic effect on the atrial muscle. In the frog heart the cause of this effect was attributed to the shortened action potential caused by an increase in g_K of the cell membrane. Recently, a reduction in I_{Ca} by ACh was suggested (Giles and Tsien, 1975; Ikemoto and Goto, 1975). This chapter presents evidence of this action of ACh discovered by use of voltage-clamp technique with double gap method. Further experiments were conducted to examine the intracellular effects of cAMP and cGMP by microelectrophoresis.

METHOD

The preparation used was freshly isolated atrial muscle of the bullfrog. In double gap experiments, the chamber in which the preparation was mounted and the electrical apparatus used were the same as previously described by Goto, Wada, and Saito (1974). The composition of normal Ringer solution in mM was: NaCl, 105.0; KCl, 2.5; CaCl$_2$, 1.8; glucose, 5.0; and Tris-Cl, 10.0. The pH of the solution was adjusted to 7.4. In contracture experiments, solution bath volume was 0.3 ml, and the solution was changed by rapid and constant perfusion of 0.5

ml per sec. Na-free contracture solution was prepared by replacing NaCl with Tris-Cl and K-excess contracture solution, simply by adding 100 mM KCl to the Ringer solution. The preparations were driven at a rate of 0.1 per sec and the clamp pulses were applied at the same frequency.

In experiments of electrophoresis, double-barrel microelectrodes were prepared, one barrel of which was filled with 3 M KCl (resistance between 40 and 100 MΩ) and the other with 50 mM cAMP or cGMP. With the former, action potential was recorded, and through the latter the drugs were injected electrophoretically into the cell. The actual phoresis current was measured by I-V converter of an OP amp. Ca concentration of the perfusing solution was lowered to 0.18 mM in order to avoid vigorous contraction. The preparations were stimulated at a rate of 10 per min and the electrophoretic current pulses of 600 msec were applied with a delay of 1.5 sec. All experiments in this report were performed at room temperature of around 17° C.

RESULTS

ACh (10^{-6} g/ml) shortened the action potential and exerted a negative inotropic effect, as expected. It must be noted that the overshoot of the action potential diminished appreciably (6 mV, $n = 7$) with unaltered gap resting potential. This observation suggests a reduction of the slow inward current during depolarization, and we examined the behavior of the muscle under voltage clamp.

The twitch tension was greatly reduced by ACh, despite the fixed configuration of the depolarizing clamp pulse (100 msec, 70 mV). The reduction was more prominent for depolarizing pulses of lower amplitude and shorter duration, but the time to peak tension was not affected under these conditions. ACh diminished the slow inward currently markedly, and the reduction was also evident in the tail current, where the membrane voltage was repolarized back to the resting potential level (−70 mV) and where anomalous rectification diminished. The peak time of the slow inward current and τ_d of 40 msec were not influenced by ACh. Furthermore, ACh did not alter the time constant of restoration of the slow inward current.

Steady-state activation curves were obtained by measuring the tail currents after 100-msec pulses of different amplitude in the presence of tetrodotoxin (10^{-6} g/ml). The maximal tail current was reduced to about 60% by ACh. The reduction corresponds to a decrease in $\bar{g}_{Ca}$. Normalization of these plots gives the steady-state activation variable d_∞, which was not greatly affected by ACh. Steady-state inactivation curves of g_{Ca} were determined by measuring the tail currents of 120-msec pulses (always depolarized to 0 mV), and by applying a conditioning prestep of 1 sec duration to different potentials. This inactivation curve was also shifted downward by ACh, with the maximal reduction of about 45%. Again, there was no appreciable change in the normalized plot of this curve, f_∞ (Figure 1).

As for the effects on contractile tension, ACh decreased only the phasic component, which was attributed to the slow inward current. The tonic component, which did not depend on I_{Ca}, was slightly enhanced, and the contracture tensions elicited by K-excess or Na-free Ringer solutions were augmented by ACh and reduced by adrenaline (10^{-6} g/ml).

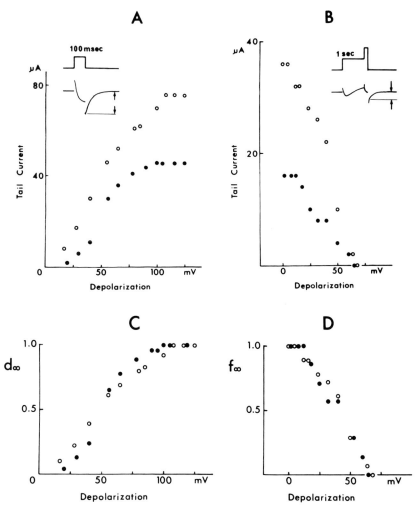

Figure 1. Activation and inactivation variables: Relationship between amplitude of tail of slow inward current and depolarizing step in the presence of tetrodotoxin (10^{-6} g/ml). *A,* activation, and *B,* inactivation of g_{Ca}, measured at −70 mV holding potential. 1: control, •: 8–12 min after application of ACh (10^{-6} g/ml). ACh reduced g_{Ca}. *C* and *D* are the normalized plots (d_∞) and (f_∞) of *A* and *B,* respectively. *Filled circles* show data after ACh. ACh did not influence d_∞ and f_∞.

Finally, we examined the effects of intracellularly injected cyclic nucleotides on the resting and action potentials of the atrial muscle. cAMP increased the overshoot and the plateau level without any change in the resting membrane potential and the action potential duration. However, cGMP decreased the overshoot and the plateau level without affecting the resting potential or the action potential duration (Figure 2).

DISCUSSION

In the present results it has been show that only the phasic component of contractile tension was reduced by ACh, indicating a decrease in I_{Ca}. Reuter described the slow inward current as follows:

$$I_{Ca} = g_{Ca} \cdot (E_m - E_{Ca})$$
$$g_{Ca} = \bar{g}_{Ca} \cdot d \cdot f.$$

He elucidated that catecholamine increased $\bar{g}Ca$ without affecting the other parameteres (Reuter, 1974). We have now presented evidence of reduction in

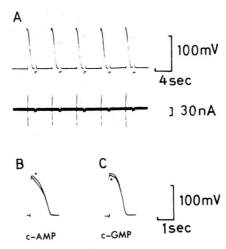

Figure 2. Effects of electrophoretically injected cyclic nucleotides on the action potential of bullfrog atrium. *A:* A slow paper record of cAMP injection. The preparation was driven at a rate of 10 per min and the electrophoretic current pulses were applied with a delay of 1.5 sec. The *lower trace* shows the current measurement by an OP amp. The overshoot is increasing appreciably. *B* and *C:* Superimposed tracings of paper records before and after 10–20 current pulses of several nanoamperes (●). *B,* cAMP increased the overshoot and the plateau level (5 mV, *n* = 14) without altering the resting membrane potential and the action potential duration. In *C,* cGMP decreased the overshoot and the plateau level (4 mV, *n* = 7), whereas the resting potential and the action potential duration were not affected. Throughout a single run continuous impalement of a single cell was maintained.

$\bar{g}_{Ca}$ without alteration in d_∞ and f_∞. These two drugs are known to exert physiologically antagonistic actions on heart, and they seem to have an antagonistic action on the kinetics of the slow inward current. ACh increased contracture tensions, whereas adrenaline decreased them. It is well known that catecholamines produce a prominent elevation of myocardial cAMP concentration, which has been reported to promote relaxation by accelerating Ca uptake into SR (Kirchberger et al., 1972). On the other hand, there are many reports indicating that ACh causes a significant increase in concentration of cGMP (George, Wilkerson, and Kadowitz, 1973). In the microelectrophoresis experiments, we have shown opposite effects of these two cyclic nucleotides on the action potential. cAMP increased the overshoot and the plateau level, and cGMP decreased them. It is known that in frog heart the rising phase of action potential has two components and that the second slow component is related to the slow inward current. Therefore, the reduction in I_{Ca} by ACh and that of the overshoot and the plateau level by cGMP suggest that ACh reduced the slow inward current through an increase in concentration of intracellular cGMP.

REFERENCES

CORABOEUF, E. 1974. Membrane electrical activity and double component contraction in cardiac tissue. J. Mol. Cell. Cardiol. 6:215–225.

GEORGE, W. J., WILKERSON, R. D., and KADOWITZ, P. J. 1973. Influence of acetylcholine on contractile force and cyclic nucleotide levels in the isolated perfused rat heart. J. Pharmacol. Exp. Ther. 184:228–235.

GILES, W., and TSIEN, W. 1975. Effects of acetylcholine on membrane currents in frog atrial muscle. J. Physiol. 246:64p–66p.

GOTO, M., WADA, Y., and SAITO, M. 1974. Tension components and tension fall of the bullfrog atrial muscle during depolarization. Jpn. J. Physiol. 24:359–375.

IKEMOTO, Y., and GOTO, M. 1975. Nature of the negative inotropic effect of acetylcholine on the myocardium: An elucidation on the bullfrog atrium. Proc. Jap. Acad. 51:501–505.

KIRCHBERGER, M. A., TADA, M., REPKE, D. I., and KATZ, A. M. 1972. Cyclic adenosine 3':5' monophosphate-dependent protein kinase stimulation of calcium uptake by canine cardiac microsomes. J. Mol. Cell. Cardiol. 4:673–680.

REUTER, H. 1974. Localization of beta adrenergic receptors, and effects of noradrenaline and cyclic nucleotides on action potentials, ionic currents and tension in mammalian cardiac muscle. J. Physiol. 242:429–451.

Mailing address:
Y. Ikemoto,
Department of Physiology,
Faculty of Medicine,
Kyushu University, Fukuoka City 812 (Japan).

Recent Advances in Studies on
Cardiac Structure and Metabolism, Volume 11
Heart Function and Metabolism
Edited by T. Kobayashi, T. Sano, and N. S. Dhalla
Copyright 1978   University Park Press   Baltimore

CONTRIBUTION OF AN ELECTROGENIC SODIUM PUMP TO THE RESPONSE OF SINOATRIAL NODE CELLS TO ACETYLCHOLINE

K. NISHI, Y. YOSHIKAWA, and F. TAKENAKA

Department of Pharmacology, Kumamoto University
Medical School, Kumamoto, Japan

SUMMARY

ACh (10^{-7} – 10^{-6} g/ml) induced hyperpolarization in pacemaker cells in the sinoatrial (SA) node of the rabbit heart varied inversely with the level of the maximal diastolic potential of the pacemaker cells. The hyperpolarization induced by ACh was completely abolished at $4°$–$6°$ C. Ouabain (10^{-6} g/ml) markedly depressed or abolished the hyperpolarizing response. The response was also depressed in K-free solution, but not abolished. In Ca-free or low-Na solution, the sino atrial node cell responded well to ACh, showing marked hyperpolarization. Present results indicate that the hyperpolarization induced by ACh is at least in part due to an electrogenic Na pump activated by ACh.

INTRODUCTION

The basic mechanism of changes in membrane characteristic of pacemaker cells in the sinoatrial node in the mammalian heart on application of acetylcholine (ACh) has been believed to be an increase in K^+ permeability (Trautwein and Dudel, 1958; Toda and West, 1967). However, the explanation of the effect of ACh on the sinoatrial node cell was predicted from the results obtained in the atrial tissue. In fact, the pacemaker cells in the sinoatrial node differ in many ways from other cardiac cells (see Brooks and Lu, 1972). Therefore, it was felt necessary to reinvestigate the effect of exogenously applied ACh on the pacemaker cell in the sinoatrial node in the mammalian heart in an attempt to clarify the ionic mechanism involved in the ACh response.

METHOD

The right atrium with the sinoatrial node region of the rabbit's heart was excised and superfused with well-oxygenated Tyrode solution ($36°$–$37°$ C) of the following composition in mM: NaCl, 136.8; KCl, 2.68; CaCl$_2$, 1.80; MgCl$_2$, 1.08; NaH$_2$PO$_4$, 0.26; NaHCO$_3$, 10.0; and glucose, 5.56. Transmembrane potentials were recorded with microelectrodes filled with 3 M KCl through a conventional high-input impedance amplifier. The output of the amplifier was displayed on both a cathode-ray oscilloscope and a polygraph recorder. When ACh was applied, the superfusion was stopped and the drug (dissolved in saline solution) was directly added to the bathing solution. g-Strophanthin (ouabain) was dissolved in the superfusing solution. Final concentrations of the drugs were expressed in grams per milliliter. Low-Na solution was prepared by substituting Na for sucrose. Cooling the tissue was done by superfusing the preparation with well-oxygenated solution previously cooled at temperatures desired.

RESULTS

Sample records of original transmembrane potentials at different stages and continuous records before and after application of ACh obtained from different sinoatrial node cells are illustrated in Figure 1. The configuration and amplitude

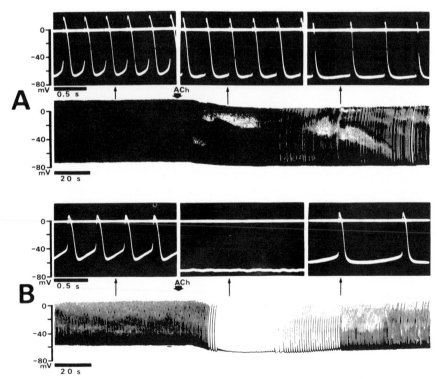

Figure 1. Effects of ACh on pacemaker cells in the SA node of the rabbit's heart. Sample photographic records of action potentials in the upper column in *A* and *B* were taken at the points indicated by *thin arrows* in the continuous record in the lower column. ACh (10^{-6}g/ml in *A,* and 10^{-7}g/ml in *B*) was applied at *thick arrows.* (Nishi, Yoshikawa, and Takenaka, unpublished observation.)

of action potentials during the control period were identical to those of a typical true pacemaker type potential (Hoffman and Granefield, 1960; Brooks and Lu, 1972). Effects of ACh on pacemaker cells varied considerably depending upon the level of the maximal diastolic potential. When the maximal diastolic potential was large (−74 mV), as shown in Figure 1A, ACh (10^{-6}g/ml) decreased the speed of the diastolic potential, hyperpolarized the cell membrane (−78 mV), and reduced both the amplitude and duration of the action potential. In other cells, where the maximal diastolic potential was relatively low (−57 mV), ACh, even at a low dose (10^{-7}g/ml), induced marked hyperpolarization (−76 mV), accompanied by transient abolition of action potentials (Figure 1B). In 33 cells in the sinoatrial node examined, ACh hyperpolarized the cell membrane to the level ranging from −68 mV to −97 mV (mean, −77; 6 ± 2.3 mV). The amount of hyperpolarization induced by ACh was inversely related to the level of the maximal diastolic potential (Figure 2).

When the preparation was cooled to about $10°$ C, the spontaneously appearing action potentials were abolished and the cell membrane was depolarized to the lower level, ranging from −30 mV to −40 mV. The response to ACh was completely blocked at $4°–6°$C, and at relatively low temperatures ($17°–23°$C) the hyperpolarizing response was small compared with that at the control temperature (Figure 3).

Ouabain (10^{-6} g/ml) gradually decreased the amplitude and the frequency of spontaneous action potentials in the sinoatrial node cell, and finally the action potential was abolished, the membrane being depolarized to about −30 mV. ACh applied at this stage did not produce hyperpolarization anymore. The effect of ouabain on the ACh response was reversible, since the cell responded well to ACh after washing ouabain out.

In K-free solution the maximal diastolic potential gradually decreased and only the oscillatory potential remained. The ACh response progressively decreased in the K-free solution; the magnitude of the hyperpolarization was markedly depressed at 30-min superfusion with the K-free solution, but not completely abolished. In the absence of external K^+ ions there was no clear relationship between the level of the maximal diastolic potential and the amount of the hyperpolarization induced by ACh (Figure 2).

In Ca-free or low-Na solution the pacemaker cell responded well to ACh, showing marked hyperpolarization.

DISCUSSION AND CONCLUSION

Present experiments have demonstrated that ACh induces hyperpolarization that is inversely related to the level of the maximal diastolic potential of the pacemaker cell in the rabbit's heart. The hyperpolarization induced by ACh or by vagal stimulation might be due to an increase in K^+ permeability (Trautwein and Dudel, 1958; Toda and West, 1967). In fact, Toda and West (1967) reported

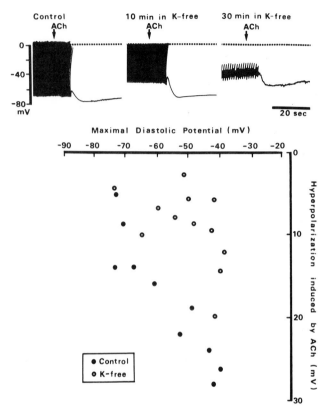

Figure 2. Effects of K-free solution on the ACh responses of pacemaker cells in the SA node. *Upper records* show the ACh responses of the same pacemaker cell before and after the superfusion with K-free solution. ACh (10^{-6}g/ml) was applied at *arrows.* The *lower chart* indicates the relationship between the magnitude of the hyperpolarization induced by ACh (10^{-6}g/ml) and the level of the maximal diastolic potential of pacemaker cells in normal K solution (*closed circle*) and in K-free solution (*open circle*). (Nishi, Yoshikawa, and Takenaka. Unpublished observation.)

that the amount of hyperpolarization resulting from vagal stimulation was an inverse function of the external potassium ions. However, in the K-free solution the hyperpolarizing response was markedly reduced, indicating that the presence of the external potassium ions is essential in eliciting the response. Furthermore, the hyperpolarization was about −77 mV, which greatly deviated from the potassium equilibrium potential predicted by DeMello (1960). Thus, the hyperpolarization resulting from application of ACh on the pacemaker cells in the sinoatrial node cannot be explained solely by an increase in K^+ permeability in the pacemaker cell membrane. Other factors may contribute to eliciting the hyperpolarizing response in the cells. In this regard, it is interesting to note that

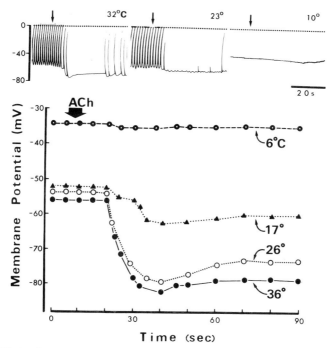

Figure 3. Effects of temperatures on the ACh responses of pacemaker cells in the SA node. Upper records show effects of various temperatures on the ACh responses of the same pacemaker cell. ACh (10^{-6} g/ml) was applied at *arrows.* The lower chart illustrates the time course of changes in the transmembrane potentials after ACh (10^{-6} g/ml) in different pacemaker cells at various temperatures. ACh was applied at a *thick arrow.* (Nishi, Yoshikawa, and Takenaka, unpublished observation.)

the response was abolished 1) at low temperatures and 2) by ouabain, which is known as the most specific inhibitor of Na^+-K^+-dependent ATPase, and was depressed in K-free solution. The results are consistent with the general concept of an electrogenic sodium pump (see Glynn and Karlish, 1975). It seems likely that active Na^+ extrusion by the electrogenic sodium pump activated by ACh is at least in part responsible for producing the hyperpolarization in the pacemaker cell. Recently, the presence of the electrogenic sodium pump activity has been suggested in pacemaker cell of the rabbit sinoatrial node (Noma and Irisawa, 1974).

REFERENCES

BROOKS, C. McC., and LU, H. H. 1972. The Sinoatrial Pacemaker of the Heart. Charles C Thomas, Springfield, Ill.

DeMELLO, W. C. 1960. Some aspects of the interrelationship between ions and electrical activity in specialized tissue of the heart. *In* P. de Carvallo, W. C. DeMello, and B. F. Hoffman (eds.), The Specialized Tissue of the Heart, pp. 95–107. Elsevier, New York.

GLYNN, I. M., and KARLISH, S. J. D. 1975. The sodium pump. Annu. Rev. Physiol. 35:13–53.

HOFFMAN, B. F., and GRANEFIELD, P. 1960. Electrophysiology of the Heart. McGraw-Hill, New York.

NOMA, A., and IRISAWA, H. 1974. Electrogenic sodium pump in rabbit sinoatrial node cell. Pfluegers Arch. 351:177–182.

TODA, N., and WEST, T. C. 1967. Interaction of K, Na, and vagal stimulation in the S-A node of the rabbit. Amer. J. Physiol. 212:416–423.

TRAUTWEIN, W., and DUDEL, J. 1958a. Zum Mechanismus der Membranewirkung des Acetylcholin an der Herzmuskelfaser. Pfluegers Arch. 266:324–334.

TRAUTWEIN, W., and DUDEL, J. 1958b. Hemmende und "erregende" Wirkungen des Acetylcholin am Warmblüterherzen. Zur Frage der spontanen Erregungs bildung. Pfluegers Arch. 266:653–664.

Mailing address:
K. Nishi, M. D.,
Associate Professor of Pharmacology,
Department of Pharmacology,
Kumamoto University Medical School,
Honjo 2-2-7, Kumamoto City (Japan).

Recent Advances in Studies on
Cardiac Structure and Metabolism, Volume 11
Heart Function and Metabolism
Edited by T. Kobayashi, T. Sano, and N. S. Dhalla
Copyright 1978   University Park Press   Baltimore

SELECTIVE EFFECTS OF TTX AND VERAPAMIL ON THE UPSTROKE COMPONENTS OF THE ACTION POTENTIAL FROM THE ATRIOVENTRICULAR NODE

E. RUIZ-CERETTI, A. PONCE ZUMINO, and O. F. SCHANNE

Department of Biophysics, Faculty of Medicine, University of Sherbrooke,
Sherbrooke, Quebec, Canada

SUMMARY

The upstroke of the nodal action potential shows a fast initial depolarization followed by a slower depolarizing phase. TTX depressed the fast depolarization selectively, whereas verapamil inhibited the slow phase.

INTRODUCTION

The upstroke of the nodal action potential presents two depolarizing phases with different rates of rise. They are differently affected by changes in extracellular sodium and calcium (Ruiz-Ceretti and Ponce Zumino, 1976). In order to investigate whether these two phases result from the activation of a fast and a slow inward current, the effect of specific inhibitors of the ionic conductances was tested.

METHOD

Perfused rabbit hearts were exposed to TTX (0.5 μM) or verapamil (1.1 μM). The transmembrane potential was recorded with flexibly mounted microelectrodes. The different fiber types (atrial, atrionodal, and nodal) were characterized according to the anatomical location of the impalement, the action potential and its first time derivative (V). Under control conditions the upstroke

RESULTS

Figure 1*a* shows the effects of TTX and verapamil on the atrionodal action potential and its first time derivative ($\dot{V}$). Under control conditions, the upstroke

---

Supported by the Medical Research Council and the Québec Heart Foundation.

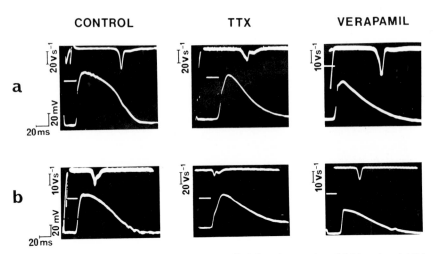

CONTROL   **TTX**   **VERAPAMIL**

Figure 1. Effects of TTX (0.3 μM) and verapamil (1.1 μM) on atrionodal (a) and nodal (b) action potentials. *Upper traces,* first time derivative; *lower traces,* potential.

was composed of a fast depolarizing phase (phase I) followed by a slow depolarization (phase II). These two components were also evident in the $\dot{V}$ recording. Tetrodotoxin decreased the amplitude and the maximum depolarization rate of phase I. The amplitude of phase II increased and its $\dot{V}_{max}$ did not change. Verapamil depressed phase II considerably without altering the amplitude or the $\dot{V}_{max}$ of phase I.

Figure 1*b* shows that under control conditions the first time derivative of the nodal action potential was composed of two distinctive peaks. Under TTX the amplitude of the first peak decreased drastically, and a marked reduction of phase I occurred. A time lag appeared between phase I and phase II, and the amplitude of the latter increased. The action potential amplitude did not change. Verapamil abolished phase II. The second deflection in the $\dot{V}$ recording disappeared.

The results of all the measurements performed in nodal action potentials are presented in Table 1. Verapamil increased the resting potential. This effect cannot be explained in the light of what is known about the action of this inhibitor. The action potential amplitude did not change under TTX because the relative contribution of phase II to the upstroke increased. In atrionodal fibers (not shown) the increase in the amplitude of phase II did not offset completely the decrease in phase I. Consequently, the action potential amplitude decreased under TTX. Verapamil reduced the nodal action potential amplitude by a mean amount of 17 mV. The maximum rate of rise of phase I decreased under TTX, whereas the deflection of the $\dot{V}$ recording corresponding to phase II of the upstroke became nonmeasurable under verapamil.

Table 1. Effects of TTX and verapamil on nodal action potentials*

Condition	RP (mV)	APA (mV)	Phase I		Phase II	
			(mV)	(V/s)	(mV)	(V/s)
Control	−63	62	36	10	25	5
	±1.5	±1.4	±1.9	±1.0	±1.4	±0.4
	(16)	(19)	(16)	(18)	(16)	(13)
TTX	−61	61	29	8	30	6
	±1.1	±1.1	±1.3††	±0.5**	±1.0***	±0.5
	(18)	(25)	(23)	(22)	(23)	(16)
Verapamil	−69	45	38	10	nonmeasurable	nonmeasurable
	±1.2††	±2.9§	±2.75	±0.9		
	(18)	(18)	(18)	(18)		

*All values are means ±S.E.M. Number of impalements in parentheses. RP, resting potential; APA, action potential amplitude. Under phase I and phase II, their amplitudes and maximum rate of rise.
**$p < 0.05$.
***$p < 0.02$.
††$p < 0.005$.
§$p < 0.001$.

DISCUSSION

Our previous observations (Ruiz-Ceretti and Ponce Zumino, 1976) showed that a decrease in extracellular sodium depressed phase I of the nodal action potential, but this finding was not conclusive because Na^+ as well as Ca^{2+} may act as charge carriers for the slow current (Rougier et al., 1969). However, the configurational changes of atrionodal and nodal action potentials under TTX are similar to those observed in low sodium medium (Ruiz-Ceretti, Ponce Zumino, and Parisii, 1971). This indicates that the sodium dependence of phase I is determined by the fast sodium system. As in frog ventricle (Hagiwara and Nakajima, 1966), TTX reduced the V_{max} of phase I but did not change the action potential amplitude or the overshoot of the nodal action potential. This reflects the larger contribution of the slow inward current to the total depolarizing current in nodal cells. Although the amplitude of phase II increased under TTX, this inhibitor did not affect the maximum slow current because the $\dot{V}_{max}$ of phase II did not change. The insensitivity of $\dot{V}_{max}$ of phase I to verapamil indicates that this phase arises from the activation of an ionic channel other than the slow inward channel. Based on the voltage dependence of the $\dot{V}_{max}$ in nodal cells (Shigeto and Irisawa, 1974) and the results of Kreitner (1975), we postulate that failure to detect a TTX-sensitive component in the nodal action potential (Zipes and Mendez, 1973) may result from membrane depolarization.

CONCLUSION

In summary, our results indicate that the two systems for inward current described in cardiac muscle are present in nodal cell membranes and their relative contribution to the excitation process may depend on the resting potential.

Acknowledgments The authors acknowledge the technical help of Mr. D. Chartier and the secretarial assistance of Mrs. M. Godbout and Miss L. Denault.

REFERENCES

HAGIWARA, S., and NAKAJIMA, S. 1966. Differences in Na and Ca spikes as examined by application of tetrodotoxin, procaine, and manganese ions. J. Gen. Physiol. 49: 793–806.

KREITNER, D. 1975. Evidence for the existence of a rapid sodium channel in the membrane of rabbit sinoatrial cells. J. Mol. Cell. Cardiol. 7:655–662.

PAES de CARVALHO, A., HOFFMAN, B. F., and DE PAULA CARVALHO, M. 1969. Two components of the cardiac action potential. I. Voltage-time course and the effect of acetylcholine on atrial and nodal cells of the rabbit heart. J. Gen. Physiol. 54:607–635.

ROUGIER, O., VASSORT, G., GARNIER, D., GARGOUIL, Y. M., and CORABOEUF, E. 1966. Existence and role of a slow inward current during the frog atrial action potential. Pfluegers Arch. 308:91–110.

RUIZ-CERETTI, E., PONCE ZUMINO, A., and PARISII, I. M. 1971. Resolution of two components in the upstroke of the action potential in atrioventricular fibers of the rabbit heart. Can. J. Physiol. Pharmacol. 49:642–648.

RUIZ-CERETTI, E., and PONCE ZUMINO, A. 1976. Action potential changes under varied $[Na]_o$ and $[Ca]_o$ indicating the existence of two inward currents in cells of the rabbit atrioventricular node. Circ. Res. 39:326–336.

SHIGETO, N., and IRISAWA, H. 1974. The effect of polarization on the action potentials of the rabbit AV nodal cells. Jpn. J. Physiol. 24:605–616.

ZIPES, D. P., and MENDEZ, C. 1973. Action of manganese ions and tetrodotoxin on atrioventricular nodal transmembrane potentials in isolated rabbit hearts. Circ. Res. 32:447–454.

Mailing address:
E. Ruiz-Ceretti,
Department of Biophysics,
Faculty of Medicine,
University of Sherbrooke,
Sherbrooke, Quebec J1H 5N4 (Canada).

Recent Advances in Studies on
Cardiac Structure and Metabolism, Volume 11
Heart Function and Metabolism
Edited by T. Kobayashi, T. Sano, and N. S. Dhalla
Copyright 1978   University Park Press   Baltimore

DUAL EFFECTS OF FLUORIDE ON THE ACTION POTENTIAL, CONTRACTION, AND MEMBRANE CURRENTS IN FROG ATRIAL MUSCLE

Y. ABE, M. AOMINE, and M. GOTO

Department of Physiology, School of Health Science and Faculty of Medicine,
Kyushu University, Fukuoka, Japan

SUMMARY

The effects of NaF ($10^{-7}-10^{-2}$ M) on the membrane potential, current, and contractile tension in bullfrog atrial muscle were investigated under voltage-clamped or unclamped conditions. NaF showed two opposite actions, positive and negative inotropic effects, depending on the concentration of the drug. NaF in lower concentrations produced a marked increase in contractility, a moderate prolongation of action potential, an augmentation of calcium response, and an increase of I_{Ca}-dependent tension. Contrarily, NaF in higher concentrations produced an inhibition of contractile tension associated with a shortening of action potential, an increase in potassium conductance, and an inhibition of calcium response. These results indicate that NaF affects the contractile response by dual mechanisms.

INTRODUCTION

A number of recent studies suggest that the adenyl cyclase systems mediate the positive inotropic actions in cardiac and skeletal muscles (Murad and Vaughan, 1969; Gold *et al.*, 1970; Reuter, 1974), and the activity of adenyl cyclase is stimulated by several hormones (Rodbell, 1967; Weiss, 1969; McNeill and Muschek, 1972). Fluoride is also known to stimulate the adenyl cyclase activity (Sutherland, Rall, and Menon, 1962; Oka *et al.*, 1973), while it inhibits the activity of (Na,K)-ATPase (Kishner, 1964; Opit, Potter, and Charnock, 1966; Farias, Goldember, and Trucco, 1970). Correspondingly, positive and negative inotropic effects of fluoride have been reported in cardiac muscle of various species (Loewi, 1955; Covin and Berman, 1959; Rice and Berman, 1961; Berman, 1966). However, details of the mechanism of the inotropic actions of fluoride are still unknown. In order to clarify the mechanism, the present study on the effects of fluoride on the membrane potential, current, and contractile tension of the atrial muscle under voltage-clamped or unclamped conditions was undertaken.

METHOD

Atrial muscle bundles, 4–5 mm in length and 0.5 mm in diameter, isolated from the bullfrog heart, were set up in a double sucrose-gap apparatus and stimulated at a constant frequency of 0.1 c/sec. In voltage-clamp experiments the membrane potential, current, and tension were measured simultaneously. The normal Ringer's solution was at the following composition (mM): NaCl, 111; KCl, 2.1; $CaCl_2$, 1.0; Tris-Cl, 2.4; and glucose, 5.6. The solution was equilibrated with 100% oxygen gas and the pH was adjusted to 7.4. All experiments were carried out at 16–18° C. Solutions containing fluoride and/or manganese were prepared by the addition of NaF (final concentration, 10^{-7}–10^{-2} M) and/or $MnCl_2$ (3 × 10^{-3} M) to the normal Ringer's solution. For Na-free solutions, NaCl of the solution was replaced by sucrose isosmotically.

RESULTS

The contractile force was markedly augmented by the addition of low concentrations of NaF. Similar positive inotropic effects were observed even at a concentration as low as 10^{-7} M, and a maximal effect was obtained at 10^{-5} or 10^{-4} M. The increase in tension amplitude began within 1 min, and the full effects were attained within 10–20 min and then gradually depressed by longer perfusion. On the other hand, in higher concentrations of NaF up to 10^{-2} M, positive inotropic effect did not appear at all, or disappeared within a few minutes, and the twitch tension rapidly diminished.

As for the membrane potential, NaF in a lower concentration (10^{-4} M) produced a transient prolongation of the duration of action potential (Figure 1A). A higher concentration of NaF (10^{-2} M), on the other hand, elicited a marked shortening of action potential and a depression of the plateau phase. However, no appreciable alteration of the resting potential and the amplitude of action potential was noticed (Figure 1B), although the electrotonic potentials produced by externally applied constant current became small. Under voltage clamp in normal and Mn solutions there was no significant effect of NaF on the fast sodium current until 15 min of exposure, even at higher concentrations. Since the rising phase of action potential depends on the fast sodium current, this result agrees with the data observed in action potential. The measurements of outward potassium current in Na-free solution containing 3 mM Mn showed that at lower concentrations of NaF the potassium currents showed no appreciable change, but at higher concentrations both the leaky membrane current and the delayed outward current were increased, reducing the anomalous rectification. These facts may account for the shortening of duration of action potential at higher concentrations. The calcium current, which was determined under voltage-clamp condition in Na-free solution, was virtually unaffected or slightly

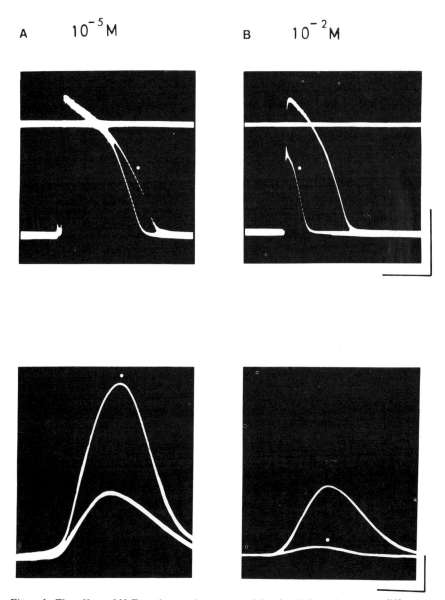

Figure 1. The effect of NaF on the membrane potential and twitch tension at two different concentrations. The responses in control and NaF solution are superimposed, the latter being labeled with *white dots. A,* in 10^{-5}; *B,* in 10^{-2} M NaF. *Vertical bars* are calibration of 50 mV and 100 mg. *Horizontal bar* is a calibration of 500 msec.

increased when the muscle was perfused with lower concentrations of NaF. In contrast, the current was decreased or completely abolished at higher concentrations. The time required for complete suppression was a function of the concentration used. The slow calcium responses in Na-free solution under current clamp conditions also showed that the lower concentrations of NaF, ranging from 10^{-7} to 10^{-4} M, increased the amplitude of slow calcium response. The addition of 10^{-3} or 10^{-2} M NaF, however, depressed the calcium response and finally abolished it completely. The effects of NaF on I_{Ca}-dependent and independent tensions were examined by paired step pulses. The I_{Ca}-dependent tension produced by the short (0.15 sec) and small pulse (70 mV) was markedly augmented at lower concentrations of NaF, while the I_{Ca}-independent tension with the long (1 sec) and large pulse (120 mV) tended to increase slightly (Figure 2). The rate of fall in I_{Ca}-independent tension, however, was markedly depressed in this condition.

DISCUSSION

The present experiments have disclosed that NaF has two opposite effects, positive and negative inotropic actions. These two effects appeared in different degrees and time courses, depending on the concentration of the drug. NaF at lower concentrations produced a marked increase in the contractility, a moderate prolongation of action potential, and an enhancement of calcium response, and an augmentation of I_{Ca}-dependent tension. These effects accord well with the fact that NaF stimulates adenyl cyclase systems and increases the intracellular level of cAMP (Drummond and Duncan, 1966; Robison, Butcher, and Sutherland, 1968). However, the positive inotropic action of NaF was not inhibited by a β-adrenergic blocker, propranolol, and the observation suggests that NaF may stimulate the adenyl cyclase or the contractile systems by

A   **B**

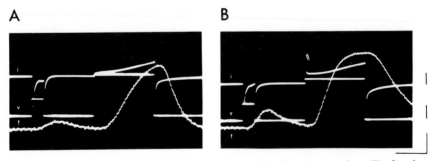

Figure 2. The effect of NaF on the I_{Ca}-dependent and independent tensions. The I_{Ca}-dependent tension was elicited by a short and small depolarizing pulse (0.15 sec, 120 mV). *A,* in control; *B,* after 30 min in 10^{-5} M NaF. *Vertical bars* are calibrations of 10^{-5} A, 50 mV, and 100 mg for the membrane current (i), voltage (v), and tension records (t), respectively. *Horizontal bar* is a calibration of 500 msec.

mechanisms different from those of catecholamine. Moreover, the membrane (Na,K)-ATPase is known to be inhibited by fluoride (Kishner, 1964; Opit *et al.*, 1966; Farias *et al.*, 1970). It is possible that the positive inotropic effect of NaF is also associated with an inhibition of the membrane (Na,K)-ATPase, as in the case of ouabain (Glynn, 1964; Lee and Klaus, 1971). NaF may increase the contractility not only by a stimulation of adenyl cyclase systems but also by an inhibition of membrane (Na,K)-ATPase.

The cause of the negative inotropic action is still uncertain. A relatively simple explanation of the negative inotropic effect is to suppose that the decrease of developed tension is due to the shortening of duration of action potential caused by an increase of potassium conductance, as observed. However, the magnitude of tension elicited by voltage-clamp pulses was reduced markedly even when a long depolarizing pulse was used during action of excess NaF. Therefore, the action of NaF as a metabolic inhibitor may dominate at higher concentrations.

REFERENCES

BERMAN, D. A. 1966. Effect of calcium, strontium and magnesium on the positive inotropic action of fluoride. J. Pharmacol. Exp. Ther. 152:75–80.

BIRNBAUMER, L., POHL, S. L., and RODBELL, M. 1969. Adenyl cyclase in fat cells. I. Properties and the effects of adrenocorticotropin and fluoride. J. Biol. Chem. 244: 3468–3476.

COVIN, L. I., and BERMAN, D. A. 1959. Metabolic aspects of the positive inotropic action of fluoride on rat ventricle. J. Pharmacol. Exp. Ther. 125:137–141.

DRUMMOND, G. I., and DUNCAN, L. 1970. Adenyl cyclase in cardiac tissue. J. Biol. Chem. 245:976–983.

FARIAS, R. N., GOLDEMBER, A. L., and TRUCCO, R. E. 1970. The effect of fat deprivation of the allosteric inhibition by fluoride of the (Mg^{2+})-ATPase and $(Na^+ + K^+)$-ATPase from rat erythrocytes. Arch. Biochem. Biophys. 139:38–44.

GLYNN, I. M. 1964. The action of cardiac glycosides on ion movements. Pharmacol. Rev. 16:381–407.

GOLD, H. K., PRINDLE, K. H., LEVEY, G. S., and EPSTEIN, S. E. 1970. Effects of experimental heart failure on the capacity of glucagon to augment myocardial contractility and activate adenyl cyclase. J. Clin. Invest. 49:999–1006.

KISHNER, L. B. 1964. Fluoride inhibition of sodium extrusion from erythrocytes and metabolic correlation. Arch. Biochem. Biophys. 106:57–64.

LEE, K. S., and KLAUS, W. 1971. The subcellular basis for the mechanism of inotropic action of cardiac glycosides. Pharmacol. Rev. 23:193–261.

LOEWI, O. 1955. On the mechanism of the positive inotropic action of fluoride, oleate, and calcium on the frog's heart. J. Pharmacol. Exp. Ther. 114:90–99.

McNEILL, J. H., and MUSCHEK, L. D. 1972. Histamine effects on cardiac contractility, phosphorylase and adenyl cyclase. J. Mol. Cell Cardiol. 4:611–624.

MURAD, F., and VAUGHAN, M. 1969. Effect of glucagon on rat adenyl cyclase. Biochem. Pharmacol. 18:1053–1059.

OKA, H., KANEKO, T., YAMASHITA, K., SUZUKI, S., and ODA, T. 1973. The glucagon and fluoride sensitive adenyl cyclase in plasma membrane of rat liver. Endocrinol. Japon. 20:263–270.

OPIT, L. J., POTTER, H., and CHARNOCK, J. S. 1966. The effect of anions on $(Na^+ + K^+)$-activated ATPase. Biochim. Biophys. Acta 120:159–161.

REUTER, H. 1974. Localization of beta adrenergic receptors, and effects of noradrenaline and cyclic nucleotides on action potentials, ionic currents and tension in mammalian cardiac muscle. J. Physiol. 242:429–451.

RICE, L. I., and BERMAN, D. A. 1961. Malonate and fluoride effects on metabolism and contraction of electrically stimulated heart strips. Amer. J. Physiol. 20:727–731.

ROBISON, G. A., BUTCHER, R. W., and SUTHERLAND, E. W. 1968. Cyclic AMP. Annu. Rev. Biochem. 37:149–174.

RODBELL, M. 1967. Metabolism of isolated fat cells. V. Preparation of 'ghosts' and their properties; adenyl cyclase and other enzymes. J. Biol. Chem. 242:5744–5750.

SUTHERLAND, E. W., RALL, T. W., and MENON, T. 1962. Adenyl cyclase. I. Distribution, preparation and properties. J. Biol. Chem. 237:1220–1227.

WEISS, B. 1969. Similarities and differences in the norepinephrine and sodium fluoride-sensitive adenyl cyclase system. J. Pharmacol. Exp. Ther. 166:330–338.

Mailing address:
Y. Abe
Department of Physiology,
School of Health Science and Faculty of Medicine,
Kyushu University, Fukuoka (Japan).

Recent Advances in Studies on
Cardiac Structure and Metabolism, Volume 11
Heart Function and Metabolism
Edited by T. Kobayashi, T. Sano, and N. S. Dhalla
Copyright 1978   University Park Press   Baltimore

EFFECTS OF ANOXIA AND METABOLIC INHIBITORS ON REACTION OF THE FAST SODIUM SYSTEM

T. SANO, M. HIRAOKA, and T. SAWANOBORI

Institute for Cardiovascular Diseases, Tokyo Medical
and Dental University, Tokyo, Japan

SUMMARY

The effects of anoxia and metabolic inhibitors on inactivation and reactivation of the fast Na system of dog ventricular muscle fibers were studied by examining $(dV/dt)_{max}$ of the action potential upstroke. Anoxia for 60 min, dinitrophenol (DNP) (2.0 mM), and sodium azide (2.0 mM) depressed markedly steady-state $(dV/dt)_{max}$ at each membrane potential produced by changing $[K]_o$. Anoxia tended to prolong recovery slightly, but DNP and azide changed little the time course of recovery of the $(dV/dt)_{max}$, which was studied by applying double pulses to elicit action potential at different intervals. It is concluded that anoxia, DNP, and azide caused prominent depression of the maximum Na conductance but had less influence on its recovery kinetics.

INTRODUCTION

The effects of anoxia, DNP, and sodium azide on inactivation and reactivation of the fast Na system were studied by a method similar to that of Gettes and Reuter (1974), examining $(dV/dt)_{max}$ of the action potential upstroke. Haas, Kern, and Einwächter (1970) examined similar effects of DNP on frog atria, but the effects of DNP were reexamined on dog ventricles for comparison.

METHOD

Right ventricular papillary or trabecular muscles were isolated from dog hearts and were perfused with normal Tyrode solution at $36°$ C, and gassed with 95% O_2 and 5% CO_2 in the control. The preparation was stimulated at a basic rate of 0.5 cycle per second. The $(dV/dt)_{max}$ of the action potential upstroke was obtained by an electronic differentiator. A single test stimulus was introduced between two conditioning action potentials and the diastolic interval was progressively decreased. The diastolic interval was defined as the interval between the completely (within 3 mV) repolarized conditioning action potential and the onset of the following test action potential.

Anoxia was introduced by gassing with 95% nitrogen and 5% of CO_2. In examination of metabolic inhibitors, DNP or sodium azide was added in the Tyrode solution at the final concentration of 2.0 mM each.

RESULTS AND DISCUSSION

When anoxia was introduced, the duration of the action potential shortened gradually and the resting potential was decreased slightly. After 60 min of anoxia the steady-state $(dV/dt)_{max}$ and the time course of the recovery of the $(dV/dt)_{max}$ were examined (Figure 1). Each representative case in which action potential was recorded from the same cell during continuous monitoring is shown in Figures 2 and 3.

As is shown in Figure 2, the absolute value of the steady-state $(dV/dt)_{max}$ was decreased in anoxia, showing the decrease of membrane conductance. The normalized curves show, however, that voltage-dependency and slope of the curves were the same in both curves.

The recovery of the $(dV/dt)_{max}$ in anoxia did not show a marked change from the control (Figure 3). In anoxia there seems to be some delay of the time constant with which the $(dV/dt)_{max}$ in the test responses regained the steady-state value. The time constants of the recovery of $(dV/dt)_{max}$ in the control and

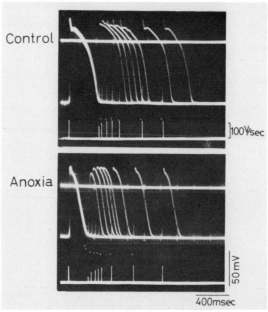

Figure 1. An example of the effect of 60 min of anoxia, demonstrating the method of measurement of the time course of recovery of $(dV/dt)_{max}$ and the steady-state $(dV/dt)_{max}$.

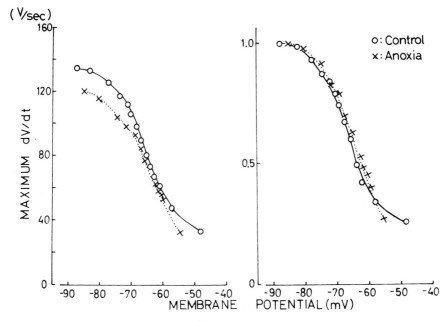

Figure 2. Change of the steady state $(dV/dt)_{max}$ after 60 min of anoxia. *Left:* absolute values. *Right:* normalized curves.

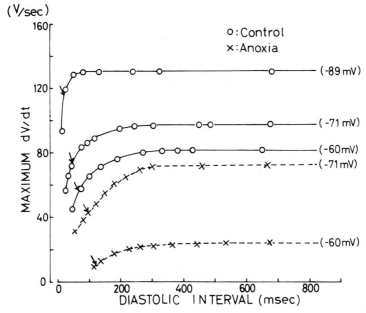

Figure 3. Change of the recovery of $(dV/dt)_{max}$ after 60 min of anoxia. *Arrows* show the time constant with which the $(dV/dt)_{max}$ in test responses regained the steady-state value.

in anoxia, when the resting potential was between −81 mV and −90 mV, were 31.3 ± 13.8 msec ($n = 14$) and 31.5 ± 12.7 ($n = 5$), respectively. Those between −66 mV and −80 mV were 45.7 ± 9.1 ($n = 7$) and 63.0 ± 24.3 ($n = 9$), respectively, and those between −50 mV and −65 mV were 66.4 ± 17.7 ($n = 8$) and 84.4 ± 26.0 ($n = 12$), respectively. These values support such a tendency, but the difference is not statistically significant. In relatively high resting potentials the onset of the responses was about the same in control and anoxia (e.g., curves of −71 mV in Figure 3). But in lower resting potentials there was a delay in the onset of the responses in anoxia (e.g., curves of −60 mV in Figure 3).

The effects of DNP and sodium azide were similar to, but larger than, those of anoxia as far as the examined conditions were concerned. DNP showed the most marked decrease of the steady-state $(dV/dt)_{max}$ (Figure 4). Similarly, with anoxia both DNP and azide did not shift the normalized curve. In the recovery of $(dV/dt)_{max}$ there is no difference in time constant and the onset of test responses between control and DNP and also between azide and control (Figure 5).

The results show that anoxia, DNP, and azide caused prominent depression of the maximum Na conductance but had less influence on its recovery kinetics. The decrease of $(dV/dt)_{max}$ indicates the decrease of the conduction velocity. In usual anoxia, although the diastolic interval of the onset of the responses is

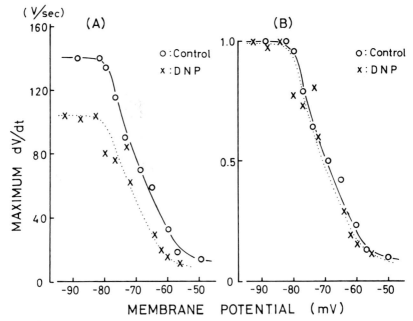

Figure 4. Change of the steady-state $(dV/dt)_{max}$ after addition of DNP in the Tyrode solution to the final concentration of 2.0 mM. *A:* absolute values. *V:* normalized curves.

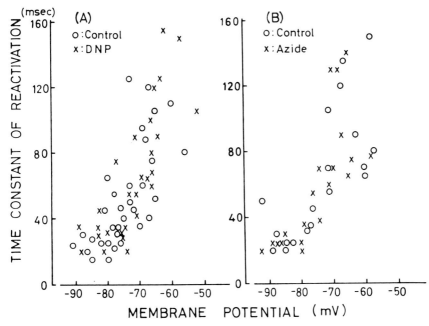

Figure 5. Time constants of all the recovery curves of $(dV/dt)_{max}$ of control and after addition of DNP and sodium azide at a final concentration of 2.0 mM each. *A:* addition of DNP. *B:* addition of sodium azide.

little affected, the duration of the action potentials shortens markedly. It is presumed, therefore, that the effective refractory period is markedly shortened, and thus re-entry is likely to occur. In the area where the anoxia is so marked as to induce a marked reduction of the resting potential, the diastolic interval of the onset of the responses shows a prolongation. The effective refractory period will then increase and may induce conduction block.

REFERENCES

GETTES, L. S., and REUTER, H. 1974. Slow recovery from inactivation of inward currents in mammalian myocardial fibers. J. Physiol. 240:703–724.
HAAS, H. G., KERN, R., and EINWÄCHTER, H. M. 1970. Electrical activity and metabolism in cardiac tissue: an experimental and theoretical study. J. Membr. Biol. 3: 180–209.

Mailing address:
T. Sano, M. D.,
Institute for Cardiovascular Diseases,
Tokyo Medical and Dental University,
No. 5-45, 1-chome, Yushima,
Bunkyo-ku, Tokyo (Japan).

Recent Advances in Studies on
Cardiac Structure and Metabolism, Volume 11
Heart Function and Metabolism
Edited by T. Kobayashi, T. Sano, and N. S. Dhalla
Copyright 1978   University Park Press   Baltimore

INTRAVENTRICULAR CONDUCTION DISTURBANCE DUE TO DELAYED RECOVERY FROM VENTRICULAR INACTIVATION IN CHLORPROMAZINE-TREATED DOGS

M. ARITA, Y. NAGAMOTO, and T. SAIKAWA

Department of Physiology, Faculty of Medicine,
Kyushu University, Fukuoka, Japan

SUMMARY

In *in situ* canine hearts, chlorpromazine induced a time (preceding cycle length)-dependent decrease in conduction velocity within the ventricle. Thus, QRS duration of nonpremature beats was lengthened at rapid pacing rates while QRS duration of atrial premature beats was lengthened at short coupling intervals. These slow conductions were not due to reduced take-off potential of ventricular action potentials but to drug-induced slow recovery of the rapid Na^+ system. The phenomenon may be responsible for reported QRS prolongation and fatal ventricular arrhythmias encountered in patients receiving phenothiazines.

INTRODUCTION

The duration of QRS complex of electrocardiogram (ECG) in patients treated with phenothiazine derivatives is prolonged (Leestma and Koenig, 1968), especially when the sinus tachycardia is present (Arita and Surawicz, 1973). The QRS prolongation could be a prodromal sign of reported fatal ventricular arrhythmias. Hence we studied the effect of chlorpromazine on the ventricular conduction at various cardiac cycle lengths produced by changing heart rate or by introducing premature excitations. Our results suggest that chlorpromazine suppresses ventricular conduction velocity, primarily due to delayed recovery of rapid sodium channel, and hence the prolongation of QRS complex is more marked at rapid heart rates or at short coupling intervals.

METHODS

Twenty-six mongrel dogs (7—15 kg) were anesthetized with pentobarbital (40 mg/kg I. P.) and open-chested under artificial respiration. Lead II ECG and ventricular monophasic action potential were recorded by use of a suction electrode, simultaneously with arterial blood pressure and left atrial electrogram, displayed on an ink-writing recticorder (paper speed, 200 mm/sec). The heart rate was changed by combination of atrial pacing and vagal stimulation. In some experiments a premature atrial or ventricular excitation was introduced to change the cycle length. After the recording of control data, chlorpromazine hydrochloride (1, 5, and 20 mg/kg) was injected intravenously within 5 min and the recording was repeated.

RESULTS

Figure 1 shows an experiment demonstrating ECG (II), ventricular action potential, and left atrial electrogram before (*A* and *B*) and 5 min after injection of the drug, 20 mg/kg (*C* and *D*) at two different atrial pacing rates (150 and 230/min). In the control records (*A* and *B*), QRS duration was virtually the same (46 and 47 msec) at both pacing rates. After drug injection, however, QRS durations at both pacing rates were significantly different from each other. The duration increased by 9 msec (from 55 to 64 msec) when the rate was increased from 150 (*C*) to 230/min (*D*). This prolongation was not due to incomplete repolarization of the preceding action potential because the action potential terminated well before the upstroke of subsequent action potential (Figure 1*C*). Interatrial conduction time was also prolonged with increasing heart rate after treatment with the drug (Figure 1*C* and *D*).

Figure 2 summarizes the results of this kind of experiment obtained from 20 dogs treated with three different chlorpromazine concentrations. It is obvious that the QRS duration prolonged as the heart rate was increased, and that the statistical significance of the correlation between heart rate and QRS duration was increased as the injected dose was increased.

The prolongation of WRS complex may indicate decreased conduction velocity of the excitation within the ventricular myocardium. Thus, in Figure 3 the conduction velocity of ventricular premature impulses originated at the anterior base of left ventricule, and transmissions to the apex were measured with varying coupling intervals before and after application of the drug. An additional reason for using these ventricular premature beats was to eliminate A-V conduction delay, thus making it possible to elicit a premature response immediately after termination of preceding ventricular action potential. In the control (○) the conduction velocity of premature beats was constant unless the upstroke of action potential encroached on phase 3 of the preceding action potential. The time of full repolarization of the preceding action potential was indicated by an arrow. During the drug action (●), however, the conduction velocity decreased progressively with shortening of coupling intervals, even when the premature excitation was elicited during phase 4 of the preceding action potential (time-dependent conduction delay). This time-dependent suppression of conduction

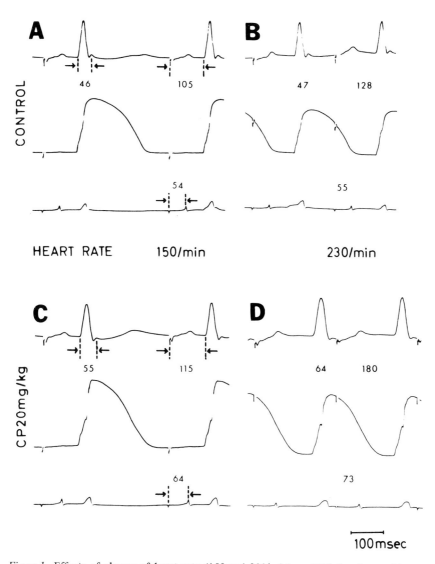

Figure 1. Effects of change of heart rate (150 and 230/min) on QRS duration and inter-atrial conduction time before (*A* and *B*) and after injection of chlorpromazine 20 mg/kg (*C* and *D*). Each panel, from top to bottom, shows lead II ECG, monophasic action potential from left ventricle, and surface electrogram from left atrium. Each number below QRS-complexes shows the QRS duration in msec; the number above the bottom trace shows impulse conduction time from right to left atrium (interatrial conduction time) in msec. Note that the QRS duration and the interatrial conduction time are longer at rapid (*D*) than at slow pacing rate (*C*) after treatment with the drug.

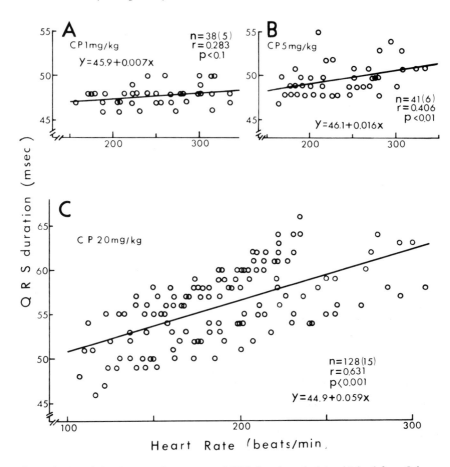

Figure 2. Correlation between heart rate and QRS duration. *A,* data obtained from 5 dogs after injection of chlorpromazine (1 mg/kg); *B,* from 6 dogs injected with the drug (5 mg/kg); *C,* from 15 dogs injected with the drug (20 mg/kg). A *straight line* in each panel indicates the least squares linear regression line.

velocity was reversible and became less pronounced at 60 min after the injection (▲). The same results were obtained from the other 5 dogs tested.

DISCUSSION

Phenothiazine derivatives reduced the maximum rate of rise of action potentials in isolated ventricular tissue when the cycle length was shortened, and the effect was attributed to delayed recovery from inactivation of the rapid sodium system

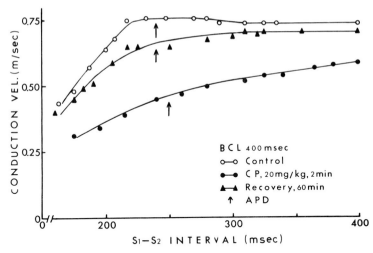

Figure 3. Relation between the coupling interval of ventricular premature beats measured as an interval from basic (S_1) to premature stimulus (S_2) and the conduction velocity within the ventricle. *Circles* indicate control; *dots,* 2–5 min, and *triangles,* 60 min after chlorpromazine injection (20 mg/kg). *Arrows* indicate the time of full repolarization of preceding nonpremature action potential.

(Arita and Surawicz, 1972). In the present study it has been evidenced that chlorpromazine induced slow conduction also in *in situ* canine hearts paced with a comparable program of stimulation. Prolongation of QRS complex induced by this mechanism, i.e., slow recovery of rapid Na^+ channel, has never been reported earlier, either in man or in experimental animals. The mechanism seems to explain the fact that the QRS prolongation in phenothiazine-treated patients could be normalized by a concomitant administration of a β-blocker, propranolol, by reducing the heart rates considerably (Arita and Mashiba, 1970). The patients treated with phenothiazine drugs may be vulnerable to premature excitations, causing ventricular tachycardia or fibrillation due to re-entry, because, as is shown in Figure 3, the conduction velocity of premature beat was markedly reduced when the coupling interval was relatively short. The result also suggests that a ventricular vulnerable period may be prolonged far across the T wave in ECG in phenothiazine-treated patients.

REFERENCES

ARITA, M., and MASHIBA, H. 1970. Effects of phenothiazine and propranolol on ECG. The effects of propranolol on the electrocardiographic abnormalities induced by phenothiazine derivatives. Jpn. Circ. J. 34:391–400.

ARITA, M., and SURAWICZ, B. 1973. Electrophysiologic effect of phenothiazines on canine cardiac fibers. J. Pharmacol. Exp. Ther. 184:619–630.
LEESTMA, J. E., and KOENIG, K. L. 1968. Sudden death and phenothiazines. A current controversy. Arch. Gen. Psychiat. 18:137–148.

Mailing address:
M. Arita, M.D.,
Associate Professor.
Department of Physiology,
Faculty of Medicine,
Kyushu University, Fukuoka 812 (Japan).

Biophysical Aspect

Recent Advances in Studies on
Cardiac Structure and Metabolism, Volume 11
Heart Function and Metabolism
Edited by T. Kobayashi, T. Sano, and N. S. Dhalla
Copyright 1978 University Park Press Baltimore

CALCIUM ION IN CARDIAC CONTRACTILITY

S. EBASHI, T. KITAZAWA,[1] K. KOHAMA, and P.-C. VAN EERD[2]

Department of Pharmacology, Faculty of Medicine,
University of Tokyo, Bunkyo-ku, Tokyo, Japan

SUMMARY

Under physiological conditions where the intracellular Ca ion concentration does not exceed 3×10^{-6} M, the sarcoplasmic reticulum plays a major role in the relaxation process of cardiac muscle; mitochondria do not take up a significant amount of Ca ion during this process. If cardiac muscle undergoes maximum contraction, in which the intracellular Ca ion concentration should reach 10^{-4} M, the role of mitochondria in reducing intracellular Ca ion becomes appreciable. The relationship of the tension developed by cardiac glycerinated muscle fibers to the Ca ion concentration resembles the relationship of the amount of bound Ca of cardiac troponin to the Ca ion concentration, being less steep in its slope compared with those of fast and slow skeletal muscles. This gentle slope seems to reflect the great diversity of affinities for Ca ion of the two Ca-binding sites of cardiac troponin, one being about 100 times that of the other.

ROLE OF CARDIAC MITOCHONDRIA IN REGULATING INTRACELLULAR CALCIUM ION CONCENTRATION

There is no doubt that the intracellular Ca ion required for contraction of fast white skeletal muscle is solely controlled by the sarcoplasmic reticulum (SR) (cf. Ebashi and Endo, 1968). However, the situation is not so simple in cardiac muscle, because the amount of mitochondria in cardiac muscle is quite large, and the capacity of cardiac SR for Ca ion is small compared with that of fast skeletal muscle (Harigaya and Schwartz, 1969). This chapter reports our experiments that investigated whether or not mitochondria would play a significant role in the Ca metabolism of cardiac SR.

The methods and materials used were the same as described in the paper of Kitazawa (1976); they were briefly described in the legends to the figures. In

---

Supported in part by research grants from the Muscular Dystrophy Associations of America, Inc., the Ministry of Education, Japan, the Ministry of Health and Welfare, Japan (No. 216), the Iatrochemical Foundation, the Toray Science Foundation, and the Mitsubishi Foundation.
[1] Present address: Department of Pharmacology, Tohoku University School of Medicine, Sendai, Japan.
[2] Present address: Pharmakologisches Institut der Universität Zürich, Gloriastrasse 32, 8006 Zürich, Switzerland.

addition to chicken heart used in that article, we also examined dog heart and obtained essentially the same results. The following experiments were carried out at pH 6.8 unless otherwise stated.

The apparent binding constant of cardiac SR for Ca, viz., 2×10^6 M^{-1}, is two-thirds that of white skeletal muscle, and its capacity, ~ 60 nmol/mg protein, about a quarter of that of fast skeletal muscle. The rate constant of Ca uptake at quasi-steady state, i.e., the rate at several seconds after addition of ATP, is about 4,100 M^{-1} sec^{-1} at higher Ca concentrations around 10^{-4} M, but 24,000 M^{-1} at lower Ca concentrations less than 10^{-6} M.

The relationship between the amount of Ca uptake and Ca ion concentrations was complicated and could not be approximated by a single binding constant; half-maximum uptake was attained at 9×10^{-4} M Ca ion. The rate of Ca uptake by mitochondria under massive loading condition, which was considered to be more physiological than limited loading condition, was fairly well expressed as that of a second-order reaction (Figure 1).

If cardiac mitochondria or SR was incubated with a specified amount of Ca ion for a certain time and then applied to the glycerinated fibers, the resulting contraction corresponded well to the amount of free Ca ion calculated by using the rate constants above.

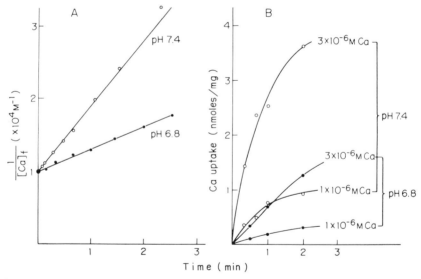

Figure 1. Time course of Ca uptake by cardiac mitochondria under massive loading conditions. *A:* at a high Ca ion concentration plotted as a second-order reaction. *B:* at low Ca ion concentrations. Reaction mixtures contained: 0.1 M KCl, 20 mM Tris-maleate (pH 6.8) or 20 mM TES (pH 7.4), 5 mM MgCl$_2$, 2 mM ATP, 4 mM pyruvate, 4 mM malate, 4 mM phosphate, 0.7 mg/ml of mitochondria, and specified concentrations of Ca ion, viz., 100 μM in *A* or those noted in *B*. Temperature: 28°C.

We then compared the calculated time course of relaxation of cardiac glycerinated fibers induced by cardiac SR or mitochondria in the presence of 100 μM Ca (Figure 2) with the actual data, taking the rate constants above and the affinity of troponins for Ca ion into account. In the case of the SR the extent of relaxation was just as calculated, but the time course of relaxation was nearly ten times slower than calculated. Since the application of the same concentration of cardiac SR to fast skeletal glycerinated fibers showed about three times faster relaxation, and EGTA (ethylene glycol bis(β-aminoethyl ether)-N, N'-tetraacetic acid, GEDTA) exhibited almost the same time course as calculated, the discrepancy between calculated and actual data may be largely explained by a simple diffusion problem. In the case of mitochondria, no relaxation was actually seen under the condition as described in the legend to Figure 2. Perhaps a high concentration of mitochondria would have induced their aggregation, and, consequently, the difficulty in diffusion would be aggravated.

Since the discrepancy between calculated and actual data may be explained, at least in the case of the SR, by the diffusion problem, we then calculated the time course of relaxation in living cardiac fibers, as is illustrated in Figure 3.

Under ordinary conditions, cardiac muscle reaches only 25% of maximum tension, which is obtained by 2×10^{-6} M Ca (Figure 4). In this condition, mitochondria do not take up a significant amount of Ca when a complete relaxation has already been produced by the SR (lower curves in Figure 3). Even if we increase the tension up to 50% of maximum, which is seen at 3×10^{-6} M

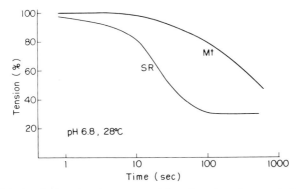

Figure 2. Calculated relaxation time course of glycerinated cardiac muscle fibers induced by cardiac SR or mitochondria. Rate constants of Ca uptake by the SR or mitochondria shown in the text of Figure 1 were used. Calculation was made under the assumptions that Ca release from troponin is not rate-limiting, and the SR or mitochondria are located in their original positions. Cardiac SR, 1.7 mg/ml; mitochondria, 14 mg/ml. Initial Ca ion concentration was 0.1 mM. The experiments to be compared with this calculation were made under the conditions: 0.12 M KCl, 20 mM Tris-maleate (pH 6.8), 5 mM $MgCl_2$, 4 mM ATP, 10 mM phosphoenolpyruvate, 3,000–4,000 units pyruvate kinase, 8 mM pyruvate, and 4 mM malate at 28°C.

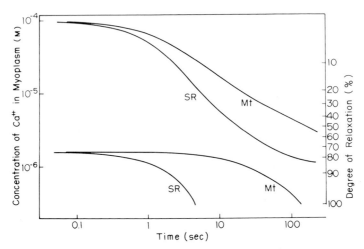

Figure 3. Calculated time course of relaxation of cardiac muscle fibers under physiological contraction or maximum contraction. *Lower curves:* relaxation of physiologically contracted fibers. *Upper curves:* relaxation of maximally contracted fibers. Mt: mitochondria. Calculation was made under the assumptions: SR, 3.5 mg/ml, having a capacity of 60 nmol Ca per mg protein and a rate constant described in the text; mitochondria, 100 mg/ml, which have rate constants shown in Figure 1; temperature, 28° C. (Quoted from Kitazawa, 1976.)

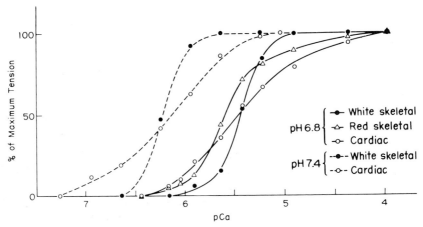

Figure 4. Isometric tension developed by glycerinated cardiac, slow (red) skeletal and fast (white) skeletal muscle fibers as a function of Ca ion concentrations at different pHs. pH 6.8 (*solid lines*): 0.12 M KCl, 20 mM Tris, 20 mM maleate, 4 mM MgCl$_2$, 4 mM ATP, 4 mM EGTA, specified concentrations of CaCl$_2$ to give the required concentrations of free Ca at pH 6.8. At room temperature (23–25° C). pH 7.4 (*dotted lines*): the same as above except for 0.13 M KCl and 40 mM Tris instead of 0.12 M KCl and 20 mM Tris plus 20 mM maleate. (Quoted from Kitazawa, 1976.)

Ca, the situation is not significantly different from the above. Therefore, mitochondria do not appear to play an appreciable role in taking up intracellular Ca ion to induce relaxation.

If we increase the Ca ion concentration up to such an unphysiological concentration as 100 μM, which gives rise to maximum tension, the SR cannot afford to induce full relaxation and requires the collaboration of other Ca uptake systems, e.g., mitochondria.

One might argue that even at lower Ca concentrations mitochondria should play a more significant role at higher pH, e.g., 7.4, where the rate of Ca uptake is several times higher than that at pH 6.8 (Figure 1). As shown in Figure 4, however, the sensitivity of contractile system to Ca ion increases sharply with increase in pH, almost ten times with increase in pH by 0.6. As a result, the time course of relaxation at pH 7.4 due to mitochondrial Ca uptake does not differ from that at pH 6.8. Since the capability of the SR is very weak at this pH (Nakamaru and Schwartz, 1970), cardiac muscle may not have any powerful Ca uptake system at alkaline pH.

In the above we disregarded the role of Ca efflux from cardiac cells, probably due to Ca-Na exchange reaction (Reuter, 1973), but this may not substantially alter the conclusion illustrated in Figure 3.

ROLE OF CALCIUM BINDING SITES
OF TROPONIN IN CONTRACTILE PROCESSES

The main purpose of this section is to discuss the role of each Ca binding site of cardiac troponin in comparison with that of fast and slow skeletal troponins.

Troponins were bound to Sepharose 4 B according to the method of March, Parikh, and Cuatrecasas (1974). Determinations of Ca and Sr were made by isotope technique and atomic absorption method. The whole troponin, not troponin C, was used, because troponin C bound to the gel resulted in a decrease in the number of Ca binding sites. Treatment of gel-bound troponin with sodium dodecyl sulfate released almost stoichiometric amount of troponin C and minute amounts of troponin I and T, indicating that troponin was bound to the gel through troponin I and/or troponin T. The molar ratio of troponin C to parent cardiac troponin was shown to be one to one.

As shown in Table 1, the number of Ca binding sites of fast skeletal troponin coincided well with previous data (Potter and Gergely, 1975). Ca binding sites of slow skeletal and cardiac troponin did not exceed two moles per mole (according to our preliminary experiments using equilibrium dialysis method, the amount of Ca binding to cardiac troponin C was 2.0–2.4 mol/mol).

The whole amino acid sequence of cardiac troponin C was determined, and, in comparison to the sequence of fast skeletal troponin C, the number of Ca binding sites were estimated to be three (van Eerd and Takahashi, 1975, 1976),

Table 1. Binding capacity of troponins for divalent cations (mol/mol)*

	Muscle		
Cation	Cardiac	Fast skeletal	Slow skeletal
Ca	1.5	3.6	1.4
	(1.8×10^{-6})	(1.2×10^{-6})	(4.6×10^{-7})
Sr	1.3	3.4	1.7
	(2.2×10^{-5})	(2.5×10^{-5})	(5.5×10^{-6})
Mg	~4	~7	~3

*Reaction mixtures contained: 0.1 M KCl, 1.3 mM MgCl$_2$, 20 mM Tris-maleate (pH 6.8) and a specified concentration of troponin-bound Sepharose 4B, approximately 30 mg/troponin/g gel. Figures in parentheses indicate the molar concentrations of divalent cations to give half saturation. For the others, see the text.

rather in disagreement with the actual value. It is not decided at present whether one of these possible sites cannot actually bind Ca in spite of its plausible structure, or one of them is inaccessible for Ca ion when troponin C is involved in the parent troponin.

As indicated in Figure 4, the slope of the curve representing the relationship between the developed tension and the Ca ion concentration is less steep in cardiac muscle than the slopes in fast and slow skeletal muscle, irrespective of pH. This is also the case of the relationship between the tension and the Sr ion concentration (Figure 5).

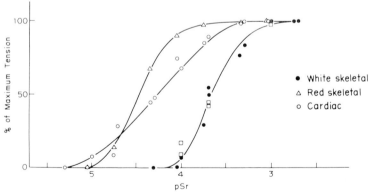

Figure 5. Isometric tension developed by glycerinated cardiac, slow (red) skeletal and fast (white) skeletal muscle fibers as a function of Sr ion concentration. (Quoted from Kitazawa, 1976.) Experimental conditions: 0.12 M KCl, 20 mM Tris, 20 mM maleate, 4 mM MgCl$_2$ 4 mM ATP, 10 mM EGTA, specified concentrations of SrCl$_2$ at pH 6.8. At room temperature (23–25° C). □, white skeletal muscle under the same condition as that of *filled circle* except for omitting EGTA.

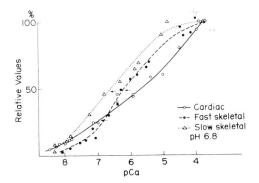

Figure 6. The relationship between the Ca ion concentration and the amounts of Ca bound to troponins. Determinations were made in a solution containing 0.1 M KCl, 1.3 mM MgCl$_2$, and 20 mM Tris-maleate (pH 6.8). *Arrows* in the figure indicate the threshold concentrations of Ca ion for contraction shown in Figure 4 with corrections due to the difference in Mg concentration. For further explanations, see the text.

In Figures 6 and 7 the relationships between the amounts of bound Ca or Sr and the concentrations of Ca or Sr ion are illustrated. The slope exhibited by cardiac troponin is also less steep than the slopes of slow and fast skeletal troponins. This may indicate that the mode of Ca binding of respective troponin, not the property of the myosin-actin system, is responsible for the Ca-tension relationship.

The higher sensitivity of glycerinated fibers of cardiac muscle to Sr ion compared to that of fast skeletal muscle (Figure 4) was in good agreement with the results derived from superprecipitation of their myosin B (Ebashi, Kodama, and Ebashi, 1968). In the case of slow skeletal muscle, the high affinity of its troponin for Sr ion corresponded well to the high sensitivity of its contractility

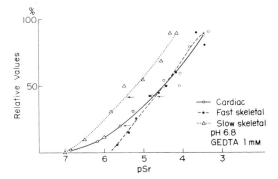

Figure 7. The relationship between the Sr ion concentration and the amounts of Sr bound to troponins. For explanation, see the legend to Figure 6. (The threshold concentrations indicated by *arrows* were derived from Figure 5.)

to Sr ion. However, the relationship of the amount of bound Sr to the Sr ion concentration in cardiac troponin was not so much different from that in fast skeletal troponin, especially if we consider the half maximum concentration (Table 1), which is in agreement with the results of Berson (1974). This may suggest that the high affinity site of fast skeletal troponin would not be utilized in the contractile cycle.

The contraction of fast skeletal glycerinated fibers does not start until nearly half of their four Ca or Sr binding sites per mole troponin are saturated (indicated by arrows in Figures 6 and 7). Furthermore, the first binding site of fast skeletal troponin has a high apparent binding constant for Ca, i.e., 3×10^7 M^{-1} even in the presence of 1.3 mM Mg, so that it is very likely that the site has already been saturated by Ca ion in the ordinary resting state. Thus the idea that the first binding site may not be working in ordinary contractile process is substantiated in many ways.

In contrast with this, the high affinity site of cardiac troponin, of which the apparent binding constant is about 10^7 M^{-1} in the presence of 1.3 mM Mg ion, seems to be playing a more important role than the low affinity site, which has an apparent binding constant less than 10^5 M^{-1}.

REFERENCES

BERSON, G. 1975. Ca^{2+}, Sr^{2+} and Ba^{2+} sensitivity of tropomyosin-troponin complex from cardiac and fast skeletal muscles. *In* W. Drabikowski *et al.* (eds.), Ca Binding Proteins, pp. 197–201. Elsevier Scientific Publishing Co., Amsterdam, and PWN-Polish Scientific Publishers, Warszawa.

EBASHI, S., and ENDO, M. 1968. Calcium ion and muscle contraction. *In* J.A.V. Butler and D. Noble (eds.), Progress in Biophysics and Molecular Biology, Vol. 18, pp. 123–183. Pergamon Press, Oxford.

EBASHI, S., KODAMA, A., and EBASHI, F. 1968. Troponin, I. Preparation and physiological function. J. Biochem. 64:465–477.

HARIGAYA, S., and SCHWARTZ, A. 1969. Rate of calcium binding and uptake in normal animal and failing human cardiac muscle. Circ. Res. 21:781–794.

KITAZAWA, T. 1976. Physiological significance of Ca-uptake by mitochondria in heart in comparison with that by cardiac sarcoplasmic reticulum. J. Biochem. 80:1129–1147.

MARCH, S. C., PARIKH, I., and CUATRECASAS, P. 1974. Simplified method for cyanogen bromide activation of agarose for affinity chromatography. Anal. Biochem. 60:149–152.

NAKAMARU, Y., and SCHWARTZ, A. 1970. Possible control of intracellular calcium metabolism by H^+: sarcoplasmic reticulum of skeletal and cardiac muscle. Biochem. Biophys. Res. Commun. 41:830–836.

POTTER, J. D., and GERGELY, J. 1975. The calcium and magnesium binding sites on troponin and the role in the regulation of myofibrillar adenosine triphosphatase. J. Biol. Chem. 250:4628–4633.

REUTER, H. 1973. Exchange of calcium in the mammalian myocardiums. Circ. Res. 34:599–605.

VAN EERD, J.-P., and TAKAHASHI, K. 1975. The amino acid sequence of bovine cardiac troponin-C. Biochem. Biophys. Res. Commun. 64:122–127.
VAN EERD, J.-P., and TAKAHASHI, K. 1976. Determination of the complete amino acid sequence of bovine cardiac troponin C. Biochemistry 15:1171–1180.

Mailing address:
Dr. S. Ebashi,
Department of Pharmacology,
Faculty of Medicine,
University of Tokyo,
7-3-1 Hongo, Bunkyo-ku,
Tokyo (Japan).

Recent Advances in Studies on
Cardiac Structure and Metabolism, Volume 11
Heart Function and Metabolism
Edited by T. Kobayashi, T. Sano, and N. S. Dhalla
Copyright 1978   University Park Press   Baltimore

BINDING OF DIVALENT CATIONS BY CANINE CARDIAC MYOSIN: DIFFERENCES IN NORMAL RIGHT AND LEFT VENTRICLES DEPENDENT UPON NUMBER OF LIGHT CHAINS

J. WIKMAN-COFFELT and D. T. MASON

Section of Cardiovascular Medicine, Department of Medicine,
University of California, Davis, School of Medicine, Davis, California, USA

SUMMARY

The moles of calcium bound by the left ventricle were 1.5 ± 0.1, while those of the right ventricle were 2.9 ± 0.2. The calcium binding constants were the same between myosins of the two cardiac ventricles. The Ca^{2+} binding constants were approximately 1.1×10^5 M^{-1} for both left and right ventricular myosins. Left ventricular myosin bound 1.3 ± 0.1 mol of Mn^{2+}, whereas right ventricular myosin bound 2.8 ± 0.1 mol of Mn^{2+}. The divalent cation Mn^{2+} only partially competed out Ca^{2+} (50%). Because of the partial competition, it seemed that Ca^{2+} and Mn^{2+} had some sights in common. These studies demonstrate a twofold difference in divalent cation binding (Ca^{2+}, Mn^{2+}) between left and right ventricular myosins. This variation in cation binding between the two ventricles is reflected in similar differences in myosin ATPase activity between the two ventricles.

INTRODUCTION

Because myosin, particularly the myosin light chains, binds calcium, Morimoto and Harrington (1974) proposed that skeletal muscle myosin may also have a Ca^{2+}-dependent activation mechanism in contraction. A myosin-linked calcium regulation has been shown in vertebrate smooth muscle (Bremel, 1974). Margossian, Lowey, and Barshop (1975) showed that the myosin light chains bound Ca^{2+} and that elevated Ca^{2+} concentrations weakened actomyosin interactions. The studies described here were undertaken to analyze the myosin-Ca^{2+} complex in enzymatically active cardiac myosin, the number of Ca^{2+}-myosin sites, and the degree of displacement of Ca^{2+} with other divalent cations, including Mg^{2+} and Mn^{2+}.

Myosins from the two canine cardiac ventricles were used for these studies, since these myosins were different, based on alterations in myosin ATPase activities (Wikman-Coffelt et al., 1975c) and differences in chemical (Wikman-Coffelt et

---

Supported in part by Research Program Project Grants HL 14780 and AMDD 16716 from the National Institutes of Health, Bethesda, Maryland, and a Research Grant from the California Chapter of the American Heart Association.

al., 1975c) and physical (Smith, Mason, and Wikman-Coffelt, 1974) properties, including variations in the amount of light chains present (Wikman-Coffelt *et al.*, 1975c).

PROCEDURES

Purification of Ca^{2+}-Free Myosin

To obtain myosin from canine cardiac ventricles, only the free wall of each was used; the septum was not analyzed. All glassware used in the following studies was acid washed and then rinsed extensively in ion-free distilled water. Myosin was purified, as described earlier (Wikman-Coffelt *et al.*, 1973, 1975c), except for the addition of extra chelating agents (Wikman-Coffelt *et al.*, 1975e).

Equilibrium Dialysis

^{45}Ca (10.5 mCi/mg), ^{54}Mn (carrier-free), and Omnifluor were purchased from New England Nuclear. Equilibrium dialysis was carried out at 4° in slowly rotating cells, as described earlier (Wikman-Coffelt *et al.*, 1975e).

RESULTS

Cation Binding Sites and
Enzymatic Activity in Right versus Left Ventricular Myosins

Right ventricular canine cardiac myosin (RVM) bound 2.9 ± 0.20 mol of calcium (Figure 1*A*), and left ventricular myosin (LVM) bound 1.5 ± 0.1 mol of calcium (Figure 1*B*) ($p < 0.001$). The calcium binding affinity constants for both myosins were the same (1.1×10^5 M^{-1}). Ca^{2+}-activated myosin ATPase was also different between left and right ventricular myosins (Table 1). Another divalent cation, Mn^{2+}, which activates myosin ATPase (Wikman-Coffelt *et al.*, 1975d) and ITPase activity, complexed to myosin: (RVM: 2.8 ± 0.1 M Mn^{2+}/mol myosin; LVM: 1.3 ± 0.1 M Mn^{2+}/mol myosin) (Figure 2). The average affinity binding values of the two ventricular myosins for Mn^{2+} were similar but slightly greater than for Ca^{2+} (RVM: 1.4×10^5 M^{-1}; LVM: 1.9×10^5 M^{-1}). Mn^{2+}-activated myosin ITPase activity was also different between left and right ventricular myosins (Table 1). Mn^{2+} caused only a partial displacement of Ca^{2+} from myosin (50%) (Figure 3), whereas Mg^{2+} displaced Ca^{2+} to an even lesser degree (Figure 4).

DISCUSSION

Left versus Right
Ventricular Myosins—Cation Binding and Enzymatic V_{max} Values

The differences noted here in the number of Ca^{2+} and Mn^{2+} myosin binding sites in the two canine cardiac ventricles reflect the molecular differences (Wikman-

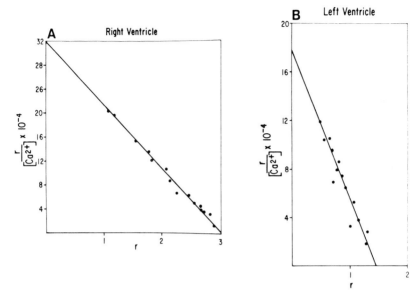

Figure 1. Scatchard plots for the binding of Ca^{2+} by (*A*) right ventricular myosin and (*B*) left ventricular myosin. Binding parameters were calculated from least squares regression lines for Scatchard plots using a Wang 720 C computer (Langer, 1973). The molecular weights for right and left ventricular myosin, established by sedimentation, equilibrium studies (Langer, 1973), were used for these experiments. (*A*) $n = 3.0$; $k = 1.05 \times 10^{-5}$. (*B*) $n = 1.4$; $k = 1.09 \times 10^{-5}$. (Representative plots are shown.) The addition of the analogue of ATP adenyl-5'-ylimododiphosphate (AMP-P(NH)P), ranging in concentration from 0.2×10^{-5} M to 2×10^{-5} M, to the dialysis equilibrium did not significantly affect the degree of Ca^{2+} binding of myosin, using conditions described in this report.

Table 1. Myosin activity*

Substrate	Cation activator	Enzymatic V_{max} values (μmol PO_4/mg myosin, min^{-1})	
		Left ventricle	Right ventricle
ATP	Ca^{2+}	1.03 ± 0.04	0.75 ± 0.03
ITP	Ca^{2+}	2.50 ± 0.05	1.90 ± 0.04
ITP	Mn^{2+}	2.20 ± 0.04	1.55 ± 0.06

*Purification of myosin and enzymatic incubation conditions for substrate saturation curves were as described earlier (Fenner *et al.*, 1973) except myosin ATPase activity was assayed at $37°$ (Bing *et al.*, 1971). For Mn^{2+}-activated ITPase activity, similar concentrations of ITP, as compared to ATP, were used (Fenner *et al.*, 1973).

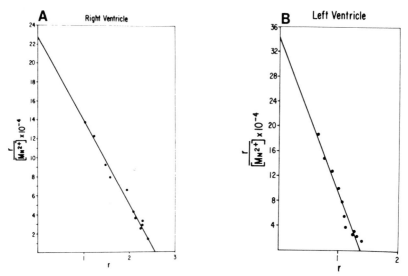

Figure 2. Scatchard plots of Mn²⁺ binding by (*A*) right ventricular myosin and (*B*) left ventricular myosin. Analyses are as described in Figure 1. (*A*) $n = 2.5; k = 9.0 \times 10^{-4}$. (*B*) $n = 1.4; k = 2.4 \times 10^{-5}$. The intercepts were determined by least squares analyses using a Wang 720 C computer. (Representative plots are shown.)

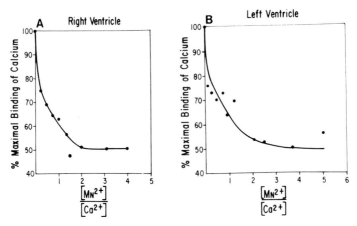

Figure 3. Percent inhibition of calcium binding with increasing concentrations of manganese for (*A*) right ventricular myosin and (*B*) left ventricular myosin. Calcium concentration was 5×10^{-5} M and manganese concentration ranged from 0.2×10^{-5} M to 25×10^{-5} M.

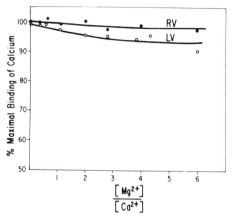

Figure 4. Effects of increasing magnesium concentration on calcium binding using left ventricular myosin (LV) and right ventricular myosin (RV). Calcium concentration was 5 × 10^{-5} M, and magnesium concentration ranged from 1 to 40 × 10^{-5} M. (A representative plot is shown.)

Coffelt *et al.*, 1975c) and the variation in Ca^{2+}- and Mn^{2+}-activated enzymatic V_{max} values between these two cardiac myosins. The differences in left and right ventricular myosins are related to the differences in the workload of the two ventricles. When the workload placed on the ventricles was altered by surgical intervention, the myosins changed relative to enzymatic V_{max} values (Wikman-Coffelt *et al.*, 1975a,d and 1976), chain proportions (Wikman-Coffelt *et al.*, 1975b, 1976), and calcium binding (Wikman-Coffelt *et al.*, 1975e, 1976). Force of contraction has been associated with myosin ATPase activity (Chandler *et al.*, 1967; Bing *et al.*, 1971; Langer, 1973), and this in turn inversely related to the degree of Ca^{2+} binding (Vitali-Mazza *et al.*, 1972; Wikman-Coffelt *et al.*, 1975e). Ca^{2+} influx is associated with contractile force, specifically in heart failure (Ito, Suko, and Chidsey, 1974), where myosin ATPase activity and the binding of calcium by myosin are altered (Wikman-Coffelt *et al.*, 1975b,e). The myosin light chains appear to bind Ca^{2+} (Morimoto and Harrington, 1974; Werber and Oplatka, 1974; Margossian *et al.*, 1975) and weaken the actin-myosin interaction (Margossian *et al.*, 1975).

In view of the work of Margossian *et al.* (1975) we propose that the left ventricle in dogs has stronger actomyosin interactions than the right ventricle, since canine left ventricular myosin binds less Ca^{2+} at 10^{-5} M Ca^{2+} concentrations. When the right ventricle is subjected to a mild pressure overload, right ventricular myosin increases in enzymatic V_{max} values, and decreases in both moles of light chains and a number of Ca^{2+} binding sites; the number of Ca^{2+}-myosin sites decreases from 3.0 to 1.8 (Wikman-Coffelt *et al.*, 1975b). Recent studies show that when pressure overload or volume overload become too severe, when pCO_2 is elevated, and contractility is decreased, then myosin decreases in enzymatic V_{max} values, but increases in both moles of light chains and number of Ca^{2+} binding sites (Wikman-Coffelt et al., 1975e, 1976). For an undefined reason, just when stronger actomyosin interactions are needed these interactions become weaker and thereby heart failure ensues.

REFERENCES

BING, O. H. L., MATSUCHITA, S., FANBURG, B. L., and LEVINE, H. J. 1971. Mechanical properties of rat cardiac muscle during experimental hypertrophy. Circ. Res. 28: 234–245.

BREMEL, R. D. 1974. Myosin linked calcium regulation in vertebrate smooth muscle. Nature 252:405–407.

CHANDLER, B. M., SONNENBLICK, E. H., SPANN, J. F., and POOL, P. E. 1967. Association of depressed myofibrillar adenosine triphosphate and reduced contractility in experimental heart failure. Circ. Res. 21:717–725.

FENNER, C., MASON, D. T., ZELIS, R., and WIKMAN-COFFELT, J. 1973. Regulatory properties of myocardial myosin. Proc. Natl. Acad. Sci. USA 70:3205–3209.

ITO, Y., SUKO, J., and CHIDSEY, C. A. 1974. Intracellular calcium and myocardial contractility. V. Calcium uptake of sarcoplasmic reticulum fractions in hypertrophied and failing rabbit hearts. J. Mol. Cell. Cardiol. 6:237–247.

LANGER, G. A. 1973. Heart: Excitation-contraction coupling. Annu. Rev. Physiol. 35: 55–86.

MARGOSSIAN, S. S., LOWEY, S., and BARSHOP, B. 1975. Effect of DTNB light chain on the interaction of vertebrate skeletal myosin with actin. Nature 258:163–166.

MORIMOTO, K., and HARRINGTON, W. F. 1974. Evidence for structural changes in vertebrate thick filaments induced by calcium. J. Mol. Biol. 88:693–709.

SMITH, A., MASON, D. T., and WIKMAN-COFFELT, J. 1974. Molecular weight studies on canine cardiac myosins. FEBS Lett. 43:104–106.

VITALI-MAZZA, L., ANVERSA, P., TEDESCHI, F., MASTANDREA, R., MAVILLAR, V., and VISIOLI, O. 1972. Ultrastructural basis of acute left ventricular failure from severe acute aortic stenosis in the rabbit. J. Mol. Cell. Cardiol. 4:661–671.

WERBER, M. M., and OPLATKA, A. 1974. Physico-chemical on the light chains of myosin III. Evidence for a regulatory role of a rabbit myosin light chain. Biochem. Biophys. Res. Commun. 57:823–830.

WIKMAN-COFFELT, J., FENNER, C., COFFELT, R. J., SALEL, A., KAMIYAMA, T., and MASON, D. T. 1975a. Chronological effects of mild pressure overload on myosin ATPase activity in the canine right ventricle. J. Mol. Cell. Cardiol. 7:219–224.

WIKMAN-COFFELT, J., FENNER, C., McPHERSON, J., ZELIS, R., and MASON, D. T. 1975b. Alterations of subunit composition and ATPase activity of myosin in early hypertrophied right ventricles of dogs with mild experimental pulmonic stenosis. J. Mol. Cell. Cardiol. 7:513–522.

WIKMAN-COFFELT, J., FENNER, C., SMITH, A., and MASON, D. T. 1975c. Comparative analyses of the kinetics and subunits of myosins from canine skeletal muscle and cardiac tissue. J. Biol. Chem. 250:1257–1262.

WIKMAN-COFFELT, J., FENNER, C., WALSH, R., SALEL, A., KAMIYAMA, T., and MASON, D. T. 1975d. Comparison of mild vs severe pressure overload on the enzymatic activity of myosin in the canine ventricles. Biochem. Med. 14:139–146.

WIKMAN-COFFELT, J., SMITH, A., WALSH, R., FENNER, C., KAMIYAMA, T., SALEL, A., and MASON, D. T. 1975e. Activity and molecular changes in right and left ventricular myosins during right ventricular volume overload. Biochem. Med. 14:33–41.

WIKMAN-COFFELT, J., SMITH, A., WALSH, R., FENNER, C., KAMIYAMA, T., SALEL, A., and MASON, D. T. 1976. Effects of severe hemodynamic pressure overload on the properties of canine left ventricular myosin: Mechanism by which myosin ATPase activity is lowered during chronic increased hemodynamic stress. J. Mol. Cell. Cardiol. 8:263–268.

WIKMAN-COFFELT, J., ZELIS, R., FENNER, C., and MASON, D. T. 1973. Comparative purification of myocardial myosin and antigenic specificity of the two light chains. Prep. Biochem. 3:439–449.

Mailing address:
Joan Wikman-Coffelt, Ph.D.,
Section of Cardiovascular Medicine, Department of Medicine,
University of California, Davis, School of Medicine,
Davis, California 95616 (USA).

Recent Advances in Studies on
Cardiac Structure and Metabolism, Volume 11
Heart Function and Metabolism
Edited by T. Kobayashi, T. Sano, and N. S. Dhalla
Copyright 1978 University Park Press Baltimore

PHOSPHORYLATION OF CARDIAC
MYOFIBRILLAR PROTEINS

H. A. COLE, N. FREARSON, A.J.G. MOIR, S. V. PERRY, and R. J. SOLARO

Department of Biochemistry, University of Birmingham,
Birmingham, England

SUMMARY

The P light chain of cardiac myosin is phosphorylated and dephosphorylated by highly specific enzymes. These reactions take place in the beating rabbit heart and there is evidence that dephosphorylation of the light chain occurs during the inotropic response produced by adrenaline. The extent of phosphorylation of cardiac troponin I is determined by the functional state of the beating heart. During perfusion of the rabbit heart the basal phosphate content of troponin I increased from the basal level of about 1.5 moles P per mole to about 2.7 moles P per mole at the height of the inotropic response to adrenaline. The three sites of phosphorylation on troponin I are probably located in the N terminal cyanogen bromide peptide of 48 residues.

INTRODUCTION

Three of the proteins of the myofibril, myosin, troponin I, and troponin T, can be phosphorylated by enzymes present in the muscle cell (Table 1) at sites that are well defined for white skeletal muscle (Perrie, Smillie, and Perry, 1973; Huang *et al.,* 1974; Moir, Wilkinson, and Perry, 1974; Moir, Cole, and Perry, 1977). The cardiac proteins have been studied in less detail, but the information available indicates that similar phosphorylation sites can be identified on them. There are, however, certain differences in enzyme levels and in the nature of the sites, particularly in the case of troponin I, that suggest that phosphorylation of the myofibrillar proteins may be of particular significance for cardiac function.

PHOSPHORYLATION OF MYOSIN

All muscles so far examined contain a highly specific enzyme, myosin light-chain kinase, that phosphorylates the light chain of molecular weight 18,000–20,000,

This work was supported in part by research grants from the Medical Research Council and the British Heart Foundation, and was carried out during the tenure by Dr. R. J. Solaro of a British American Research Fellowship of the American Heart Association and the British Heart Foundation.

Table 1. Phosphorylated proteins of the rabbit cardiac myofibril†

Protein	Molecular weight	Main phosphorylated sites (no./mole)	Enzymes involved	
			Phosphorylation	Dephosphorylation
Myosin P light chain	19,000	1	Myosin light chain-kinase	Myosin light-chain phosphatase
Troponin I	23,000[1]	3	cAMP-dependent protein kinase	Troponin I phosphatase*
			Phosphorylase kinase	Troponin I phosphatase*
Troponin T	40,500[2]	3*	Phosphorylase kinase	Troponin T phosphatase*

† Data marked with an asterisk are presumptive.
[1] From sequence studies of Grand *et al.*, 1976.
[2] Apparent from polyacrylamide gel electrophoresis in sodium dodecyl sulphate (Greaser *et al.*, 1972).

the P light chain, present in all vertebrate myosins (Pires, Perry, and Thomas, 1974; Frearson and Perry, 1975; Frearson, Focant, and Perry, 1976). When myosin is freshly prepared from heart, particularly if the extraction buffers contain phosphate, the P light chain of molecular weight 19,000 usually migrates in polyacrylamide gel electrophoresis in 8 M urea, pH 8.6, as four closely spaced bands, the P light chain, the "satellite" P light chain (a modified form of the light chain that is formed spontaneously during preparation), and the phosphorylated derivatives of both these forms of the P light chain (Frearson and Perry, 1975). The "satellite" form is less readily formed in myosin prepared from hearts of some species than of others.

Dephosphorylation is catalyzed by another highly specific enzyme, myosin light-chain phosphatase, of molecular weight about 70,000, in skeletal muscle (Morgan, Perry, and Ottaway, 1976a,b). Like the kinase, the phosphatase from cardiac tissue has been studied in less detail, but both enzymes seem very similar to their skeletal counterparts, possibly differing slightly in physical properties.

In mammalian striated and smooth muscles the phosphatase is roughly similar in activity per gram wet weight, whereas the kinase activity varies widely, with the lowest amount in cardiac muscle when tested against the whole light chain fraction from white skeletal muscle myosin (Frearson et al., 1976). The enzymic levels in cardiac muscle are such that a relatively small change in the activity of either enzyme would lead to a rapid change from the phosphorylated to the dephosphorylated form of myosin. In the case of skeletal muscle the relative enzyme concentrations are strongly in favor of phosphorylation of the P light chain. Phosphorylation-dephosphorylation processes involving the P light chain occur in the beating heart, for after perfusion with modified Krebs-Henseleit solution containing $^{32}P_i$ for 15 min by the Langendorff procedure the phosphate on the P light chain became labeled.

Studies on the perfused heart also indicate that under normal control conditions of perfusion the P light chain is almost fully phosphorylated. When light chains were rapidly isolated after homogenization of the heart (in 9 M urea, 75 mM Tris-HCl, pH 8.0, 1 mM $CaCl_2$, 15 mM β-mercaptoethanol), at the point at which maximum force was developed after addition of adrenaline, a fall in the extent of phosphorylation could be demonstrated. The extent of dephosphorylation paralleled the increase in force obtained at the different adrenaline concentrations used until, at maximum inotropic effect, the P light-chain fraction was about 50% dephosphorylated. When the inotropic effect was prevented by prior addition of propranolol to the perfusate, dephosphorylation of the P light chain was much reduced. Thus it appears that the increased force of contraction of the myocardium that is produced by adrenaline is accompanied by dephosphorylation of the P light chain of cardiac myosin. The increased intracellular concentration of Ca^{2+} that results from the action of adrenaline on the myocardium would be expected to favor phosphorylation rather than dephosphorylation of the P light chain, as myosin light kinase requires Ca^{2+} for activity (Pires *et al.*, 1974). Preliminary studies on the enzymic and actin-combining properties of myosin from white skeletal muscle do not indicate that phosphorylation of the P light chain has a marked effect on these properties *in vitro* (Morgan *et al.*, 1976a,b). There is, however, some evidence suggesting that the P light chain may be involved in the interaction of myosin with actin (Margossian, Lowey, and Barshop, 1976; Morgan *et al.*, 1976b). Phosphorylation results in the addition of two negative charges at a specific site on each molecule of P light chain and would clearly have some effect on the binding forces involved.

PHOSPHORYLATION OF TROPONIN

Troponin T and troponin I can be phosphorylated by phosphorylase kinase, although in both cases the rates are low compared to those obtained with phosphorylase b as substrate. Troponin I is also phosphorylated by cAMP-dependent protein kinase, but troponin T is not phosphorylated at a significant rate by this enzyme. These properties apply to troponin components isolated from both skeletal (Perry and Cole, 1974) and cardiac muscle (Cole and Perry, 1975).

Troponin T

Cardiac troponin T has a slightly higher molecular weight than skeletal troponin T, in which 3 sites of phosphorylation have been identified (Moir *et al.*, 1977). One site, close to the N terminus, is usually about 70% phosphorylated when troponin T is isolated from skeletal muscle. When isolated, cardiac troponin T contains about 0.3 mole P_i per mole, which by analogy with the protein from skeletal muscle is presumably located at the N-terminal site. There is, as yet, no clear indication of the role of phosphorylation of troponin T, although there is evidence that the serine residues that can be phosphorylated are located close to the sites of interaction with troponin C and tropomyosin (Moir *et al.*, 1977).

Troponin I

The primary sequence of rabbit cardiac troponin I is similar to fast skeletal troponin I with an additional 26 residue N-terminal peptide containing a serine residue at position 20 (Grand, Wilkinson, and Mole, 1976). Residues 27 to 206 of cardiac troponin I show a high degree of homology with fast skeletal muscle troponin I, and regions similar to those identified in fast skeletal troponin I as involved in binding troponin C and actin (Syska *et al.*, 1976) can be recognized. Serine residues at positions 37 and 146 appear to be analogous to threonine 11 and serine 118, which have been shown in fast skeletal troponin I to be the main sites of phosphorylation by phosphorylase kinase and cAMP-dependent protein kinase, respectively. With the latter enzyme, cardiac troponin I is phosphorylated 20–30 times faster than white skeletal troponin I due to rapid phosphorylation of the additional site at serine 20, although phosphorylation also occurs more slowly at serine 146.

When isolated by affinity chromatography from heart immediately after death, troponin I contains 2–3 moles P per mole, whereas fast skeletal muscle troponin I isolated under similar conditions contains only 0.5–1.0 mole P per mole. After 15–20 min perfusion with modified Krebs-Henseleit solution by the Langendorff procedure the phosphate content of rabbit heart troponin I fell to about 1.5 moles per mole and remained at this value during perfusion for up to 100 min. $^{32}P_i$ was taken up from the perfusate by the troponin I and found to be located almost exclusively ($> 80\%$) at serine 20.

The increase in contractile force developed by the rabbit heart on addition of adrenaline to the perfusate was paralleled by a rise in the phosphate content of troponin I (Figure 1). The maximum force usually developed 10–15 sec after addition of the adrenaline to the perfusate. At that point the heart was rapidly removed from the perfusion apparatus, immediately homogenized in buffered 9 M urea and troponin I isolated by affinity chromatography. If perfusion was continued with adrenaline-free medium after the response to adrenaline had taken place the phosphate content of the troponin fell to the original value of about 1.5 moles P per mole. Preincubation with 1 μM propranolol inhibited the inotropic response to adrenaline as well as the rise in the phosphate content of troponin I. In general, the greater the increase in contractile force resulting from the perfusion with adrenaline, the higher the phosphate content of the troponin I. The maximum force was obtained on addition of 2 μM adrenaline to the perfusate and corresponded to the maximum phosphate content of about 3.0 moles P_i per mole of troponin I. These results confirm and extend the findings of England (1975) with the perfused rat heart and suggest that most of the increase in contractile force of the perfused rabbit heart resulting from adrenaline treatment occurred when the troponin I phosphate content increased from 2–3 moles per mole protein.

The distribution of phosphate in the troponin I molecule was investigated by perfusing the heart with $^{32}P_i$ and fractionating the peptides obtained on CNBr digestion of the purified ^{32}P-labeled troponin I. After addition of adrenaline, a much greater incorporation of ^{32}P into troponin I was obtained compared with controls perfused without added hormone. When troponin I was isolated either at the peak of the inotropic response or during perfusion without adrenaline, practically all the ^{32}P incorporated was localized in the N terminal CNBr peptide consisting of residues 1–48 (Grand et al., 1976). Because troponin I contains about 3 moles P per mole at maximum inotropic response, these preliminary results suggest that all three main sites of phosphorylation are situated in the N-terminal CNBr peptide. One of these sites is serine 20, which is normally partially phosphorylated in hearts perfused under control conditions.

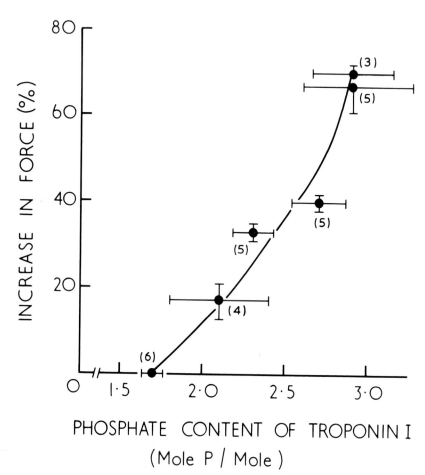

Figure 1. Relation between the phosphate content of troponin I and the increase in force developed in the perfused rabbit heart. Force changes were induced by adding 0.3 to 4.0 μM adrenaline to modified Krebs-Henseleit buffer (118 mM NaCl, 4.7 mM KCl, 2.5 mM $CaCl_2$, 1.2 mM $MgSO_4$, 0.2 mM KH_2PO_4, 0.5 mM Na_2 EDTA, 25 mM $NaHCO_3$, and 5 mM glucose) equilibrated with 95% O_2 : 5% CO_2 at 37° C, pH 7.4. Hearts were first perfused for a 15-min equilibration period with normal buffer and then switched to buffer containing adrenaline. At the peak of the force change the hearts were rapidly homogenized in buffered 9 M urea and troponin I isolated as described in the text. P content calculated from total phosphate and nitrogen contents measured in duplicate samples of trichloroacetic acid-washed troponin I as described by Perry and Cole (1974) using a molecular weight of 23,000 and a nitrogen content of 16% for cardiac troponin I. Figures in parentheses indicate number of hearts analyzed.

The others have not been identified, but there are four serine and two threonine residues in this peptide in addition to serine 20 (Grand *et al.,* 1976). A serine located at position 37 is in an analogous position to threonine 11 of white skeletal troponin I and would be expected to be a site for phosphorylation catalyzed by phosphorylase kinase. Our studies do not yet enable us to decide if this site is being labeled during perfusion.

The correlation between the increase in contractile force obtained with adrenaline in the perfused heart and the degree of phosphorylation of troponin I is good. A similar increase in phosphorylation in response to adrenaline probably also occurs *in vivo.* When isolated immediately after death by stunning, rabbit cardiac troponin I usually contained 2–3 moles P per mole. If, however, the hearts of animals anesthetized with pentobarbital were frozen *in situ* with Wollenberger clamps chilled with liquid nitrogen, the troponin I isolated contained 1.5 ± 0.2 moles P per mole. This suggests that the phosphate content of the cardiac troponin I in the resting heart is very similar to the basal value obtained after 10–15 min perfusion of the isolated heart.

It is significant that most of the phosphorylation that results from treatment with adrenaline occurs in the N-terminal region. A number of lines of evidence (Cole and Perry, 1975; Syska *et al.,* 1976) indicate that this part of the molecule is the region that interacts with troponin C. As has been suggested elsewhere (Cole and Perry, 1975), the introduction of negative charges in this region, which has a net positive charge, would be expected to weaken the interaction with troponin C.

There is evidence that interaction with troponin I modifies the affinity of troponin C for Ca^{2+} (Potter and Gergely, 1975). If this is the case, it would be expected that modification of the binding constant of troponin I for troponin C, for example by phosphorylation of the former protein, would lead to a change of the binding constants of troponin C for Ca^{2+}. The inotropic effect of adrenaline could be explained by assuming that the increased phosphorylation of troponin I that accompanies it leads to an increase in the affinity of troponin C for Ca^{2+}. This would lead to activation of the actomyosin ATPase at a lower Ca^{2+} concentration and presumably increased contractile force. The report of Rubio, Bailey, and Villar-Palasi (1975) that the ATPase is activated at lower Ca^{2+} concentrations when the troponin I component in natural actomyosin from cardiac muscle is phosphorylated by cAMP-dependent protein kinase would suggest that this is the case. In our laboratory, however, we have been unable to confirm the findings of Rubio *et al.* (1975), either with natural actomyosin or myofibrils from bovine heart or with desensitized actomyosin from skeletal muscle regulated by cardiac troponin that was phosphorylated to known levels by prior incubation with bovine cardiac cAMP-dependent kinase (Figure 2). In all cases phosphorylation reduced the sensitivity of the system to Ca^{2+} (Figure 2). Thus the results of the effect of phosphorylation of troponin I on the Ca^{2+}

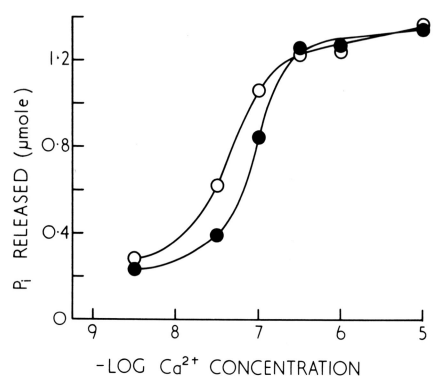

Figure 2. Effect of phosphorylation of troponin I on the ATPase activity of cardiac natural actomyosin at varying Ca²⁺ concentrations. Natural actomyosin (5 mg/ml) prepared from bovine heart by a modification of the method of Reddy and Honig (1972) incubated with 50 mM Tris-HCl, (pH 7.5) 2.5 mM $MgCl_2$, 2.5 mM dithiothreitol, 0.05 mM bovine cardiac cAMP-dependent protein kinase (0.04 mg/ml) 2.5 mM Na ATP. Final vol = 10 ml incubated 10 min at 25° C and chilled. For the control incubation, protein kinase and cAMP were omitted and ATP added after chilling. Using $[\gamma\text{-}^{32}P]$ATP in these conditions it was shown that the natural actomyosin contained 1 nmol P per mg after incubation with enzyme, whereas the control natural actomyosin contained 0.1 nmol P per mg after incubation. After polyacrylamide gel electrophoresis in sodium dodecyl sulphate at pH 7.0 (Weber and Osborn, 1969), of the incubated actomyosin, virtually all ^{32}P was in the band corresponding to an apparent molecular weight of 28,000. ATPase determination was carried out under the following conditions: 50 mM Tris-HCl (pH 7.5), 2.5 mM $MgCl_2$, 2.5 mM dithiothreitol, 2.5 mM ATP, 1 mM EGTA + $CaCl_2$ to give pCa^{2+} shown (K_a = 3.7 × 10⁷; Sillen and Martell, 1964), 0.4 ml of incubate prepared as described above. Final vol = 2 ml incubated 7 min at 25° C. For blanks which were deducted preincubated natural actomyosins added after 1 ml 15% trichloroacetic acid used to stop the ATPase reaction. ○, control natural actomyosin (~ 0.1 nmol P per mg actomyosin). ●, phosphorylated natural actomyosin (~ 1.0 nmol P per mg actomyosin).

regulation of myofibrillar ATPase appear at the moment to be equivocal. It would seem, however, that a role in which phosphorylation reduces the sensitivity of the contractile apparatus to Ca^{2+} makes good biological sense. If, due to its action at the membrane, adrenaline leads to an increased intracellular Ca^{2+} concentration, there would be little advantage in making troponin C more sensitive to Ca^{2+} at the same time. A smoother response would follow if the accompanying phosphorylation of troponin I led to a reduction in Ca^{2+} sensitivity of the myofibrillar ATPase—in effect a negative feedback system to smooth out the response.

In a number of enzymic systems, phosphorylation leads to a dramatic change in activity. The role of phosphorylation-dephosphorylation processes in myofibrillar function does not appear to involve a mechanism in which covalent modification is essential for activity. All the evidence would suggest that phosphorylation or dephosphorylation per se is not essential for myofibrillar function, but that by changing the net charge at important sites of interaction between the myofibrillar proteins these processes can modulate the contractile response and its regulation.

Note added in proof

Further study of the phosphorylation of troponin I in the perfused rabbit heart has indicated that there was a systematic error in the phosphate determinations presented above. This has led to an over-estimation of the amounts present, although the pattern of change remains the same. The revised figure for the phosphate content of troponin I from the perfused equilibrated rabbit heart is 1.2 ± 0.05 mol P per mol. On treatment with adrenaline the phosphate content increased to about 1.9 mol P per mol and returned to the lower value after removal of adrenaline from the perfusate. These results suggest that, in addition to serine 20, one, rather than two, sites in the N terminal 48 residue peptide is also phosphorylated.

REFERENCES

COLE, H. A., and PERRY, S. V. 1975. The phosphorylation of troponin I from cardiac muscle. Biochem. J. 149:525–533.

ENGLAND, P. 1975. Correlation between contraction and phosphorylation of the inhibitory subunit of troponin in perfused rat heart. FEBS Lett. 50:57–60.

FREARSON, N., and PERRY, S. V. 1975. Phosphorylation of the light chain components of myosin from cardiac and red skeletal muscle. Biochem. J. 151:99–107.

FREARSON, N., FOCANT, B. W. W., and PERRY, S. V. 1976. Phosphorylation of a light chain component of myosin from smooth muscle. FEBS Lett. 63:27–32.

GRAND, R. J. A., WILKINSON, J. M., and MOLE, L. E. 1976. The amino acid sequence of rabbit cardiac troponin I. Biochem. J. 159:633–641.

GREASER, M. L., YAMAGUCHI, M., BREKKE, C., POTTER, J., and GERGELY, J. 1972. Troponin subunits and their interactions. Cold Spring Harbor Symp. Quant. Biol. 37:235–244.

HUANG, T. S., BYLUND, D. B., STULL, J. T., and KREBS, E. G., 1974. The amino acid sequences of the phosphorylated sites in troponin I from rabbit skeletal muscle. FEBS Lett. 42:249–252.

MARGOSSIAN, S. S., LOWEY, S., and BARSHOP, B. 1975. Effects of DTNB light chain on the interaction of vertebrate skeletal myosin with actin. Nature 258:163–166.

MOIR, A. J. G., COLE, H. A., and PERRY, S. V. 1977. The phosphorylation sites of troponin T from white skeletal muscle and the effects of interaction with troponin C on their phosphorylation by phosphorylase kinase. Biochem. J. 161:371–382.

MOIR, A. J. G., WILKINSON, J. M., and PERRY, S. V. 1974. The phosphorylation sites of troponin I from white skeletal muscle of the rabbit. FEBS Lett. 42:253–256.

MORGAN, M., PERRY, S. V., and OTTAWAY, J. 1976a. A new protein phosphatase from skeletal muscle: Myosin light-chain phosphatase. Biochem. Soc. Trans. 4:351–352.

MORGAN, M., PERRY, S. V., and OTTAWAY, J. 1976b. Myosin light chain phosphatase. Biochem. J. 157:687–697.

PERRIE, W. T., SMILLIE, L. B., and PERRY, S. V. 1973. A phosphorylated light chain component of myosin from skeletal muscle. Biochem. J. 135:151–164.

PERRY, S. V., and COLE, H. A. 1974. Phosphorylation of troponin and the effects of interactions between the components of the complex. Biochem. J. 141:733–743.

PIRES, E., PERRY, S. V., and THOMAS, M. A. W. 1974. Myosin light chain kinase, a new enzyme from striated muscle. FEBS Lett. 41:292–296.

POTTER, J. D., and GERGELY, J. 1975. The calcium and magnesium binding sites on troponin and their role in the regulation of myofibrillar adenosine triphosphatase. J. Biol. Chem. 250:4628–4633.

REDDY, Y. S., and HONIG, C. L. 1972. Ca^{2+}-binding and Ca^{2+}-sensitizing functions of cardiac native tropomyosin, troponin and tropomyosin. Biochim. Biophys. Acta 275:453–463.

RUBIO, R., BAILEY, C., and VILLAR-PALASI, C. 1975. Effects of cyclic AMP-dependent protein kinase on cardiac actomyosin: Increase in Ca^{++} sensitivity and possible phosphorylation of troponin I. J. Cyc. Nuc. Res. 1:143–150.

SILLEN, L. G., and MARTELL, A. E. 1964. Stability constants of metal-ion complexes. Chemical Society. Special Publication No. 17. pp. 697–698.

SYSKA, H., WILKINSON, J. M., GRAND, R. J. A., and PERRY, S. V. 1976. The relationship between biological activity and primary structure of troponin I from white skeletal muscle of the rabbit. Biochem. J. 163:375–387.

WEBER, K., and OSBORN, M. 1969. The reliability of molecular weight determinations by dodecyl sulphate polyacrylamide gel electrophoresis. J. Biol. Chem. 244:4406–4412.

Mailing address:
Professor S. V. Perry,
Department of Biochemistry,
University of Birmingham,
P. O. B. 363, Birmingham B15 2TT (England).

Recent Advances in Studies on
Cardiac Structure and Metabolism, Volume 11
Heart Function and Metabolism
Edited by T. Kobayashi, T. Sano, and N. S. Dhalla
Copyright 1978   University Park Press   Baltimore

FREQUENCY-DEPENDENT CHANGES IN THE ELECTROMECHANICAL AND (Na$^+$, K$^+$)-ATPase ACTIVITY OF CARDIAC MUSCLE

K. PRASAD, P. K. SINGAL, and J. C. KHATTER

Department of Physiology, College of Medicine,
University of Saskatchewan, Saskatoon, Saskatchewan, Canada

SUMMARY

Influence of certain interventions on the frequency-dependent changes in the electromechanical activity of papillary muscles from monkey's heart was investigated. Also, the effect of frequency of stimulation on the Mg^{2+}-dependent (Na$^+$, K$^+$)-ATPase of isolated sarcolemmal fractions from dog's heart was studied. An increase in the rate of stimulation from 15 to 30, 60, and 90/min produced frequency-dependent increases in the contractility and shortening of the duration of action potential (APD) in papillary muscles. Ouabain and KCl-free Krebs-Ringer solution, well-known ATPase inhibitors, prevented the frequency-dependent positive inotropy and converted the response from positive to negative. However, epinephrine (4.5×10^{-8} M) and quinidine (1.3×10^{-5} M), which are supposedly not ATPase inhibitors, did not affect the frequency-dependent positive inotropy. Rate-dependent shortening of the APD was greater in the presence of ATPase inhibitors than in the presence of quinidine. There was a frequency-dependent inhibition of the (Na$^+$, K$^+$)-ATPase of the isolated sarcolemmal fraction from the dog's heart. These results suggest that the frequency-dependent positive inotropy and shortening of the APD in cardiac muscle are most likely mediated through the inhibition of the Mg^{2+}-dependent, Na$^+$-K$^+$-stimulated sarcolemmal ATPase.

INTRODUCTION

It is known that a change in the rate of stimulation alters the force of contraction in an isolated piece of cardiac muscle (Katzung, Rasin, and Scheider, 1957; Blinks and Koch-Weser, 1961) as well as in the perfused heart (Lendrum *et al.*, 1960). This frequency-force relationship in cardiac muscle varies from species to species (Henderson *et al.*, 1961) and from normal to diseased heart (Buckley, Penefsky, and Litwalk, 1972). Similar to cardiac glycosides, an increase in the frequency of stimulation has been reported to produce an increase in the rate of tension development and a reduction in time to peak tension

This work was supported by a grant from Saskatchewan Heart Foundation and by a Post-doctoral Fellowship from Medical Research Council to Dr. P. K. Singal.

(Blinks and Koch-Weser, 1961; Koch-Weser and Blinks, 1963). Since it has been suggested that the positive inotropic effect of cardiac glycosides is mediated through an inhibition of Mg^{2+}-dependent, Na^+-K^+-activated sarcolemmal ATPase (Akera, Larsen, and Brody, 1970; Besch *et al.,* 1970; Prasad and Callaghan, 1969; Prasad, 1972, 1974, 1975), it is possible that frequency-dependent increase in the contractility in cardiac muscle might be mediated through an inhibition of the membrane ATPase. Inhibition of active transport of Na^+ and K^+ has been suggested to be somehow related to an increased efflux of K^+ and an increased influx of Ca^{2+}, resulting, respectively, in shortening of the action potential duration and an increase in the cardiac contraction (Prasad and Callaghan, 1969; Prasad, 1970, 1972, 1974).

If this is the case, then the frequency-dependent increases in the contractility and shortening of the duration of action potential should be associated with an inhibition of the sarcolemmal (Na^+, K^+)-ATPase, and should be reduced or abolished in the presence of ATPase inhibitors.

It was therefore decided to study the effects of certain ATPase inhibitors on the frequency-dependent changes in the contractility and action potential. Also, the effects of frequency of stimulation on the isolated sarcolemmal ATPase from cardiac muscle were investigated.

MATERIALS AND METHODS

Papillary muscles (thickness never more than 0.75 mm) were obtained from the right ventricle of the monkey under pentobarbital anesthesia. The methods for recording action potential and contraction were the same as those used by Prasad (1974). The muscles were tied horizontally in a jacketed 100-ml constant temperature bath at $37°$ C containing Krebs-Ringer solution. One end of the muscle was tied to a fixed holder, and the other end to a Grass FT-03 force displacement transducer through a movable holder in such a way as to permit isometric contraction. The Krebs-Ringer solution used had the following composition in mEq/liter: Na, 146.8; K, 5; Ca, 5.31; HCO_3, 20.14; PO_4, 4.36; Cl, 137.14; and glucose, 45 mM. The solution in the bath was constantly bubbled with 95% oxygen and 5% carbon dioxide. The resting tension was set about halfway up the length tension curve. The muscle was stimulated supramaximally with square wave stimuli of 5 msec duration at desired rate by a Grass stimulator through platinum electrodes placed at one end of the muscle.

Single-cell electrical activity was recorded with flexibly mounted glass microelectrodes of tip diameter less than 5 μm filled with 3 M KCl having a resistance of 5 to 10 MΩ. Potential measurements were made through a Medistor negative capacitance electrometer. Action potential and contraction were monitored on a Tektronix 564A storage oscilloscope and photographed on Polaroid film. The muscles were equilibrated in Krebs-Ringer solution for at least one hour before normal action potential and contraction were recorded.

Relatively pure sarcolemma from cardiac muscle of dog was prepared using the method of Kidwai *et al.* (1971). The methods for ATPase estimation were the same as used earlier by Prasad (1975). For electrical stimulation of the isolated sarcolemmal fraction, the reaction mixture without ATP was placed in a special tube, fitted at the base with platinum electrodes such that both the electrodes were submerged in the mixture medium. The electrodes were connected to the stimulator for stimulation of the mixture media at different frequencies. The mixtures were incubated at 37° C. Reaction was started by the addition of ATP while at the same time the complete mixture was stimulated at a desired frequency (0, 15, 30, 60, or 120/min) for 5 min duration. The reaction was terminated by addition of 10% trichlor acetic acid.

The statistical analysis of the results was done using Student's *t* test.

RESULTS

Frequency-Force Relationship

After equilibration the muscles were stimulated at the rate of 15/min. In all the experiments the basal rate of stimulation was 15/min. An increase in the rate of stimulation from 15/min to 30, 60, or 90/min produced a frequency-dependent increase in the force of contraction, and shortening of the duration of action potential in eight papillary muscles. A representative recording is shown in Figure 1, and the results for force of contraction are summarized in Figure 2. The shortening of the duration of action potential was observed at all levels of repolarization. There was a decrease in the amplitude of action potential also. The results for the changes in the duration of action potential are summarized in Figure 3.

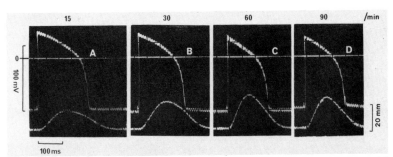

Figure 1. Effect of rate of stimulation on the simultaneously recorded action potential and contraction in single papillary muscle of monkey. Numerals at the top of each tracing are the rates of stimulation. In each tracing, the *upper recording* is the action potential and the *lower recording* is the force of contraction. Calibrations are indicated in the figure.

K. Prasad, P. K. Singal, and J. C. Khatter

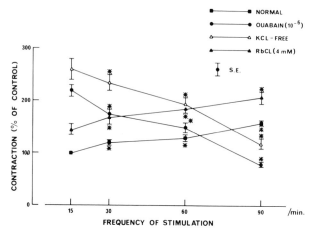

Figure 2. The influence of ouabain, KCl-free solution, and substitution of rubidium chloride on the frequency-dependent changes in the contractility. *Asterisk* indicates that the results are significant when compared to the value for stimulation at 15/min normal, in the normal Krebs-Ringer solution.

Effect of ATPase Inhibitors on Frequency-Force Relationship

If the frequency-dependent positive inotropy is mediated through an inhibition of sarcolemmal (Na^+, K^+)-ATPase, then this effect of frequency should be either reduced or absent when the sarcolemmal ATPase is already inhibited. It was, therefore, decided to study the effects of increasing frequency of stimulation on the myocardial contractility in the presence of ouabain or in KCl-free Krebs-Ringer solution, which are supposed to inhibit sarcolemmal ATPase.

Ouabain $(10^{-6}$ M) increased the force of contraction by 220% ± 10% in five papillary muscles stimulated at a rate of 15/min. Figure 4 is a representative

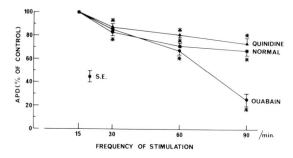

Figure 3. The influence of quinidine and ouabain on the frequency-dependent changes in the duration of action potential (APD) at 50% level of repolarization. *Asterisk* values are significantly different from control.

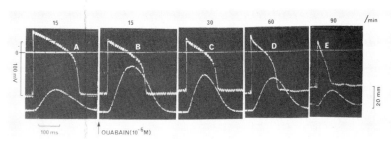

Figure 4. Influence of ouabain on the frequency-dependent changes in the simultaneously recorded contractility (*lower tracing*) and duration of action potential (*upper tracing*). At the *arrow* mark the muscle was exposed to ouabain, and *B* is the tracing after 20 min exposure to ouabain. The numerals at the top of each tracing are the rate of stimulation. Calibrations are indicated in the figure.

recording from one such experiment. After a steady level of contraction, which was attained after 15–20 min of ouabain, the muscle was stimulated at different frequencies (30, 60, or 90/min). The rate-dependent increase in the contractility was absent in the presence of ouabain (Figures 2 and 4). However, a negative inotropic effect was apparent that was greater at higher frequency of stimulation (Figures 2 and 4). The quality of the rate-dependent change in duration of action potential remained unchanged. However, the shortening of the duration of action potential at the frequency of 60 and 90/min in the presence of ouabain was greater than that in the absence of ouabain (Figures 2 and 3).

Five papillary muscles, after equilibration in normal Krebs-Ringer solution, were exposed to a KCl-free Krebs-Ringer solution. Muscles exposed to KCl-free Krebs-Ringer solution and stimulated at 15/min showed a marked increase in the contractility (Figure 2). After the steady-state contraction (260 ± 20% of control) was established, the muscles were stimulated at the frequency of 30, 60, or 90/min. In these muscles, also, no positive inotropy was observed in response to an increase in the rate of stimulation. Rather, a negative inotropy was observed that was frequency-dependent (Figure 2).

Frequency-Force and Rubidium

Rubidium has been reported to replace potassium for stimulation of Mg^{2+}-dependent, Na^+-K^+-activated sarcolemmal ATPase in cardiac muscle (Prasad, 1974). If this is the case, and if the rate-dependent positive inotropy is mediated through an inhibition of sarcolemmal ATPase, then rubidium should be able to reverse the effect of KCl-free Krebs-Ringer solution on the frequency-dependent decrease in the contractility. The muscles were first exposed to KCl-free Krebs-Ringer solution and the rate-dependent decreases in the contractility were recorded. Rubidium chloride was then added in the bath to give final concentrations of either 4 mM (3 experiments) or 8 mM (2 experiments). Rubidium chloride markedly decreased the contractility in the papillary muscles stimulated at a rate of 15/min (Figure 2). An increase in the rate of stimulation in the presence of rubidium, however, produced a frequency-dependent increase in the contractility (Figure 2). The latter was dependent upon concentration of rubidium in the solution.

Frequency-Force and Epinephrine

The possibility that the positive inotropic agents might affect the frequency-dependent increase in cardiac contractility, even if they do not inhibit the membrane ATPase, exists. It was therefore decided to study the influence of epinephrine (4.5×10^{-8} M), which is known not to inhibit membrane ATPase, on the frequency-dependent changes in the contractility in papillary muscles. Epinephrine increased the contractility in five papillary muscles stimulated at the rate of 15/min (Figure 5). Frequency-dependent increase in contractility similar to that recorded in the absence of any interventions was observed in the presence of epinephrine in all the experiments (Figure 5).

Frequency-Force and Quinidine

Quinidine (1.3×10^{-5} M), a negative inotropic agent that has been shown not to inhibit membrane ATPase (Ells, 1964; Harrow and Dhalla, 1975), was used in

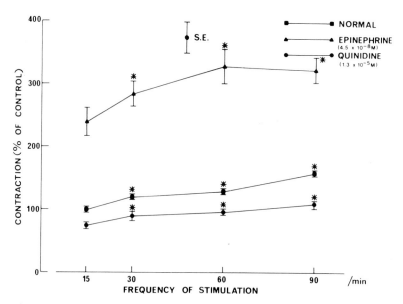

Figure 5. Influence of quinidine and epinephrine on the frequency-dependent changes in the contractility of the papillary muscle. *Asterisk* values are significantly different from the control.

four experiments. It produced a decrease in the contractility in the muscles stimulated at the rate of 15/min (Figures 5 and 6). However, an increase in the rate of stimulation produced a frequency-dependent increase in contractility (Figures 5 and 6). The frequency-dependent changes in the duration of action potential in the presence of quinidine were qualitatively similar to those recorded in its absence. However, the shortening of the duration of action potential in response to an increase in the rate of stimulation was less as compared to that observed in the absence of quinidine (control).

Frequency of Stimulation and Sarcolemmal ATPase

Experiments were conducted in which the sarcolemmal fractions from dog hearts were stimulated (stimulus strength of 0.5 V and 5 msec duration) at a frequency of 0, 15, 30, 60, or 120/min for a duration of 5 min, and the sarcolemmal ATPase activity was determined. The results are summarized in Figure 7. The sarcolemmal ATPase activity for unstimulated fraction incubated for 5 min was found to be 12.15 ± 0.28 μmol/mg protein/hr. The sarcolemmal ATPase was inhibited at all frequencies of stimulation.

DISCUSSION

The present results indicate that the frequency-dependent increase in the cardiac contractility was absent when the sarcolemmal ATPase was preinhibited with ouabain or KCl-free Krebs-Ringer solution. Rubidium, which is supposed to replace potassium in stimulating sarcolemmal (Na^+, K^+)-ATPase (Skou, 1965; Prasad, 1974), returned the frequency-dependent positive inotropy in muscles that previously lacked this property in KCl-free Krebs-Ringer solution. Also, there was an inhibition of (Na^+, K^+)-ATPase in isolated sarcolemmal fraction from dog's heart in response to an increase in the frequency of stimulation.

It has been suggested earlier by Prasad and Callaghan (1969) and Prasad, (1974) that an increase in the contractility of human papillary muscle in KCl-free

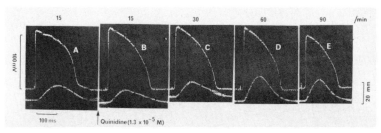

Figure 6. Influence of quinidine on the frequency-dependent changes in the simultaneously recorded action potential (*upper tracing*) and contraction (*lower tracing*) in the papillary muscle. At the *arrow* mark the muscle was exposed to quinidine, and *B* is 20 min after exposure to quinidine. *A* is control in Krebs-Ringer solution. The numerals at the top of each tracing are the rates of stimulation of the muscle. Calibrations are indicated.

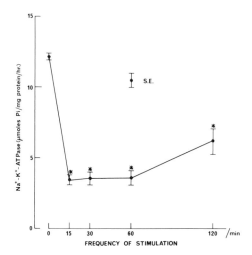

Figure 7. Effect of frequency of stimulation on the Mg^{2+}-dependent, Na^+-K^+-activated sarcolemmal ATPase. *Asterisk* calues are significantly different from those without stimulation.

Krebs-Ringer solution might be associated with an inhibition of the membrane (Na^+, K^+)-ATPase. They also suggested that the rubidium-induced decrease in the contractility might be associated with the stimulation of this enzyme system.

In the present investigation, other agents that either increase or decrease the contractility but do not inhibit the sarcolemmal ATPase were used to see if they also modify the frequency-dependent increase in the contractility. Reportedly, quinidine, a negative inotropic agent, does not inhibit (Na^+, K^+)-ATPase in the rat myocardium even in the concentration of 10^{-3} M (Harrow and Dhalla, 1975). Lack of ATPase inhibition by low dose of quinidine has also been reported by Ells (1964). It is therefore unlikely that the quinidine (1.3×10^{-5} M) used in the present study would inhibit membrane ATPase. Although quinidine showed a negative inotropic effect, the frequency-dependent positive inotropy was still observed, suggesting that if ATPase is not inhibited this frequency-dependent change will occur.

It can be argued that positive inotropic agents (ouabain, KCl-free solution) may alter the muscle cell response to increased stimulation rate without inhibiting the membrane ATPase. However, our experiments using epinephrine, a positive inotropic agent, do not support this contention. As in the presence of epinephrine, unlike ouabain and KCl-free solution, frequency-dependent positive inotropy was still present. Epinephrine at a concentration of 10^{-6} M depresses the ATPase activity of guinea pig heart by only 20% (Lee and Yu, 1963). A lower concentration, 4.5×10^{-8} M, used in the present study might not have affected the sarcolemmal ATPase. In the isolated sarcolemmal fraction, an increase in the stimulation rate resulted in a rate-dependent inhibition of the Mg^{2+}-dependent, Na^+-K^+-activated sarcolemmal ATPase. This observation strongly supports the hypothesis that the frequency-dependent increase in the cardiac contractility might be associated with an inhibition of sarcolemmal ATPase.

Frequency-dependent changes in the duration of action potential have also been reported in dog by Prasad and Kidwai (1974). A correlation between the shortening of the duration of action potential and the inhibition of the sarcolemmal ATPase in human papillary muscle has also been observed (Prasad, 1974).

The following question arises: How does this inhibition in the sarcolemmal ATPase increase the contractility and shorten the duration of action potential in cardiac muscle? It has been suggested by Prasad (1970, 1974) and Prasad and Callaghan (1969) that an inhibition of active transport of Na^+ and K^+ is somehow related to an increased efflux of K^+ and an increased influx of Ca^{2+}, resulting, respectively, in shortening of the duration of action potential and in an increase in the cardiac contractility. If this is so, then there should be a loss of K^+ and gain of Na^+ and Ca^{2+} in the cell. A net loss of K^+ (Hajdu, 1953) and a net gain of Ca^{2+} (Langer, 1965) have been observed with frequency-dependent increases in the contractility. However, in a study of frequency-force relationship, Koch-Weser and Blinks (1963) suggested that the resultant contraction is the sum total of positive inotropic effect of activation (PIEA) and negative inotropic effect of activation (NIEA). The nature of the PIEA and NIEA is not known. The present study shows that the PIEA appears to be mediated through an inhibition of the sarcolemmal ATPase. Negative inotropic effect of activation might be operational through some other mechanism.

The present results strongly suggest that the frequency-dependent positive inotropy might be mediated through an inhibition of Mg^{2+}-dependent, Na^+-K^+-activated sarcolemmal ATPase in cardiac muscle.

REFERENCES

AKERA, T., LARSEN, F. S., and BRODY, T. M. 1970. Correlation of cardiac sodium and potassium-activated adenosine triphosphatase activity with ouabain induced inotropic stimulation. J. Pharmacol. Exp. Ther. 173:145–151.

BESCH, H. R., ALLEN, J. C., GLICK, G., and SCHWARTZ, A. 1970. Correlation between the inotropic action of ouabain and its effects on subcellular enzyme systems from canine myocardium. J. Pharmacol. Exp. Ther. 171:1–12.

BLINKS, J. R., and KOCH-WESER, J. 1961. Analysis of the effects of changes in rate and rhythm upon myocardial contractility. J. Pharmacol. Exp. Ther. 134:373–389.

BUCKLEY, N. M., PENEFSKY, Z. J., and LITWALK, R. S. 1972. Comparative force-frequency relationships in human and other mammalian ventricular myocardium. Pfluegers Arch. 332:259–270.

ELLS, H. A. 1964. Inhibition of muscle cell membrane ATPase by quinidine. Proc. Soc. Exp. Biol. Med. 115:324–325.

HAJDU, S. 1953. Mechanism of staircase and contraction in ventricular muscle. Amer. J. Physiol. 174:371–380.

HARROW, J. A. C., and DHALLA, N. S. 1975. Subcellular and functional effects of quinidine, procainamide and lidocaine on rat myocardium. Can. J. Physiol. Pharmacol. 53:1058–1064.

HENDERSON, A. M., BRUTSAERT, B. L., PARMLEY, W. W., and SONNENBLICK, E. H. 1961. Myocardial mechanics in papillary muscles of rat and cat. Amer. J. Physiol. 217:1273–1279.

KATZUNG, B., RASIN, H., and SCHEIDER, F. 1957. Frequency-force relationship in the rabbit auricle and its modification by some metabolic inhibitors. J. Pharmacol. Exp. Ther. 120:324–333.

KIDWAI, A. M., RADCLIFFE, M. A., DUCHON, G., and DANIEL, E. E. 1971. Isolation of plasma membrane from cardiac muscle. Biophys. Res. Commun. 45:901–910.

KOCH-WESER, J., and BLINKS, J. R. 1963. Influence of the interval between beats on myocardial contractility. Pharmacol. Rev. 15:601–652.

LANGER, G. A. 1965. Calcium exchange in dog ventricular muscle: Relation to frequency of contraction and maintenance of contraction. Circ. Res. 17:78–89.

LEE, K. A., and YU, D. H. 1963. A study of the sodium and potassium-activated adenosine-triphosphatase activity of heart microsomal fraction. Biochem. Pharmacol. 12:1253–1264.

LENDRUM, B., FEINBERG, H., BOYD, E., and KATZ, L. N. 1960. Rhythm effects on contractility of the beating isovolumic left ventricle. Amer. J. Physiol. 199:1115–1120.

PRASAD, K. 1970. Influence of energy supply and calcium on the low sodium-induced changes in the transmembrane potential and contraction of guinea pig papillary muscle. Can. J. Physiol. Pharmacol. 48:241–253.

PRASAD, K. 1972. Transmembrane potential, contraction and ATPase activity of human heart in relation to ouabain. Jpn. Heart J. 13:59–72.

PRASAD, K. 1974. Membrane Na^+-K^+-ATPase and electromechanics of human heart. In N. S. Dhalla (ed.), Recent Advances in Studies on Cardiac Structure and Metabolism, Vol. 4: Myocardial Biology, pp. 91–105, University Park Press, Baltimore.

PRASAD, K. 1975. Glucagon-induced changes in the action potential, contraction, and Na^+-K^+-ATPase of cardiac muscle. Cardiovasc. Res. 9:355–365.

PRASAD, K., and CALLAGHAN, J. C. 1969. Effect of replacement of potassium by rubidium on the transmembrane action potential and contractility of human papillary muscle. Circ. Res. 24:157–166.

PRASAD, K., and KIDWAI, A. M. 1974. Frequency-dependent changes in contractility, action potential duration and membrane N^+-K^+-ATPase in cardiac muscle. Proc. Can. Fed. Biol. Soc. 17:16 (Abstract).

SKOU, J. C. 1965. Enzymatic basis for active transport of Na^+ and K^+ across cell membrane. Physiol. Rev. 45:596–617.

Mailing address:
K. Prasad, M.B.B.S. (Hons.), M.D., Ph.D., F.A.C.C.
Department of Physiology,
College of Medicine,
University of Saskatchewan,
Saskatoon, Saskatchewan (Canada).

Recent Advances in Studies on
Cardiac Structure and Metabolism, Volume 11
Heart Function and Metabolism
Edited by T. Kobayashi, T. Sano, and N. S. Dhalla
Copyright 1978   University Park Press   Baltimore

POSSIBLE MECHANISM OF RATE-DEPENDENT CHANGE OF CONTRACTION IN DOG VENTRICULAR MUSCLE: RELATION TO CALCIUM MOVEMENTS

Y. SAEKI and A. KAMIYAMA

Department of Physiology, Yokohama City University,
School of Medicine, Urafune-cho, Minami-ku, Yokohama, Japan

SUMMARY

The effects of stimulation interval (0.5–10 sec) on action potential and isometric contraction were studied in the right subepicardial muscle under various solutions in order to analyze the staircase phenomenon. In the normal Tyrode solution (control condition), the rate of second slow depolarization (RSD) after the initial rapid depolarization of action potential increased with the decrease of stimulation interval. However, in most preparations the strength of contraction first decreased to a low level, then increased as the stimulation interval was shortened progressively. In contrast, the RSD decreased with a decrease of stimulation interval in Tyrode solution containing 4 mg/liter of verapamil. Although no significant change in RSD was found at the stimulation interval of 10 sec, the second slow depolarization was completely abolished at stimulation intervals of 0.5 and 1 sec. The strength of contraction decreased with the decrease of RSD and disappeared at shorter stimulation intervals, over which the second slow depolarization was abolished. In Tyrode solution containing 0.06 mg/liter of ouabain, no significant change of action potential configuration was found at the early stages of the drug's effect (after 100 min). However, it was observed that the positive inotropic effect was increased as the stimulation interval was lengthened. The effect of verapamil on action potential in the ouabain-pretreated preparations was qualitatively similar to the effect on the normal (untreated) preparation. However, the effect on contraction was different in that a small but finite contraction was observed in spite of the abolition of the second slow depolarization of the action potential. These results suggest that the strength of contraction at higher contraction rates depends primarily on the calcium influx associated with the action potential, whereas at lower contraction rates the strength also depends on the electroneutral calcium influx, which seems to become greater under circumstances of inadequate metabolic support.

INTRODUCTION

In most mammalian cardiac muscles, it is well established that the strength of contraction varies with the interval between contractions (the staircase phenomenon) (Koch-Weser and Blinks, 1963). However, no clear relationship has been demonstrated between the external calcium as the source of intracellular free calcium ions and the interval-dependent change of contraction. Many investigators have proposed dual pathways of calcium ions across the surface membrane. There is electrogenic calcium influx associated with the depolarization of action potential (Matsubara and Matsuda, 1969; Beeler *et al.*, 1970) and electroneutral calcium influx coupled with sodium efflux (Na-Ca exchange) (Langer, 1973). The purpose of the present study is to identify each role of the dual calcium pathways in the strength of contraction/interval of contraction.

METHODS

Muscle strips were obtained from the epicardial surface of the canine right ventricle and cut to approximately 10–15 mm long, 4–5 mm wide, and 0.5–0.7 mm thick. One half of the strip was pinned onto a paraffin block by several stainless-steel pins, with the epicardial surface upwards. The other half of the strip was connected to the core of a mechano-electrical transducer. Using conventional techniques, action potential and isometric contraction were recorded simultaneously on an ink-writer and photographed from an oscilloscope. All measurements were made after a steady-state value of the contraction for a particular interval of stimulation (0.5–10 sec) had been reached.

RESULTS

Contractile responses of 17 preparations to the changes in stimulation interval showed different patterns. These patterns could be classified on a qualitative basis into the following three types:

1. In four muscles, the strength of contraction increased with a decrease in stimulation interval.
2. In two muscles, the strength of contraction decreased with a decrease in stimulation interval.
3. In eleven muscles, the strength of contraction first decreased with a decrease in stimulation interval from 10 to 1 sec, then increased, but with a further decrease to 0.5 sec. By contrast, RSD progressively increased with the decrease of stimulation interval in all preparations (Figure 1, *upper panel*).

After the administration of 4 mg/liter verapamil into the bath solution, the preparations stimulated at the interval of 1 sec showed a gradual decrease of contractile strength and a gradual decrease of RSD. These effects reached a steady state within 30 min, the strength of contraction decreasing to almost zero, and the second slow depolarization of action potential being abolished completely. However, the effect of verapamil on the contraction greatly depended on the rate of contraction. For example, at an interval of 10 sec the strength of contraction was not affected at all (Figure 1, *lower panel*). Under the influence of verapamil the relationship between the stimulation interval and the RSD was also reversed by verapamil from the control relationship (Figure 1).

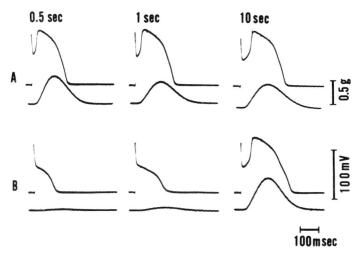

Figure 1. Action potentials and contractions at stimulation intervals 0.5, 1, and 10 sec. *Upper trace:* action potential. *Lower trace:* contraction. *A,* control. *B,* 30 min after administration of verapamil (4 mg/liter).

The administration of 0.06 mg/liter of ouabain produced positive inotropic effects at all the intervals. The relative increase of contractile strength was greater at longer intervals. The RSD showed only a slight and uniform decrease over all the intervals at the early stages of the drug's effect (after 100 min) (Figure 2B). In some experiments, effects of verapamil were studied on preparations pretreated with 0.06 mg/liter of ouabain. Verapamil showed an interval-dependent effect in these ouabain-pretreated preparations similar to that observed in the untreated preparation. However, the contractile strength was not altered at longer stimulation intervals and maintained a certain value at shorter stimulation intervals in spite of the disappearance of the second slow depolarization of action potential. Typical examples from these experiments are illustrated in Figure 2D.

DISCUSSION

It has been reported in several studies on cardiac muscles that calcium influx during membrane excitation contributes to the plateau component of action potential (Nidergerke and Orkand, 1966; Matsubara and Matsuda, 1969; Kamiyama and Saeki, 1974). Fleckenstein (1971) has found that verapamil selectively blocks the slow inward calcium current, but does not affect the initial fast inward sodium current. Therefore, the present results (Figure 1), indicating that verapamil clearly abolished the second slow depolarization of action potential and the contractile response at shorter stimulation intervals, can be interpreted

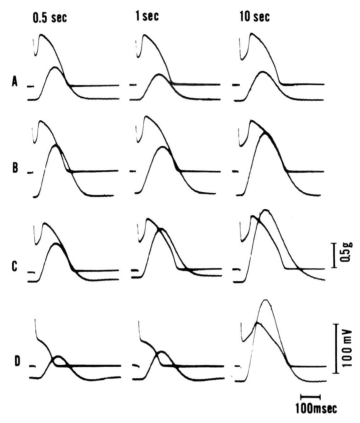

Figure 2. Action potentials and contractions at stimulation intervals 0.5, 1, and 10 sec. *Upper trace:* action potential. *Lower trace:* contraction. *A,* control. *B,* 100 min after, and *C,* 170 min after administration of ouabain (0.06 mg/liter). *D,* 30 min after addition of verapamil (4 mg/liter) to *C.*

to mean that the strength of contraction at higher contraction rates depends mainly on the calcium influx during depolarization of action potential.

Langer (1972) has explained the positive inotropic action of cardiac glycosides by their augmentatory effect on the Na-Ca exchange mechanism. This explanation is supported by the present evidence that ouabain increased the contractile strength of the preparation without significant changes in action potential at an early stage of the drug effect (after about 100 min). In the ouabain-pretreated muscles, verapamil affected the action potential in a way similar to its effect on the untreated muscles. However, the contractile strength was not altered at longer stimulation intervals and maintained a small but finite value at shorter stimulation intervals, in spite of the disappearance of the second slow depolarization of action potential.

Based on these findings, it is suggested that ouabain-induced positive ino-tropic action is caused by calcium influx through the electroneutral phe-nomenon, such as Na-Ca exchange. The fact that the positive inotropic effect of ouabain is greater at lower contraction rates suggests that ouabain increases calcium influx through the electroneutral phenomenon in proportion to the length of diastolic interval.

The mechanisms of rate-dependent action of verapamil that affect the plateau component of action potential still remain to be investigated using other methods, such as voltage-clamp techniques. However, in normal Tyrode solution RSD decreased with the increase in stimulation interval (monophasic pattern). On the other hand, the contractile strength-interval relationship showed various patterns (usually a biphasic pattern).

Accordingly, both calcium influx associated with action potential and the electroneutral calcium influx seem to contribute to the staircase phenomenon. It is suggested that the former is predominant at higher contraction rates, and that the latter becomes predominant at the lower contraction rates, in particular under circumstances of inadequate metabolic support.

REFERENCES

BEELER, G. W., JR., and REUTER, H. 1970. Membrane calcium current in ventricular myocardial fibres. J. Physiol. 207:191–209.

FLECKENSTEIN, A. 1971. Specific inhibitors and promoters of calcium action in the excitation-contraction coupling of heart muscle and their role in the prevention or production of myocardial lesions. In P. Harris and L. Opie (eds.), Calcium and the Heart, pp. 135–188. Academic Press, New York.

KAMIYAMA, A., and SAEKI, Y. 1974. Myocardial action potential of right- and left-subepicardial muscles in the canine ventricle and effects of manganese ions. Proc. Jap. Acad. 50:771–774.

KOCH-WESER, J., and BLINKS, J. R. 1963. The influence of the interval between beats on myocardial contractility. Pharmacol. Rev. 15:601–652.

LANGER, G. A. 1972. The effects of digitalis on myocardial ionic exchange. Circulation 46:180–187.

LANGER, G. A. 1973. Heart: Excitation-contraction coupling. Annu. Rev. Physiol. 35: 55–86.

MATSUBARA, I., and MATSUDA, K. 1969. Contribution of calcium current to the ventricular action potential of dog. Jpn. J. Physiol. 19:814–823.

NIDERGERKE, R., and ORKAND, R. K. 1966. The dual effect of calcium on the action potential of the frog's heart. J. Physiol. 184:291–311.

Mailing address:
Dr. Y. Saeki
Department of Physiology,
Yokohama City University, School of Medicine,
Urafune-cho, Minami-ku, Yokohama (Japan).

Recent Advances in Studies on
Cardiac Structure and Metabolism, Volume 11
Heart Function and Metabolism
Edited by T. Kobayashi, T. Sano, and N. S. Dhalla
Copyright 1978 University Park Press Baltimore

SODIUM-CALCIUM EXCHANGE
IN REGULATION OF CARDIAC CONTRACTION

M. HORACKOVA and G. VASSORT

Department of Physiology and Biophysics, Dalhousie University,
Halifax, Nova Scotia, Canada; and Laboratoire de Physiologie Comparée,
Université Paris XI, Centre d'Orsay, France

SUMMARY

The origin and possible regulatory mechanism of tonic tension (I_{Ca}-independent component of active contractile activity) were investigated in frog atrial muscle under voltage-clamp conditions. Replacement of NaCl by LiCl resulted in a fast decrease in tonic tension; a similar fast decrease of this contractile component was induced by Ca-free solution. When low Na Ringer's solution was applied, tonic tension increased transiently and then decreased to a steady amplitude; at return to normal Ringer's, a further, substantial decrease in tonic tension occurred before the original level was reached. Similar behavior of tonic tension was observed when both $[Na]_o$ and $[Ca]_o$ were lowered, but the ratio $[Ca]_o/[Na]_o^2$ remained constant; the transient changes were prevented by using low Ca and Na solutions and keeping the ratio of $[Ca]_o/[Na]_o^5$ constant. The significance of Na-Ca exchange in regulating tonic tension and the possibility that this exchange may be electrogenic are discussed.

INTRODUCTION

The mechanical activity in frog heart can be separated into two components: 1) the phasic component, which is directly related to the Ca inward current; and 2) the tonic component, which accounts for the contraction observed in the absence of Ca inward current and is therefore dependent on some other source of Ca ions. It has been shown (Vassort, 1973) that this tonic tension is regulated by membrane potential, is strongly dependent on the extracellular presence of Na ions, and could be modified by $[Na]_i$. However, the origin and regulative mechanism(s) involved in the development of this component of tension are not yet understood.

There is increasing evidence that the transport of Ca in various tissues involves a carrier-mediated transmembrane exchange of Na ions for Ca ions (reviewed by Blaustein, 1974). Glitsch, Reuter, and Scholz (1970) suggested that in cardiac muscle such a Na-Ca exchange transport mechanism could be

This study was supported by Medical Research Council, Canada, and DGRST, France.

important in determining the intracellular Ca concentration and thereby the contractility.

In this study we investigated the possible role of Na-Ca exchange mechanism in regulating tonic tension. Details of the experimental technique and composition of the Ringer's solutions were the same as those described previously (Horackova and Vassort, 1974).

RESULTS AND DISCUSSION

The mechanical activity was recorded under voltage clamp from frog (*Rana pipiens*) atrial bundles that were depolarized by pulses of 160 mV; at this membrane potential the contractile force consists mainly of tonic tension, since the Ca current and phasic tension are negligible (Vassort, 1973). Thus, effects of various changes in $[Na]_o$ and $[Ca]_o$ on this tension could be observed directly.

In the presence of veratrine, the tonic component of tension is increased severalfold consequent to an increase in $[Na]_i$ (Horackova and Vassort, 1974). Figure 1 shows that the application of Ca-free Ringer's solution abolished this tonic tension (i.e., the large positive inotropic effect) in 60 sec. Figure 1 also shows that when Na-free Ringer's was applied, the tonic tension decreased again very rapidly, while contracture developed. The return of Ca ions resulted in fast return of tonic tension; the return from Na-free Ringer's was slower, reflecting the return of $[Na]_i$ to its original level. Similar results were obtained in the absence of veratrine, tonic tension of the same amplitude being elicited by longer (400 msec) depolarizing pulses (unpublished data).

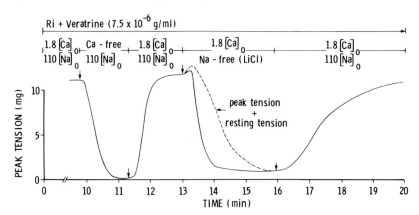

Figure 1. Effects of Ca- and Na-free (LiCl) Ringer's solution on peak tonic tension (*full line*) in the presence of veratrine. Mechanical responses were elicited by 160-mV and 100-msec depolarizing clamp pulses at a frequency of 15/min. (*Arrows* indicate time application of various Ringer's solutions; $[Na]_o$ and $[Ca]_o$ in control Ri are 110 mM and 1.8 mM, respectively. Application of Na-free Ringer's solution resulted in the development of contracture, represented by the difference between the *dotted line* and the *full line*.)

The short time needed to observe noticeable effects on tonic tension amplitude when removing the extracellular Ca or Na ions suggested regulatory importance of external sites, as would be expected with the Na-Ca exchange as the
regulating mechanism. This hypothesis was further supported by experiments in
low Na media. In these solutions, we anticipated the following behavior of Na-Ca
exchange (Na efflux linked to Ca influx), based essentially on the findings of
Baker *et al.* (1969): their results clearly indicated that the rate of Na efflux
linked to Ca influx is determined by $[Na]_o$, $[Na]_i$, and also by the transmembrane gradient for these ions. Thus, switching to low Na media would result in a
transient decrease of Na gradient, thereby facilitating Na efflux and Ca influx
(which should transiently increase tonic tension); with time, as $[Na]_i$ decreases
in low Na media, the rate of the exchange would decrease below the control
level also.

Figure 2 shows the result of such an experiment where $[Na]_o$ was lowered
to 30 mM. As expected, the peak amplitude of tonic tension transiently
increased and then decreased; by analogy, on return to normal Ringer's due to
transient large increase in Na gradient, the Na efflux is hindered, thereby
reducing Ca influx and resulting in a further substantial decrease of tonic tension
that precedes recovery to the initial amplitude (similar results were obtained in
the presence of veratrine (unpublished data)). Furthermore, Figure 2 shows
tonic tension, when the $[Ca]_o$ and $[Na]_o$ were decreased simultaneously, so
that the ratio of $[Ca]_o/[Na]_o^2$ was kept constant; the tonic tension again
increased transiently upon switching to low Na and low Ca solutions, and
transiently decreased (Figure 3) on return to normal Ringer's. This result

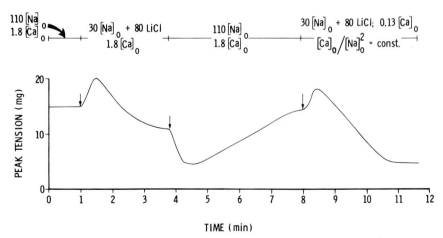

Figure 2. Peak tonic tension elicited by 400-msec and 160-mV depolarizing clamp pulses at
a frequency of 15/min. *Arrows* indicate the time of application of Ringer's solutions with
various $[Na]_o$ and $[Ca]_o$ (concentrations [mM] shown above the curve).

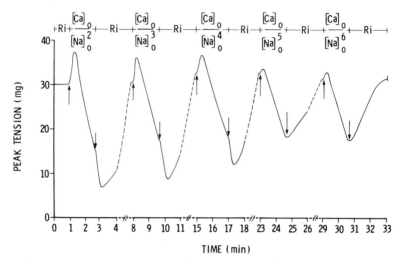

Figure 3. Peak tonic tension elicited by 400-msec and 160-mV depolarizing clamp pulses at a frequency of 15/min. *Arrows* indicate the time of application of normal Ringer's solution (Ri) and solutions with various constant ratios $[Ca]_0/[Na]_0^x$ (x = 2,3,4,5,6, respectively). In these Ringer's solutions the $[Ca]_0 = 10^{-2}$ mM (buffered with 4 mM EGTA) and $[Na]_0$ was (mM): 8.4, 19.4, 30.8, 39.9, 46.8 for x = 2 to 6, respectively. (LiCl was used as a replacement for NaCl.) These solutions were buffered with 25 mM Tris to pH 7.2 – 7.4.

suggests that the Na-Ca exchange is not electroneutral. If it were, i.e., exchanging 2 Na⁺ for 1 Ca²⁺, using low Na and Ca media and keeping $[Ca]_0/[Na]_0^2$ constant (according to the law of mass action), we should not observe any transient change in tension, because the decrease in Na gradient that facilitates Na extrusion would be compensated for by less tendency for Ca ions to enter the cell. Moreover, the competition of external Ca and Na ions for the carrier's binding sites should remain unchanged.

However, regardless of the decreased absolute values of $[Na]_0$ and $[Ca]_0$, application of such solutions with constant $[Ca]_0/[Na]_0^2$ always induced transient increase and/or decrease of tonic tension when these low Na and Ca solutions were introduced and replaced by normal Ringer's, respectively. Such transient changes of tonic tension were prevented when $[Na]_0$ was decreased less, i.e., using solutions with constant ratio $[Ca]_0/[Na]_0^5$ or $[Ca]_0/[Na]_0^6$, as is shown in Figure 3. Results similar to those in this experiment were obtained also with higher $[Ca]_0$ and $[Na]_0$ ($[Ca]_0$, 0.5 mM; $[Na]_0$, 58–78 mM) (unpublished data). In agreement with data of Baker *et al.* (1969) these results suggested that more than 2 (perhaps 4–5) exciting Na ions exchange for each Ca ion entering the cell; this, however, indicates electrogenicity of such Na-Ca exchange (i.e., net transfer of electrical charge across the membrane per each coupled transport).

Thus, our experiments indicated that tonic tension in frog myocardium and the positive inotropic effect of veratrine are regulated by a Na-Ca exchange mechanism (Na-dependent Ca influx); similarly, as proposed recently in squid axon by Mullins and Brinley (1975), this exchange may be electrogenic and thus influenced by the membrane potential. Moreover, during cardiac action potential at the plateau level, such an electrogenic pump would generate an outward current that could be one of the numerous currents involved in the repolarization process.

REFERENCES

BAKER, P. F., BLAUSTEIN, M. P., HODGKIN, A. L., and STEINHARDT, R. A. 1969. The influence of calcium on sodium efflux in squid axons. J. Physiol. (Lond.) 200:431–458.

BLAUSTEIN, M. P. 1974. The interrelationship between sodium and calcium fluxes across cell membranes. Rev. Physiol. Biochem. Pharmacol. 70:34–82.

GLITSCH, H. G., REUTER, H., and SCHOLZ, H. 1970. The effect of the internal sodium concentration on calcium fluxes in isolated guinea pig auricles. J. Physiol. (Lond.) 209:25–43.

HORACKOVA, M., and VASSORT, G. 1974. Excitation-contraction coupling in frog heart; effect of veratrine. Pfluegers Arch. 352:291–302.

MULLINS, L. J., and BRINLEY, F. J., JR. 1975. Sensitivity of calcium efflux from squid axons to changes in membrane potential. J. Gen. Physiol. 65:135–152.

VASSORT, G. 1973. Influence of sodium ions on the regulation of frog myocardial contractility. Pfluegers Arch. 339:225–240.

Mailing address:
Dr. M. Horackova,
Department of Physiology and Biophysics,
Faculty of Medicine,
Dalhousie University,
Halifax, B3H 4H7 Nova Scotia (Canada).

Recent Advances in Studies on
Cardiac Structure and Metabolism, Volume 11
Heart Function and Metabolism
Edited by T. Kobayashi, T. Sano, and N. S. Dhalla
Copyright 1978 University Park Press Baltimore

RELAXATION OF FROG MYOCARDIUM

G. VASSORT, M. J. ROULET, K. MONGO, and R. CLAPIER-VENTURA

Laboratoire de Physiologie Comparée,
Université Paris-Sud F-91405, Orsay, France

SUMMARY

Tension fall of frog heart contraction was analyzed under voltage-clamp conditions. It appears mostly exponential. The rate of relaxation depends upon the extracellular and intracellular Na concentrations. This suggests that the relaxation is under the control of Na-Ca exchange. The speeding up of relaxation by adrenaline in frog heart is revealed by low Na solution, while it is hidden by the primordial Na-Ca exchange in Ringer's solution.

INTRODUCTION

Very few studies were recently devoted to the mechanism of relaxation, while the origin of Ca ions involved in tension development is extensively analyzed, thanks to the voltage-clamp technique. It is demonstrated that the increase in the intracellular Ca concentration, $[Ca]_i$, partly results from the Ca current. To prevent Ca overloading, the Ca influx is shown to be compensated by a Ca-Na exchange mechanism that extrudes Ca ions as a consequence of a linked Na influx (Reuter and Seitz, 1968; Baker, 1972). However, tracer studies in mammalian heart (Jundt *et al.*, 1975) suggest that the Ca efflux is too slow to account for the relaxation of a contraction, although relaxation is slowed up in low Na solution.

METHOD

To further investigate the effects of Na ions in the relaxation process, experiments were performed on small trabeculae isolated from the frog (*Rana esculenta*) auricles. Under voltage-clamp conditions using the double sucrose-gap method (Vassort and Rougier, 1972), the tension fall (relaxation) of an elicited contraction is analyzed after the membrane is returned to the resting potential.

Supported by contract Délégation Générale à la Recherche Scientifique et Technique: 74. 7. 0275.

RESULTS AND DISCUSSION

In Ringer solution (mM: NaCl, 110; KCl, 2.4; CaCl$_2$, 1.8; NaHCO$_3$, 2.4) the relaxation, after a delay less than 200 msec, appears mostly exponential (Goto *et al.*, 1972; Vassort, 1973). Its time constant, determined by semi-logarithmic plot (Figure 1*A*) or by a mini-computer (Plurimat-S, Intertechnique), is 190 msec. This value differs markedly on different trabeculae—from 140 to 220 msec—but extreme values of 75 and 280 msec were also obtained. The relaxation rate was independent of the amplitude of contraction and of the amplitude and duration of the triggering depolarization, but was modified by the membrane potential, since relaxation is then mixed with tonic tension, thus requiring the use of a voltage-clamp technique.

The relaxation is markedly slowed up in Na-free solution. The time constant is about 10 times larger, reaching 2 sec (Figure 1*B*). Using intermediate Na concentrations in the external solution, intermediate values of time constant of relaxation were determined.

The noticeable effect of external Na ions suggests that these ions are involved in the relaxation process, possibly in relation to the Na-Ca exchange mechanism. The involvement of Na-Ca exchange is supported by demonstrating that an increase in [Na]$_i$, which is supposed to slow the Ca efflux, decreases the rate of relaxation.

Veratrine was shown to inhibit the Na-inactivation process, leading thus to a large entry of Na ions and to an increase in [Na]$_i$ (Horackova and Vassort, 1974). In the illustrated experiment (Figure 2), the [Na]$_o$ has been reduced to 30 mM, a Na concentration that slows the relaxation and facilitates the observation. After addition of veratrine (7.5 × 10^{-6} g/ml) the tension is enhanced and the time constant of relaxation increases from 300 msec to 420 msec (stimulation frequency 0.2 sec^{-1}).

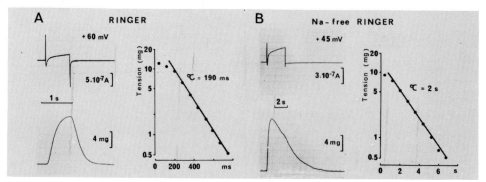

Figure 1. Original records of currents and tensions under voltage-clamp conditions and semilogarithmic plot of tension fall in Ringer solution (*A*) and in Na-free solution (*B*).

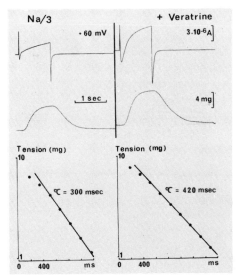

Figure 2. Decrease in relaxation rate of tension induced by veratrine (*middle traces*) and further evidence given by its semilogarithmic plot (*lower traces*). This decrease is consequent to an increase in [Na]$_i$ due to inhibition of inactivation of the Na current (*upper traces*) by the drug.

The involvement of the Na-Ca exchange in the relaxation process is further supported by the analysis of the transitory effects following application of different Na-containing solutions. The above observations were made at steady state after 2 to 3 min. However, this steady state is not reached in a monotonic way. When switching from Ringer's solution to a Na-poor solution (Na : 30 mEq) the time constant increases transitorily from 140 msec in Ringer's to 320 msec after one minute in low Na solution and then reaches a steady value at about 250 msec (Figure 3). Switching back to Ringer's solution, a transitory decrease in the time constant to 75 msec is observed. These results are better explained by assuming that, when switching to a low Na solution, the Na gradient is reduced and, correlatively, the Ca efflux; however, a low Na solution induces a decrease in [Na]$_i$, which thus partially restores the Na gradient and the Ca efflux. Similarly, on switching back to Ringer's solution, the Na gradient is then the largest and the time constant the smallest.

The primary involvement of Na-Ca exchange in the regulation of [Ca]$_i$ in frog heart in addition to intracellular Ca-binding and uptake is reinforced by the following result. Adrenaline is known to increase the contractile force in mammalian heart and simultaneously to accelerate the relaxation (Reiter, 1972). This increase in rate of relaxation is thought to be consequent upon an increased binding on the sarcoplasmic reticulum mediated by cAMP (Kirchberger *et al.,* 1974).

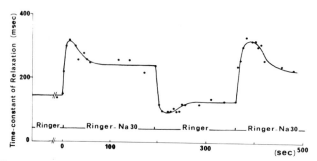

Figure 3. Time course of variation in the time constant of relaxation after a contraction induced by a given depolarization when switching from Ringer's solution to low-Na (30 mM) solution (and back).

Adrenaline enhances the contractile force in frog heart as well, but it does not significantly modify the relaxation rate in normal Na-containing solution. However, when decreasing $[Na]_o$, thus decreasing the Ca efflux consequent to the Na-Ca exchange, a marked effect of adrenaline is observed. The time constant of relaxation, which was 1.5 sec in Na-free solution, is decreased to 1.1 sec after addition of adrenaline (Figure 4). It can be said that, in normal solution, adrenaline is similarly effective in frog and mammalian heart in facilitating internal Ca binding; however, its effect is hindered in frog heart because most of the regulation of $[Ca]_i$ is controlled by the Ca-Na exchange mechanism.

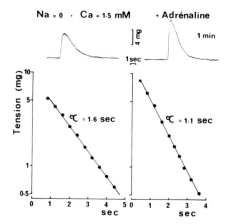

Figure 4. Increase in relaxation rate of tension induced by adrenaline (10^{-5} g/ml) in a Na-free solution.

CONCLUSION

In conclusion, the above results suggest that, in opposition to the time- and voltage-dependent Ca influx, a large Na-dependent Ca efflux occurs during each cardiac cycle, thus accounting for the immediate control of heartbeat by the external Na and Ca concentrations.

REFERENCES

BAKER, P. F. 1972. Transport and metabolism of calcium ions in nerve. Prog. Biophys. Mol. Biol. 24: 177–223.

GOTO, M., KIMOTO, Y., SAITO, M., and WADA, Y. 1972. Tension fall after contraction of bullfrog atria muscle examined with the voltage clamp technique. Jpn. J. Physiol. 22:637–650.

HORACKOVA, M., and VASSORT, G. 1974. Excitation-contraction coupling in frog heart. Effect of veratrine. Pfluegers Arch. 352:291–302.

JUNDT, H., PORZIG, H., REUTER, H., and STUCKI, J. W., 1975. The effects of substances releasing intracellular calcium ions on sodium-dependent calcium efflux from guinea-pig auricles. J. Physiol. (Lond.) 246:229–253.

KIRCHBERGER, M. A., TADA, M., REPKE, D. I., and KATZ, A. M. 1974. AMPc-dependent protein kinase catalyzed phosphorylation reaction and its reaction to calcium transport in cardiac S. R. J. Biol. Chem. 249:6166–6173.

REITER, M. 1972. Differences in the inotropic cardiac effects of noradrenaline and dihydro-ouabain. Naunyn Shmiedebergs Arch. Pharmacol. 275:243–250.

REUTER, H., and SEITZ, N. 1968. The dependence of calcium efflux from cardiac muscle on temperature and external ion composition. J. Physiol. (Lond.) 195:451–470.

VASSORT, G. 1973. Influence of sodium ions on the regulation of frog myocardial contractility. Pfluegers. Arch. 339:225–240.

VASSORT, G., and ROUGIER, O. 1972. Membrane potential and slow inward current dependence of frog cardiac mechanical activity. Pfluegers Arch. 331:191–203.

Mailing address:
Dr. G. Vassort,
Laboratoire Physiologie Comparée,
Université Paris-Sud,
F-91405 Orsay (France).

Recent Advances in Studies on
Cardiac Structure and Metabolism, Volume 11
Heart Function and Metabolism
Edited by T. Kobayashi, T. Sano, and N. S. Dhalla
Copyright 1978   University Park Press   Baltimore

DYNAMICS OF CONTRACTION
WITH SPECIAL REFERENCE TO CALCIUM

H. MASHIMA

Department of Physiology, School of Medicine,
Juntendo University, Tokyo, Japan

SUMMARY

Using a new method for tetanizing frog ventricle muscle, the tension-length, force-load-velocity, and load-extension relations were determined under the steady active state. On the basis of these experiments a mechanochemical model was developed. Time courses of internal calcium concentration, the rates of release, and uptake of calcium during isometric twitches were calculated by the model.

INTRODUCTION

Previous studies of the dynamics in cardiac muscles were difficult because of an inability to tetanize the muscle. During twitch it was hard to measure velocity under different loads at the same active state. Forman, Ford, and Sonnenblick (1972) described the method for tetanizing cat papillary muscle with repetitive electrical pulses at 12 Hz in the presence of 10 mM caffeine and 10 mM calcium. In the present study a new method for tetanizing frog ventricle muscle was developed and the fundamental mechanical properties under the steady active state were investigated.

METHODS

Material used was the muscle strip prepared from frog ventricle, about 10 mm in length and less than 1 mm in diameter. The muscle was mounted horizontally in a polystyrol bath that contained 10 ml of Ringer's solution. One end of the muscle was tied to an isometric lever and the other end to an isotonic one. The compliance of the apparatus was about 5 μm/g. A pair of platinum foil electrodes were placed on the opposite walls of the bath in parallel with the muscle. Thus, the muscle was stimulated transversely by the electric field between the electrodes. The solution was bubbled with a 5% CO_2 and 95% O_2 gas mixture and the temperature was maintained at $20°$ C. If necessary, a quick release apparatus or a velocity controller was attached to the isotonic lever. Tension and displacement were displayed on an ink-writing rectigraph or sometimes on a cathode-ray oscilloscope.

RESULTS AND DISCUSSION

Tetanic Contraction of the Cardiac Muscle

When the muscle was stimulated by alternating current (AC) from a high current stimulator, tetanic contraction was observed. As seen in Figure 1, the complete tetanus was obtained at 10 Hz within 3 sec but the tension decreased at more than 20 Hz. The tension increased with increasing field strength up to 17 V/cm, but it decreased at more than 20 V/cm. Repetitive square pulses also produced the same tetanic contraction at 10 Hz, 6 V/cm in field strength. The tetanic tension and its rate of rise increased with an increase in the external calcium concentration up to 9 mM, but little increase was observed at more than 10 mM. From these results, AC of 20 V/cm, 10 Hz for 5 sec was employed as the optimum stimulus in the solution containing 9 mM calcium. The maximum tetanic tension thus obtained was several times larger than the twitch tension. Upon repetition of the stimulus at 2-min intervals, the muscle generated exactly

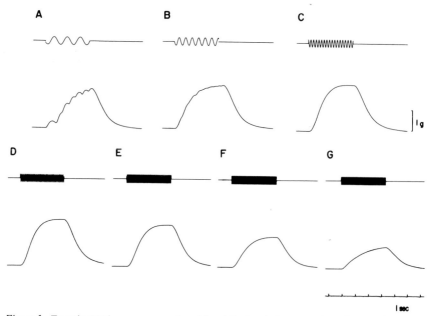

Figure 1. Tetanic tension curves produced by AC stimulation at various frequencies. Frog ventricle, 20°C, *upper:* stimulus; field strength, 20 V/cm; *lower:* tension, *A:* 1 Hz, *B:* 2 Hz, *C:* 5 Hz, *D:* 10 Hz, *E:* 20 Hz, *F:* 40 Hz, *G:* 80 Hz.

the same tensions many times. Moreover, in the potassium-rich solution, containing 8 mM potassium, various tetanic tensions less than the maximum tension were obtained by reducing the intensity of AC.

When 10^{-6} g/ml of adrenaline was added to the external solution, the twitch tension was markedly potentiated but the maximum tetanic tension was unchanged, although the rate of rise of tension increased.

Tension-Length Relation

The isometric tetanic tension of the frog cardiac muscle and also the peak twitch tension were measured at various muscle lengths. The results are shown in Figure 2. After the physiological measurement, the preparation was fixed at the length L_m, at which the maximum tension, F_m, was obtained, and examined with an electron microscope. Usually, L_m was about 2.0–2.2 μm in sarcomere length. The tension-length relation of cardiac muscle is similar to that of skeletal muscle. However, in the region at shorter lengths the force of cardiac muscle falls almost linearly. In addition, it was difficult to stretch the muscle beyond 130% L_m, because of the rupture of the preparation.

Force-Load-Velocity Relation

During the plateau of isometric tetanus, where the active state is steady, controlled quick release, described by Mashima *et al.* (1972), was made, and the shortening or lengthening velocity against the load was measured. The initial length was fixed at 0.9 L_m, where the resting tension was sufficiently small. The relation between the load, P, and the velocity, V, was determined at various isometric tetanic tensions, F_i (i = 1–5), as shown in Figure 3. Of course, F

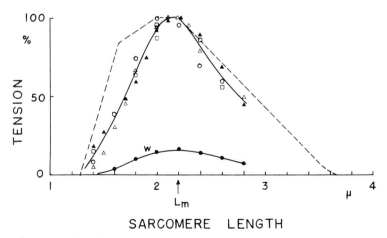

Figure 2. Tension-length curve for the tetanic contraction of the cardiac muscle. Frog ventricle, 20°C, *curve w:* peak twitch tension; *broken line:* skeletal muscle.

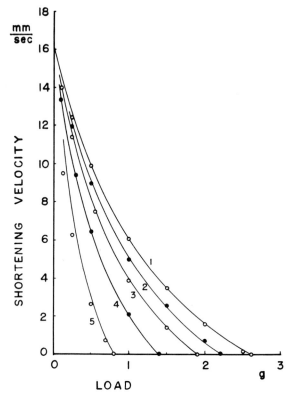

Figure 3. Load-velocity curves at various tetanic forces. Frog ventricle, 20° C, initial length: 10 mm (0.9 L_m).

represents the force of the contractile component under the isometric condition. Each relation can be described by a hyperbolic equation:

$$(P + a_i)(V + b_i) = b_i(F_i + a_i) \tag{1}$$

or

$$F_v = F_i - P = (F_i + a_i)\frac{V}{V + b_i} \tag{2}$$

where a_i and b_i are constants and F_v is the viscous-like force. All curves in Figure 3 were drawn by taking $a_i/F_i = a/F_m$ and $b_i = b$, as all curves converge to a common maximum velocity V_m, on the V-axis, where a and b are the dynamic constants at the maximum tension. The measured points fit well to these curves. Only at smaller load in curve 5 are measured points slightly below the curve, probably because the noncontractile structure in the preparation becomes effective as extra-load at such a small force. Therefore, Equation 2 can be generalized as follows:

$$F_v = F - P = F(1 + \frac{a}{F_m}) \frac{V}{V + b} \tag{3}$$

The average values of constants in 10 cases are $a/F_m = 0.62$, $b/L_m = 0.98$/sec, $F_m = 3$–5 g/mm^2, $V_m = 1.56$ L_m/sec at 20°C. It is apparent from Equation 3 that the viscous-like force is not only a function of the velocity but also a linear function of the force. This fact suggests that each crossbridge has proper force and viscosity, as described by Mashima et al. (1972) in the frog skeletal muscle.

When the load was larger than the force, the muscle was lengthened by the load. The relation between the load and the lengthening velocity was also expressed as follows:

$$F_v = P - F = F(1 + \frac{a'}{F_m}) \frac{V}{V + b} \tag{4}$$

where $a'/F_m = 0.40$, $b'/L_m = 0.98$/sec at 20° C. By changing the force by decreasing the external calcium concentration, it was confirmed that the load-velocity relations always satisfied these equations at 0.9 L_m.

However, when the muscle length decreased, measured load-velocity curves systematically deviated from calculated curves, as if some internal load or viscosity increased at shorter lengths. The internal load, P_{in}, defined as the difference between measured and calculated F_vs, increased almost linearly with increasing velocity and decreasing muscle length. Therefore, we obtain

$$P_{in} = V(-cL + d) \tag{5}$$

where c and d are constants. The nature of the internal load is not clear.

Load-Extension Relation of the Series Elastic Component

During the plateau of isometric tetanus, controlled quick release was made, and the small shortening immediately after the release was measured against the load. The initial length was fixed to 0.9 L_m. The load-extension curves of the series elastic component (SEC) under various isometric tensions are shown in Figure 4.

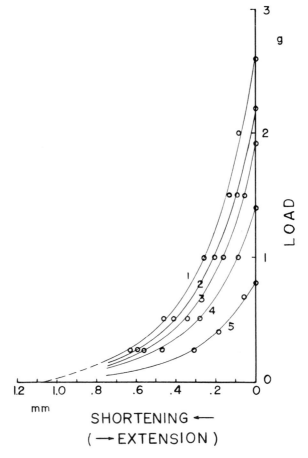

Figure 4. Load-extension curves of the series elastic component at various tetanic forces. Frog ventricle, 20° C, initial length: 10 mm (0.9 L_m).

The curves 2–5 were drawn by multiplying the ordinate of curve 1 by F_i/F_1 ($i =$ 2–5). Measured points fit well to these curves. Therefore, the following equation will be obtained,

$$P = \frac{F}{F_m} f(x) \qquad (6)$$

where x is the extension and P is the load. The fact that the tension of SEC for a given extension is proportional to the isometric force may suggest that the series elasticity resides mainly in the crossbridge. The function $f(x)$ cannot be described with a simple exponential equation; therefore, we approximated the tension with a third-power function of the extension for computer calculation.

Mechanochemical Model of the Cardiac Muscle

A mechanochemical model of the skeletal muscle described by Akazawa *et al.* (1976) was applied to the cardiac muscle. The model consists of three subsystems: 1) the regulatory mechanism of contraction by calcium ion, 2) the crossbridge cycle coupled with actin-myosin interaction, and 3) the dynamics of contraction.

Subsystem 1   The rate of increase in the number of active sites on the thin filament, N^*, is expressed by

$$N^* = \frac{dD([Ca])}{d[Ca]} [\dot{Ca}] L_p \tag{7}$$

$$[\dot{Ca}] = \dot{c}_r - \dot{c}_u \tag{8}$$

where $\dot{c}_r$ is the rate of release of calcium from the store; $\dot{c}_u$ is the rate of uptake to the store; time courses of both rates are assumed to be exponential; $D([Ca])$ is the density of active sites, which is a function of the internal calcium concentration, $[Ca]$; and L_p is the overlap length of thick and thin filaments, which is a constant during isometric contraction.

Subsystem 2   Five states are considered in the crossbridge cycle: that is, state R is the resting state, state 1 the activation phase by calcium ion, state 2 the force-generating phase on attaching to the thin filament, state 3 the sliding phase, and state 4 the detachment phase of the crossbridge. When the site is activated by calcium ions, the state changes immediately from state R to 1, and then cyclic reactions of $1 \rightarrow 2 \rightarrow 3 \rightarrow 4 \rightarrow 1$ continue. If the calcium concentration decreases below the threshold, state 4 turns back to state R. It was assumed that the rate constant from state 2 to 3 is proportional to the sliding velocity.

Subsystem 3   The dynamic properties of cardiac muscle are described above.

All parameters of this model were determined from the results of experiments or by computer simulation. Using the identical parameters, the tension curves of isometric twitches under various conditions were calculated by giving $\dot{c}_r$ and $\dot{c}_u$ as inputs. One of the results is shown in Figure 5. The time constants of $\dot{c}_r$ and $\dot{c}_u$ were selected so as to obtain best fit for the calculated tension curve to the experimental one. Consequently, $\dot{c}_r$, $\dot{c}_u$, and $[Ca]$ curves during the control and potentiated twitches were determined as seen in Figure 5.

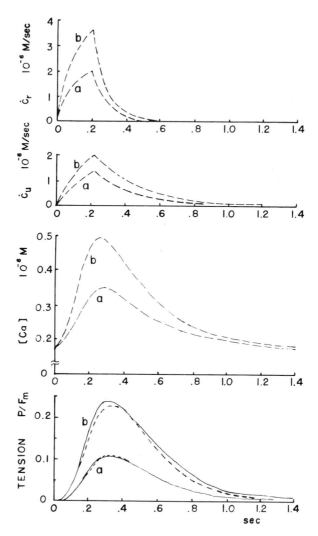

Figure 5. Time courses of $\dot{c}_r$, $\dot{c}_u$, $[Ca]$ and tension during isometric twitch. *Solid line:* experimental tension curve of the frog ventricle, 20° C; *a:* control; *b:* potentiated by 1 × 10^{-6} g/ml adrenaline; *broken lines:* calculated by the model.

REFERENCES

AKAZAWA, K., YAMAMOTO, M., FUJII, K., and MASHIMA, H. 1976. A mechanochemi-cal model for the steady and transient contractions of the skeletal muscle. Jpn. J. Physiol. 26:9–28.

FORMAN, R., FORD, L. E., and SONNENBLICK, E. H. 1972. Effect of muscle length on the force-velocity relationship of tetanized cardiac muscle. Circ. Res. 31:195–206.

MASHIMA, H., AKAZAWA, K., KUSHIMA, H., and FUJII, K. 1972. The force-load-velocity relation and the viscous-like force in the frog skeletal muscle. Jpn. J. Physiol. 22:103–120.

Mailing address:
Dr. H. Mashima,
Professor of Physiology,
Department of Physiology, School of Medicine,
Juntendo University, Bunkyo-ku Hongo 2-1-1,
Tokyo (Japan).

Recent Advances in Studies on
Cardiac Structure and Metabolism, Volume 11
Heart Function and Metabolism
Edited by T. Kobayashi, T. Sano, and N. S. Dhalla
Copyright 1978   University Park Press   Baltimore

ISOMETRIC DYNAMIC RESPONSE OF MAMMALIAN HEART MUSCLE DUE TO STEP CHANGES IN THE CALCIUM CONCENTRATION OF THE PERFUSING MEDIUM

M. O. TOLL

Department of Physiology, University College London,
London, England

SUMMARY

The isometric tension transient response of isolated kitten papillary muscle was found to exhibit direction-dependent dynamics when subjected to step changes in the calcium concentration of the bathing medium. The tension transient curves could be resolved into a minimum of two to three exponential components, which could be considered to indicate different calcium compounds or compartments within the muscle. However, a model relating calcium diffusion across the muscle to the dose-response curve indicates that the exponential components of the tension transient curves are due to the properties of calcium diffusion through the extracellular space, and that the direction-dependent dynamics are caused by the nonlinearity of the dose-response curve.

INTRODUCTION

It is an established fact that the extracellular calcium concentration $[Ca^{2+}]_o$ can modulate myocardial contractility (e.g., Ringer, 1883). It has also been shown that calcium moves across the sarcolemma during the plateau phase of the action potential and that the magnitude of this calcium current is dependent upon $[Ca^{2+}]_o$ (Wood, Heppner, and Weidmann, 1969; Beeler and Reuter, 1970a,b). Using skinned cardiac cells, Fabiato and Fabiato (1975) have shown that the activation of the myofilaments is directly dependent upon the free intracellular calcium concentration $[Ca^{2+}]_i$.

Unlike skeletal muscle, cardiac muscle requires extracellular calcium for tension development. Thus, in cardiac muscle there appears to be a movement of Ca^{2+} from the extracellular space across the membrane into the intracellular

This work was supported in part by an Athlone Fellowship provided by the Department of Trade and Industry (U. K.), by a Canadian Heart Foundation Fellowship, and by the British Heart Foundation in the form of an operating grant to Dr. B. R. Jewell of University College London.

space and back into the extracellular space. In addition, internal stores of Ca^{2+} are released from the sarcoplasmic reticulum (SR) to assist in tension development (Fabiato and Fabiato, 1975). However, the exact kinetics of these cellular calcium movements are unknown.

METHODS

Papillary muscles (mean diameter ± S.D.; 0.7 ± 0.1 mm, $n = 9$) from the right ventricles of kittens anesthetized with chloroform were dissected and stabilized in the muscle apparatus using the procedure described by Jewell and Rovell (1973). The muscles were mounted in a vertical isometric muscle apparatus and a superfusion system was used for muscle perfusion (Toll and Jewell, 1975). With this superfusion system the speed of switching between any two solutions of different calcium concentration was on the order of 10 msec.

For these experiments the isolated kitten papillary muscles were stimulated using platinum punctate electrodes (Blinks, 1965) at a rate of 20 min^{-1} and were maintained at a temperature of 30 ± 0.1° C. The muscles were then subjected to step changes in the calcium concentration of the perfusate $[Ca^{2+}]_p$ over the range of 0.5–4.5 mM. The resulting isometric tension transient curves were measured in real time and on a beat-to-beat basis using a LINC-8 computer (Jewell and Toll, 1972).

RESULTS

When the muscles were subjected to step changes in the $[Ca^{2+}]_p$ the isometric tension transient responses exhibited different dynamics depending upon whether the $[Ca^{2+}]_p$ was increased or decreased (Figure 1). This difference in dynamics has been called "direction-dependent dynamics."

An analysis of the peak isometric tension transient curves indicated that these curves could be resolved into a minimum of two to three exponential components. These components could then be related to the cellular compartments, as proposed by Langer (1971), or they could be considered different cardiac calcium compounds, as postulated by Chapman and Niedergerke (1970).

Steady-state dose-response curves of peak isometric tension (P_{max}) as a function of $[Ca^{2+}]_o$ were found to be highly nonlinear (Figure 2), and within the region studies ($[Ca^{2+}]_o = 0.5$–4.5 mM) they could be fitted by an exponential equation of the form:

$$P_{max} = A_{sat} - B \exp(-[Ca^{2+}]_o/T_c) \tag{1}$$

where P_{max} is the peak isometric tension (mN–mm^{-2}), A_{sat} is the saturation value of P_{max} (mN–mm^{-2}), B is a coefficient (mN–mm^{-2}), $[Ca^{2+}]_o$ is the

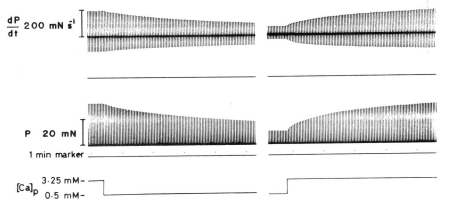

Figure 1. The isometric tension response, *P,* of a kitten papillary muscle subjected to step changes in the external calcium concentration [Ca]$_p$. Note the direction-dependent dynamics for a step decrease and a step increase in the calcium concentration. The separation between records represents a time interval of 12 min. This muscle was at a temperature of 30° C and was stimulated at a rate of 20 min^{-1}. Equivalent muscle diameter = 1.0 mm.

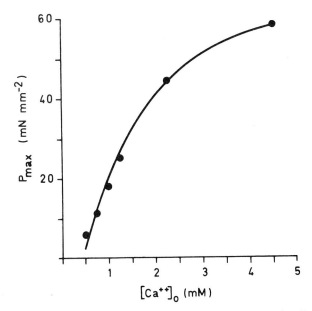

Figure 2. The steady-state dose-response curve of peak isometric tension P_{max} versus the extracellular calcium concentration $[Ca^{2+}]_o$ for a single muscle. The continuous curve represents the exponential curve that best fits the experimental data. Rate of muscle stimulation, 20 min^{-1}; temperature, 30 ± 0.1° C; equivalent diameter, 0.76 mm.

calcium concentration in the extracellular space (mM), and T_c is a "calcium constant" (mM).

DISCUSSION

Papillary Muscle Model

Since isolated papillary muscle preparations were used, diffusion must be regarded as the main mechanism by which calcium can enter or leave the extracellular space from the surface of the muscle. The complexity of the extracellular space may then be expected to influence the diffusion of the calcium ions through this space (Page, 1962).

In order to develop the diffusion model, two simplifying assumptions must be made. The first assumption is that the muscle is cylindrical in shape with an equivalent diameter, D (mm), computed from $2 (M/\pi L_{max})^{0.5}$, where M is the muscle mass (mg) and L_{max} is the optimum length (mm) of the muscle. The second assumption is that the muscle is homogeneous.

Clearly, this latter assumption is not true, but it is necessary if one is to use the diffusion equations of Hill (1928) to describe diffusion through a homogeneous cylinder of tissue.

Hill (1928) showed that diffusion through a homogeneous cylinder of tissue could be described by two equations. One equation described the concentration at any radius through the muscle as a function of time after a step change in concentration had been applied to the surface of the tissue. The other equation described the average concentration throughout the cylinder as a function of time only.

Both equations consisted of an infinite sum of exponential terms, with the time constants a function of the radius of the cylinder and the diffusion constant of the substance under consideration.

Based on these two equations, a computer program was developed to calculate the average calcium concentration as well as the instantaneous concentration distribution throughout the muscle, both as a function of time. These calcium concentration values were then related to the experimentally derived dose-response curves to simulate the peak isometric tension transient curves.

Diffusion Model Evaluation

Implementation of the average concentration equation is quite straightforward, as there is only one independent variable, time. However, the equation describing the concentration distribution throughout the muscle cross-section is more complex because it has two independent variables, time and distance. This added complexity required that the muscle be divided into a number of concentric shells (10) in order to calculate the concentrations at the boundaries of these shells.

In testing the muscle model, the two diffusion equations were used in conjunction with linear and nonlinear dose-response curves, which were coincident at $[Ca^{2+}]_o = 0.5$ and 4.5 mM. Theoretical tension transient curves were then computed for both a step increase and a step decrease in calcium concentration at the surface of the muscle.

Figure 3a shows that, with a linear dose-response curve, the use of both diffusion equations gives identical tension transient curves, both for a step increase and a step decrease in calcium concentration. Furthermore, both sets of curves have identical time constants.

However, when the linear dose-response curve was replaced by the nonlinear curve and the calculations repeated, the transient curves were significantly altered (Figure 3b). The most notable change was the appearance of direction-dependent dynamics. In addition, the transient curves differed when the average concentration equation and the shell equation were used. Analysis also showed that 10 shells were sufficient for transient curve calculations.

The reason that a nonlinear dose-response curve causes direction-dependent dynamics can be better appreciated from Figure 4. In this figure, the time course of calcium concentration, when the external level is switched from A to B, is assumed to be identical to that when the concentration is switched from C to D, i.e., the fractional or percentage change in concentration at any time is identical in the two directions.

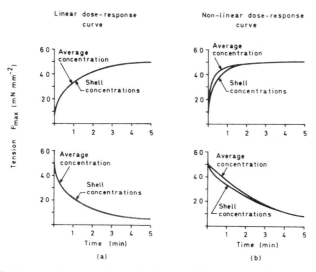

Figure 3. Theoretical tension transients based on linear and nonlinear dose-response curves and on calculations of extracellular calcium concentrations using the average concentration equation and the shell method of analysis. Concentration changes are between 0.5 and 4.5 mM.

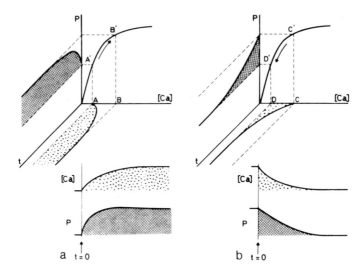

Figure 4. A schematic representation of the influence of a nonlinear dose-response curve on tension transients. See text for a detailed discussion of this figure.

It can be seen (Figure 4*a*) that initially an increase in concentration from A to B causes a rapid climb up the dose-response curve as the tension moves from A′ to B′. This is because the slope of the dose-response curve is quite steep at A′. If the concentration is returned to its original level, after tension equilibrium has been reached, the tension does not decrease as rapidly as it moves from C′ to D′ (Figure 4*b*). This is because the slope of the dose-response curve at C′ is not as steep as it is at D′.

Thus, the amount by which the dynamics differ is governed by the degree of nonlinearity present in the dose-response curve over the region of interest. For a linear curve, there is no difference in dynamics (Figure 3*a*), but for a nonlinear curve there can be a marked difference (Figure 3*b*).

Comparison of Theoretical and Experimental Step Responses

Using experimentally derived dose-response curves and the theoretical considerations presented earlier, step-responses were computed for a number of muscles. These predicted transient curves were then compared with the experimentally measured curves under the same conditions (Figure 5).

In the process of matching these curves, the value of the diffusion constant, k, was varied until a reasonable, by eye, fit was achieved. This was because the rate at which a substance diffuses through the extracellular space is taken to be about one-quarter the free solution value, and is not known exactly (see Conclusion). For the transient curves analyzed, the average value of k was found to be $1.5\ (\pm 0.3) \times 10^{-6}\ cm^2\ sec^{-1}$ (S.D. of 10 measurements).

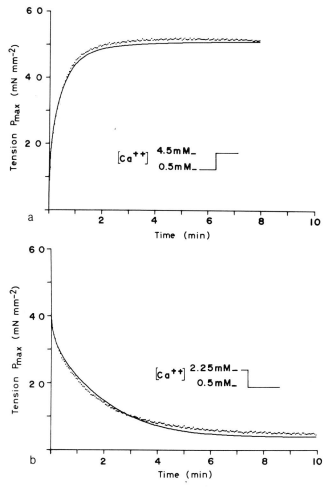

Figure 5. Comparisons between the theoretical peak isometric tension transients (*continuous curve*) and the experimental data (*individual points*). The calcium concentration was varied from 0.5 – 4.5 mM in Figure 5a and from 2.25 – 0.5 mM in 5b. The muscle was at 30° C and was stimulated at a rate of 20 min[-1]. Equivalent muscle diameter was 0.6 mm.

CONCLUSION

If diffusion dominates the step response of isolated papillary muscles, as has been postulated, then a number of important observations can be made.

For a change in $[Ca^{2+}]_p$ at the surface of the isolated muscle to influence the tension produced by the individual cells within the muscle, the Ca^{2+} must first diffuse through the extracellular space, and only at equilibrium does $[Ca^{2+}]_o = [Ca^{2+}]_p$ throughout the muscle.

For isolated kitten papillary muscles the rate of diffusion for calcium in the extracellular space was found to be about one-fifth the free solution value of 7.78×10^{-6} cm^2 sec^{-1} (Wang, 1954). This reduction is attributed to the obstruction of cells, and to the tortuosity of the pathway that a substance diffusing through the extracellular space must follow. Similar results have been reported for sodium diffusing through the extracellular space of frog skeletal muscle. Here, however, the diffusion constant was found to be reduced to about one-quarter the free solution value (Harris and Burn, 1949; Johnson, 1955).

The diffusion equations indicate that, for a step change in concentration at the surface of a cylindrical muscle, the concentration across the muscle can be described by an infinite sum of exponential terms. The time constants for these terms are a function of the diffusion constant for the substance under consideration and the square of the radius of the muscle.

If the peak isometric tension is considered as a measure of $[Ca^{2+}]_o$, the resulting tension transient curves will also be exponential in shape and will have time constants that are a measure of the diffusion process only. In addition, these time constants can be severely distorted if the step change in concentration takes place over the nonlinear region of the dose-response curve (Figures 3 and 4).

Studying calcium kinetics in isolated kitten papillary muscle preparations suggests that the diffusion of calcium through the extracellular space is the rate-limiting process. This masks the intracellular calcium movements and makes the identification of the cellular kinetics extremely difficult.

Acknowledgment Sincerest appreciation is expressed to Dr. B. R. Jewell for his guidance in the conduct of this work.

REFERENCES

BEELER, G. W., and REUTER, H. 1970a. Membrane calcium current in ventricular myocardial fibres. J. Physiol. 207:191–209.

BEELER, G. W., and REUTER, H. 1970b. The relation between membrane potential, membrane currents and activation of contraction in ventricular myocardial fibres. J. Physiol. 207:211–229.

BLINKS, J. R. 1964. Convenient apparatus for recording contractions of isolated heart muscle. J. Appl. Physiol. 20:755–757.

CHAPMAN, R. A., and NIEDERGERKE, R. 1970. Effects of calcium on the contraction of the hypodynamic frog heart. J. Physiol. 211:389–421.

FABIATO, A., and FABIATO, F. 1975. Contractions induced by a calcium-triggered release of calcium from the sarcoplasmic reticulum of single skinned cardiac cells. J. Physiol. 249:469–495.

HARRIS, E. J., and BURN, G. P. 1949. The transfer of Na and K between muscle and the surrounding medium. Trans. Faraday Soc. 45:508–528.

HILL, A. V. 1928. The diffusion of oxygen and lactic acid through tissues. Proc. Royal Soc. [B] 104:39–96.

JEWELL, B. R., and ROVELL, J. M. 1973. Influence of previous mechanical events on the contractility of isolated cat papillary muscle. J. Physiol. 235:715–740.

JEWELL, B. R., and TOLL, M. O. 1972. Use of an on-line computer in experiments on cardiac muscle. J. Physiol. 224:17–18.

JOHNSON, J. A. 1955. Kinetics of release of radioactive sodium, sulfate and sucrose from the frog sartorius muscle. Amer. J. Physiol. 181:263–268.

LANGER, G. A. 1971. Coupling calcium in mammalian ventricle: its source and factors regulating its quantity. Cardiovasc. Res. (Suppl.) I:73–75.

PAGE, E. 1962. Cat heart muscle in vitro. III. The extracellular space. J. Gen. Physiol. 46:201–213.

RINGER, S. 1883. A further contribution regarding the influence of the different constituents of the blood on the contraction of the heart. J. Physiol. 4:29–42.

TOLL, M. O., and JEWELL, B. R. 1975. A rapid-switching superfusion system for the study of drug action on isolated tissues. Med. Biol. Eng. 13:654–661.

WANG, J. H. 1953. Tracer diffusion in liquids. IV. Self diffusion of calcium ion and chloride ion in aqueous calcium chloride solutions. J. Amer. Chem. Soc. 75:1769–1772.

WOOD, E. H., HEPPNER, R. L., and WEIDMANN, S. 1969. Inotropic effects of electrical currents. Circ. Res. 24:409–445.

Mailing address:
M. O. Toll,
Faculty of Engineering,
Memorial University of Newfoundland,
St. John's, Newfoundland (Canada).

Recent Advances in Studies on
Cardiac Structure and Metabolism, Volume 11
Heart Function and Metabolism
Edited by T. Kobayashi, T. Sano, and N. S. Dhalla
Copyright 1978   University Park Press   Baltimore

CONTRACTION DURATION AND DIASTOLIC STIFFNESS IN AGED CANINE LEFT VENTRICLE

G. H. TEMPLETON, J. T. WILLERSON, M. R. PLATT, and M. WEISFELDT

Departments of Physiology, Medicine, and Surgery at the University
of Texas Health Science Center, Dallas, Texas, USA; and Department
of Medicine at The Johns Hopkins University, Baltimore, Maryland, USA

SUMMARY

The data obtained from groups of young and old beagles demonstrate that senescent beagle hearts are characterized by lower contractile function as measured by developed pressure and maximal rate of pressure change with time, by longer contraction duration, and by increased dynamic stiffness per given pressure as measured by the sinusoidal forcing technique.

INTRODUCTION

Old age is characterized by a diminished myocardial ability to respond to stress (Lakatta *et al.,* 1975a). In an attempt to explain this relative myocardial weakness, questions have been posed as to whether aging results in structural, hemodynamic, or stiffness alterations in the heart, independent of the presence of coronary artery disease. Some investigators have found age-related changes in myocardial stiffness while others have not (Weisfeldt, Loever, and Shock, 1971; Korecky, Bernath, and Rosengarten, 1974), but the physiological relevance of these previous studies and the preciseness of their techniques have been subjects of controversy. Accordingly, we have performed a study in an inbred group of young and old beagles, using a sinusoidal forcing technique capable of sensitively measuring ventricular stiffness (Templeton, Ecker, and Mitchell, 1972; Templeton *et al.,* 1974) to try to determine whether changes in ventricular stiffness (the reciprocal of compliance) develop as a consequence of aging in this model.

Supported by Contract NO1-AG-4-2813, National Gerontology Institute, and Ischemic Heart Disease Specialized Center of Research SCOR Grant HL 17669, National Heart and Lung Institute. Dr. Willerson is an Established Investigator of the American Heart Association.

MATERIALS AND METHODS

The surgical procedure and the sinusoidal forcing technique we used for measuring ventricular stiffness have been described in detail previously (Templeton *et al.*, 1972, 1974). In the present study young ($n = 8$) and old ($n = 7$) beagle dogs were anesthetized with sodium pentobarbital and a midline thoracotomy was performed. The young beagles had a mean age of 27 ± 2.5 months; the old ones were 128 ± 20.5 months. The vena cavae were cannulated and the venous blood directed to extracorporeal circuitry consisted of an oxygenator, heart exchanger, and a pump. The warmed, oxygenated blood was returned to the carotid arteries of the animal to perfuse the coronary and systemic circulations. Heart block was obtained by ligating the bundle of His in the atrial septum and the heart was paced at 120 beats per min by electrodes implanted in the left ventricle. An isovolumic left ventricle was prepared by placing teflon buttons in the inflow and outflow tracts of the ventricle and by inserting a balloon on the end of a metal cannula into the ventricular cavity through a stab incision in the apical dimple. Once inserted, the balloon was filled with saline until a diastolic pressure of approximately 5 mm Hg and a developed pressure of approximately 100–120 mm Hg were obtained. At this time the balloon filled the ventricular cavity, with the exception of Thebesian venous blood in the space between the balloon and endocardium. Thebesian blood was not allowed to accumulate, but was drained continuously through perforations in the mitral button and around the stab incision.

To measure ventricular stiffness, a piston at the distal end of the stainless steel cannula was driven sinusoidally at 20 Hz to induce a peak volume change of 0.5 cc within the ventricular cavity. The resulting sinusoidal component of ventricular pressure was measured with a high fidelity pressure transducer. Ventricular stiffness, defined as the ratio of a change in pressure to a change in volume, could then be calculated from the peak values of the sinusoidal pressures and volume waveforms.

During the experiments the pacing artifacts, the left ventricular pressure, and the sinusoidal volume displacement were recorded on analog tape and later processed by computer (Tektronix Processing Oscilloscope, Model WP1210). Successive pressure and volume waveforms from 16 cardiac cycles were averaged together to remove nonperiodic noise. Fourier analysis was used to separate the sinusoidal component of ventricular pressure from the total waveform. The maximal values of the sinusoidal pressure and volume waveforms were then used to calculate ventricular stiffness throughout the cardiac cycle.

Previous experience in our laboratory has shown that ventricular stiffness is linearly related to pressure during the entire contraction cycle. This same linear relationship between stiffness and pressure was found in the beagles under all the experimental conditions employed; the Pearson's *r* for the relationships was always above 0.9. The existence of a linear relationship between stiffness and pressure for both groups of beagles permitted a comparison of their stiffness by using the slopes and intercepts of the relationships.

At the beginning of each experiment, a diastolic pressure volume relationship was established by a stepwise infusion of saline into the ventricular balloon. The ventricular volume of the apex of the pressure volume curve was determined, and this was the volume used during the data collection period. The difference in this diastolic volume and the associated diastolic pressure was not significantly different between the two groups of beagles. Each animal was paced at 120 beats per min and the systemic arterial pressure was set at 80 mm Hg by the extracorporeal pump rate. With the application of the sinusoidal forcing function and after the animals stabilized, ventricular pressure and volume data were recorded on analog tape. In the old beagles, norepinephrine was infused at the rate of 0.8 μg/kg/min to raise their peak left ventricular pressure.

RESULTS

The source for the beagles was Laboratory Research Enterprises (Kalamazoo, Michigan). Their medical histories were studied and all beagles were in perfect health.

To ensure against the possibility that any differences observed between the two groups of animals did not result from size differences, the size and body weights were determined for the young and senescent groups. Heart mass was 111 ± 3.8 (S.E.M.) g and 90 ± 5.6 g, and the ratios of heart mass to body weight were 10.6 ± 0.12 and 8.4 ± 0.73 g/kg for the young and old groups, respectively. Further, the hearts were studied at the volume present at the knee of the diastolic pressure volume curve. These diastolic volumes were 14 ± 1.2 cc and 15 ± 1.2 cc for the young and old groups, and the corresponding pressures were 6 ± 0.9 mm Hg and 8 ± 1.3 mm Hg; these differences are also not statistically significant.

The ventricular hemodynamic data obtained from the beagles are shown in Table 1 and include left ventricular end diastolic pressure, peak developed pressure, contraction duration, and the slope and intercept of the linear stiffness pressure relationships. These data were collected during the application of the sinusoidal forcing function to the left ventricle. The left ventricular end diastolic pressures were not different for the two groups, but the maximal developed pressure of the left ventricle was significantly lower in the old beagles, indicating a lower level of cardiac function in this group. Furthermore, the older beagles were characterized by a longer contraction duration, even though the developed left ventricular pressure was reduced. Contraction duration is defined as the time from the rise of left ventricular pressure above its end diastolic value to its fall during relaxation to one-half of its maximal value. Ventricular stiffness measured

Table 1. Influence of aging on ventricular parameters*

Parameter	Young beagles (27 ± 2.5 months) $n = 8$	Old beagles (128 ± 20.5 months) $n = 7$
End diastolic pressure (mm Hg)	3.8 ± 0.20	3.1 ± 0.54
Peak pressure (mm Hg)	124 ± 6.6	78 ± 8.4[a]
Contraction duration (msec)	256 ± 3.1	341 ± 12.4[b]
Slope of stiffness-pressure relationship (ml)$^{-1}$	0.086 ± 0.0059	0.106 ± 0.0093[a]
Intercept of stiffness-pressure relationship (mmg Hg/ml)	1.31 ± 0.763	4.75 ± 0.647[b]

*Data are presented as mean values ±S.E.M. Superscripts in the second column note significant differences between young and old groups as determined by Student's t-test for group comparisons: [a] $p < 0.01$; [b] $p < 0.001$.

with the sinusoidal forcing technique was higher for any given left ventricular pressure in the older beagles during all phases of the contraction cycle. As shown in Table 1, the slope and intercept of the linear stiffness pressure relationships were significantly higher in the older group of dogs.

DISCUSSION

The results of our study indicate that left ventricular function is impaired in older beagles, as indicated by significantly lower developed pressure in the left ventricles, a prolonged contraction duration, and by an increase in ventricular stiffness during diastole and systole. The prolonged contraction duration agrees with a previous investigation (Lakatta *et al.*, 1975b).

Previous studies of ventricular diastolic stiffness in young and old rats have led to contradictory conclusions. Weisfeldt and his associates (Weisfeldt *et al.*, 1971) found resting tension to be elevated at L_{max} in their older group (27 months) as compared to their young group (12 months), while Korecky and his co-workers (Korecky *et al.*, 1974) found no difference in the stiffness of anoxically arrested rat hearts divided into age groups of 1, 7, and 12 months.

It is interesting that Weisfeldt's data suggested that there was greater viscosity in the heart muscle from senescent rats. Our stiffness parameter contains a viscous component, which could have been responsible for the observed stiffness increase in the hearts of the older beagles. Further, the increase in contraction duration in the senescent beagles in our present study could have occurred because of an increase in the viscous component of stiffness.

There may be species differences and age extremes that will determine whether changes in ventricular stiffness are found as a consequence of age, but the data obtained in the present study demonstrate that aging is associated with increased ventricular stiffness and decreased developed left ventricular pressure in beagle hearts.

REFERENCES

KORECKY, B., BERNATH, P., and ROSENGARTEN, M. 1974. Effect of age on the passive stress-strain relationship of the rat heart. Fed. Proc. 33:321. (Abstr.)

LAKATTA, E. G., GERSTENBLITH, G., ANGELL, C. S., SHOCK, N. W., and WEIS-FELDT, M. L. 1975a. Diminished inotropic response of aged myocardium to catecholamines. Circ. Res. 36:262–269.

LAKATTA, E. G., GERSTENBLITH, G., ANGELL, C. A., SHOCK, N. W., and WEIS-FELDT, M. L. 1975b. Prolonged contraction duration in aged myocardium. J. Clin. Invest. 55:61–68.

TEMPLETON, G. H., ECKER, R. R., and MITCHELL, J. H. 1972. Left ventricular stiffness during diastole and systole; the influence of changes in volume and inotropic state. Cardiovas. Res. 6:95–100.

TEMPLETON, G. H., WILDENTHAL, K., WILLERSON, J. T., and REARDON, W. C. 1974. Influence of temperature on the mechanical properties of cardiac muscle. Circ. Res. 39:624–634.

WEISFELDT, M. L., LOEVER, W. A., and SHOCK, N. W. 1971. Resting and active mechanical properties of trabeculae cornae from aged male rats. Amer. J. Physiol. 220:1921–1927.

Mailing address:
G. H. Templeton, Ph.D.,
Department of Physiology,
University of Texas Health Science Center,
5323 Harry Hines Boulevard,
Dallas, Texas 75235 (USA).

Recent Advances in Studies on
Cardiac Structure and Metabolism, Volume 11
Heart Function and Metabolism
Edited by T. Kobayashi, T. Sano, and N. S. Dhalla
Copyright 1978   University Park Press   Baltimore

DELAY IN DIASTOLIC RESTITUTION OF FULL MYOCARDIAL CONTRACTILITY IN GUINEA PIG ATRIUM

H. REICHEL and K. BAUMANN

Physiologisches Institut der Universität Hamburg, West Germany

SUMMARY

In an isolated perfused left atrium of guinea pig, pressure amplitudes were recorded at $37°$ C and a stimulation rate of 240/min with interposed variable resting pauses. After prolonged intervals the preparation develops maximum pressure, which does not depend on perfusion time or on any positive inotropic intervention. The latter is found to shorten the time needed for restitution of full contractility. Nifedipine (5×10^{-7}M) exerts its negative inotropic effect mainly by a delay in restitution time; acetylcholine (2×10^{-7}M), by a concomitant reduction of all pressure amplitudes over the whole range of stimulus intervals. The latter effect is similar to that of lowering $[Ca^{2+}]_o$.

INTRODUCTION

Isometric force development in cardiac muscle can be varied by positive or negative inotropic interventions. In spite of this property a heart muscle cannot raise its isometric force beyond a certain limit, which may be determined either by the number of simultaneous interactions between the myosin- and actin-filaments or by the amount of calcium available for the activation of the contractile proteins (Katz, 1970). Attempts have been made to assess maximum force in papillary muscles or other ventricular and atrial preparations by paired stimulation and elevation of Ca^{2+} concentration in the bathing fluid (Nayler, 1961; Kavaler, Fisher, and Stuckney, 1965). Both interventions are supposed to act via an increase in available Ca^{2+} (Suko, Ueba, and Chidsey, 1970). It is also suggested that calcium availability rises with time during a prolonged resting pause (Manring and Hollander, 1971; Tritthart *et al.*, 1973; Kaufmann *et al.*, 1974). Thus, a prolongation of stimulus interval after a series of rhythmical contractions is a further suitable method for determination of maximum contractile response (Wood, Heppner, and Weidmann, 1969). On the other hand, negative inotropic actions on rhythmical contractions might be explained by a delaying effect on the process that restitutes the amount of Ca^{2+} needed for a certain force development (McCans *et al.*, 1974; Bayer *et al.*, 1975). In the present study we attempted to define maximum contractile response at physiological

175

conditions by resting potentiation and other interventions and to differentiate the negative inotropic effects of various agents in respect to their delaying action on the restitution process during stimulus intervals of variable duration.

METHODS

The preparation was a left atrium of guinea pig, perfused through its cavity with Krebs-Henseleit solution (temperature $37°$ C pH 7.4) (for detail, see Baumann and Reichel, 1974). The recording system for isovolumetric pressure, taken by a Statham P 23 Gb pressure transducer, a pen consists of ultraviolet optical recorder and storage oscilloscope. The stimulation system was a quartz digital impulse generator adapted for interruption of rhythmical stimulation (rates 120 and 240/min) by precisely adjustable single intervals ("test intervals") of 0.1 to 8.0 sec. Square wave stimuli were twice the threshold intensity and 1 msec duration. Interventions were a variation of $[Ca^{2+}]_o$ in a range of 0.5 to 5.0 mM (control, 2.5 mM), application of acetylcholine (2×10^{-7}M), or of the Ca^{2+} antagonist nifedepine (5×10^{-7}M). In these concentrations either agent was found to depress rhythmical steady-state pressure amplitude to about half of control recorded before and after the intervention. For a comparison of values obtained in different experiments, pressure amplitudes are expressed as a percentage of maximum pressure amplitudes (test contractions after prolonged resting pauses during rhythmical contraction of 240/min) at the beginning of each experiment. For statistical evaluations, Student's t-test is used.

RESULTS AND DISCUSSION

Figure 1 depicts the contractile response to stimuli interposed into a series of rhythmical contractions at a rate of 240/min. Pressure amplitude of test contractions increases with the duration of the interval between the last rhythmical stimulus and the test stimulus. At control conditions ($[Ca^{2+}]_o = 2.5$ mM) maximum pressure is developed after a test interval of about 2.0 sec (Figure 1a). All interventions known to exert positive inotropic effects on rhythmical contractions, such as an elevation of $[Ca^{2+}]_o$ (to 5.0 mM), application of noradrenaline (10^{-6}M) and paired stimulation (120 double stimuli per min), shorten the test interval required for maximum pressure development and make the pressure-test interval curve steeper. Maximum pressure development itself remains unaffected. An example is shown in Figure 1a. In spite of the strong potentiating effect of a rise in $[Ca^{2+}]_o$, maximum pressure development is not enhanced, but is achieved within a shorter test interval.

The opposite, i.e., a retardation of full pressure development and a shift of the pressure-test interval curve to longer test intervals, is affected by nifedepine (5×10^{-7}M), lowering rhythmical amplitude to about half of control (Figure 1b).

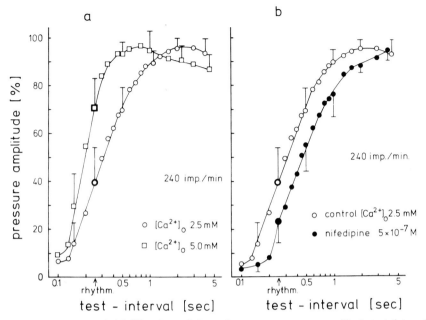

Figure 1 a. Effect of $[Ca^{2+}]_0$ from 2.5 to 5 mM on pressure amplitude-test interval relationship. *Ordinate* is percentage of maximum pressure development during the first hour of control perfusion. (100 % = 13.4 ± 2.9 cm H_2O; mean ± S.D. of 14 experiments.) Records taken during the fourth hour of perfusion. *b*, Effect of nifedipine (5 × 10^{-7}M) on pressure amplitude-test interval relationship. (Mean values of the same experiments as in Figure 1*a*.)

Again, maximum pressure development remains unaffected. The same negative inotropic effect on rhythmical pressure development is exerted by acetylcholine in a concentration of 2 × 10^{-7}M. The pressure-test interval curve is flattened and reaches its maximum at longer test intervals than controls. However, in contrast to the effect of nifedepine, the level of maximum pressure development is depressed significantly ($p < 0.001$). Almost the same significant deviations from control are obtained by lowering $[Ca^{2+}]_0$ to a concentration (1 mM) that reduces rhythmical pressure amplitude to half of control (Figure 2*b*).

In the preparation used in these experiments, maximum pressure development signifies the upper limit of contractility, which cannot be further enhanced by any positive inotropic interventions. This means that the positive inotropic effect on the amplitude of rhythmical steady-state contractions is mainly due to a shortening of the process that is responsible for the restitution of full contractility during prolonged stimulus intervals. The effect might be interpreted as an acceleration of reactions enhancing Ca^{2+} availability for the contractile proteins (Wood *et al.*, 1969; Tritthart *et al.*, 1973). The opposite effect is induced by nifedepine, which exerts negative inotropic action on rhythmical

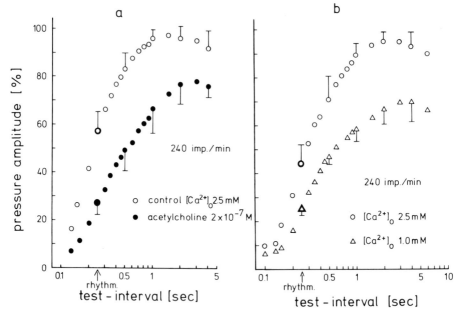

Figure 2 a. Effect of acetylcholine (2 × 10⁻⁷ M) on pressure amplitude-test interval relationship. *Ordinate* is percentage of maximal pressure development during the first hour of control perfusion. (100 % = 14.2. ± 4.2 cm H₂O; mean ± S.D. of 6 experiments.) Records taken during the third hour of perfusion. *b,* Effect of lowering [Ca²⁺]₀ from 2.5 to 1 m on pressure amplitude-test interval relationship. *Ordinate* is percentage of maximal pressure development during the first hour of control perfusion. (100 % = 15.7 ± 2.8 cm H₂O; mean ± S.D. of 9 experiments.) Records taken during the fourth hour of perfusion.

pressure amplitude mainly by delaying restitution of full contractility. Thus far, the results are in accordance with the findings of Bayer *et al.* (1975) on the Ca²⁺ antagonist verapamil (Fleckenstein, 1971). In the concentrations used in the present experiments, nifedepine does not impair maximum pressure development. Application of acetylcholine and reduction of [Ca²⁺]₀—the concentration of both being adjusted to a comparable negative inotropic effect—retards not only restitution but also depresses pressure amplitudes over the whole range of stimulus intervals. It is reasonable that lowering [Ca²⁺]₀ also reduces the amount of intracellular available Ca²⁺ for pressure development even after a prolonged test interval. Opposite to the so-called Ca²⁺ antagonists described as inhibitors of Ca²⁺ permeability of the membrane (Kohlhardt *et al.,* 1972), acetylcholine appears to affect total Ca²⁺ availability from intracellular stores, possibly induced by its known shortening effect on the duration of the action potential (Furchgott, Sleator, and de Gubareff, 1960).

REFERENCES

BAUMANN, Kl., and REICHEL, H. 1974. Time dependence of frequency potentiation in the isolated guinea-pig's atrium. Pfluegers Arch. 350:69–80.

BAYER, R., HENNEKES, R., KAUFMANN, R., and MANNHOLD, R. 1975. Inotropic and electrophysiological actions of verapamil and D 600 in mammalian myocardium. Naunyn Schmiedebergs Arch. Pharmacol. 290:49–68.

FLECKENSTEIN, A. 1971. *In* P. Harris and L. Opie (eds.), Calcium and the Heart, p. 235. Academic Press, New York.

FURCHGOTT, R. F., SLEATOR, W., and DE GUBAREFF, T. 1960. Effects of acetyl-choline and epinephrine on the contractile strength and action potential of electrically driven guinea pig atria. J. Pharmacol. Exp. Ther. 129:405–416.

KATZ, A. M. 1970. Quantification of myocardial contractility. Amer. J. Cardiol. 26: 331–332.

KAUFMANN, R., BAYER, R., FÜRNISS, T., KRAUSE, H., and TRITTHART, H. 1974. Calcium-movement controlling cardiac contractility II. Analog computation of cardiac excitation-contraction coupling on the basis of calcium kinetics in a multi-compartment model. J. Mol. Cell. Cardiol. 6:543–559.

KAVALER, R., FISHER, V. J., and STUCKNEY, J. H. 1965. The potentiated contraction and ventricular "contractility." Bull. N. Y. Acad Med. 41:592–601.

KOHLHARDT, M., BAUER, B., KRAUSE, H., and FLECKENSTEIN, A. 1972. Differentiation of the transmembrane Na and Ca channels in mammalian cardiac fibres by the use of specific inhibitors. Pflugers Arch. 335:309–322.

MANRING, A., and HOLLANDER, P. B. 1971. The interval-strength relationship in mammalian atrium: A calcium exchange model. Biophys. J. 11:483–501.

McCANS, J. L., LINDENMAYER, G. E., MUNSON, R. G., EVANS, R. W., and SCHWARTZ, A. 1974. A dissociation of positive staircase (bowditch) from ouabain-induced positive inotropism. Circ. Res. 35:439–447.

NAYLER, W. G. 1961. The importance of calcium in poststimulation potentiation. J. Gen. Physiol. 44:1059–1072.

SUKO, J., UEBA, Y., and CHIDSEY, C. A. 1970. Intracellular calcium and myocardial contractility. II. Effects of postextrasystolic potentiation in the isolated rabbit heart. Circ. Res. 27:227–234.

TRITTHART, H., KAUFMANN, R., VOLKMER, H. P., BAYER, R., and KRAUSE, H. 1973. Ca-movement controlling myocardial contractility. I. Voltage-, current- and time-dependence of mechanical activity under voltage clamp conditions (cat papillary muscles and trabeculae). Pfluegers Arch. 338:207–231.

WOOD, E. H., HEPPNER, R. L., and WEIDMANN, S. 1969. Inotropic effects of electric currents. I. Positive and negative effects of constant electric or current pulses applied during cardiac actions potentials. II. Hypotheses: Calcium movements, excitation-contraction coupling and inotropic effects. Circ. Res. 24:409–445.

Mailing address:
H. Reichel,
Professor of Physiology,
University of Hamburg,
Physiological Institute,
Martinistrasse 52,
2000 Hamburg 20 (West Germany).

Recent Advances in Studies on
Cardiac Structure and Metabolism, Volume 11
Heart Function and Metabolism
Edited by T. Kobayashi, T. Sano, and N. S. Dhalla
Copyright 1978   University Park Press   Baltimore

EFFECT OF RAPID COOLING ON
TOAD AND GUINEA PIG CARDIAC MUSCLES

S. KURIHARA and T. SAKAI

Department of Physiology,
The Jikei University School of Medicine,
Minatoku, Tokyo, Japan

SUMMARY

When bathing solution temperature was lowered rapidly to below $5°$ C, contracture was observed in toad and guinea pig cardiac muscles (Rapid Cooling Contracture, RCC). RCC in toad cardiac muscle was observed even in the presence of TTX and Mn, and enhanced by reducing $[Na]_0$ and caffeine. RCC in guinea pig cardiac muscle showed two components; phasic component was dependent on stimulation frequency before cooling, stimulation period, $[Ca]_0$, and $[Na]_0$; tonic component was not dependent on these factors, but was enhanced by reducing $[Na]_0$ and in high $[K]_0$ solution. From these results, the possible role of Ca ion accumulated at intracellular sequestered sites in cardiac muscle was discussed in relation to excitation-contraction (E-C) coupling.

INTRODUCTION

In frog skeletal muscle fibers treated with low concentration caffeine, contracture was observed when the temperature of the bathing solution was lowered rapidly to below $5°$ C. Rapid cooling contracture of skeletal muscle fibers is considered to be induced by Ca ion release, especially from the sarcoplasmic reticulum (Sakai, Geffner, and Sandow, 1971; Sakai and Kurihara, 1974b). Recently it was reported that rapid cooling contracture was observed in the toad cardiac muscle in which the sarcoplasmic reticulum was not well developed (Sakai and Kurihara, 1974a). On the other hand, important roles of the sarcoplasmic reticulum in mammalian cardiac muscles are suggested by Allen, Jewell, and Wood (1976), Edman and Jóhannsson (1976), and Fabiato and Fabiato (1975). In the present experiment, the possible dependence of E-C coupling of guinea pig cardiac muscle on the sarcoplasmic reticulum was studied by using a rapid cooling technique.

METHODS AND MATERIALS

Guinea pigs of either sex, weighing 250–300 g, were stunned and bled. Papillary muscles of the right ventricle were used. With 50 μm silver wire, one end of the preparation was attached to a glass rod and the other was fixed to a mechanotransducer. The preparation was placed in a 0.1-ml lucite chamber and continuously irrigated with modified Krebs solution at 36.5 ± 0.5° C. The temperature of the solution was lowered from 36.5° C to below 5° C within 10 sec by flowing precooled solution. The temperature of the solution was monitored continuously by a thermister thermometer placed within 1 mm above the preparation. Electrical stimulation was applied through Pt-black electrodes using square 2-msec pulses at various frequencies (0.1–3 Hz).

RESULTS AND DISCUSSION

Effects of Electrical Stimulation on Rapid Cooling Contracture

When the temperature of the Krebs solution was lowered from 36.5°C to below 5° C within 10 sec, a slight, relatively rapid initial tension and a slowly developed tonic tension, leveling off within 7 min, were observed in the nonstimulated guinea pig papillary muscle (rapid cooling contracture). Rewarming the preparation produced a small step, followed by gradual relaxation of tonic contraction back to resting tension. If rapid cooling was preceded by electrical stimulation, and initiated within 5 sec after cessation of the stimulation, the initial transient contraction increased (phasic contraction). Phasic contraction amplitude was directly dependent on stimulation period, for periods up to 5 min, after which it leveled out. This effect was stable enough to be observable and constant throughout experiments lasting 3 to 4 hr in good preparations. However, during the same 3 to 4 hr twitch response amplitude gradually diminished. If electrical stimulation was continued throughout cooling, twitch tension showed a large potentiated response at the onset, disappeared during, and restarted upon termination of cooling. Meanwhile, tonic contraction approximated control conditions. These results suggest that phasic contraction differs from twitch, which is triggered by action potential. Examination of membrane potential change during cooling (which was not a part of this experiment) might elucidate this suggestion.

Phasic contraction was small if rapid cooling was initiated 5 sec after cessation of short period stimulation. The longer the stimulation period (up to 5 min), the larger the phasic contraction. It did not increase any further, however, if the stimulation period exceeded 5 min. Phasic contraction was also dependent on stimulation frequency, increasing with frequency from 0.1 to 3 Hz. Tonic contraction was influenced slightly by frequency. If the period between cessation of the 5-min electrical stimulation and the onset of cooling was increased from 5 sec to 2 min, the resultant phasic contraction amplitude was inversely proportional to the delay interval.

Effect of $[Ca]_0$ and $[Na]_0$ on Rapid Cooling Contracture

Change of $[Ca]_0$ from 2.5 mM to concentrations up to 10 mM for 5 to 10 min in nonstimulated preparations did not affect rapid cooling contracture. However, in stimulated preparations, twitch and phasic contraction increased with increase of $[Ca]_o$. Tonic contraction increased very slightly, but contraction amplitude fluctuation appeared. Phasic and tonic contractions of stimulated preparation were potentiated by reducing $[Na]_o$ from normal concentration to 25% of normal, and wavy contractions were also recognized. In nonstimulated preparations, RCC was not enhanced by reduction of $[Na]_o$ by as much as 50%. However, rapid cooling itself could initiate phasic and tonic contractions, even in nonstimulated preparations, when $[Na]_o$ was reduced to below 25% for longer than 20 min. The relationship between peak tension of rapid cooling contracture and $[Ca]_o/[Na]_o$ was a sigmoid curve.

Rapid Cooling Contracture in Depolarized Muscle

After addition of 200 mM KCl as a solid, resting tension increased slightly and RCC was observed. This extent of depolarization produced very great phasic and tonic contractions. Five minutes after the immersion of the preparation in Ca-free 200 mM KCl solution containing 0.5 mM EGTA (ethylene glycol bis(β-aminoethyl ether)-N,N'-tetraacetic acid), tonic contraction was markedly reduced, but phasic contraction was only slightly affected. After 10 min, both tonic and phasic contractions were decreased (Figure 1).

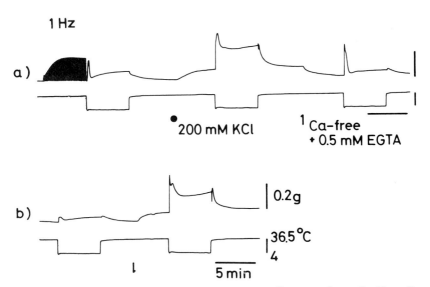

Figure 1. Rapid cooling contracture in depolarized papillary muscle. *a,* Rapid cooling contracture, after 5 min of 1 Hz stimulation. Interval from cessation of stimulation to onset of cooling was 5 sec. Five minutes after addition of 200 mM KCl as a solid, rapid cooling contracture was observed. Tonic contraction, but not phasic contraction, was greatly reduced by treatment with Ca-free + 0.5 mM EGTA solution. *b,* Phasic contraction also decreased by long exposure to Ca-free + 0.5 mM EGTA solution, and rapid cooling contracture recovered in normal concentration of CA.

These results indicate that phasic contraction induced by rapid cooling might be triggered by the Ca ion accumulated in a Ca-sequestered site, possibly the sarcoplasmic reticulum, and that tonic contraction, which probably is controlled by a portion of the sarcoplasmic Ca, may possibly be also affected by another Ca regulation mechanism.

REFERENCES

ALLEN, D. G., JEWELL, B. R., and WOOD, E. H. 1976. Studies of the contractility of mammalian myocardium at low rates of stimulation. J. Physiol. 254:1–17.

EDMAN, K. A. P., and JOHANNSSON, M. 1976. The contractile state of rabbit papillary muscle in relation to stimulation frequency. J. Physiol. 254:565–581.

FABIATO, A., and FABIATO, F. 1975. Contractions induced by a calcium-triggered release of calcium from the sarcoplasmic reticulum of single skinned cardiac cells. J. Physiol. 249:469–495.

SAKAI, T., GEFFNER, E. S., and SANDOW, A. 1971. Caffeine contracture in muscle with disrupted transverse tubules. Amer. J. Physiol. 220:712–717.

SAKAI, T., and KURIHARA, S. 1974a. The rapid cooling contracture of toad cardiac muscles. Jpn. J. Physiol. 24:649–666.

SAKAI, T., and KURIHARA, S. 1974b. A study on rapid cooling contracture from the viewpoint of excitation-contraction coupling. Jikeikai Med. J. 21:47–88.

Mailing address:
S. Kurihara,
Department of Physiology,
The Jikei University School of Medicine,
3-25-8 Nishishinbashi,
Minatoku, Tokyo (Japan).

Recent Advances in Studies on
Cardiac Structure and Metabolism, Volume 11
Heart Function and Metabolism
Edited by T. Kobayashi, T. Sano, and N. S. Dhalla
Copyright 1978   University Park Press   Baltimore

REGULATORY MECHANISM IN ARTERIAL
SMOOTH MUSCLE CONTRACTION

T. KOIZUMI, Y. ITO, and S. EBASHI

Fourth Department of Internal Medicine
and Department of Pharmacology, University of
Tokyo, Faculty of Medicine, Tokyo, Japan

SUMMARY

The regulatory mechanism in the aortic actomyosin system was studied. Superprecipitation of desensitized aortic myosin B was not exhibited even in the presence of Ca^{2+}, but was observable only in the presence of native tropomyosin and Ca^{2+}. Reconstituted actomyosin composed of pure aortic myosin and pure skeletal actin did not show superprecipitation. Addition of aortic native tropomyosin and Ca^{2+} caused a marked superprecipitation. The ATPase of reconstituted actomyosin was enhanced three- or fourfold by aortic native tropomyosin and Ca^{2+}. The extent of superprecipitation of aortic myosin B did not show a biphasic type of response to Mg-ATP concentration. Thus, aortic native tropomyosin induces a real activation of the myosin, actin, and ATP system in the presence of Ca^{2+}, in contrast with the case of skeletal native tropomyosin, which induces the depression of skeletal myosin-actin-ATP interaction in the absence of Ca^{2+}.

INTRODUCTION

The regulatory mechanism of contraction in arterial smooth muscle had generally been considered to be the same as that represented by skeletal muscle. Recently, however, a new type of regulatory mechanism of contraction has been shown in gizzard and bovine stomach smooth muscle (Ebashi *et al.*, 1975a; Ebashi *et al.*, 1976). This type of regulation is substantially different from that of skeletal muscle. The present studies were performed to clarify the regulatory mechanism of contraction in arterial smooth muscle.

METHODS

Preparation methods of various proteins of bovine aortic muscle and experimental procedures were carried out by the methods of Ebashi (Ebashi and Ebashi, 1964; Ebashi, 1976). However, to prepare pure aortic myosin slight modifications were needed, i.e., actin fraction was precipitated by twice-repeated ultracentrifugation ($1.4 \times 10^5 \times g$, $2.2 \times 10^5 \times g$, respectively) from myosin B dissolved in Mg-ATP solution. ATPase activities were estimated by measuring liberated inorganic phosphates according to the method of Youngburg and Youngburg (1930).

RESULTS

As shown in the patterns of SDS-polyacrylamide gel electrophoresis (Figure 1), we obtained fairly pure preparations in the case of myosin and tropomyosin, but native tropomyosin was contaminated with a small amount of actin and other proteins. Separation of troponin from aortic native tropomyosin was not yet fully successful, but three main bands (mol. wt. 80,000, 18,000, and 17,000) of aortic troponin were the same as those of gizzard troponin (Ebashi et al., 1975b).

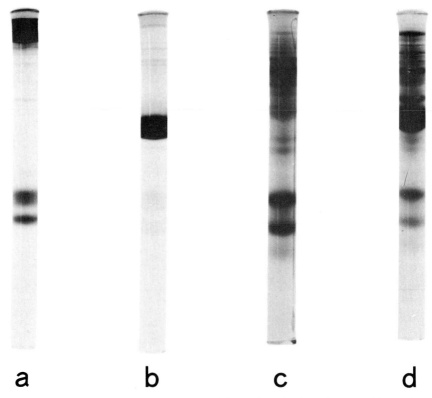

a   b   c   d

Figure 1. Patterns of SDS-polyacrylamide gel electrophoresis of aortic contractile proteins. *a*, myosin; *b*, tropomyosin; *c*, crude troponin; *d*, native tropomyosin. 10% polyacrylamide gel was used.

In order to make clear the regulatory mechanism of contraction, desensitization of aortic myosin B was the first step of our studies. Using successful preparations, it was found that desensitized myosin B did not show significant superprecipitation even in the presence of Ca^{2+}. A marked superprecipitation was exhibited only by addition of aortic native tropomyosin and Ca^{2+} (Figure 2). This finding is quite different from that of skeletal muscle. As is well known, desensitized myosin B of skeletal muscle exhibits a marked superprecipitation irrespective of the presence or absence of Ca^{2+}, and skeletal native tropomyosin induces the depression of skeletal myosin-actin-ATP interaction in the absence of Ca^{2+} (Ebashi and Endo, 1968; Ebashi, 1974).

The results above must be confirmed by using a much simpler system, i.e., reconstituted actomyosin. Since we have not yet successfully prepared aortic actin, the reconstituted actomyosin used in our experiments was composed of relatively pure aortic myosin and pure skeletal actin. Superprecipitation of this reconstituted actomyosin was not observable. Tropomyosin itself was not effective on this system. However, addition of native tropomyosin and Ca^{2+} caused a marked superprecipitation (Figure 3).

The Mg-ATPase activities of reconstituted actomyosin system fairly coincided with the results of superprecipitation above, i.e., the highest activation of the actomyosin ATPase was observed in the presence of native tropomyosin

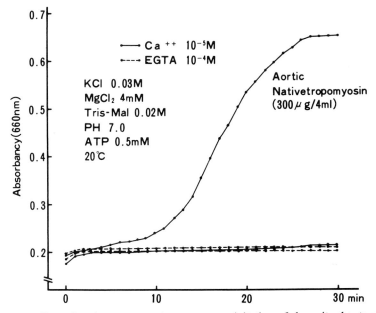

Figure 2. Effect of native tropomyosin on superprecipitation of desensitzed actomyosin. Desensitized aortic myosin B, 1.8 mg/4 ml. The reaction was started by adding ATP.

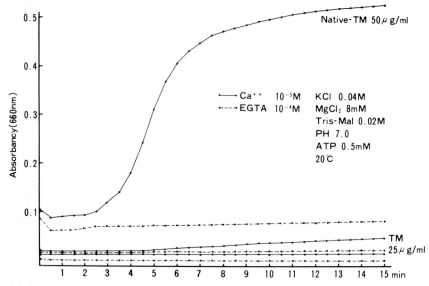

Figure 3. Effect of aortic native tropomyosin on superprecipitation of reconstituted acto-myosin. Aortic myosin, 0.3 mg/ml; skeletal actin, 0.15 mg/ml. Native-TM, aortic native tropomyosin; TM, aortic tropomyosin. The reaction was started by adding ATP.

and Ca^{2+} (Table 1). Activation of aortic myosin ATPase by skeletal actin alone was very weak, and addition of tropomyosin alone did not also activate the actomyosin ATPase. However, native tropomyosin enhanced the ATPase of the reconstituted actomyosin three- or fourfold in the presence of Ca^{2+}. Unexpectedly, native tropomyosin affected the enhancement of the ATPase activity of the actomyosin moderately even in the absence of Ca^{2+} (Table 1). This is different from the case of gizzard (Ebashi *et al.,* 1976); perhaps the use of skeletal actin in place of aortic actin is one of the reasons for this discrepancy.

Table 1. Mg-ATPase activities of reconstituted actomyosin and the effect of native tropomyosin on this system*

	My	My + Ac	My + Ac + TM	My + Ac + NTM
2×10^{-4} M GEDTA	1.8 ± 0.04	3.0 ± 0.08	3.6 ± 0.04	7.9 ± 0.28
2×10^{-5} M Ca^{2+}	1.9 ± 0.07	3.5 ± 0.11	4.5 ± 0.07	12.0 ± 0.41

*The activities were expressed as nmol Pi $min^{-1} \cdot mg^{-1} \cdot$ myosin $\pm$ S.E. My = aortic myosin, 0.5 mg/ml; Ac = skeletal actin, 0.25 mg/ml; TM = aortic tropomyosin, 25 μg/ml; NTM = aortic native tropomyosin, 50 μg/ml. The reactive conditions are: KCl, 0.05 M; $MgCl_2$, 8 mM; Tris-maleate buffer, 0.02 M, pH 6.8; ATP, 1.0 mM, 25°C.

Thus it is clear that aortic native tropomyosin induces a real activation of the myosin, actin, and ATP system in the presence of Ca^{2+}.

The extents of superprecipitation relative to those of maximum turbidity are shown in Figures 4 and 5, respectively. The results clearly indicated that there was no tendency of dissociation or relaxation at higher concentrations of ATP in the presence of Ca^{2+}. Thus, unlike the case of skeletal muscle, myosin B of aortic muscle does not show biphasic response to Mg-ATP concentration.

Accordingly, our results were in good agreement with those of gizzard muscle (Ebashi et al., 1976).

DISCUSSION

The second type of regulation by the troponin-tropomyosin system has recently been revealed in gizzard and bovine stomach smooth muscle (Ebashi et al., 1975a; Ebashi et al., 1976). This type of regulation now appears to be also the case of arterial smooth muscle contraction. In view of this, it was expected that physicochemical properties of contractile proteins of arterial muscle should be similar to those of gizzard contractile proteins. Indeed, aortic myosin is highly soluble even in low ionic strength (0.05–0.1 M KCl), and the fine structure of bovine aortic tropomyosin paracrystal is almost the same as that of bovine

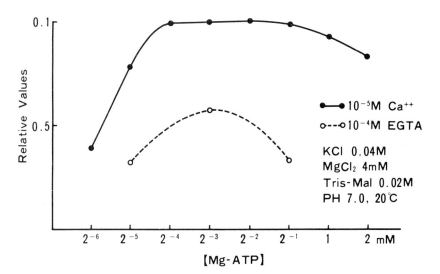

Figure 4. Extent of superprecipitation of aortic myosin B at varied Mg-ATP concentrations. Relative values of optical absorbancies at final state of superprecipitation were plotted against Mg-ATP concentrations. The highest value is shown at 2^{-4}mM Mg-ATP and almost no change can be seen until 2 mM in the presence of Ca^{2+}.

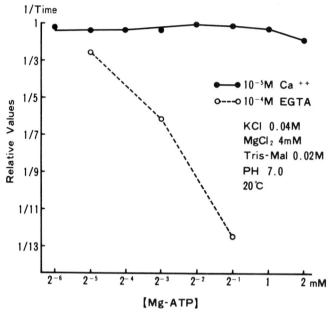

Figure 5. Rates of superprecipitation of aortic myosin B at varied Mg-ATP concentrations. The rates of turbidity increase, expressed as the reciprocal of the time to reach half maximum turbidity relative to that of the fastest superprecipitation, were plotted against Mg-ATP concentrations. The values are almost constant at all Mg-ATP concentrations in the presence of Ca^{2+}.

stomach tropomyosin (Y. Nonomura, personal communication). These observations are favorable for the consideration that smooth muscle-type of regulatory mechanism is common among all kinds of smooth muscle.

In conclusion, regulatory mechanism in arterial smooth muscle is very similar to that of gizzard and bovine stomach smooth muscle (Ebashi *et al.,* 1976), i.e., superprecipitation of actomyosin is observed only in the presence of native tropomyosin and Ca^{2+}; in other words, Ca^{2+} acts as the real activator in arterial smooth muscle, in contrast with skeletal muscle, in which Ca^{2+} acts as a kind of derepressor.

Essentially the same results were independently obtained by N. Ito and K. Hotta (personal communication).

Acknowledgments The authors are grateful to Associate Professor Y. Nonomura for useful discussion. We also thank Dr. Y. Kira and Mrs. T. Kuroda for their technical assistance.

REFERENCES

EBASHI, S., and EBASHI, F. 1964. A new protein component participating in the superprecipitation of myosin B. J. Biochem. 55:604–613.

EBASHI, S. 1974. Regulatory mechanism of muscle contraction with special reference to the Ca- troponin- tropomyosin system. *In* P. N. Campbell and F. Dickens (eds.), Essays in Biochemistry, Vol. 10, pp. 1–36. Academic Press, London.

EBASHI, S. 1976. A simple method of preparing actin-free myosin from smooth muscle. J. Biochem. 79:229–231.

EBASHI, S., and ENDO, M. 1968. Calcium ion and muscle contraction. Prog. Biophys. Mol. Biol. 18:123–183.

EBASHI, S., NONOMURA, Y., KITASAWA, T., and TOYO-OKA, T. 1975a. Troponin in tissues other than skeletal muscle. *In* E. Carafoli, F. Clementi, W. Drabikowski, and A. Margreth (eds.), Calcium Transport in Contraction and Secretion, pp. 405–414. North-Holland Publishing Company, Amsterdam.

EBASHI, S., NONOMURA, T., TOYO-OKA, T., and KATAYAMA, E. 1976. Regulation of muscle contraction by the calcium-troponin-tropomyosin system. *In* C. Duncan (ed.), Calcium in Biological System, 30th Symposium organized by the Society for Experimental Biology, pp. 349–360.

EBASHI, S., TOYO-OKA, T., and NONOMURA, Y. 1975b. Gizzard troponin. J. Biochem. 78:859–861.

YOUNGBURG, G. E., and YOUNGBURG, M. V. 1930. J. Lab. Clin. Med. 16:158.

Mailing address:
T. Koizumi, M.D.,
Fourth Department of Internal Medicine
(Tokyo University Branch Hospital),
Faculty of Medicine, University of Tokyo,
3-28-6 Mejirodai, Bunkyo-ku, Tokyo (Japan).

Biochemical Aspect

Recent Advances in Studies on
Cardiac Structure and Metabolism, Volume 11
Heart Function and Metabolism
Edited by T. Kobayashi, T. Sano, and N. S. Dhalla
Copyright 1978 University Park Press Baltimore

MODULATION OF CALCIUM IN THE HEART

A. SCHWARTZ, G. S. LEVEY,[1] M. L. ENTMAN,
E. G. EZRAILSON, W. B. VAN WINKLE,
E. P. BORNET, and B. J. R. PITTS

Departments of Cell Biophysics and Medicine,
Baylor College of Medicine and The Methodist Hospital,
Texas Medical Center, Houston, Texas, USA

The control of cardiac contraction has been the subject of numerous investigations for many years. It is now clear that a number of enzymatically active structures must participate in either the beat-to-beat control and/or relatively long-range maintenance of tension. These include the sarcolemma, the T system, the lateral cisternae, the longitudinal sarcoplasmic reticulum, mitochondria, and contractile proteins. Investigators in our laboratory have concentrated on the (Na^+, K^+)-ATPase, an enzyme presumably associated with sarcolemma, sarcoplasmic reticulum (SR), mitochondria, and, more recently, troponin C and myosin light chains in heart muscle, both from normal and diseased animals. Figure 1 is a schematic depiction of the various "calcium sinks."

We have developed procedures for isolation, purification, and characterization of (Na^+, K^+)-ATPase and have recently been successful in isolating the enzyme from dog heart that exhibits a specific activity (μmol inorganic phosphate/mg protein/hr) in excess of 400, and binds 600–800 pmol of $[H^3]$ ouabain/mg protein. We have found that phospholipids associated with the (Na^+, K^+)-ATPase may contain sites for calcium binding and that these regions appear to be affected by treatment with ouabain, which produces changes in calcium affinity. It may be that the (Na^+, K^+)-ATPase membrane system plays a role not only in the control of Na and K, but also in the delivery of calcium to the cardiac muscle cell. It has been known since the late 1800s that heart muscle, in contrast to skeletal muscle, requires an external source of calcium. It is possible, therefore, that the cell membrane of heart muscle is different from the membrane from skeletal muscle.

We have isolated sarcoplasmic reticulum from cardiac muscle, from fast and slow muscle, and from a variety of species, including cat, dog, and beef. We have

---

[1] Department of Medicine, Division of Endocrinology, University of Miami, Miami, Florida, USA

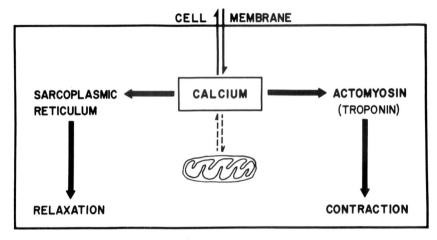

Figure 1. Schematic depiction of calcium "sinks" in cardiac muscle.

found that the energy-linked accumulation of calcium *in vitro* is consistent in terms of rapidity and quantity with the process of muscle relaxation. Both cAMP-dependent protein kinase and also phosphorylase b kinase phosphorylate all of the SR preparations, but only the cardiac muscle and slow skeletal muscle preparations contains a 19–21,000-dalton component that is phosphorylated. In fact, fast skeletal muscle SR does not contain a 20,000-dalton component.

Nevertheless, both enzymes cause a significant augmentation of calcium uptake (that is, the transport of calcium in the presence of oxalate) in all of the SR preparations studied. We have also found that the SR from cardiac muscle as well as skeletal muscle contains almost the entire glycogenolytic complex, including glycogen, adenylate cyclase, protein kinase, phosphorylase b kinase, phosphorylase b, and "debrancher" enzyme. The SR preparations derived from all of the muscles are responsive to hormones, including catecholamines, and our recent results suggest that the SR, therefore, may not only modulate contraction and relaxation by controlling the level of calcium, but it may also regulate carbohydrate metabolism. The possibility that the SR is contaminated with, or contains in some way, fragments of cell membrane and perhaps other structures should be a consideration in interpreting results. All of the SR preparations are undoubtedly "dirty" in this respect. In particular, the presence of a "latent" (Na^+ K^+)-ATPase, a putative cell membrane marker has been discussed in this meeting by Dr. H. R. Besch, Jr., and in our preliminary experiments we have repeated his findings, i.e., that cardiac SR contains more (Na^+ K^+)-ATPase activity than was heretofore appreciated. However, in a SR preparation derived from almost pure white fast skeletal muscle, we have not been able to find any (Na^+ K^+)-ATPase, even after detergent treatment, and yet this preparation responds in a manner similar to those described above. Therefore, it would appear that the adenylate cyclase, as well as the other enzymes we find, may in fact be associated with the internal membrane system. Whether these enzymes are associated with the T system and/or lateral cisternae that cosediment with the longitudinal sarcoplasmic reticulum is not at this time known. However, the amount of (Na^+, K^+)-ATPase is either low or absent in many of the preparations we have studied.

We and others have discussed in the literature for some years the postulate that (Na^+, K^+)-ATPase is the pharmacological receptor for cardiac glycosides. If this is true, the mechanism linking the interaction between the drug and the (Na^+, K^+)-ATPase and the final release of calcium from a membrane pool is and has been unknown. Currently, there are a number of suggestions about the characteristics of this mechanism, e.g., there is an electroneutral sodium-calcium exchange system that operates in concert with the (Na^+, K^+)-ATPase such that, whenever there is an increase in internal sodium, a carrier system is activated that brings enough calcium in from the extracellular space to augment contraction. The (Na^+, K^+)-ATPase may also function as some kind of calcium sink itself, as we have described above. Another possibility, and a most intriguing one, is that the adenylate cyclase in some way "oscillates." This has been suggested by the most interesting experiments of Dr. Gary Brooker, by Dr. Albert Wollenberger, and others, which essentially show that alterations of cAMP and cGMP levels may be associated with changes in contraction in heart muscle. In collaboration with Dr. Gerald Levey from the University of Miami, we have been using a partially purified inhibitor of adenylate cyclase whose

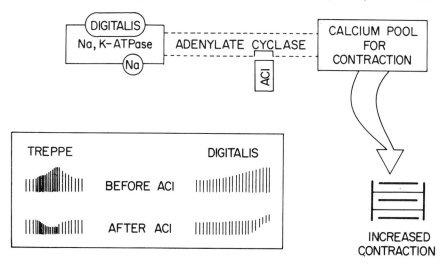

Figure 2. Suggested role of adenylate cyclase in modulating calcium in heart. ACI = adenylate cyclase inhibitor. *Insert:* traces of isolated, stimulated atrial preparation from guinea pig.

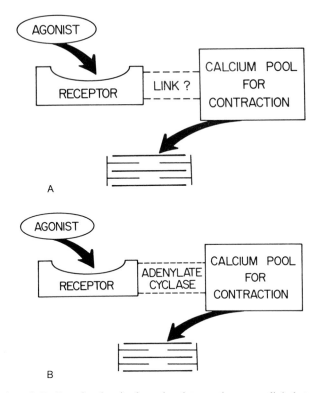

Figure 3. A and *B,* Postulated role for adenylate cyclase as a link between receptor activation and release of calcium.

molecular weight is apparently low enough that it can affect the cell membrane of isolated beating atrial and ventricular preparations. We have shown that treatment of the heart muscle with this inhibitor causes an obliteration of the positive staircase phenomenon. In addition, it appears to separate a "therapeutic" from a "toxic" action of cardiac glycosides. This is summarized in Figures 2, 3*A*, and 3*B*.

Mailing address:
Dr. Arnold Schwartz,
Department of Pharmacology and Cell Biophysics,
University of Cincinnati,
College of Medicine,
231 Bethesda Avenue, Cincinnati, Ohio 45267 (USA).

Recent Advances in Studies on
Cardiac Structure and Metabolism, Volume 11
Heart Function and Metabolism
Edited by T. Kobayashi, T. Sano, and N. S. Dhalla
Copyright 1978   University Park Press   Baltimore

QUENCH-FLOW MEASUREMENTS
OF INITIAL RATES OF Ca²⁺ ACCUMULATION
BY ISOLATED CARDIAC SARCOPLASMIC RETICULUM

H. WILL, J. BLANCK, G. SMETTAN, and A. WOLLENBERGER

Central Institute of Heart and Circulatory Regulation,
Research and Central Institute of Molecular Biology,
Academy of Sciences of the DDR, 1115 Berlin-Buch,
German Democratic Republic

SUMMARY

Using a quench-flow technique, the initial velocity of Ca^{2+} accumulation by isolated cardiac sarcoplasmic reticulum was estimated at free Ca^{2+} ion concentrations in the range encountered in the myoplasm during the cardiac contraction cycle. With cardiac microsomes exhibiting a Ca^{2+} accumulative capacity of 25.6 nmol Ca^{2+}/mg protein, initial rates were found to increase from 3.7 to 33.4 nmol Ca^{2+}/mg protein/sec, when the free Ca^{2+} ion concentration was raised from 0.2 to 18.0 μM. Preincubation of the cardiac microsomes with a partly purified soluble cardiac protein kinase, MgATP, and cAMP led to a significant increase in the initial Ca^{2+} accumulation rate.

INTRODUCTION

It is believed that in mammalian myocardium the ability of the sarcoplasmic reticulum to accumulate Ca^{2+} ions provides the principal means for effecting relaxation (Katz and Repke, 1967; Solaro and Briggs, 1974). Studies of the Ca^{2+} accumulation process have in the past concentrated on the relatively slow linear oxalate-supported uptake of the ion, at the comparative neglect of the fast short-lasting initial phase. In fact, this phase, which presumably is the one most pertinent to the relaxation process, has not yet been studied at low, physiologically relevant free Ca^{2+} ion concentrations. Therefore, a kinetic investigation of Ca^{2+} accumulation by cardiac microsomal vesicles derived chiefly from sarcoplasmic reticulum was undertaken utilizing a quench-flow technique, which allows us to follow the fast process of Ca^{2+} accumulation over the whole range of Ca^{2+} ion concentrations encountered in the myoplasm during the cardiac contraction cycle.

METHODS

The quench-flow method involved rapid mixing of the cardiac microsomes with ATP and Ca^{2+} and rapid quenching of Ca^{2+} binding by and transport into the microsomal vesicles by 10 to 50 mM EGTA (Will *et al.*, 1977) (see legend of Figure 1 and Table 1).

RESULTS AND DISCUSSION

The time course of Ca^{2+} accumulation as measured with the present technique is shown in Figure 1. Initial Ca^{2+} accumulation rates estimated from the experimental curves at different free Ca^{2+} ion concentrations can be compared with the quantities of the ion that need to be removed for induction of relaxation at

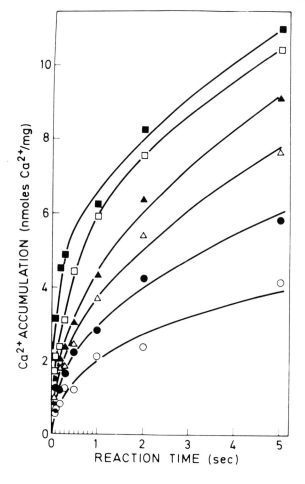

different levels of tension activation (Solaro and Briggs, 1974) and are then found to be consistent with the concept of a predominant role of the sarcoplasmic reticulum in cardiac relaxation (Will *et al.*, 1977). Figure 2 represents in a double reciprocal plot the initial velocity and the Ca^{2+} accumulative capacity as functions of the free Ca^{2+} ion concentration. Ca^{2+} accumulation capacity exhibits a linear dependence on the Ca^{2+} ion concentration in the range of 0.2–18.9 μM (Figure 2B). From the intercepts in Figure 2B the maximal amount of Ca^{2+} that can be accumulated by the vesicles within the indicated Ca^{2+} ion concentration range is estimated to be 25.6 nmol/mg and the $K_{0.5}$ value is calculated to be 0.28 μM.

For the initial Ca^{2+} accumulation velocity, a quasi-linear dependence, with a $K_{0.5}$ value of 0.34 μM, was observed at Ca^{2+} ion concentrations varying from 0.2 μM to 4.2 μM. A marked deviation from linearity is found at higher Ca^{2+} ion concentrations (Figure 2A). This is due to a further increase in the rate of Ca^{2+} transport that is incompatible with a simple Michaelis-Menten mechanism.

In previous investigations from this and other laboratories (LaRaia and Morkin, 1974; Tada *et al.*, 1974; Will *et al.*, 1977) oxalate-promoted Ca^{2+} uptake was found to be accelerated after phosphorylation of a microsomal protein by a cAMP-dependent protein kinase. With the quench-flow method a relatively small but reproducible increase in Ca^{2+} accumulation during the first 0.3 sec of the reaction could be demonstrated after preincubation of the microsomal membranes with a partly purified protein kinase, MgATP, and cAMP

Figure 1. (*at left*)   Time course of Ca^{2+} ion accumulation by isolated cardiac sarcoplasmic reticulum at 22° C and pH 6.8. The kinetic data were estimated with a quench-flow method using a Durrum model 134 multimixing apparatus. Syringe A contained rabbit heart microsomes (0.4–0.6 mg/ml) and syringe B contained 50 or 100 μM ^{45}[Ca]Cl$_2$ (specific activity: 8–32 μCi/nmol), 10 mM Tris-ATP, and 0–0.59 mM EGTA. The solutions in both syringes were buffered wtih 40 mM histidine-HCl of pH 6.8 or 7.2 and contained 120 mM KCl and 5 mM Mg Cl$_2$. The solution in syringe C consisted of 10 to 50 mM EGTA, 120 mM KCl, and 40 mM histidine-HCl, pH 6.0 or 5.8. The mixing ratio of syringe A, B, and C was 1:1:2, the pH after mixing was 6.37. Samples of 0.4 ml of the mixed solutions were collected and immediately filtered through type GS (0.22 μm pore size) Millipore filters. No significant change in the distribution of $^{45}Ca^{2+}$ between the microsomes and the mixed solutions occurred during the time intervening between quenching and termination of Millipore filtration (Will *et al.*, 1977). The amount of $^{45}Ca^{2+}$ retained on the filters was estimated by liquid scintillation spectrometry, using a Mark II spectrometer of Nuclear Chicago. Blank values, measured in the absence of ATP, were subtracted from total Ca^{2+} accumulation. For measurements of Ca^{2+} accumulation at time intervals greater than 10 sec, the reaction was started and terminated without the mixing apparatus. Free Ca^{2+} ion concentrations, calculated by equations similar to those derived by Katz *et al.* (1970) were 0.2 μM (-○-), 0.5 μM (-●-), 2.0 μM (-△-), 4.22 μM (-▲-), 9.45 μM (-□-), and 18.9 μM (-■-). Ca^{2+} accumulation at steady state, i.e., the amounts of Ca^{2+} taken up by the vesicles at the above free Ca^{2+} ion concentrations in 5 min, amounted to 10.7, 17.4, 20.0, 22.0, 23.3, and 28.2 nmol Ca^{2+}/mg, respectively. The experimental data were fitted by Spline third-order functions (Reinsch, 1967), using an ES 1010 computer, and the initial velocities were estimated as the first derivative of the smoothed curves at time zero. They amounted to 3.67, 5.27, 9.01, 9.26, 18.7, and 33.4 nmol/mg·sec, respectively. (From Will *et al.*, 1977.)

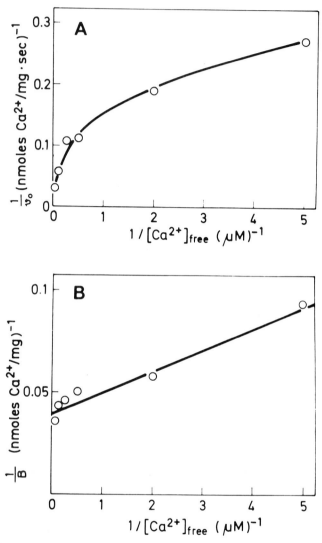

Figure 2. A, Double reciprocal plot of the initial Ca²⁺ accumulation velocity (V_0). B, Double reciprocal plot of Ca²⁺ accumulative capacity (B). For experimental details, see Figure 1. (From Will *et al.*, 1977.)

(Table 1). This preincubation had peviously been shown to result in the in-corporation of about 2 nmol of inorganic phosphate per mg of membrane protein (Will *et al.*, 1977). As has been observed before (LaRaia and Morkin, 1974; Tada *et al.*, 1974; Will *et al.*, 1977), steady-state Ca²⁺ accumulation by isolated cardiac sarcoplasmic reticulum is not changed by such preincubation of

Table 1. Enhancement of Ca^{2+} accumulation by cardiac microsomes after incubation of the microsomal membranes with a partly purified cAMP-dependent protein kinase and cAMP*

Reaction time (sec)	Ca^{2+} accumulation (nmol/mg)	
	Control membranes	Phosphorylated membranes
Without oxalate		
0.3	0.70 ± 0.23	1.02 ± 0.23**
5.0	2.68 ± 0.82	3.04 ± 0.79
300.0	8.0 ± 2.30	7.93 ± 2.00
2.5 mM oxalate		
200.0	11.15 ± 6.20	45.30 ± 18.75***

*Rabbit heart microsomes, 0.4–0.8 mg protein per ml of a solution containing 120 mM KCl, 5 mM $MgCl_2$, 5 mM Tris-ATP, and 40 mM histidine-HCl buffer of pH 6.8, were incubated for 3 min at 25°C in the presence (phosphorylated membranes) and absence (control membranes) of 5 μM cAMP and 0.2 mg/ml of partly purified soluble calf heart protein kinase having a specific activity of 12.0 nmol of inorganic phosphate/mg · min, with histone as substrate. The microsomal membranes were subsequently washed with 50 mM KCl–20 mM Tris-HCl solution of pH 6.8. The amount of Ca^{2+} accumulated by control and phosphorylated membranes in 300 msec was measured by the quench-flow technique at pH 7.2 and at total concentrations of Ca^{2+} and EGTA of 50 μM and 127 μM, respectively. The data represent means ±S.D. from 8 experiments.
  **$p < 0.05$
  ***$p < 0.01$

the membrane. Although the stimulation of the initial Ca^{2+} accumulation amounted to only 46%, it exceeds, reckoned in absolute terms of nmol of Ca^{2+} accumulated per mg protein per sec, the four-fold enhancement of the rate of oxalate-promoted Ca^{2+} uptake by protein kinase and cAMP, which was measured in a time interval of minutes (Table 1). The observed stimulation of the fast process of initial Ca^{2+} accumulation after preincubation of cardiac microsomes with protein kinase, MgATP, and cAMP strengthens the conclusion drawn from the reported acceleration of the relatively slow linear oxalate-supported Ca^{2+} uptake following cAMP-dependent phosphorylation of membrane protein (LaRaia and Morkin, 1974; Tada *et al.*, 1974; Will *et al.*, 1977), namely, that this phosphorylation forms part of the biochemical mechanism whereby cAMP-raising catecholamines accelerate relaxation in the myocardium.

REFERENCES

KATZ, A. M., and REPKE, D. I. 1967. Quantitative aspects of dog cardiac microsomal calcium binding and calcium uptake. Circ. Res. 21:153–162.

KATZ, A. M., REPKE, D. I., UPSHAW, J. E., and POLASCIK, M. A. 1970. Characterization of dog cardiac microsomes. Use of zonal centrifugation to fractionate fragmented sarcoplasmic reticulum, $(Na^+ + K^+)$-activated ATPase and mitochondrial fragments. Biochim. Biophys. Acta 205:473–490.

LARAIA, P. J., and MORKIN, E. 1974. Adenosine 3',5'-monophosphate-dependent membrane phosphorylation. Circ. Res. 35:298–306.

REINSCH, C. H. 1967. Smoothing by Spline function. Numer. Math. 10:177–183.

SOLARO, R. J., and BRIGGS, F. N. 1974. Estimating the functional capabilities of sarcoplasmic reticulum in cardiac muscle. Circ. Res. 34:531–540.

TADA, M., KIRCHBERGER, M. A., REPKE, D. I., and KATZ, A. M. 1974. The stimulation of calcium transport in cardiac sarcoplasmic reticulum by adenosine 3':5'-monophosphate-dependent protein kinase. J. Biol. Chem. 249:6174–6180.

WILL, H., BLANCK, J., SMETTAN, G., and WOLLENBERGER, A. 1977. A quench-flow kinetic investigation of calcium ion accumulation by isolated sarcoplasmic reticulum. Dependence of initial velocity on free calcium ion concentration and influence of preincubation with a protein kinase, MgATP, and cyclic AMP. Biochim. Biophys. Acta 449:295–303.

Mailing address:
Dr. H. Will
Central Institute of Heart
and Circulatory Regulation Research,
Academy of Sciences of the DDR,
1115 Berlin-Buch (German Democratic Republic).

Recent Advances in Studies on
Cardiac Structure and Metabolism, Volume 11
Heart Function and Metabolism
Edited by T. Kobayashi, T. Sano, and N. S. Dhalla
Copyright 1978   University Park Press   Baltimore

CALCIUM TRANSPORT AND RELEASE BY THE SARCOPLASMIC RETICULUM

A. M. KATZ[1], M. SHIGEKAWA[1], D. I. REPKE, W. HASSELBACH

Division of Cardiology, Department of Medicine, Mount Sinai
School of Medicine, New York, New York, USA and
Abteilung Physiologie, Max-Planck-Institut für Medizinishe
Forschung, Heidelberg, West Germany

SUMMARY

The slow rate of calcium transport by cardiac sarcoplasmic reticulum vesicles, compared to those prepared from skeletal muscle, is due mainly to a lesser density of transport sites and a lower Ca^{2+} affinity. Because the turnover rate of the cardiac sarcoplasmic reticulum calcium pump is similar to that of comparable skeletal muscle preparations, the cardiac sarcoplasmic reticulum seems able to effect the slower relaxation of the heart. Calcium permeability of skeletal sarcoplasmic reticulum vesicles is increased when the Ca^{2+} concentration outside the vesicles is increased, or when that inside the vesicles is decreased.

INTRODUCTION

The ability of the sarcoplasmic reticulum of muscle, an intracellular membrane system that surrounds the contractile proteins, to transport and store calcium allows these membranes to participate in the processes of excitation-contraction coupling. The sarcoplasmic reticulum of the mammalian heart plays an additional role in the regulation of myocardial contractility, both by controlling the amount of activator calcium released at the onset of systole, and by varying the rate at which this cation becomes dissociated from the calcium receptor protein of the contractile apparatus (Katz and Repke, 1973). An ATP-dependent calcium pump has been clearly identified in membrane vesicles derived from the sarcoplasmic reticulum of skeletal (Hasselbach, 1964; Weber, Herz, and Reiss, 1966; Ebashi and Endo, 1968) and cardiac (Hasselbach, 1961; Abe *et al.*, 1963; Carsten, 1964; Inesi, Ebashi, and Watanabe, 1964; Fanburg and Gergely, 1965;

Supported in part by a Grant-in-Aid from the New York Heart Association and Grants from the National Institute of Health (HL-13191, HL-18801, and A-00316). A portion of this work was done while Dr. Katz was recipient of a Senior U. S. Scientist Award from the Alexander von Humboldt Foundation of the Federal Republic of Germany.
[1] Present address: University of Connecticut, Farmington, Connecticut 06032, USA.

Katz and Repke, 1967; Weber, Herz, and Reiss, 1966; Harigaya and Schwartz, 1969) muscle, although the rates of both calcium transport and the associated Ca^{2+}-dependent ATPase activity are less in the cardiac sarcoplasmic reticulum. A number of recent studies have shown that calcium transport by skeletal sarcoplasmic reticulum involves a phosphoprotein intermediate (Hasselbach, 1972; Inesi, 1972; Martonosi, 1972; Tonomura, 1972) that is responsible for the transport of 2 moles of calcium per mole ATP hydrolyzed. A similar phosphoprotein intermediate has been found in cardiac sarcoplasmic reticulum (Namm, Woods, and Zucker, 1972; Fanburg and Matsushita, 1973; Pang and Briggs, 1973; Shigekawa, Finegan, and Katz, 1976; Suko and Hasselbach, 1976), in which calcium transport also proceeds through a tightly coupled calcium pump that transports 2 moles of calcium per mole ATP hydrolyzed (Tada *et al.*, 1974). These findings, while providing important insights about the role of the cardiac sarcoplasmic reticulum in excitation-contraction coupling, leave unanswered a number of important questions regarding the mechanisms by which this membrane system participates in the regulation of myocardial contractility. The present article will address briefly two of these questions: First, why is the rate of calcium transport into sarcoplasmic reticulum vesicles slower in cardiac than in skeletal preparations, and can the slow transport of calcium by the former account for relaxation in the intact heart? Second, what mechanisms might be responsible for the release of calcium from the sarcoplasmic reticulum at the onset of contraction?

SLOW CALCIUM UPTAKE BY CARDIAC SARCOPLASMIC RETICULUM

There is universal agreement that calcium uptake velocity is less in cardiac than in skeletal sarcoplasmic reticulum; for example, we (Repke and Katz, 1972; Katz and Repke, 1973) found that calcium uptake velocity in canine cardiac sarcoplasmic reticulum was approximately one-tenth that of the sarcoplasmic reticulum of rabbit fast skeletal muscle when both were measured under identical conditions at low (< 1 μM) Ca^{2+} concentrations. In a recent study (Shigekawa *et al.*, 1976) the mechanisms responsible for these differences have been examined.

Density of Calcium Transport Sites

The number of calcium transport sites in sarcoplasmic reticulum preparations can be estimated by measurements of the concentration of the phosphorylated ATPase intermediate. Maximum values for acyl-phosphoprotein levels in cardiac sarcoplasmic reticulum made by the method of Harigaya and Schwartz (1969) were found to be approximately 1.3 nmol per mg protein, compared to approximately 4.9 nmol per mg protein in similar preparations of skeletal sarcoplasmic reticulum (Shigekawa *et al.*, 1976). These findings agree with earlier measurements in cardiac (Pang and Briggs, 1973) and skeletal (Panet, Pick, and Selinger, 1971; Martonosi, 1972; Tonomura, 1972) sarcoplasmic reticulum. The lower concentration of the phosphoprotein intermediate in cardiac sarcoplasmic reticulum reflects partly the well-known heterogeneity of these membrane preparations (e.g., Katz *et al.*, 1970). However, it is now clear that the sarcoplasmic reticulum serves a more complex regulatory function in cardiac muscle than it does in skeletal muscle (Katz and Repke, 1973; Katz, Tada, and Kirchberger, 1975), so that the lower density of calcium transport sites in the cardiac preparations can also be attributed to the presence in the membranes themselves of regulatory systems not found in skeletal muscle preparations.

ATP- and pH-Dependence of Calcium Transport

Slight differences between the apparent ATP affinities of cardiac and skeletal sarcoplasmic reticulum at high ATP concentrations have been found (Shigekawa *et al.*, 1976), but these probably contribute little to the large differences in calcium transport velocity described above. The pH-dependences of the Ca^{2+}-activated ATPase activities of cardiac and skeletal sarcoplasmic reticulum also differ slightly, the pH optimum of the cardiac preparations being at a slightly more alkaline level than that of comparable preparations from skeletal muscle (Shigekawa *et al.*, 1976). This difference contributes slightly to the lower activities found in most studies of the cardiac sarcoplasmic reticulum, which are usually carried out at levels of pH well below the optimum of approximately 8.0 found in the cardiac preparations.

Ca^{2+}-Dependence of Calcium Transport

The Ca^{2+}-dependence of acyl-phosphoprotein formation and the calcium transport ATPase activity are the same when both activities are compared in the sarcoplasmic reticulum of either cardiac or skeletal muscle. However, when the cardiac and skeletal preparations are compared with each other, the Ca^{2+}-dependence of these activities differs (Shigekawa *et al.*, 1976; Figure 1). These tissue-specific differences are most marked in the physiological range of Ca^{2+} concentration; for example, the Ca^{2+}-activated ATPase activity of the skeletal preparation at 1 μM Ca^{2+} is approximately half of the maximal activity at saturating Ca^{2+} concentrations, whereas that of the cardiac preparation is less than one-fifth maximal at 1 μM Ca^{2+}. Similar differences are also seen in the Ca^{2+} dependence of phosphorylation of the ATPase intermediates in cardiac and skeletal sarcoplasmic reticulum at 1 μM Ca^{2+} (Figure 1). Values for K_{Ca} are approximately 4.7 μM for cardiac and 1.3 μM for skeletal sarcoplasmic reticulum (Shigekawa *et al.*, 1976). The lower Ca^{2+} affinity of the calcium pump of the cardiac sarcoplasmic reticulum thus contributes significantly to the slower rate of calcium transport by cardiac sarcoplasmic reticulum when studies are carried

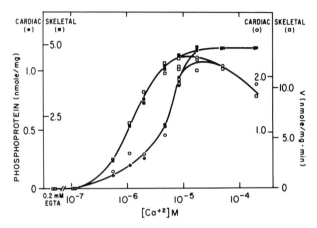

Figure 1. Ca^{2+} dependence of ATPase activity and phosphoprotein level in cardiac and skeletal microsomes. Reactions were carried out for 30 sec at 0° C with 0.52 mg per ml of cardiac microsomes (● ○) or 0.32 mg per ml of skeletal microsomes (■ □) in 25 μM [γ-^{32}P]ATP, 2 mM MgCl$_2$, 50 mM Tris-maleate (pH 6.8), 120 mM KCl, and 0.2 mM EGTA, or 0.15 to 3.2 mM EGTA and 0.15 mM CaCl$_2$. For Ca^{2+} concentrations above 50 μM, only CaCl$_2$ was added to the reaction medium. The Ca^{2+}-dependent portions of ATPase activity (○ □) and phosphoprotein level (● ■) are plotted in the figure. (Modified from Shigekawa *et al.*, 1976.)

out at physiological concentrations of Ca^{2+} (e.g., Repke and Katz, 1972; Katz and Repke, 1973).

Maximum Turnover Rates of the Calcium Pump

Calculations of the ratio between maximal Ca^{2+}-activated ATPase activity and the maximal number of phosphorylated calcium transport sites showed no significant differences between cardiac and skeletal sarcoplasmic reticulum (Shigekawa *et al.*, 1976), indicating that the turnover rates of the phosphorylated ATPase intermediates are the same in both types of sarcoplasmic reticulum.

Physiological Significance

The finding that the slower rate of calcium transport by cardiac sarcoplasmic reticulum reflects primarily a 3- to 4-fold lower concentration of calcium transport sites and an approximately 3-fold lower Ca^{2+} affinity of these sites, but not a slower turnover rate of the calcium pump, is in accord with the view that relaxation in mammalian cardiac muscle can be effected by the sarcoplasmic reticulum, as it is well known that the rate of relaxation in the heart is more than an order of magnitude slower than that of skeletal muscle.

CALCIUM RELEASE BY THE SARCOPLASMIC RETICULUM

In contrast to the many detailed studies of the mechanism by which calcium is transported into the sarcoplasmic reticulum (see above), relatively little is known of the mechanisms by which calcium is released from this intracellular membrane system to initiate contraction. Studies of the sarcoplasmic reticulum in "skinned" muscle fibers have shown that transient calcium release can be induced when the level of ionized Ca^{2+} in the medium is elevated ("Ca-triggered calcium release," Endo, Tonaka, and Ogawa, 1970; Ford and Podolsky, 1970), or when a permanent anion is substituted for a nonpermeant anion ("depolarization," Endo and Nakajima, 1973). Most attempts to demonstrate comparable phenomena in sarcoplasmic reticulum vesicles studies *in vitro* have not, however, been successful.

A number of observations of skeletal sarcoplasmic reticulum vesicles indicate that calcium permeability in these membranes is not constant, but varies when the concentrations of ionized Ca^{2+} inside (Ca_i) and outside (Ca_o) the vesicles are changed. Weber *et al.* (1966) found that when oxalate-supported calcium uptake reaches a steady state the level of Ca_o increases when relatively more calcium is presented to these vesicles, and that the rate of calcium exchange at a steady state of calcium storage in the absence of calcium precipitating anions increases with increasing Ca_o. Hasselbach *et al.* (1969) found that the rate of calcium efflux from vesicles in which Ca_i was held constant by a calcium oxalate precipitate increases 50- to 100-fold when Ca_o is elevated after a small, initial step of calcium uptake, findings that were confirmed by Makinose (1973), who reported that an increase in Ca_o increases the rate of calcium release at the same time that the added calcium is transported into vesicles that had previously taken up a small amount of calcium in the presence of oxalate. These reports provide evidence that calcium permeability of the membranes of the sarcoplasmic reticulum depends in a complex manner on both Ca_i and Ca_o. In a recent study of the control of calcium permeability in the sarcoplasmic reticulum, we (Katz *et al.,* 1976) have obtained evidence that the calcium permeability of these membranes correlates with the ratio Ca_i/Ca_o (Ca^{2+} concentration inside the vesicles divided by Ca^{2+} concentration in the medium).

Spontaneous Calcium Release after
Oxalate-Supported Calcium Uptake Reaches a Steady State

When either cardiac or skeletal sarcoplasmic reticulum vesicles take up calcium in the presence of a large excess of this cation, i.e., when the total calcium:protein ratio exceeds the "capacity" of the vesicles, the cessation of calcium uptake is followed by a significant spontaneous calcium release. In contrast, when the total calcium:protein ratio is low, the uptake of calcium slows as the vesicles fill, but spontaneous calcium release is not seen. This difference can be shown not to reflect the absolute protein or total calcium concentrations, but instead arises from an effect of high Ca_O to increase calcium permeability (Katz *et al.*, 1977a).

Effect of Ca_O on Calcium Efflux Rate

Calcium efflux rate can be measured in paired reactions, the first of which is started with radioactive calcium, while the second is carried out in exactly the same manner, except that nonradioactive instead of radioactive calcium is used. The first reaction allows net calcium uptake and release to be followed, while addition of a very small amount of radioactive calcium ("tracer") to the second reaction allows the rate of calcium influx to be determined. *Calcium efflux* can then be calculated as the sum of calcium influx *plus* net calcium release, or as calcium influx *minus* net calcium uptake at the time of tracer addition. If there is neither uptake nor release of calcium at the time of tracer addition, calcium efflux is equal to calcium influx. *Calcium permeability* can be calculated by dividing calcium efflux rate by the Ca^{2+} concentration inside the vesicles (Ca_i).

In studies where Ca_i was maintained by different concentrations of the calcium-precipitating anions, oxalate and phosphate, calcium permeability was found to increase with increasing Ca_O, and to decrease with increasing Ca_i (Katz *et al.*, 1976, 1977a). A close correlation between the calcium concentration

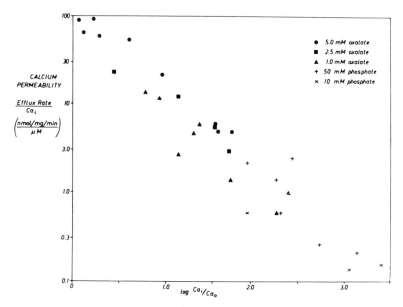

Figure 2. Relationship between calcium permeability and the ratio Ca_i/Ca_O, Ca_i was 4 μM (5.0 mM oxalate, ●), 8 μM (2.5 mM oxalate, ■), 20 μM (1.0 mM oxalate, ▲), 150 μM (50 mM phosphate, +) or 750 μM phosphate, x). (Modified from Katz *et al.*, 1976.)

gradient, Ca_i/Ca_o, and calcium permeability was found (Figure 2). The ability of elevated Ca_o to increase the calcium permeability of sarcoplasmic reticulum vesicles is similar to the phenomenon of "calcium-triggered calcium release" seen in mechanically "skinned" muscle fibers (Ford and Podolsky, 1970; Endo *et al.*, 1970).

The findings might be explained if calcium permeability were inversely proportional to an electrical potential related to the Ca^{2+} concentration gradient across the membrane. More recently, however, we have found that the ability of increasing Ca_o to promote calcium efflux resembles a saturable process, and that the calcium pump ATPase may play a major role in controlling calcium release from the sarcoplasmic reticulum (Katz *et al.*, 1977b).

REFERENCES

ABE, H., TAKAUJI, M., TAKAHASHI, H., and NAGAI, T. 1963. Uber das erschlaffungsftorsystem der herzmusklatur. Biochim. Biophys. Acta 71:7–14.

CARSTEN, M. E. 1964. The cardiac calcium pump. Proc. Natl. Acad. Sci. (USA) 52: 1456–1462.

EBASHI, S., and ENDO, M. 1968. Calcium ion and muscle contraction. Prog. Biophys. 18:123–183.

ENDO, M., and NAKAJIMA, Y. 1973. Release of calcium induced by "depolarization" of the sarcoplasmic reticulum membrane. Nature (NB) 246:216–218.

ENDO, M., TANAKA, M., and OGAWA, Y. 1970. Calcium induced release of calcium from the sarcoplasmic reticulum of skinned skeletal muscle fibers. Nature (Lond.) 228:34–36.

FANBURG, B., and GERGELY, J. 1965. Studies on adenosine triphosphate-supported calcium accumulation by cardiac subcellular particles. J. Biol. Chem. 240:2721–2728.

FANBURG, B., and MATSUSHITA, S. 1973. Phosphorylated intermediate of ATPase of isolated cardiac sarcoplasmic reticulum. J. Mol. Cell. Cardiol. 5:111–115.

FORD, R. E., and PODOLSKY, R. J. 1970. Regenerative calcium release within muscle cells. Science 167:58–59.

HARIGAYA, S., and SCHWARTZ, A. 1969. Rate of calcium binding and uptake in normal animal and failing human cardiac muscle. Circ. Res. 24:781–794.

HASSELBACH, W. 1961. Kontraktile strukturen des Herzmuskels und Kontraktionszyklus. Verh. Dtsch. Ges. Kreislaufforsch 27:114–125.

HASSELBACH, W. 1964. Relaxing factor and relaxation of muscle. Prog. Biophys. 14: 167–222.

HASSELBACH, W. 1972. The sarcoplasmic calcium pump. *In* H. H. Weber (ed.), Molecular Bioenergetics and Macromolecular Biochemistry, pp. 149–171. Springer-Verlag, Berlin.

HASSELBACH, W., FIEHN, W., MAKINOSE, M., and MIGALA, A. J. 1969. Calcium fluxes across isolated sarcoplasmic membranes in the presence and absence of ATP. *In* D. C. Toteson (ed.), The Molecular Basis of Membrane Function, pp. 299–316. Prentice-Hall, Inc., Englewood Cliffs, N.J.

INESI, G. 1972. Active transport of calcium ion in sarcoplasmic membranes. Annu. Rev. Biophys. Bioeng. 1:191–210.

INESI, G., EBASHI, S., and WATANABE, S. 1964. Preparation of vesicular relaxing factor from bovine heart tissue. Amer. J. Physiol. 207:1339–1344.

KATZ, A. M., DUNNETT, J., REPKE, E. I., and HASSELBACH, W. 1976. Control of calcium permeability in the sarcoplasmic reticulum. FEBS Letters 67:207–208.

KATZ, A. M., and REPKE, D. I. 1967. Quantitative aspects of dog cardiac microsomal calcium binding and calcium uptake. Circ. Res. 21:153–162.

KATZ, A. M., and REPKE, D. I. 1973. Calcium transport by rabbit skeletal muscle microsomes ("Fragmented sarcoplasmic reticulum"). Biochim. Biophys. Acta 298: 270–278.

KATZ, A. M., and REPKE, D. I. 1973. Calcium-membrane interactions in the myocardium: Effects of ouabain, epinephrine and 3':5'-cyclic adenosine monophosphate. Amer. J. Cardiol. 31:193–201.

KATZ, A. M., REPKE, D. I., DUNNETT, J., and HASSELBACH, W. 1977a. Dependence of calcium permeability of sarcoplasmic reticulum vesicles on external and internal calcium ion concentrations. J. Biol. Chem. 252:1950–1956.

KATZ, A. M., REPKE, D. I., FUDYMA, G., and SHIGEKAWA, M. 1977b. Control of calcium efflux from sarcoplasmic reticulum vesicles by external calcium. J. Biol. Chem. 252:4210–4214.

KATZ, A. M., REPKE, D. I., UPSHAW, J. E., and POLASCKI, M. A. 1970. Characterization of dog cardiac microsomes. Use of zonal centrifugation to fractionate fragmented sarcoplasmic reticulum, (Na$^+$-K$^+$)-activated ATPase and mitochondrial fragments. Biochem. Biophys. Acta 205:473–490.

KATZ, A. M., TADA, M., and KIRCHBERGER, M. A. 1975. Control of calcium transport in the myocardium by cyclic AMP-protein kinase system. *In* G. I. Drummond, P. Greengard, and G. A. Robison (eds.), Advances in Cyclic Nucleotide Research, Volume 5, pp. 453–472. Raven Press, New York.

MAKINOSE, M. 1973. Possible function states of the enzyme of the sarcoplasmic calcium pump. FEBS Lett. 37:140–143.

MARTONOSI, A. 1972. Biochemical and clinical aspects of sarcoplasmic reticulum function. *In* F. Bronner and A. Kleinzeller (eds.), Current Topics in Membranes and Transport, Volume 3, pp. 83–197. Academic Press, New York.

NAMM, D. H., WOODS, E. L., and ZUCKER, J. L. 1972. Incorporation of the terminal phosphate of ATP into membranal protein of rabbit cardiac sarcoplasmic reticulum. Correlation with active calcium transport and study of effects of cyclic AMP. Circ. Res. 31:308–316.

PANET, R., PICK, U., and SELINGER, Z. 1971. The role of calcium and magnesium in the adenosine triphosphate reaction of sarcoplasmic reticulum. J. Biol. Chem. 246: 7349–7356.

PANG, D. C., and BRIGGS, F. N. 1973. Reaction mechanism of the cardiac sarcotubule calcium. (II) Dependent adenosine trophosphatase. Biochemistry 12:4905–4911.

REPKE, D. I., and KATZ, A. M. 1972. Calcium-binding and calcium-uptake by cardiac microsomes: A kinetic analysis. J. Mol. Cell. Cardiol. 4:401–416.

SHIGEKAWA, M., FINEGAN, J. -A., and KATZ, A. M. 1976. Calcium transport ATPase of canine cardiac sarcoplasmic reticulum: A comparison with that of rabbit fast skeletal muscle sarcoplasmic reticulum. J. Biol. Chem. 251:6894–6900.

SUKO, J., and HASSELBACH, W. 1976. Characterization of cardiac sarcoplasmic reticulum ATP-ADP phosphate exchange and phosphorylation of the calcium transport adenosine trophosphatase. Eur. J. Biochem. 64:123–130.

TADA, M., KIRCHBERGER, M. A., REPKE, D. I., and KATZ, A. M. 1974. The stimulation of calcium transport in cardiac sarcoplasmic reticulum by adenosine 3':5'-monophosphate-dependent protein kinase. J. Biol. Chem. 249:6174–6180.

TONOMURA, Y. 1972. The Ca$^+$-Mg^{2+}-dependent ATPase and the uptake of Ca^{2+} by the fragmented sarcoplasmic reticulum. Muscle Proteins, Muscle Contraction and Cation Transport, pp. 305–356. University of Tokyo Press, Tokyo.

WEBER, A., HERZ, R., and REISS, J. 1966. Study of the kinetics of calcium transport by isolated fragmented sarcoplasmic reticulum. Biochem. Z. 345:329–369.

Mailing address:
Dr. Arnold M. Katz,
Division of Cardiology,
Department of Medicine,
University of Connecticut,
Farmington, Connecticut
06032 (USA)

Recent Advances in Studies on
Cardiac Structure and Metabolism, Volume 11
Heart Function and Metabolism
Edited by T. Kobayashi, T. Sano, and N. S. Dhalla
Copyright 1978   University Park Press   Baltimore

SUBSTITUTION OF PHOSPHATE FOR OXALATE IN THE STUDY OF CALCIUM ACCUMULATION AND RELEASE BY CARDIAC MICROSOMAL FRACTIONS

J. DUNNETT and W. G. NAYLER

Cardiothoracic Institute, University of London,
London, England

SUMMARY

Phosphate-supported calcium uptake by guinea pig cardiac sarcoplasmic reticulum has been shown to exhibit a pattern different from that of oxalate-supported calcium uptake. Ionophore-induced calcium release has been demonstrated following phosphate-supported calcium uptake. Rat cardiac sarcoplasmic reticulum has been shown to differ from the guinea pig in its sensitivity to ionophore.

INTRODUCTION

Various agents have been shown to increase the rate at which calcium is released from the sarcoplasmic reticulum following calcium binding in the absence of precipitating anions. These include a sudden increase in pH (Nakamura and Schwartz, 1970, 1972) and adding either Salygran (Martinosi and Feretos, 1964) or ionophoric agents (Entman *et al.,* 1972a and b).

None of these agents induced appreciable release of calcium following oxalate-supported calcium uptake.

Experiments have been carried out in which phosphate has been substituted for oxalate and release has been induced by the ionophore A 23187, which is a specific carrier for divalent cations.

METHODS

Microsomal fractions rich in sarcoplasmic reticulum were isolated from guinea pig and rat hearts, as described previously (Nayler, Dunnett, and Berry, 1975). Protein was estimated by the method of Lowry *et al.* (1951) and standardized against crystalline bovine serum albumin.

These investigations were supported by grants in aid from the Medical Research Council of Great Britain and the British Heart Foundation.

Calcium accumulation was measured by the spectrophotometric method, using murexide as indicator.

The incubated medium contained 100 mM KCl, 11 mM MgCl$_2$, 20 mM Tris-maleate (pH 6.8), 1 mM Na$_2$ ATP, 30 or 60 μM CaCl, 60 μM murexide, and 0.25 mg/ml microsomal protein. Where indicated, 5 mM K phosphate or 5 mM K oxalate were included. The reaction was carried out at 37° C and was started by adding ATP. The ionophore A 23187 was dissolved in alcohol. After completion of Ca^{2+} accumulation, but before the onset of any spontaneous release, ionophore was added to a final concentration of 0.1 − 2 μM (0.22 − 4.4 μg/mg protein). Alcohol controls were included, and allowance was made for any deflection caused by ATP or ionophore.

Because the ionophore-induced release of calcium is extremely rapid, no attempt was made to measure the rate of Ca^{2+} release. The results are expressed in terms of total amounts of Ca accumulated and released, in nmol Ca^{2+}/mg microsomal protein. Results are means ± S.E.M. The results were analyzed for significance either by the Students t-test, or, where applicable, the paired t-test, using $p = 0.05$ as the limit of significance.

RESULTS

Under the conditions used in the present experiments, guinea pig microsomes bound 45 ± 2 nmol Ca^{2+}/mg protein. Some of this Ca^{2+} was eventually released spontaneously, but at a relatively slow rate (7.4 ± 0.63 nmol Ca^{2+}/mg protein/min).

In the presence of 5 mM K oxalate, guinea pig microsomes took up Ca^{2+} to a much larger extent. This uptake process characteristically showed three different phases—an initial rapid rate, probably representing Ca^{2+} binding, a slower lag phase, and a third linear rate of Ca^{2+} accumulation representing the precipitation of Ca^{2+} as calcium oxalate within the vesicles of the sarcoplasmic reticulum. When guinea pig microsomes accumulate Ca^{2+} in the presence of 5 mM K phosphate, although more Ca^{2+} is accumulated than by the binding process (76.4 ± 1.2 nmol/mg), the three-phase pattern of accumulation seen in the presence of oxalate was not observed.

A rapid release of Ca^{2+} following Ca^{2+} binding was observed on addition of A 23187. Ca^{2+} was also released by the ionophore after Ca^{2+} uptake in the presence of 5 mM K phosphate. However, very little release was observed after uptake of Ca^{2+} in the presence of 5 mM K oxalate, even at relatively high concentrations of the ionophore. The results given in Figure 1 show the percentage of accumulated Ca^{2+} released by various concentrations of ionophore.

At a concentration of ionophore of 2 μM, all the accumulated Ca^{2+} is released after Ca^{2+} binding, and after Ca^{2+} uptake with 5 mM K phosphate.

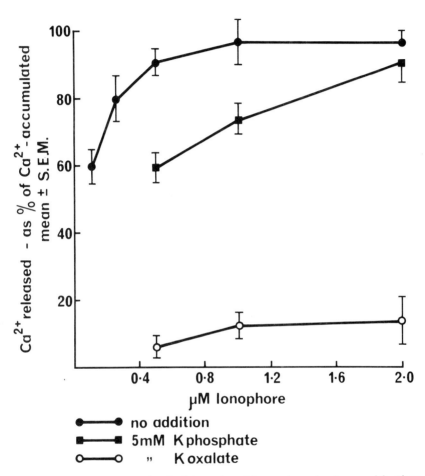

IONOPHORE-INDUCED Ca²⁺ RELEASE FROM GUINEA PIG CARDIAC MICROSOMES

Figure 1. Percentage of accumulated calcium released from guinea pig microsomal fractions by varying concentration of the ionophore A 23187 after calcium binding, and phosphate- or oxalate-supported calcium uptake, as indicated. Experimental conditions as described in the text.

However, only a very small percentage of Ca^{2+} taken up in the presence of 5 mM K oxalate is released, and this is subsequently reaccumulated. The amount of Ca^{2+} taken up and subsequently released by A 23187 in the presence of K phosphate is not affected by increasing the phosphate concentration up to 20 mM phosphate. Increasing the Ca^{2+} concentration did not significantly increase the amount of Ca^{2+} taken up and released in the presence of phosphate. However, uptake in the presence of oxalate was greatly increased by doubling the Ca^{2+} concentration, but the amount of Ca^{2+} released by the ionophore was the same at both Ca^{2+} concentrations.

In the rat cardiac microsomal fraction, Ca^{2+} binding is rapid and is followed by the early onset of a relatively rapid spontaneous release phase. Phosphate-supported Ca^{2+} uptake is similar to Ca^{2+} binding in this species, but the release phase, although slower, is still present. The rat microsomal fraction also

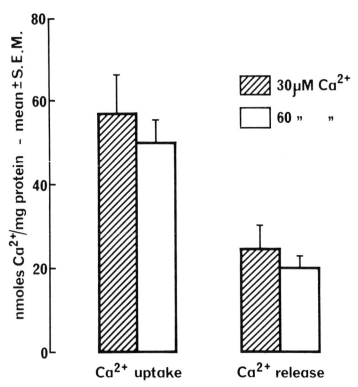

UPTAKE AND RELEASE OF Ca^{2+} BY *RAT* CARDIAC MICROSOMES IN PRESENCE OF 5mM K OXALATE

Figure 2. Oxalate-supported calcium uptake by rat cardiac microsomal fractions, and calcium release following oxalate-supported uptake induced by the ionophore 23187 at a concentration of 2 μM (4.4 μg/mg protein). Calcium concentration 30 or 60 μM, as indicated. Other experimental conditions as described in the text.

has a very limited ability to accumulate Ca^{2+} in the presence of oxalate, and the three-phase pattern of uptake seen in the guinea pig microsomal fraction is absent. The rat microsomal fraction responds in a similar way to A 23187. Calcium accumulated by the binding process and by phosphate-supported calcium uptake is completely and rapidly released at low ionophore concentrations. Of calcium taken up in the presence of oxalate, 43.3% is released by 2 μM ionophore, which is similar in amount to that released in the guinea pig (Figure 2).

DISCUSSION

The absence of a three-phase pattern of phosphate-supported calcium uptake probably represents the higher solubility product of calcium phosphate compared to calcium oxalate, which would prevent the precipitation of calcium phosphate inside the sarcoplasmic reticulum. This could also account for the more rapid release of calcium after phosphate-supported calcium uptake, indicating that the calcium is in a more releasable form than when uptake is supported by oxalate. The very limited calcium release after oxalate-supported calcium uptake may also reflect the low outside calcium concentration.

The altered ability of the rat sarcoplasmic reticulum to accumulate calcium may reflect differences in the permeability of the rat cardiac sarcoplasmic reticulum compared to the guinea pig, or it may be due to an impairment of the transport mechanism.

Acknowledgment   We thank Eli Lilly for the gift of the ionophore.

REFERENCES

ENTMAN, M. L., ALLEN, J. C. BORNET, E. P., GILLETTE, P. C., WALLICK, E. T., and SCHWARTZ, A. 1972a. Mechanisms of calcium accumulation and transport in cardiac relaxing system (sarcoplasmic reticulum membranes): Effects of verapamil, D600, X537A and A 23187. J. Mol. Cell. Cardiol. 4:681–687.

ENTMAN, M. L., GILLETTE, P. C., WALLICK, E. T., PRESSMAN, B. C., and SCHWARTZ, A. 1972b. A study of calcium binding and uptake by isolated cardiac sarcoplasmic reticulum: The use of a new ionophore (X537A). Biochem. Biophys. Res. Commun. 48:847–853.

LOWRY, O. H., ROSEBOUGH, N. J., FARR, H. L., and RANDALL, R. J. 1951. Protein measurement with folin phenol reagent. J. Biol. Chem. 193:265–275.

MARTINOSI, A., and FERETOS, R. 1964. Sarcoplasmic reticulum I. The uptake of Ca^{2+} by sarcoplasmic reticulum fragments. J. Biol. Chem. 239:648–658.

NAKAMURA, Y., and SCHWARTZ, A. 1970. Possible control of intracellular calcium metabolism by $[H^+]$. Sarcoplasmic reticulum of skeletal and cardiac muscle. Biochem. Biophys. Res. Commun. 41:830–836.

NAKAMURA, Y., and SCHWARTZ, A. 1972. The influence of hydrogen ion concentration on calcium binding and release by skeletal muscle sarcoplasmic reticulum. J. Gen. Physiol. 59:22–32.

NAYLER, W. G., DUNNETT, S. J., and BERRY, D. 1975. The calcium accumulating activity of subcellular fractions isolated from rat and guinea pig heart muscle. J. Mol. Cell. Cardiol. 7:275–285.

Mailing address:
J. Dunnett,
Cardiothoracic Institute,
University of London,
2 Beaumont Street,
London, W1N 2DX (England).

Recent Advances in Studies on
Cardiac Structure and Metabolism, Volume 11
Heart Function and Metabolism
Edited by T. Kobayashi, T. Sano, and N. S. Dhalla
Copyright 1978   University Park Press   Baltimore

INTACT VESICLES OF MEMBRANES IN CARDIAC MICROSOMES: EVIDENCE FROM VECTORIAL PROPERTIES OF INTEGRAL ENZYMES

H. R. BESCH, JR., L. R. JONES, and A. M. WATANABE

Departments of Pharmacology and Medicine and the Krannert Institute of Cardiology,
Indiana University School of Medicine, Indianapolis, Indiana, USA

SUMMARY

The orientation and relative impermeability of vesicles of cardiac membranes were studied using microsomes isolated from tissue homogenized in dilute bicarbonate solutions (H_2O microsomes). Ouabain (10^{-7} to 10^{-3} M), which inhibits (Na^+,K^+)-ATPase from the extracellular face of the cardiac cell membrane, prevented only 5–10% of the stimulation of ATPase activity induced by optimal Na plus K concentrations, which reached 15–23 μmol Pi/mg protein/hr. Furthermore, K^+-stimulated phosphatase activity of ~ 1.0 μmol Pi/mg protein/hr was present, and was 85% ouabain-sensitive. Treatment of the microsomal vesicles with increasing concentrations of the detergent SDS increased the distribution space of [^{14}C]inulin to a greater extent than it increased that of [^{3}H]H_2O and rendered the Na^+,K^+-stimulated ATPase activity increasingly sensitive to ouabain without markedly diminishing the absolute magnitude of Na^+,K^+ stimulation. For example, after 0.25 mg SDS/ml, the Na^+,K^+ stimulation was 80 ± 5% ouabain-inhibitable ($\bar{X}$ ± S.E.M.; n = 4 preparations) whereas the absolute magnitude was decreased only 14%. Qualitatively similar effects were produced by deoxycholate. Activation of Na^+,K^+-stimulated ATPase in intact vesicles was stimulated by low concentrations of Ca^{2+}, the threshold for this effect being less than 10^{-7} M Ca^{2+}, and maximal effect occurring at about 15 μM Ca^{2+}. Detergent treatments abolished this Ca^{2+} effect but left the inhibitory influence of 0.1–10 mM Ca^{2+} concentrations intact. These results suggest that both right-side out and inside out vesicles of cardiac membranes are present in cardiac microsomes. Furthermore, augmentation of ouabain sensitivity of the (Na^+, K^+)-ATPase by detergents probably results from opening of permeability-intact vesicles.

INTRODUCTION

Canine cardiac microsomes have been prepared from sucrose homogenates and have been shown to contain enzymic activity from several different subcellular membranes (Katz *et al.*, 1970). A microsomal preparation made from dilute bicarbonate homogenates of cardiac muscle has been shown to be highly en-

Supported by Grants HL 06308, HL 14159, HL 05363, and HL 05749 from the National Heart and Lung Institute, by the American Heart Association, Indiana Affiliate, and by the Herman C. Krannert Fund. Dr. Besch is supported by the Showalter Research Trust Fund.

riched in sarcoplasmic reticular membranes (Harigaya and Schwartz, 1969). Such membrane fragments must assume the form of relatively intact vesicles of low passive Ca^{2+} permeability in order to exhibit high Ca^{2+} binding and uptake activities. If spherical vesicles of sarcolemma were also present in such a microsomal preparation, and if the membrane remained relatively impermeable to passive diffusion of ions, they might be suitable for studies of vectorial ion transport uncomplicated by intracellular membrane systems.

To search for such membrane vesicles, we looked for the putative sarcolemmal marker (Na^+,K^+)-ATPase, an integral protein that spans the membrane (Kyte, 1974), utilizing its known sidedness properties (Figure 1) to detect even the latent form of activity. Direct confirmation of the presence of latent (Na^+,K^+)-ATPase activity was achieved by unmasking the activity by judicious incubations with detergents.

METHODS

Membrane vesicles were prepared according to the method of Harigaya and Schwartz (1969), as modified for dog hearts (Besch *et al.* 1970). High Ca^{2+}

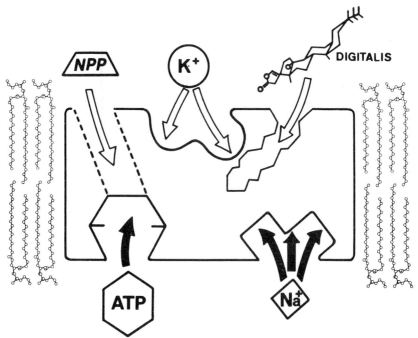

Figure 1. Heuristic model of (Na^+,K^+)-ATPase in a lipid bilayer membrane. Sites for interaction of NPP (*p*-nitrophenylphosphate), K^+ (potassium ions), and digitalis glycosides are oriented toward the exterior of the enzyme, whereas Na^+ (sodium ions) and ATP must interact with the interior face, sidedness being referenced to the intact cell.

binding activity was confirmed spectrophotometrically using murexide and/or arsenazo III, as previously described (Harigaya and Schwartz, 1969; Besch *et al.,* 1970; Besch and Watanabe, 1975; Besch, Jones, and Watanabe, 1976). Potassium-stimulated *para*-nitrophenylphosphatase (K^+-pNPPase) activity was measured as described by Skou (1974). For experiments in which the membrane vesicles were preincubated with the detergents sodium dodecyl sulfate (SDS) or deoxycholate (DOC), the method of Jorgensen (1975) was used. Basal Mg^{2+}-ATPase activity was defined as the rate of Pi release at $37°$ C in a basal buffer consisting of 3 mM $MgCl_2$, 50 mM DL-histidine (pH 7.5) and 3 mM Tris-ATP. The (Na^+,K^+)-ATPase activity was the difference between the basal Mg^{2+}-ATPase and that in the presence of 100 mM NaCl plus 10 mM KCl. Ouabain inhibitability of K^+-NPPase and of (Na^+,K^+)-ATPase activities were defined using 1 mM ouabain in the presence of maximally activating concentrations of cations.

RESULTS AND DISCUSSION

Broken segments of sarcolemma formed into relatively sealed membrane vesicles should not exhibit typical ouabain-inhibitable (Na^+,K^+)-ATPase activity, because both sides of the enzyme (Figure 1) would not be simultaneously exposed to the activating ions, substrate, and ouabain added to the incubating solution. However, such membrane vesicles [if formed right-side out (RO) with respect to the membrane in intact tissue] should be capable of hydrolyzing p-nitrophenylphosphate; this hydrolysis should be activated by K^+ and inhibited by ouabain. Such K^+-pNPPase activity was, in fact, found in the membrane vesicle preparations (Figure 2).

The substantial portion of K^+-pNPPase activity of up to 3.5 μmol Pi/mg protein/hr suggested that latent (Na^+,K^+)-ATPase activity should also be present. Moreover, ATPase activity of membrane vesicles formed inside out (IO) with respect to intact tissue should be stimulated by Na^+ alone, if K^+ is present within the vesicle interior. Consistent with this postulate, Na^+ alone stimulated ATP hydrolysis by about twofold over basal Mg^{2+}-ATPase activity (Table 1). This extra activity was largely insensitive to ouabain, presumably because this polar cardiac glycoside had poor access to its receptor site within the interior of IO membrane vesicles. It should be noted that a variable component of the activity stimulated by Na^+ plus K^+ (100 and 10 mM, respectively) was sensitive to EGTA (0.8 mM), suggesting that this may represent alkali metal cation stimulation of Ca^{2+}-activated ATPase. Sufficient contaminating Ca^{2+} (up to 15 μM) to support such activity was consistently found in this preparation.

If the Na^+,K^+-sensitive activity were a manifestation of (Na^+,K^+)-ATPase activity of IO membrane vesicles of sarcolemma, destruction of membrane integrity might allow full expression of ouabain inhibitability. Furthermore, simultaneous exposure of the interior of RO vesicles should provide increments in ouabain-inhibitable (Na^+,K^+)-ATPase activity. To render the membrane

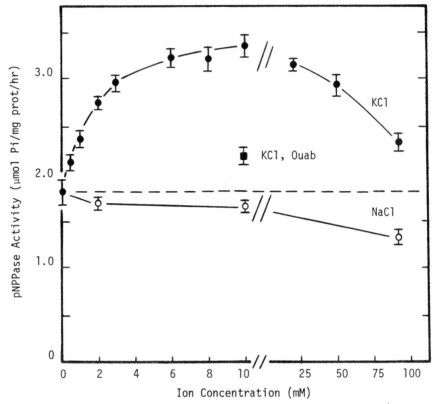

Figure 2. pNPPase activity in membrane vesicles, showing typical activation by K$^+$ (●), lack of activation by Na$^+$ (0), and ouabain inhibitability (■). Abbreviations used are pNPPase = *para*-nitrophenylphatase, and ouab = ouabain, the latter added at a final concentration of 1 mM.

Table 1. ATPase activity of membrane vesicles

Addition*	ATPase activity** (μmol Pi/mg protein/hr)
Mg^{2+} (Basal)	24.6 ± 0.6
+ Na$^+$	44.4 ± 0.7
+ Na$^+$,K$^+$	46.0 ± 0.8
+ Na$^+$,K$^+$ + Ouabain	43.8 ± 0.7

*The constituents and their final concentrations are: Basal: DL-histidine (pH 7.5), 50 mM; MgCl$_2$, 3 mM; Tris-ATP, 3 mM; NaCl$_2$, 100 mM; K$^+$, 10 mM; ouabain, 1 nM.

**Values given are means and S.D. of triplicate determinations.

vesicles leaky, preincubations with detergent were carried out and then aliquots were removed and assayed for both Na$^+$,K$^+$ stimulation and ouabain
inhibitability.

Increasing concentrations of SDS diminished the Mg^{2+} level of activity and
increased the percentage of the monovalent cation-stimulated activity inhibitable
by ouabain (Figure 3). Similarly, detergent pretreatment destroyed most of the
basal Mg^{2+}-dependent pNPPase activity. In contrast to the *apparent* destruction
of (Na$^+$,K$^+$)-ATPase activity of SDS preincubation, this detergent treatment
increased the total amount of K$^+$-pNPPase activity by about twofold (data not
shown). The increased activity (as well as most of the original K$^+$-stimulated
activity) was completely inhibitable by ouabain.

In summary, the presence of (Na$^+$,K$^+$)-ATPase activity in a cardiac microsomal preparation highly enriched in sarcoplasmic reticulum fragments has been

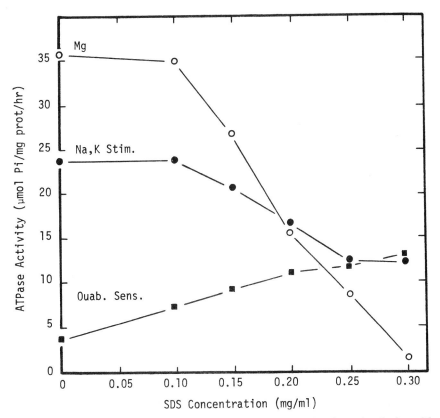

Figure 3. ATPase activity in membrane vesicles, showing activation by preincubation with
sodium dodecyl sulfate (SDS). Mg^{2+} activity, Na$^+$,K$^+$ stimulation, and ouabain sensitivity
(ouab. sens.) are defined in the text.

confirmed. Before pretreatment with SDS (or DOC, data not shown) the activity is almost entirely latent, expressing neither ATP hydrolysis nor [^{3}H] ouabain binding (Allen *et al.*, 1970). Consistent with these previous results, we have recently confirmed that in membrane vesicles prepared from hearts of dogs given lethal doses of ouabain there is no manifest (Na$^+$,K$^+$)-ATPase activity and it is not possible to activate (Na$^+$,K$^+$)-ATPase activity with simple SDS preincubation (Jones, Besch, and Watanabe, 1977). The results further suggest that latency of activity may be due to the presence of sealed, relatively impermeable vesicles of sarcolemma, if (Na$^+$,K$^+$)-ATPase activity is, in fact, a sufficient marker for sarcolemma (Schwartz, Lindenmayer, and Allen, 1975). The ratios of enzymic activities before and after activation are consistent with a ratio of inside out to right-side out vesicles of three.

Acknowledgments   We gratefully acknowledge the excellent technical assistance of Klaus Haisch, Bruce Henry, and Carol Robideau, and the secretarial assistance of Carol Holliday.

REFERENCES

ALLEN, J. C., BESCH, H. R., JR., GLICK, G., and SCHWARTZ, A. 1970. The binding of tritiated ouabain to sodium- and potassium-activated adenosine triphosphatase and cardiac relaxing system of perfused dog heart. Mol. Pharmacol. 6:441–443.

BESCH, H. R., JR., ALLEN, J. C., GLICK, G., and SCHWARTZ, A. 1970. Correlation between the inotropic action of ouabain and its effects on subcellular enzyme systems from canine myocardium. J. Pharmacol. Exp. Ther. 111:1–12.

BESCH, H. R., JR., JONES, L. R., and WATANABE, A. M. 1976. Intact vesicles of canine cardiac sarcolemma: Evidence from vectorial properties of Na$^+$,K$^+$-ATPase. Circ. Res. 39:586–595.

BESCH, H. R., JR., and WATANABE, A. M. 1975. Role of free calcium and ATP in calcium release from cardiac sarcoplasmic reticulum fragments. *In* A. Fleckenstein and N. S. Dhalla (eds.), Recent Advances in Studies on Cardiac Structure and Metabolism, Volume 5, pp. 143–149.

HARIGAYA, S., and SCHWARTZ, A. 1969. Rate of calcium binding and uptake in normal animal and failing human cardiac muscle. Circ. Res. 25:781–794.

JONES, L. R., BESCH, H. R., JR., and WATANABE, A. M. 1977. Monovalent cation stimulation of Ca^{2+}-uptake by cardiac membrane vesicles: Correlation with stimulation of Ca^{2+}-ATPase activity. J. Biol. Chem. 252:3315–3323.

JORGENSEN, P. L. 1975. Isolation and characterization of the components of the sodium pump. Quart. Rev. Biophys. 7:239–274.

KATZ, A. M., REPKE, D. I., UPSHAW, J. E., and POLASCIK, M. A. 1970. Characterization of dog cardiac microsomes: Use of zonal centrifugation to fractionate fragmented sarcoplasmic reticulum, (Na$^+$ and K$^+$)-activated ATPase and mitochondrial fragments. Biochim. Biophys. Acta 205:273–290.

KYTE, J. 1974. The reactions of sodium and potassium ion-activated adenosine triphosphatase with specific antibodies. J. Biol. Chem. 249:3652–3660.

SCHWARTZ, A., LINDENMAYER, G. E., and ALLEN, J. C. 1975. The sodium-potassium adenosine triphosphatase: Pharmacologic, physiological and biochemical aspects. Pharmacol. Rev. 27:3–134.

SKOU, J. C. 1974. Effect of ATP on the intermediary steps of the reaction of the $(Na^+ + K^+)$-dependent enzyme system. III. Effect on the p-nitrophenylphosphatase activity of the system. Biochim. Biophys. Acta 339:258–273.

Mailing address:
H. R. Besch, Jr., Ph.D.,
Departments of Pharmacology and Medicine,
Indiana University School of Medicine,
1100 West Michigan Street,
Indianapolis, Indiana 46202 (USA).

Recent Advances in Studies on
Cardiac Structure and Metabolism, Volume 11
Heart Function and Metabolism
Edited by T. Kobayashi, T. Sano, and N. S. Dhalla
Copyright 1978   University Park Press   Baltimore

SUBCELLULAR LOCALIZATION OF
CARDIAC ADENYLATE CYCLASE:
SARCOLEMMA OR SARCOPLASMIC RETICULUM?

L. R. JONES, H. R. BESCH, JR., and A. M. WATANABE

Departments of Pharmacology and Medicine and the Krannert Institute of Cardiology,
Indiana University School of Medicine, Indianapolis, Indiana, USA

SUMMARY

Adenylate cyclase was measured in cardiac microsomes prepared from dilute bicarbonate buffer (H_2O microsomes) in an attempt to determine the subcellular localization of this enzyme. Because H_2O microsomes exhibit high levels of Ca^{2+} binding but contain very low levels of ouabain-inhibitable (Na^+,K^+)-ATPase, they are commonly thought to represent a relatively purified preparation of sarcoplasmic reticulum (SR). Basal, epinephrine-stimulated (10^{-5} M), and NaF-stimulated (8×10^{-3} M) adenylate cyclase activity in H_2O microsomes from four separate preparations was 124 ± 32 ($\bar{X} \pm$ S.E.M.), 154 ± 33, and 541 ± 69 pmol/mg protein/hr, respectively. These values are comparable to those obtained with enriched fragments of sarcolemma (SL) prepared by other methods. Ca^{2+} binding in H_2O microsomes was $40-70$ nmol/mg protein, and ouabain-sensitive (Na^+,K^+)-ATPase was $0.5-1.5$ μmol Pi/mg protein/hr. Na^+,K^+ stimulation of basal Mg^{2+}-ATPase, however, was $15-20$ μM Pi/mg protein/hr, and the ouabain-sensitive component of this stimulation was increased from the original $5-10\%$ to 100% by treatment with detergent. The level of ouabain-sensitive (Na^+,K^+)-ATPase obtained after detergent treatment was twofold higher than the values commonly obtained from purified SL. Therefore, assuming that (Na^+,K^+)-ATPase is localized to the SL, lack of ouabain-sensitive ATPase activity from subcellular fractions clearly is not sufficient proof of the absence of SL from the fractions. The precise subcellular localization of adenylate cyclase must thus await purer preparations of SL and SR.

INTRODUCTION

The question of the subcellular locus of physiologically important membrane enzymes in myocardium has been addressed in several recent studies. Of special importance is the membrane-bound enzyme adenylate cyclase, which has been postulated to reside both in sarcolemma (Tada *et al.,* 1972; McNamara *et al.,* 1974; Watanabe and Besch, 1974; Tada *et al.,* 1975) and sarcoplasmic reticulum

This work was supported by grants HL 06308, HL 14159, HL 05363, and HL 05749 from the National Heart and Lung Institute, by the American Heart Association, Indiana Affiliate, and by the Herman C. Krannert Fund. Dr. Besch is supported by the Showalter Research Trust Fund.

(Sulakhe and Dhalla, 1973; Katz et al., 1974). We have measured the adenylate cyclase activity of cardiac microsomes in an attempt to determine the subcellular localization of this enzyme, by comparing its activity with the activity of (Na^+,K^+)-ATPase.

METHOD

Cardiac membrane vesicles were prepared from dog heart in dilute bicarbonate buffer according to a minor modification of the method of Harigaya and Schwartz (1969), as previously described (Besch et al., 1970). Ca^{2+} binding, adenylate cyclase activity, and ATPase activity were assayed as we have described previously (Besch, Jones, and Watanabe, 1976). The protocol for sodium dodecyl sulfate (SDS) activation of the (Na^+,K^+)-ATPase activity of membrane vesicles was identical to that previously used, the activating concentration of SDS being 0.30 mg/ml. In some experiments the membrane vesicles were further subfractionated by centrifugation through discontinuous sucrose in an SW27 swinging bucket rotor (Beckman Instruments, Inc.). Fraction A was collected at the 0.25 M/0.6 M interface, fraction B was recovered in the remainder of the 0.6 M sucrose solution, including all material to the 0.8 M sucrose interface, and fraction C was collected from the 0.8 M/1.0 M sucrose interface.

RESULTS AND DISCUSSION

Consistent with the results of others (Sulakhe and Dhalla, 1973; Katz et al., 1974), we have found cardiac membrane vesicles to exhibit high levels of Ca^{2+} binding, in the range of 50–80 nmol/mg protein. Figure 1 depicts the various manifest ATPase activities that we have identified in the same membrane vesicle preparation. In Buffer System A (optimal buffer for measurement of Ca^{2+}-ATPase activity) slightly more than half of the total ATPase activity was inhibited by EGTA, which demonstrated that the membrane vesicles contained high Ca^{2+}-ATPase activity (41.3 μ mol Pi/mg protein/hr, which was EGTA sensitive). Also measured in Buffer System A was an azide-sensitive ATPase activity (23.1 μmol Pi/mg protein/hr), which suggested that mitochondrial membrane fragments were present in the preparation. In Buffer System B (optimal buffer for measurement of (Na^+,K^+)-ATPase activity) the ouabain-sensitive (Na^+,K^+)-ATPase activity was found to be only 2.5 μmol Pi/mg protein/hr, and this activity amounted to only 3% of the total ATPase activity that was measured in this buffer. Therefore, the membrane vesicle fraction as assayed in the two buffer systems of Figure 1 contained 16 times more Ca^{2+}-ATPase activity (an enzyme marker for sarcoplasmic reticulum membranes) than (Na^+,K^+)-ATPase activity (an enzyme marker for sarcolemmal membranes). These results and the results with Ca^{2+} binding suggest that the preparation was

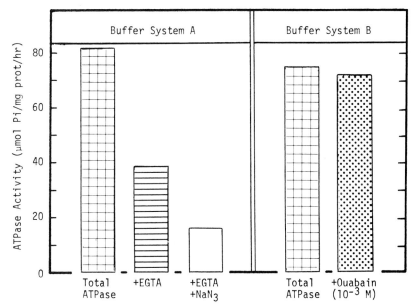

Figure 1. Manifest activity of cardiac membrane vesicles. Buffer System A contained DL-histidine, pH 7.5 (5.0 mM); MgCl$_2$ (3 mM); KCl (100 mM); and CaCl$_2$ (45 μM), with or without EGTA (0.8 mM). When used, NaN$_3$ was present at a concentration of 5 mM. Buffer System B contained DL-histidine (50 mM); MgCl$_2$ (3 mM); KCl (10 mM); and NaCl (100 mM) with or without ouabain (1 mM). Reactions were carried out at 37°C. Na$_2$ ATP was the substrate.

enriched in sarcoplasmic reticulum membranes and relatively depleted of sarcolemmal membranes.

Cardiac membrane vesicles also contained considerable adenylate cyclase activity (Figure 2). The basal activity was stimulated slightly by 10^{-5} M epinephrine and approximately fivefold by 8 mM NaF. These values of adenylate cyclase activity were similar to those found previously by us (Watanabe and Besch, 1974) and by others in various preparations designed to isolate sarcolemma (Tada *et al.,* 1972; McNamara *et al.,* 1974; Tada *et al.,* 1975). Because the membrane vesicle fraction was apparently low in sarcolemmal membranes, it is tempting to speculate that the measured adenylate cyclase activity resided in another membrane component, namely, membrane fragments derived from the sarcoplasmic reticulum (assuming that mitochondria do not contain adenylate cyclase activity). However, such a conclusion, though *perhaps* correct, we feel is premature. It is well known that (Na$^+$,K$^+$)-ATPase activity can exist as latent or masked activity (Jorgensen, 1975), and we have demonstrated previously that cardiac membrane vesicles contain considerable latent, ouabain-sensitive (Na$^+$,K$^+$)-ATPase activity (Besch, Jones, and Watanabe, 1976). This latent

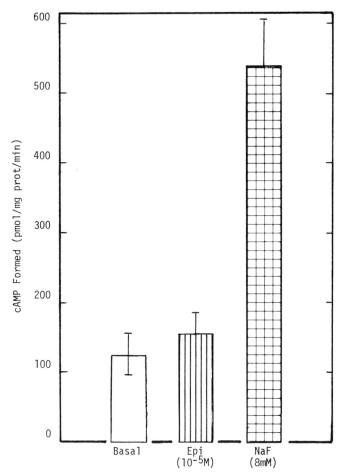

Figure 2. Adenylate cyclase activity of cardiac membrane vesicles. The incubation mixture consisted of Tris-HCl, pH 7.5 (40 mM); MgSO$_4$ (15 mM); KCl (5.5 mM) Na$_2$ATP (0.4 mM); theophylline (19 mM); phosphoenol pyruvate (20 mM); and pyruvate kinase (130 μg/ml). Reactions were carried out at 30° C. Results are $\bar{X}$ ± S.E. from six separate preparations.

(Na$^+$,K$^+$)-ATPase activity can be unmasked by treating the membrane vesicles with detergents such as SDS. Figure 3 demonstrates that before SDS exposure there was very little ouabain-sensitive (Na$^+$,K$^+$)-ATPase activity (1.9 μmol Pi/mg protein/hr) in another membrane vesicle preparation isolated identically to that used in Figure 1; after the same vesicles were exposed to SDS, however, the ouabain-sensitive activity increased eight-fold, to 16 μ mol Pi/mg protein/hr. At the same time the basal Mg^{2+}-ATPase activity was markedly inhibited. The simplest interpretation of this unmasking of latent ouabain-sensitive (Na$^+$,K$^+$)-ATPase activity by SDS is that this detergent destroys the relative impermeabil-

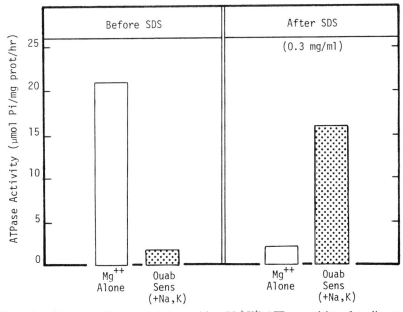

Figure 3. Activation of latent ouabain-sensitive (Na^+,K^+)-ATPase activity of cardiac membrane vesicles by SDS. Mg^{2+}-alone buffer contained DL-histidine, pH 7.5 (50 mM), $MgCl_2$ (3 mM), and Na_2ATP (3 mM). Ouabain-sensitive activity was measured in the presence of Buffer System B (see Figure 1 legend).

ity of sealed (and thus formerly unreactive) sarcolemmal vesicles. Therefore, when (Na^+,K^+)-ATPase activity is to be used as an enzyme marker for sarcolemma, all activity (manifest plus latent) should be measured to assess the content of sarcolemmal membranes.

The specific activity of the particulate (Na^+,K^+)-ATPase remaining after the vesicles had been exposed to SDS was even higher than that indicated in Figure 3, because after activation much of the total protein was solubilized and found to be devoid of measurable ATPase activity. Table 1 presents such data for another membrane vesicle preparation and also shows the effects of SDS on Ca^{2+}-ATPase activity. Before exposure to SDS, control vesicles showed 50 μmol Pi/mg protein/hr of Ca^{2+}-ATPase activity and only 3.7 μmol Pi/mg protein/hr of ouabain-sensitive (Na^+,K^+)-ATPase activity. After SDS exposure, 68% of the original protein was solubilized and released to the supernatant fraction. No Ca^{2+}-ATPase or (Na^+,K^+)-ATPase activity was demonstrable in the solubilized protein fraction. In the membrane sediment, however, ouabain-sensitive (Na^+, K^+)-ATPase activity was dramatically increased to 50.3 μmol Pi/mg protein/hr. This activity is five- to tenfold higher than (Na^+,K^+)-ATPase activities commonly reported in "purified" preparations of sarcolemma isolated from myocardium by other procedures (Stam *et al.*, 1970; Tada *et al.*, 1972; McNamara *et al.*, 1974;

Table 1. SDS enrichment of (Na^+,K^+)-ATPase activity and destruction of Ca^{2+}-ATPase activity*

Enzymic activity	Control			SDS sediment		
(Na^+,K^+)-ATPase	(−) Ouab. 38.5	(+) Quab. 34.8	Ouab. Inh. 3.7	(−) Ouab. 54.2	(+) Ouab. 3.87	Ouab. Inh. 50.3
Ca^{2+}-ATPase	(−) EGTA 75.3	(+) EGTA 25.3	Ca^{2+} Stim. 50.0	(−) EGTA 4.19	(+) EGTA 4.38	Ca^{2+} Stim. None

*One aliquot of vesicles (Control) was assayed in the usual fashion (see "Methods"). Another aliquot was preincubated in SDS (0.30 mg/ml) and centrifuged at 87,000 × g for one hour. Sixty-eight percent of the original protein was released to the supernatant and the remainder of the original protein was recovered in the sediment. Ca^{2+}-ATPase activity was assayed in Buffer System B, as described in Figure 1. Values are expressed as μmol Pi/mg protein/hr.

Watanabe and Besch, 1974; Tada *et al.*, 1975). Note that SDS completely destroyed all Ca^{2+}-ATPase activity, which was similar to the effect of this detergent on basal Mg^{2+}-ATPase activity, as depicted in Figure 3. Unfortunately, SDS preincubation also completely destroys adenylate cyclase activity in membrane vesicles.

In an attempt to determine the percentage of the total protein in the crude membrane vesicle fraction that was actually contributed by sarcolemmal membrane fragments, we have initiated studies toward purification of these latter membranes from the crude fraction (Table 2). The crude membrane vesicle fraction (MV) was centrifuged to yield subfractions A, B, and C, as described in the section entitled "Method." About 25% of the total protein applied to the gradient was recovered in these fractions. The distribution of Ca^{2+}-ATPase activity as depicted in Table 2 was not markedly enriched in any of the subfractions when their activities were compared to the activity of the crude MV fraction. These results suggested that sarcoplasmic reticulum membranes were not concentrated in those regions of the gradient that were analyzed. Ouabain-sensitive (Na^+,K^+)-ATPase activity (measured after vesicles were exposed to SDS), however, was markedly concentrated in subfraction A. The activity measured in this subfraction was 36.8 μmol Pi/mg protein/hr, or approximately 2.5-fold the activity measured in the crude MV fraction. Furthermore, the Ca^{2+}-ATPase activity of subfraction A was only 5% of the Ca^{2+}-ATPase activity of the crude MV fraction. These results suggested that subfraction A was highly enriched in membrane vesicles derived from the sarcolemma. If subfraction A were completely pure sarcolemma, then, of the total protein content of the crude MV fraction, 40% would have had to have been of plasma membrane origin (in order to account for the 2.5-fold enrichment of (Na^+,K^+)-ATPase activity that

Table 2. Partial purification of sarcolemma from cardiac membrane vesicles*

Fraction	Ca^{2+}-ATPase	(Na^+,K^+)-ATPase	
		$(-)$ SDS	$(+)$ SDS
MV	55.1	4.20	14.8
A	2.70	6.40	36.8
B	46.8	6.50	19.5
C	9.70	4.60	13.2

*Cardiac membrane vesicles (MV) and subfractions A, B, and C were prepared as described in "Methods." Ca^{2+}-ATPase activity and ouabain-sensitive (Na^+,K^+)-ATPase activity were assayed as in Figure 1. (Na^+,K^+)-ATPase activity was measured before and after membranes were exposed to SDS, as in Figure 3 (solubilized proteins were not extracted). Values are expressed as μmol Pi/mg protein/hr.

was measured in subfraction A). If subfraction A were only 50% pure with respect to sarcolemmal membrane, then 20% of the total protein content of the crude MV fraction would be contributed by sarcolemmal membrane. In either case, however, these results suggest that there is sufficient sarcolemmal membrane in the crude MV fraction to account for all adenylate cyclase activity. Techniques designed to further purify fragments of sarcoplasmic reticulum must therefore be found before it can be absolutely proven that any adenylate cyclase activity normally resides in sarcoplasmic reticulum.

Acknowledgments We gratefully acknowledge the technical assistance of Bruce Henry, Barbara Farmer, and Klaus Haisch, and the expert secretarial assistance of Carol Holliday.

REFERENCES

BESCH, H. R., JR., ALLEN, J. C., GLICK, G., and SCHWARTZ, A. 1970. Correlation between the inotropic action of ouabain and its effects on subcellular enzyme systems from canine myocardium. J. Pharmacol. Exp. Ther. 111:1–12.

BESCH, H. R., JR., JONES, L. R., and WATANABE, A. M. 1976. Intact vesicles of canine cardiac sarcolemma: Evidence from vectorial properties of Na^+,K^+-ATPase. Circ. Res. 39:586–595.

HARIGAYA, S., and SCHWARTZ, A. 1969. Rate of calcium binding and uptake in normal animal and failing human cardiac muscle. Circ. Res. 25:781–794.

JORGENSEN, P. L. 1975. Isolation and characterization of components of the sodium pump. Quart. Rev. Biophys. 7:239–274.

KATZ, A. M., TADA, M., REPKE, D. I., IORIO, J. M., and KIRCHBERGER, M. A. 1974. Adenylate cyclase: Its probable localization in sarcoplasmic reticulum as well as sarcolemma of the canine heart. J. Mol. Cell. Cardio. 6:73–78.

McNAMARA, D. B., SULAKHE, P. V., SINGH, J. N., and DHALLA, N. S. 1974. Properties of heart sarcolemmal Na^+,K^+-ATPase. J. Biochem. 75:795–803.

STAM, A. C., WEGLICKI, W. B., JR., FELDMAN, D., SHELBURNE, J. C., and SONNENBLICK, E. H. 1970. Canine myocardial sarcolemma–Its preparation and enzymic activity. J. Mol. Cell Cardiol. 1:117–130.

SULAKHE, P. V., and DHALLA, N. S. 1973. Adenylate cyclase activity of heart sarcotubular membranes. Biochim. Biophys. Acta 293:379–396.

TADA, M., FINNEY, J. O., JR., SWARTZ, M. H., and KATZ, A. M. 1972. Preparation and properties of plasma membranes from guinea pig hearts. J. Mol. Cell. Cardiol. 4:417–426.

TADA, M., KIRCHBERGER, M. A., IORIO, J. A., and KATZ, A. M. 1975. Control of cardiac adenylate cyclase and sodium, potassium-activated adenosine triphosphatase activities. Circ. Res. 36:8–17.

WATANABE, A. M., and BESCH, H. R., JR. 1974. Myocardial adenylate cyclase: Studies on the relationship of activity to purity of sarcolemmal preparation. J. Mol. Cell. Cardiol. 7:563–575.

Mailing address:
H. R. Besch, Jr., Ph.D.,
Department of Pharmacology,
Indiana University School of Medicine,
1100 West Michigan Street,
Indianapolis, Indiana 46202 (USA).

Recent Advances in Studies on
Cardiac Structure and Metabolism, Volume 11
Heart Function and Metabolism
Edited by T. Kobayashi, T. Sano, and N. S. Dhalla
Copyright 1978 University Park Press Baltimore

ISOLATION AND ENZYMATIC CHARACTERIZATION OF GUINEA PIG CARDIAC SARCOLEMMA

P. J. ST. LOUIS and P. V. SULAKHE

Department of Physiology, College of Medicine,
University of Saskatchewan, Saskatoon, Canada

SUMMARY

Sarcolemma was isolated by fractionation of salt-extracted particles on two consecutive sucrose density gradients. Salt extraction of homogenates, rather than of washed particles, was found to preserve the activities of adenylate cyclase and ouabain-sensitive $(Na^+,-K^+)$-ATPase in the isolated sarcolemmal membranes. Purified sarcolemma contained substantial adenylate cyclase and guanylate cyclase activities that were stimulable by β-adrenergic and muscarinic agonists, respectively. Significant ouabain-sensitive (Na^+,K^+)-ATPase activity as well as putative digitalis receptor activity was also present in sarcolemma. Cyclic nucleotide phosphodiesterases of sarcolemma, both cAMP- and cGMP-dependent, displayed positive cooperativity of substrate interactions; Ca^{2+} ions were found to increase the activity of the GMP-dependent enzyme.

INTRODUCTION

Numerous procedures have been used to isolate sarcolemma from cardiac tissue. Because of the relatively long periods of time required for some of these procedures, the preparations cannot be used in the study of labile activities such as adenylate cyclase and active Ca^{2+} transport, which are believed to reside in the sarcolemma. We therefore systematically investigated the possibility of developing a method for preparing cardiac sarcolemma in a high degree of purity and in which the enzymes of cyclic nucleotide metabolism as well as cyclic nucleotide/Ca^{2+} interactions could be studied. Both adenylate cyclase and (Na^+,K^+)-ATPase (ouabain-sensitive) were used as markers for sarcolemma because available data indicate that these enzymes are mainly located in the surface membranes of various tissues.

METHOD

Homogenates (10%, w/v) were prepared by mincing ventricles in 10 mM Tris-Cl, 2 mM dithiothreitol, pH 7.5 (T-D buffer), and treating with Polytron PT-10

The work reported here was supported by a grant received from the Saskatchewan Heart Foundation.

probe for 2 sec (on ice). Sarcolemma were isolated as described in Table 5. Enzyme assays were performed as described earlier (St. Louis and Sulakhe, 1976a; Sulakhe, P. V., *et al.,* 1976) and ouabain binding as described by St. Louis and Sulakhe (1976b).

RESULTS AND DISCUSSION

Extraction of Washed Particles with KCl

As shown in Table 1, recoveries as well as specific activities of (Na^+,K^+)-ATPase and adenylate cyclase were significantly better in washed particles isolated by the series II rather than by the series I method. However, extraction of either washed particle preparation by KCl caused a marked decrease in the recoveries and specific activities of these enzymes. Interestingly, substantial guanylate cyclase activity was associated with both washed and extracted particles.

Extraction of Washed Particles with LiBr

Table 2 clearly shows that brief extraction (up to 45 min) of washed particles with LiBr effected moderate purification of adenylate cyclase. Longer extraction times were less beneficial and in fact did not augment the solubilization of contractile proteins.

Extraction of Homogenate

Washed extracted particles prepared by brief KCl treatment of homogenates displayed reasonable recoveries of (Na^+,K^+)-ATPase, adenylate cyclase, and

Table 1. KCl extraction of washed particles*

	Series I	Series II		
Fraction assayed	(Na^+,K^+)-ATPase (μmol/mg/hr)	(Na^+,K^+)-ATPase (μmol/mg/hr)	Adenylate cyclase (pmol/mg/min)	Guanylate cyclase (pmol/mg/min)
H	1.63 (100)	1.49 (100)	189 (100)	44 (100)
WP	1.38 (38)	4.25 (104)	355 (79)	48 (62)
EP-A	2.27 (31)	N.A.	330 (40)	66 (40)
EP-B	2.72 (38)	3.15 (80)	321 (49)	54 (49)

*Washed particles (WP) were prepared from homogenates (H) by centrifugation at 1000, 800 and 500 (twice) $\times$ g for 10 min each with resuspension of residues in 10 vol of T-D buffer (Series I) or by centrifugation at 1500 $\times$ g for 10 min, residues being resuspended in 10, 15, and 20 (twice) vol of T-D buffer (Series II). Final residues (WP), suspended in 0.25 M sucrose in T-D buffer, were treated at 4°C with KCl to 1.25 M for 5 min (A) or to 0.5 M for 30 min (B). Preparations were then centrifuged at 40,000 $\times$ g for 1 hr and the residues washed by resuspension and centrifugation and suspended in sucrose T-D buffer to give extracted particles (EP-A and EP-B). Fractions were assayed as described in "Method." Numbers in parentheses represent percent recovery; N.A. indicates not assayed.

Table 2. Adenylate cyclase activity of LiBr-extracted particles*

Fraction	Protein (mg)	Adenylate cyclase (pmol/mg/min)	
		Basal	+ NaF
Homogenate	359 (100)	50 (100)	203 (100)
Washed particles	202 (56)	125 (140)	483 (135)
Extracted particles:			
0.32 M, 45 min	119 (33)	125 (82)	571 (93)
0.64 M, 45 min	65 (18)	169 (61)	824 (74)
0.80 M, 45 min	61 (17)	160 (54)	773 (65)
0.32 M, 4 hr	89 (25)	95 (47)	544 (67)
0.64 M, 4 hr	59 (16)	116 (38)	647 (52)
0.80 M, 4 hr	57 (16)	57 (18)	474 (37)

*Homogenate was centrifuged for 20 min at 1000 × g, residues washed twice and extracted with LiBr, final concentrations as indicated extracts were diluted to 0.2 M LiBr, centrifuged (20 min at 1500 × g), washed twice, and finally resuspended in buffer. 10 mM Tris-Cl, pH 7.5, was used throughout. Numbers in parentheses represent percent recoveries. Adenylate cyclase was measured in the presence of 8 mM NaF.

guanylate cyclase (Table 3). Furthermore, none of these enzymes showed inactivation due to salt extraction (compare Table 1). In other experiments it was observed that brief extraction of homogenates with other salts (KBr, KI, and LiBr, all 0.5 M) was equally effective.

Gradient Centrifugation

When washed particles (with or without salt extraction) were fractionated on a discontinuous sucrose gradient (40–65%, w/v) various particle zones were ob-

Table 3. Activities of particulate fractions from KCl-treated homogenates*

Fraction	(Na^+,K^+)-ATPase (μmol/mg/hr)	Adenylate cyclase (pmol/mg/min)		Guanylate cyclase (pmol/mg/min)
		Basal	+ NaF	
H	1.86 ± 0.18	129 ± 8	294 ± 31	51 ± 4
EP	5.06 ± 0.84	387 ± 23	635 ± 32	82 ± 11
	(49)	(67)	(66)	(53)

*Homogenates (H) in T-D buffer were treated with KCl (1.25 M final, 10 min, 4°). Residues were collected by centrifuging (9000 × g, 10 min) and re-extracted with 10 vol of 1.25 M KCl in T-D buffer (10 min, 4°). The suspension was centrifuged (4000 × g, 10 min) and the residues washed twice by resuspension and centrifugation and finally suspended in 0.25 M sucrose in T-D buffer to give washed extracted particles (EP). Assays were performed as indicated in "Method." Values are the mean of four experiments ±S.E.M. Numbers in parentheses indicate percent recovery where H = 100%.

tained. None of these showed selective enrichment of sarcolemmal marker enzyme activities. Washed particles prepared via KCl extraction of guinea pig ventricular homogenates gave four particle zones when fractionated on a discontinuous sucrose gradient (45–60%, w/v). The 50–55% sucrose interface fraction (F_3) showed moderate purification as well as substantial recoveries of sarcolemmal marker enzymes (Table 4). Guanylate cyclase distribution along the gradient paralleled that of adenylate cyclase and the entire procedure was equally effective with guinea pig and rabbit ventricles (Table 4) as well as with rat ventricles and dog atria and ventricles (data not shown).

We routinely used guinea pig heart and subjected F_3 to fractionation on another discontinuous sucrose gradient (50–60%) in order to increase the purification of sarcolemmal enzymes and also to decrease contamination by enzyme activities characteristic of other subcellular fractions. As described in Table 5, on the basis of marker enzyme activities the 52.5–55% sucrose interface fraction (F_{3C}) represented purified sarcolemma and was used in all our studies. With

Table 4. Enzyme activities in fractions from guinea pig and rabbit cardiac ventricles*

	Fraction	(Na^+,K^+)-ATPase (μmol/mg/hr)	Adenylate cyclase (pmol/mg/min)	Guanylate cyclase (pmol/mg/min)
A.	Guinea Pig			
	Homogenate	1.56 (100)	234 (100)	52 (100)
	Extracted particles	2.40 (56)	476 (69)	95 (59)
	Gradient fractions			
	F_1	0.75 (1.1)	119 (6)	45 (1)
	F_2	3.6 (10.1)	619 (25)	82 (17)
	F_3	4.05 (36)	904 (40)	112 (30)
	F_4	3.9 (2)	405 (3)	73 (2)
B.	Rabbit			
	Homogenate	4.38 (100)	349 (100)	58 (100)
	Extracted particles	4.52 (38)	533 (56)	95 (60)
	Gradient fractions			
	F_1	N.D.	145 (1)	34 (1)
	F_2	3.48 (5.6)	987 (20)	143 (18)
	F_3	5.61 (17.7)	831 (33)	133 (32)
	F_4	7.11 (1.2)	1018 (2)	155 (2)

*10% homogenates were treated with KCl (1.25 M) and washed extracted particles isolated as described for Table 3. Particles were applied to a discontinuous sucrose gradient (45, 50, 55, and 60% sucrose, w/v) and centrifuged at 40,000 × g for 1 hr. Fractions were removed by aspiration, diluted with T-D buffer to 10% sucrose, collected by centrifuging (15,000 × g for 15 min) and resuspended in 0.25 M sucrose in T-D buffer. Gradient fractions are designated by their interface location: F_1, sample–45%; F_2, 45–50%; F_3, 50–55%; F_4, 55–60% sucrose. Assays were performed as described in "Method." Numbers in parentheses indicate percent recovery. N.D., not detectable. Adenylate cyclase was measured in the presence of 8 mM NaF.

Table 5. Enzyme activities of isolated guinea pig cardiac sarcolemma*

A. Sarcolemmal marker enzymes

Fraction	Adenylate cyclase (nmol/mg/min)	Guanylate cyclase (pmol/mg/min)	(Na^+,K^+)-ATPase $(\mu mol/mg/hr)$	Specific ouabain binding** (pmol/mg/8 min)
H	0.24 ± 0.03	44 ± 5	2.05 ± 0.2	1.5
SL	2.80 ± 0.3	250 ± 20	10.50 ± 1.2	10.56
	(40)	(22)	(20)	

B. Other enzyme activities

Fraction	Succinate dehydrogenase $(\mu mol/mg/min)$	Cytochrome c oxidase (nmol/mg/min)	Acid phosphatase (nmol/mg/hr)	NADPH-cytochrome c reductase*** (nmol/mg/min)
H	7.04 ± 0.2	42 ± 2	426 ± 53	7.3 ± 0.40
SL	4.22 ± 0.1	25 ± 1	57 ± 7	2.5 ± 0.12
	(0.7)	(0.6)	(0.7)	(0.8)

*Homogenates (H) were extracted by treatment with KCl (1.25 M final for 10 min, 4°) and the residue obtained after centrifugation (9000 × g for 10 min) were re-extracted with 10 vol 1.25 M KCl in T-D buffer (10 min, 4°). The suspension was centrifuged (4000 × g for 10 min) and the residues washed twice by resuspension and centrifugation and finally suspended in 0.25 M sucrose in T-D buffer (sucrose T-D buffer). The washed extracted particles so obtained were fractionated by centrifugation in a discontinuous sucrose gradient (45, 50, 55, and 60% sucrose, w/v, in T-D buffer, pH 8.2) for 1 hr at 40,000 × g (see Table 4). The fraction appearing at the 50–55% sucrose interface was collected by dilution and centrifugation and further fractionated on a second discontinuous gradient (50, 52.5, 55, and 60% sucrose, w/v, in T-D buffer, pH 8.2). The fraction appearing at the 52.5–55% sucrose interface was collected by dilution and centrifugation and the final sarcolemmal pellet (SL) was resuspended in sucrose T-D buffer, pH 7.5. Values are the mean of five determinations ±S.E.M.; numbers in parentheses represent percent recoveries where homogenate = 100%. Activities for isolated mitochondria were 45.75 ± 3.0 (succinate dehydrogenase) and 189 ± 10 (cytochrome c oxidase), and, for isolated heavy microsomes, 13.2 ± 1.0 (NADH-cytochrome c reductase).
**Values are the average for two experiments and represent the $(ATP + Na^+)$-promoted binding.
***Rotenone-insensitive.

respect to adenylate cyclase activities, our procedure represents a significant improvement over other reported methods (McNamara *et al.,* 1974; Tada *et al.,* 1975; Williamson, Woodrow, and Scarpa, 1975) and is comparable to the procedure of Hui, Drummond, and Drummond (1975).

Interestingly, sarcolemmal adenylate cyclase exhibited some different kinetic properties compared to those reported by other investigators. Thus NaF decreased the affinity for ATP and increased the affinity for Mg^{2+} (St. Louis and Sulakhe, 1976a). Stimulation of sarcolemmal adenylate cyclase by β-adrenergic amines required the presence of GTP or of 5′-guanylylimidodiphosphate. Sarcolemmal guanylate cyclase revealed properties similar to those earlier described by us for the particulate cardiac enzyme (Sulakhe, P. V., *et al.,* 1976; Sulakhe,

Leung, and Sulakhe, 1976). The sarcolemmal guanylate cyclase was stimulated 35% by 10^{-9} M acetylcholine, and 10^{-5} M atropine partially blocked this stimulation. Sarcolemma contained both high and low K_m forms of cyclic nucleotide phosphodiesterases (St. Louis and Sulakhe, 1976a). Sarcolemmal phosphodiesterases displayed positive rather than negative cooperativity of substrate interactions; the cGMP-dependent form was stimulated by Ca^{2+} (St. Louis and Sulakhe, 1976a).

REFERENCES

HUI, E. C., DRUMMOND, G. I., and DRUMMOND, M. 1975. Isolation and characterization of plasma membranes enriched fractions from guinea pig heart. *In* G. I. Drummond, P. Greengard, and G. A. Robison (eds.), Recent Advances in Cyclic Nucleotide Research, Volume 5, p. 839. Raven Press, New York.

McNAMARA, D. B., SULAKHE, P. V., SINGH, J. N., and DHALLA, N. S. 1974. Properties of some heart sarcolemmal-bound enzymes. J. Biochem. 76:603–609.

ST. LOUIS, P. J., and SULAKHE, P. V. 1976a. Adenylate cyclase, guanylate cyclase and cyclic nucleotide phosphodiesterases of guinea pig cardiac sarcolemma. Biochem. J. 158:535–541.

ST. LOUIS, P. J., and SULAKHE, P. V. 1976b. Adenosine triphosphate-dependent calcium binding and accumulation in guinea pig cardiac sarcolemma. Can. J. Biochem. 54: 946–956.

SULAKHE, P. V., SULAKHE, S. J., LEUNG, N. L., ST. LOUIS, P. J., and HICKIE, R. A. 1976. Guanylate cyclase: Subcellular distribution in cardiac muscle, skeletal muscle, cerebral cortex and liver. Biochem. J. 157:705–712.

SULAKHE, S. J., LEUNG, N. L., and SULAKHE, P. V. 1976. Properties of particulate, membrane associated and soluble guanylate cyclase from cardiac muscle, skeletal muscle cerebral cortex and liver. Biochem. J. 157:713–719.

TADA, M., KIRCHBEGER, M. A., IORIO, J. M., and KATZ, A. M. 1975. Control of cardiac sarcolemmal adenylate cyclase and sodium potassium adenosine triphosphatase activities. Circ. Res. 36:8–17.

WILLIAMSON, J. R., WOODROW, M. L., and SCARPA, A. 1975. Calcium binding to cardiac sarcolemma. *In* A. Fleckenstein and N. S. Dhalla (eds.), Recent Advances in Studies on Cardiac Structure and Metabolism, Volume 5, pp. 61–71. University Park Press, Baltimore.

Mailing address:
Dr. P. V. Sulakhe,
Department of Physiology,
College of Medicine,
University of Saskatchewan,
Saskatoon, Saskatchewan, S7N OWO (Canada).

Recent Advances in Studies on
Cardiac Structure and Metabolism, Volume 11
Heart Function and Metabolism
Edited by T. Kobayashi, T. Sano, and N. S. Dhalla
Copyright 1978   University Park Press   Baltimore

CHARACTERISTICS OF HEART SARCOLEMMAL CALCIUM TRANSPORT SYSTEM AND EFFECT OF PROTEIN KINASE ON SARCOLEMMAL CALCIUM ACCUMULATION

P. V. SULAKHE and P. J. ST. LOUIS

Department of Physiology, College of Medicine,
University of Saskatchewan, Saskatoon, Canada

SUMMARY

Properties of the ATP-dependent calcium transport system of heart sarcolemma are presented. Calcium accumulation (with oxalate) in sarcolemma was increased due to cAMP-dependent protein kinase and phosphorylase b kinase. Protein kinase increased the V_{max} of the sarcolemmal calcium accumulation without any detectable effect on the affinity for Ca^{2+}. Both kinases failed to stimulate calcium binding. Protein kinase catalyzed phosphorylation of membrane proteins of molecular weights of 100,000, 25,000, and 14,000. Phosphorylase b kinase also catalyzed phosphorylation of these proteins. Protein kinase stimulated ATPase activity of sarcolemma. Sarcolemma contained endogenous protein kinase and protein phosphatase activities.

INTRODUCTION

Numerous studies have served to characterize calcium transport system of heart sarcoplasmic reticulum (SR). Although a role for sarcolemmal calcium transport system in the regulation of cardiac contractility has been suggested by many investigations, direct analysis of the ATP-dependent calcium fluxes in isolated cardiac sarcolemma (SL) is limited. Many workers have feared that contamination of isolated SL by SR is difficult to eliminate completely, and, therefore, biochemical analysis of the SL calcium transport system has been neglected for the past several years. Numerous procedures for isolation of cardiac SL are now available; however, most of these suffer from being rather harsh, and, further, many sarcolemmal activities, being labile, are inactivated or poorly preserved in the isolated membranes (Sulakhe and St. Louis, 1976). We have earlier reported isolation of cardiac SL in a high degree of purity (St. Louis, 1975; Sulakhe *et al.*, 1976a). About 40% adenylate cyclase, 22% guanylate cyclase, 20% (Na^+,K^+)-

---

The work reported here was supported by a grant received from the Saskatchewan Heart Foundation.

ATPase, and 5% cyclic nucleotide phosphodiesterases were present in the guinea pig heart SL (St. Louis, 1975; Sulakhe et al., 1976b; St. Louis and Sulakhe, 1976a). These membranes were observed to possess ATP-dependent calcium binding and accumulation activities. The kinetic properties of the SL transport system are described in this report. In addition, effects of protein kinase and phosphorylase b kinase on membrane phosphorylation, ATPase activity, and calcium accumulation in SL are presented.

MATERIALS AND METHODS

SL and SR from guinea pig heart ventricles as well as assays of calcium binding and accumulation (with oxalate), ATPase, protein kinase, and protein phosphatase are previously described (Sulakhe and Drummond, 1974; Sulakhe et al., 1976a). SL were phosphorylated by ATP in the presence of protein kinase (with and without cAMP) or phosphorylase b kinase (with and without Ca^{2+} as well as at pH 6.8 or 8.5) and the membrane proteins were separated by sodium dodecyl sulphate (SDS)–polyacrylamide gel electrophoresis (PAGE); the details of these are reported elsewhere (St. Louis and Sulakhe, 1977).

RESULTS AND DISCUSSION

Table 1 summarizes the kinetic properties of the SL and SR calcium transport systems. Besides the differences in parameters such as V_{max} and affinities for Mg^{2+} and ATP, the SR transport system can be distinguished from the SL transport system with respect to the saturability of the process. SL Ca^{2+} accumulation (oxalate-facilitated) was found to be saturable in the presence of high and low oxalate concentration in the assay, whereas SR transport system appeared to display saturation kinetics in the presence of low, but not high, oxalate concentration in the assay (St. Louis and Sulakhe, 1976b). It would be worth knowing if the differences in the permeability to oxalate in these membranes would account for these apparent differences. At any rate, our observations with guinea pig heart SR (St. Louis and Sulakhe, 1976a) confirm the reported findings of Li et al. (1974) on rabbit skeletal muscle SR.

Earlier we reported stimulation of the oxalate-facilitated calcium accumulation by protein kinase in cardiac sarcolemma (Sulakhe et al., 1976a). Here we show that phosphorylase b kinase also elicits the stimulatory effect (Figure 1). On the basis of effects of Ca^{2+} and cAMP as well as substrate (histone type II-A) specificity, phosphorylase kinase action is unlikely to be due to the presence of contaminating protein kinase (Table 2). SDS-PAGE analysis of protein kinase and phosphorylase b kinase preparations supports this view (not shown). Earlier, we reported that protein kinase–catalyzed phosphorylation of SL was hydroxylamine-insensitive (Sulakhe et al., 1976a). Table 3 shows that phos-

Table 1. Properties of ATP-dependent calcium transport systems of sarco-lemma and sarcoplasmic reticulum isolated from guinea pig heart ventricles

Parameter	Sarcolemma	Sarcoplasmic reticulum
Affinity for Ca^{2+} (μM)		
Minus oxalate	10–20	6–8
Plus oxalate (1 mM)	10–20	6–8
Plus oxalate (5 mM)	10–20	~400
V_{max} (nmol/mg/min)		
Minus oxalate	1–2	10–12
Plus oxalate (1 mM)	3–4	12–14
Plus oxalate (5 mM)	10–12	~200
Half maximal concentration of Mg^{2+} for Transport (mM)		
Minus oxalate	1–2	4–5
Plus oxalate (5 mM)	1–2	5–6
Half maximal concentration of ATP for transport (μM)		
Minus oxalate	90–100	14
Plus oxalate (5 mM)	170–180	300–400
pH Optimum		
Minus oxalate	6.8	6.5
Plus oxalate (5 mM)	7.0	6.5

phorylase kinase–catalyzed phosphorylation of SL was also mainly (75–82%) hydroxylamine-insensitive; about 18–25% of total phosphorylation represents the phosphoprotein intermediate of ATPase present in SL (Sulakhe *et al.*, 1976a). Hydroxylamine-insensitive phosphorylation of SL was also detected in the absence of exogenous kinase which was Ca^{2+}-insensitive (Table 4) and was likely to be due to the intrinsic kinase activity (Sulakhe *et al.*, 1976a). Protein kinase–catalyzed phosphorylation of SL stimulated (Ca^{2+}, Mg^{2+})-ATPase activity (Sulakhe *et al.*, 1976a); similar findings were also noted using phosphorylase kinase (not shown).

SDS-PAGE analysis of SL by Weber-Osborn as well as Fairbanks (Figure 2) procedures showed about 20 protein bands (of which six were prominent) of size ranging from 300,000 daltons to 12,000 daltons. In the presence of cAMP and protein kinase, 4 protein bands were phosphorylated; the sizes were 85,000, 60,000, 25,000, and 14,000 daltons. The 60,000-dalton band is likely to be due to the autophosphorylation of the protein kinase subunit. In the absence of cAMP, the 85,000-dalton protein was not phosphorylated. Using SDS-PAGE (6%), 200,000- and 100,000-dalton proteins were found to be phosphorylated, besides other protein bands mentioned above. Phosphorylase kinase also catalyzed phosphorylation of multiple protein bands of molecular weights

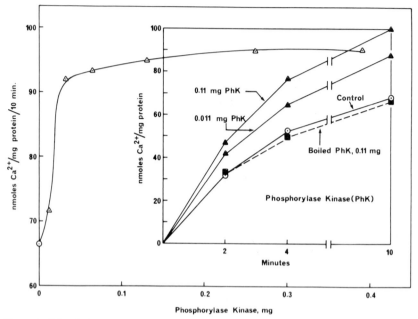

Figure 1. Stimulation of calcium accumulation by phosphorylase *b* kinase. Sarcolemma (270 µg) were preincubated in the reaction mixture (1 ml) containing 25 mM Tris-maleate (pH 6.8), 10 mM $MgCl_2$, 100 mM KCl, 5 mM K-oxalate, 5 mM sodium azide, 2 mM ATP, and varying amounts of phosphorylase kinase for 5 min at 30° C. The reaction was started by the addition of $^{45}CaCl_2$ (final 0.1 mM) and aliquots removed after 10-min incubation, filtered, washed, and counted. *Inset*—describes the time course of stimulation of calcium accumulation in sarcolemma in the presence of phosphorylase kinase.

95,000, 60,000, 40,000, and 25,000. Of these, the 95,000-dalton band was phosphorylated greater at pH 8.5 than at pH 6.8 and may represent contaminating phosphorylase *a*. However, this band was also phosphorylated at pH 6.8 and may represent phosphorylation of the ATPase molecule in SL. At pH 6.8, phosphorylation of the 95,000-dalton band was Ca^{2+}-insensitive, whereas at pH 8.5 it was stimulated (3- to 4-fold) by Ca^{2+} (50 µ M). In the absence of Ca^{2+}, phosphorylation of the 95,000-dalton band was greater at pH 6.8 than at pH 8.5.

Tada *et al.* (1975) have studied the phosphorylation of 22,000-dalton component of dog heart SR, which appears to play a modulatory role in calcium transport (Kirchberger *et al.*, 1974). Schwartz *et al.* (1976) showed that protein kinase catalyzes phosphorylation of 22,000-dalton protein in heart and slow muscle SR (also see Kirchberger and Tada, 1976). Using phosphorylase kinase, Schwartz *et al.* (1976) reported that 95,000-dalton protein in SR from all muscle types was phosphorylated and showed stimulation of Ca^{2+} accumulation. Krause *et al.* (1975) reported phosphorylation of 24,000-dalton protein in DOC-NaI-ex-

Table 2. Phosphorylation of histone by cAMP-dependent protein kinase and phosphorylase b kinase

		Phosphorylation		
Kinase	Ca^{2+}	−cAMP	+cAMP	Ratio
		(pmol of ^{32}P incorporated)		
PbK*	−	2.10	2.20	1.04**
	+	3.97 (1.89)***	2.97	0.75
PK	−	45.95	190.90	4.15
	+	31.48 (0.68)	76.16	2.42

*The reaction mixture contained 50 mM Tris-maleate, pH 6.8, 10 mM mercaptoethanol, 20 mM NaF, 5 mM EGTA, 10 mM MgCl$_2$, 100 μg histone (Type II-A), 30 μg phosphorylase b kinase (PbK) or protein kinase (PK), and 30 μM ATP (400 cpm/pmol). The reaction was started by the addition of [γ-^{32}P]ATP to the reaction mixture (preincubated at 24°C for 2 min) and was carried out for 4 min at 24°C. When added, Ca^{2+} was 50 μM (EGTA absent in the reaction mixture) and cAMP was 5 μM.

**The number denotes the ratio of activity obtained in the presence and absence of cAMP.

***The number in parentheses denotes the ratio of activity obtained in the presence and absence of Ca^{2+}.

Table 3. Phosphorylase b kinase-catalyzed phosphorylation of sarcolemma*

	Phosphorylation		
	minus Ca^{2+}	plus Ca^{2+}	Difference
	(pmol ^{32}Pi/mg sarcolemmal protein)		
Hydroxylamine-insensitive	7.62 (82)	11.53 (75)	3.91
Hydroxylamine-sensitive	1.67 (18)	3.91 (25)	2.24
Total	9.29 (100)	15.44 (100)	6.15
Total after chloroform: Methanol treatment	9.50 (102)	15.10 (98)	5.60
Total after 1 M NaOH treatment (24°C, 30 min)	3.02 (32)	3.83 (25)	0.81
Total after 1 M NaOH treatment (boil, 3 min)	0.67 (7.2)	0.92 (5.9)	0.25

*Sarcolemmal membranes (200 μg) were incubated in the reaction mixture containing 50 μg of phosphorylase kinase, 25 mM Tris-maleate (pH 6.8), 10 mM mercaptoethanol, 20 mM NaF, 10 mM MgCl$_2$, 5 mM EGTA, and 30 μM [γ-^{32}P] ATP (600 cpm/pmol) at 24°C for 5 min. When present, Ca^{2+} was 50 μM (EGTA absent). Reaction was stopped by the addition of 12% trichloracetic acid (TCA) containing 1 mM ATP and 1 mM inorganic phosphate, tubes were centrifuged, residues were washed (2X) with TCA and centrifuged and then resuspended in H$_2$O. Residues were then exposed to either 0.8 M NaCl (A) or 0.8 M hydroxylamine (B) for 30 min, reprecipitated with TCA and dissolved in 1 M NaOH and counted. The difference (A − B) represents hydroxylamine-sensitive incorporation, while that after treatment with hydroxylamine and NaCl represents insensitive and total phosphorylation, respectively. Residues were also extracted with chloroform: methanol (20:1) or exposed to NaOH, as shown.

Table 4. Phosphorylase kinase-catalyzed hydroxylamine-sensitive and hydroxylamine-insensitive phosphorylation of cardiac sarcolemma

Calcium	Phosphorylase b kinase	Phosphorylation*		
		Sensitive	Insensitive	Total
		(counts/min)		
−	+	1070	3700	4770
+	+	1900	5600	7500
−	−	1200	2050	3250
+	−	1840	2010	3850

*The details for assays were similar to those described under Table 3.

tracted microsomal preparations by the endogenous protein kinase. We have shown here that multiple proteins, including ATPase protein, are phosphorylated by both kinases. These observations clearly suggest that the mechanism(s) through which hydroxylamine-insensitive phosphorylation reactions influence Ca^{2+} accumulation in membranes are complex and will require detailed studies in the future for a better understanding. At the same time, the role of cAMP-dependent protein kinase—as well as of Ca^{2+}-stimulated phosphorylase kinase—catalyzed phosphorylation of membranes—in regulation of Ca^{2+} fluxes across membranes of heart muscle in basal and β-adrenergic amine-stimulated conditions deserves serious consideration.

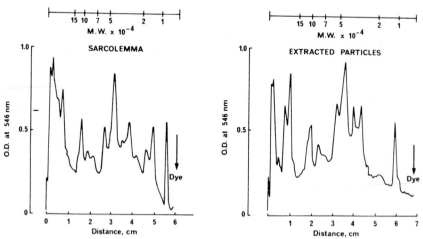

Figure 2. SDS-PAGE profiles of extracted particles and sarcolemma. Fractions were obtained by the method of Sulakhe *et al.* (1976), solubilized with SDS, and subjected to electrophoresis according to the Fairbanks method. After the run, gels were stained with coomassie blue, destained, and scanned at 546 nM.

REFERENCES

KIRCHBERGER, M. A., and TADA, M. 1976. Effects of adenosine 3',5' monophosphate-dependent protein kinase on sarcoplasmic reticulum isolated from cardiac and slow and fast contracting skeletal muscles. J. Biol. Chem. 251:725–729.

KIRCHBERGER, M. A., TADA, M., and KATZ, A. M. 1974. Adenosine 3',5' monophosphate-dependent protein kinase-catalyzed phosphorylation reaction and its relationship to calcium transport in cardiac sarcoplasmic reticulum. J. Biol. Chem. 249:6166–6173.

KRAUSE, E. -G., WILL, H., SCHIRPKE, B., and WOLLENBERGER, A. 1975. Cyclic AMP-enhanced protein phosphorylation and calcium binding in a cell membrane-enriched fraction from pig myocardium. In G. I. Drummond, P. Greengard, and G. A. Robison (eds.), Recent Advances in Cyclic Nucleotide Research, Volume 5, pp. 473–490. Raven Press, New York.

LI, H., KATZ, A. M., REPKE, D. I., and FAILOR, A. 1974. Oxalate dependence of calcium uptake kinetics of rabbit skeletal muscle microsomes (fragmented sarcoplasmic reticulum). Biochim. Biophys. Acta. 367:385–389.

SCHWARTZ, A., ENTMAN, M. L., KANIIKE, K., LANE, L. K., VAN WINKLE, W. B., and BORNET, E. P. 1976. The rate of calcium uptake into sarcoplasmic reticulum of cardiac muscle and skeletal muscle. Effects of cyclic AMP-dependent protein kinase and phosphorylase b kinase. Biochim. Biophys. Acta. 426:57–72.

ST. LOUIS, P. J. 1975. Biochemical characterization of sarcolemmal membranes (SL) of guinea pig ventricles. Proceedings of the Canadian Fed. Biol. Sci., Volume 18, p. 153.

ST. LOUIS, P. J., and SULAKHE, P. V. 1976a. Adenylate cyclase, guanylate cyclase and cyclic nucleotide phosphodiesterases of guinea pig cardiac sarcolemma. Biochem. J. 158:535–541.

ST. LOUIS, P. J., and SULAKHE, P. V. 1976b. Adenosine triphosphate-dependent calcium binding and accumulation in guinea pig cardiac sarcolemma. Can. J. Biochem. 54:946–956.

ST. LOUIS, P. J., and SULAKHE, P. V. 1977. Protein analysis of cardiac sarcolemma: Effects of membrane perturbing agents on membrane proteins and calcium transport. Biochemistry. In press.

SULAKHE, P. V., and DRUMMOND, G. I. 1974. Protein kinase-catalyzed phosphorylation of muscle sarcolemma. Arch. Biochem. Biophys. 161:448–455.

SULAKHE, P. V., LEUNG, N. L., and ST. LOUIS, P. J. 1976a. Stimulation of calcium accumulation in cardiac sarcolemma by protein kinase. Can. J. Biochem. 54:438–445.

SULAKHE, P. V., and ST. LOUIS, P. J. 1976. Biochemical properties and functions of isolated cardiac sarcolemma. In preparation.

SULAKHE, P. V., SULAKHE, S. J., LEUNG, N. L., ST. LOUIS, P. J., and HICKIE, R. A. 1976b. Guanylate cyclase: Subcellular distribution in cardiac muscle, skeletal muscle, cerebral cortex and liver. Biochem. J. 157:705–712.

TADA, M., KIRCHBERGER, M. A., and KATZ, A. M. 1975. Phosphorylation of a 22,000-dalton component of the cardiac sarcoplasmic reticulum by adenosine 3',5' monophosphate-dependent protein kinase. J. Biol. Chem. 250:2640–2647.

Mailing address:
Dr. P. V. Sulakhe,
Department of Physiology,
College of Medicine,
University of Saskatchewan,
Saskatoon, Saskatchewan, S7N OWO (Canada).

Recent Advances in Studies on
Cardiac Structure and Metabolism, Volume 11
Heart Function and Metabolism
Edited by T. Kobayashi, T. Sano, and N. S. Dhalla
Copyright 1978 University Park Press Baltimore

BINDING OF [3H]ATROPINE BY
CARDIAC PLASMA MEMBRANE-ENRICHED FRACTIONS

S. K. MA, P. V. SULAKHE, and N. L. -K. LEUNG

Department of Physiology, College of Medicine
University of Saskatchewan, Saskatoon, Canada

SUMMARY

The binding of [3H]atropine by the primary subcellular fractions and plasma membrane-enriched fractions from atria and ventricles of various species was measured by the Millipore filtration technique. Although all of the primary particulate fractions exhibited binding activities, the bulk of the total homogenate binding activity was associated with the washed particles sedimenting at the lower gravitational forces; this was observed with either atria or ventricles of dog, guinea pig, rabbit, hamster, and rat. Plasma membrane-enriched fractions isolated from the right atrium of guinea pig exhibited atropine binding activities with characteristics similar to dog atrial membranes; binding activity was moderately enriched in these membranes with respect to the starting material.

INTRODUCTION

The negative chronotropic and inotropic actions of acetylcholine are widely recognized. Furthermore, it is believed that acetylcholine initially interacts with specific muscarinic cholinergic receptors located on the surface membranes of atrial tissue. Recent studies have shown that guanosine $3':5'$-monophosphate (cGMP) levels in cardiac muscle are elevated in the presence of acetylcholine (George *et al.*, 1970; Watanabe and Besch, 1975). Some investigators (Goldberg *et al.*, 1973) have suggested that cGMP may mediate the physiological actions of acetylcholine on cardiac muscle. Investigations in our laboratory have shown the significant portions of the total homogenate guanylate cyclase activity of cardiac tissues (of various species) are present in the isolated plasma membrane-enriched fractions (St. Louis and Sulakhe, 1976a,b; Sulakhe *et al.*, 1976a) and that the stimulatory effects of acetylcholine and carbamylcholine on membrane guanylate cyclase are reduced in the presence of atropine, a muscarinic blocker. These findings suggested an involvement of muscarinic receptors in the regulation of guanylate cyclase (St. Louis and Sulakhe, 1976b). It was of interest to

The work reported here was supported by grants received from the Saskatchewan Heart Foundation and Medical Research Council of Canada.

know whether or not muscarinic cholinergic receptors are present in our membrane fractions. In this report we describe the binding of [³H]atropine to cardiac plasma membranes. The subcellular distribution of these binding sites in atria and ventricles of dog is also presented. Many physiological and pharmacological studies suggest that the density of muscarinic cholinergic receptors is greater in atria (especially right atrium) compared to ventricles (Higgins, Vatner, and Braunwald, 1973). However, negative inotropic effects of acetylcholine on rat ventricular muscle have also been reported (George, Wilkerson, and Kadowitz, 1973). The results presented in this paper show that the density of specific [³H]atropine binding sites in the right atrium is greater than in the left ventricle of various species.

MATERIALS AND METHODS

Materials

[³H]atropine (127–289 mCi per nmol) was purchased from Amersham/Searle; cholinergic agonists and antagonists from Sigma. Distilled deionized water was used to wash all glassware and plasticware.

Methods

The procedures for isolating primary subcellular fractions and plasma membrane-enriched fractions from atria and ventricles and for assaying adenylate cyclase, guanylate cyclase, and ouabain-sensitive (Na^+,K^+)-ATPase have been described in previous reports (St. Louis and Sulakhe, 1976a; Sulakhe et al., 1976a).

[³H]Atropine Binding Assay

The reaction mixture contained 116 mM NaCl, 2.1 mM KCl, 1.8 mM $CaCl_2$, 10 mM Tris-HCl (pH 7.2), cardiac particulate fractions (50–150 μg) and [³H] atropine (100–300 cpm/pmol) at the concentrations described under the appropriate table or figure. The mixture (final vol = 0.5 ml) was preincubated for 5 min at 30° C and the reaction was initiated by the addition of [³H]atropine and continued for 10 min at 30° C. Incubations were also carried out in reaction mixture containing 2 mM nonradioactive atropine. At 10 min, 0.3 ml of the reaction mixture was withdrawn and filtered through Millipore filters (0.45 μm) under mild suction. The filters were washed with 10 ml (5 ml × 2) of 1 mM atropine solution, placed in scintillation vials, dried at 60° C for two hours, covered with 10 ml of scintillation fluid and counted in a liquid scintillation spectrometer (Isocap 300A, Nuclear-Chicago). The efficiency of counting for tritium was about 35%. It was anticipated that the atropine binding by the crude particulate fractions would represent both specific and nonspecific binding. The assays were therefore carried out in the absence and presence of 2 mM (nonradioactive) atropine and the specific binding was taken as the difference in these values; all reported results refer to the specific binding. In addition, the filter discs were washed with 10 ml (5 ml × 2) of 1 mM atropine (nonradioactive) to ensure the removal of any atropine bound nonspecifically to the filters. It was established that the volume of the washing solution (1 mM atropine) must be at least 10 times greater than that of the filtered sample. Although some loss due to washing was unavoidable, this step was necessary for reproducible binding values. Using this assay procedure, the triplicates agreed within 5% under all assay conditions described in this paper; every assay was routinely carried out in triplicate.

RESULTS

The binding of [^{3}H] atropine to the particulate fractions was rapid and complete by 5 min of incubation at 30° C; this was observed with each of the various atropine concentrations tested in the assay (1 nM to 8 μM). The maximal binding was proportional to the protein concentration (up to 0.3 mg) in the assay, with both the washed particulate and membrane fractions of atria and ventricles of dog, guinea pig, rabbit, hamster, and mouse. The following observations were made with the plasma membrane-enriched fraction (F_3, see Figure 1) isolated from the right atrium of dog: Binding was optimal at a pH between 8 and 9; all assays, however, were carried out at pH 7.2. At an acidic pH, e.g., pH 5.5, atropine binding was reduced by 40%. Increasing the temperature from 0° C to 25° C increased binding from 15 to 24.5 pmol/mg/10 min (0.78 μM atropine in the assay); binding did not increase any further from 25° C to 41° C. Two binding sites were present; from the Scatchard plot, the binding constants were 2 nM and 1.5 μM for the high and low affinity sites with respective capacities of 2 and 80 pmol/mg/10 min (30° C). Bound atropine (labeled) was displaced by nonradioactive atropine; 50% displacement by 5 μM atropine (1 μM [^{3}H] atropine was present during the binding assay) while carbamylcholine, acetylcholine, norepinephrine, succinyl-, butyryl-, propionyl choline chloride, tubocurarine, and nicotine caused 50% displacement at concentrations greater than mM.

The distribution of atropine binding sites was studied in the subcellular fractions (particulate) isolated from right and left atria and right and left ventricles of various species. The results obtained with the dog heart are presented in Table 1. The specific binding was higher in the right atrial homogenate compared to the left ventricular homogenate. However, in all cases the bulk of the binding activity was present in the particulate fractions sedimenting at low gravitational force, e.g., 1000 × g; these fractions also showed modest enrichment in the specific binding activity relative to the respective homogenates. The 100,000 × g supernatant fractions contained negligible specific

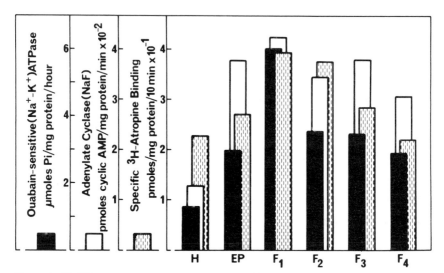

Figure 1. (Na⁺K⁺)-ATPase, adenylate cyclase, and [³H]atropine binding activities of fractions isolated from the right atrium of dog. Dog right atrial homogenate (*H*) (10%; Polytron PT-10, 6 sec, setting 9) was treated with KCl (1.25 M, 10 min at 0° C) and centrifuged at 9000 × *g* for 10 min. The residue was re-extracted with 1.25 M KCl for 10 min, centrifuged at 4000 × *g* for 10 min and washed (twice) by suspending in 10 mM Tris-HCl (pH 7.5) containing 2 mM dithiothreitol (T-D buffer) and centrifugation at 3000 × *g* × 10 min. The residue (washed extracted particles, *EP*) suspended in 0.25 M sucrose (in T-D buffer) was layered on a discontinuous gradient consisting of 7 ml each of 45%, 50%, 55%, and 60% sucrose (in T-D buffer) and the tubes were centrifuged at 40,000 × *g* for 60 min in an IEC (B-60) centrifuge (rotor # SB 110). The fractions (0.25 M − 45%; F₁; 45% − 50%, F₂; 50% − 55%, F₃; and 55% − 60%, F₄) were removed, diluted, and centrifuged at 40,000 × *g* for 60 min. The residues were suspended in 0.25-M sucrose (in T-D buffer) and assayed immediately. For adenylate cyclase, NaF was 8 mM; for atropine binding, [³H]atropine was 0.78 μ M.

atropine binding activity (not shown). The crude mitochondrial and microsomal fractions, although exhibiting atropine-binding activity, comprised altogether about 20% of the total homogenate atropine binding activity.

Plasma membrane-enriched fractions were isolated from the dog right atrium (Figure 1) and guinea pig heart (Table 2). Atropine binding activity was moderately increased in these fractions, and, as expected, these fractions showed enrichment in adenylate cyclase, ouabain-sensitive (Na⁺,K⁺)-ATPase (Figure 1, dog heart) and guanylate cyclase (not shown). We have previously described the enzymatic composition and the degree of purity of the plasma membrane fractions from the guinea pig heart (Sulakhe *et al.,* 1976b). The recovery of atropine binding activity was less than 3% in the pure (F₃C) sarcolemmal fraction (Table 2, Experiment II), containing 40% adenylate cyclase and 15% ouabain-sensitive (Na⁺,K⁺)-ATPase (not shown in the table).

Table 1. [³H] atropine binding by the primary subcellular fractions isolated from dog heart

Fraction assayed	[³H] atropine binding (pmol/mg/10 min)			
	Right atrium	Left atrium	Right ventricle	Left ventricle
Homogenate	9.07 (100)*	5.41 (100)	4.62 (100)	4.64 (100)
1,000 × g × 10 min-residue	10.24 (49.5)	6.90 (71.8)	3.15 (43.8)	5.27 (72.6)
10,000 × g × 20 min-residue	5.01 (10.5)	7.58 (16.2)	12.85 (21.0)	9.55 (17.6)
40,000 × g × 45 min-residue	4.26 (1.4)	5.73 (2.3)	8.60 (2.5)	9.77 (2.2)

*The number in the parentheses represents the percent recovery of binding sites; [³H] atropine concentration was 0.78 μM. Similar percent distributions were observed at 78 nM [³H] atropine.

Table 2. [^{3}H]atropine by the plasma membrane-enriched fraction isolated from guinea pig heart

	Experiment I		Experiment II	
Fraction	[^{3}H]atropine binding (pmol/mg/10 min)	Fraction	[^{3}H]atropine binding (pmol/mg/10 min)	
Homogenate	11.41 (100)*	Homogenate	16.74 (100)	
Extracted particles	19.88 (47.5)	F$_3$	21.13 (6.5)	
F$_1$ (0.25 M−45%)**	24.05 (1.0)	F$_{3A}$ (10%−50%)	93.92 (0.8)	
F$_2$ (45%−50%)	6.69 (4.3)	F$_{3B}$ (50%−52.5%)	29.13 (1.1)	
F$_3$ (50%−55%)	33.12 (9.8)	F$_{3C}$ (52.5%−55%)	32.70 (2.7)	
F$_4$ (55%−60%)	58.19 (0.8)	F$_{3D}$ (55%−60%)	50.62 (0.5)	

*The number in the parentheses represents the percent yield of binding sites.
**Indicates the location of the band at the sucrose interface.

DISCUSSION

We have measured [^{3}H] atropine binding by the Millipore filtration method. Our findings show that the specific binding is completed by 5 min at 30° C; nearly 70–80% of the maximal binding occurred at 2 min. We have detected two binding sites differing in affinity and binding capacity in plasma membrane fractions. For the subcellular distribution studies described, we used μM atropine in the assays, and hence these findings reflect the distribution of the low affinity sites. Although similar patterns of distribution were also observed when lower atropine concentration (10 nM) was used, the counts retained on the filters were rather low (less than 100), and hence further studies are underway, using atropine of higher specific activity and [^{3}H] quinuclidinyl benzilate (QNB), which shows a high affinity for muscarinic receptors (Yamamura and Snyder, 1974). As expected, [^{3}H] atropine binding was present in the plasma membrane-enriched fractions, although the yield of binding sites was low. Considerable loss in the recovery of binding sites was observed during the preparation of these membranes. A similar loss also occurred during the preparation of synaptic plasma membranes (unpublished observations), a finding in accord with other reports (Farrow and O'Brian, 1973).

Interestingly, the binding capacities of atrial homogenates were higher than those of ventricular homogenates of various species. These findings are in agreement with the physiological evidence concerning the relative distribution of muscarinic receptor sites in myocardial tissue. Earlier, we demonstrated an atropine-sensitive stimulation of the guinea pig cardiac sarcolemmal guanylate cyclase by acetylcholine and carbamylcholine (St. Louis and Sulakhe, 1976). In this study we show that [^{3}H] atropine binding sites are present in these membranes and suggest that these may be related to the muscarinic receptors present in cardiac sarcolemma.

REFERENCES

FARROW, J. T., and O'BRIAN, R. D. 1973. Binding of atropine and muscarone to rat brain fractions and its relation to the acetylcholine receptor. Mol. Pharmacol. 9:33–40.

GEORGE, W. J., POLSON, J. B., O'TOOLE, A. G., and GOLDBERG, N. D. 1970. Evaluation of guanosine 3',5'-cyclic phosphate in rat heart after perfusion with acetylcholine. Proc. Natl. Acad. Sci. (USA) 66:398–403.

GEORGE, W. J., WILKERSON, R. D., and KADOWITZ, P. J. 1973. Influence of acetylcholine on contractile force and cyclic nucleotide levels in the isolated perfused rat heart. J. Pharmacol. Exp. Ther. 184:228–235.

GOLDBERG, N. D., O'DEA, R. F., and HADDOX, M. K. 1973. Cyclic AMP. In P. Greengard and G. A. Robinson (eds.), Advances in Cyclic Nucleotide Research, Vol. 3, pp. 155–223. Raven Press, New York.

HIGGINS, C. B., VATNER, S. F., and BRAUNWALD, E. 1973. Parasympathetic control of the heart. Pharmacol. Rev. 25:119–155.

St. LOUIS, P. J., and SULAKHE, P. V. 1976a. Isolation of sarcolemmal membranes from cardiac muscle. Int. J. Biochem. 7:547–558.

ST. LOUIS, P. J., and SULAKHE, P. V. 1976b. Adenylate cyclase, guanylate cyclase and cyclic nucleotide phosphodiesterases of guinea pig cardiac sarcolemma. Biochem. J. 158:535–541.

SULAKHE, P. V., SULAKHE, S. J., LEUNG, N. L., ST. LOUIS, P. J., and HICKIE, R. A. 1976a. Guanylate cyclase: Subcellular distribution in cardiac muscle, skeletal muscle, cerebral cortex and liver. Biochem. J. 157:705–712.

SULAKHE, P. V., LEUNG, N. L., and ST. LOUIS, P. J. 1976b. Stimulation of calcium accumulation in cardiac sarcolemma by protein kinase. Can. J. Biochem. 54:438–445.

WATANABE, A. M., and BESCH, H. R., JR. 1975. Interaction between cyclic adenosine monophosphate and cyclic guanosine monophosphate in guinea pig ventricular myocardium. Circ. Res. 37:309–317.

YAMAMURA, H. I., and SNYDER, S. H. 1974. Muscarinic cholinergic receptor binding in the longitudinal muscle of the guinea pig ileum with [^{3}H] Quinuclidinyl benzilate. Mol. Pharmacol. 10:861–867.

Mailing address:
Dr. P. V. Sulakhe,
Department of Physiology,
College of Medicine,
University of Saskatchewan,
Saskatoon, S7N OWO (Canada).

Recent Advances in Studies on
Cardiac Structure and Metabolism, Volume 11
Heart Function and Metabolism
Edited by T. Kobayashi, T. Sano, and N. S. Dhalla
Copyright 1978   University Park Press   Baltimore

PROPERTIES OF MEMBRANE-BOUND
AND SOLUBLE GUANYLATE
CYCLASE OF CARDIAC AND SKELETAL MUSCLE

S. J. SULAKHE and P. V. SULAKHE

Department of Physiology, College of Medicine,
University of Saskatchewan, Saskatoon, Canada

SUMMARY

Kinetic properties of guanylate cyclase present in the washed particles, plasma membranes, and the soluble cytoplasm of heart and skeletal muscle are described; properties of the enzyme solubilized by Triton X-100 treatment of the particles or membrane fractions are also reported. It is apparent from the data that the membrane-bound guanylate cyclase in the cell may be regulated by acetylcholine, may exist as a metallo-protein with bound Mn^{2+} (essential for activity), and that Mg^{2+} regulates, whereas Ca^{2+} and nucleotides (especially ATP) modulate, guanylate cyclase activity. The findings also suggest that guanylate cyclase, similar to adenylate cyclase and (Na^+,K^+)-ATPase, is mainly located in the plasma membranes of heart and skeletal muscle.

INTRODUCTION

Earlier we reported that guanylate cyclase is mainly localized in the membrane fractions of heart and skeletal muscle of various species, although some activity was also present in the soluble cytoplasm (Sulakhe, P. V., *et al.*, 1976a). While both membrane-bound and soluble enzyme require Mn^{2+} for maximal activity, they exhibit several differences, e.g., number of nucleotide binding sites, effects of Mn^{2+} and Ca^{2+}, temperature, and nucleotides other than GTP as well as activation by non-ionic detergents (Sulakhe, Leung, and Sulakhe, 1976). When $MnGTP^{2-}$ concentration in the assay was held constant (but at subsaturating levels), both membrane-bound and soluble enzyme displayed similar kinetics when titrated with free Mn^{2+} (Sulakhe, S. J., *et al.*, 1976). Here we show that (1) the bulk of guanylate cyclase is particulate when the tissue is homogenized in several different ways; (2) when $MnGTP^{2-}$ and Mn^{2+} (free) concentrations in the assay are simultaneously varied, membrane-bound (but not the soluble) enzyme displays anomalous kinetic behavior; (3) pyrophosphate, an end-product of the guanylate cyclase reaction besides cGMP, stimulates the membrane-bound en-

The work reported here was supported by grants received from the Saskatchewan Heart Foundation and the Muscular Dystrophy Associations of Canada and America.

zyme; and (4) Mg^{2+} stimulates, whereas Ca^{2+} inhibits, the particulate (or Triton-dispersed) activity in the presence of low free Mn^{2+}.

MATERIALS AND METHODS

Isolation and Enzyme Assay of Fractions

The methods for the isolation of washed particles, supernatant fraction, sarco-lemma, and sarcoplasmic reticulum from heart and skeletal muscle (hind leg) of rabbit and guinea pig as well as the details of the guanylate cyclase assay, are previously described (Sulakhe, P. V., *et al.,* 1976a, 1976b; Sulakhe, S. J., *et al.,* 1976). Variations in the assay protocol are specified with the appropriate figure.

RESULTS AND DISCUSSION

The possibility that the particulate enzyme activity is due to the adsorption of the soluble enzyme was ruled out by the following observations:

1) When assayed in the absence and presence of Triton X-100 or Lubrols (P, PX, WX, etc.), 70 to 90% of the homogenate activity was present in the washed particles after the tissue (heart or muscle) was homogenized for various time periods (5 sec to 2 min) in hyper-, iso-, and hypotonic medium using Polytron (Brinkman), Omni-mixer (Sorvall), Duall or Dounce (Kontes), and Potter-type (various clearance) homogenizers. When the tissue was homogenized (Polytron, 2 min) in the buffer containing 0.1% Lubrol P-X, 75% of the homogenate activity sedimented in the 40,000 $\times$ g residue, which clearly shows that guanylate cyclase is firmly bound to the particles (membranes).
2) Kinetic properties of the particulate (or membrane) and Triton X-100 (1%)-dispersed enzyme were identical but different from the soluble enzyme (Sulakhe, S. J., *et al.,* 1976).

When titrated with varying amounts of GTP, the membrane-bound (and Triton-dispersed enzyme from membranes or washed particles) displayed anoma-lous (S-shaped) progress curves; the plots of reciprocal of velocity versus the reciprocal of (substrate)^2 were linear (Figure 1A). In contrast to this, soluble enzyme displayed Michaelis-Menten properties (Figure 1B). In these assays, both $MnGTP^{2-}$ and free Mn^{2+} were varied simultaneously. Interestingly, Mn^{2+} ions increased the V_{max} for both membrane-bound and soluble enzyme and de-creased the second-order dissociation constant for GTP of the membrane-bound (and particulate) enzyme. Similarly, when plasma membrane-bound enzyme from various tissues was titrated with Mn^{2+} in the presence of fixed GTP (total) concentrations, S-shaped curves were obtained (Figure 2); sarcoplasmic reticu-lum-bound cyclase resembled the sarcolemmal enzyme (Figure 3).

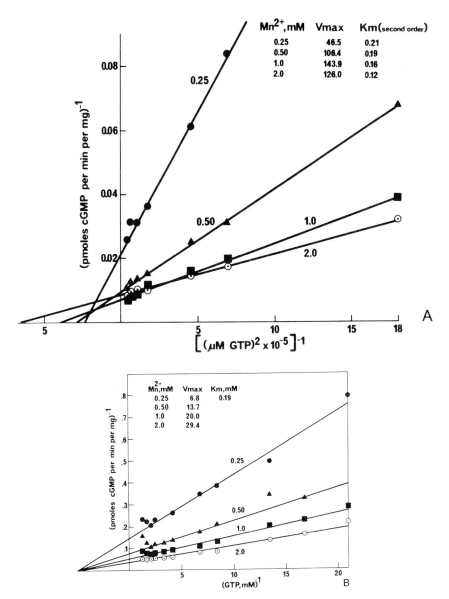

Figure 1. Titration with GTP. *A*, Solubilized fraction. *B*, Soluble fraction. Soluble (160 μg) and Triton X-100 solubilized fraction (50 μg) were incubated under standard assay conditions except that GTP concentration was varied as shown and Mn^{2+} was present at the concentration (mM) indicated by the number on each curve.

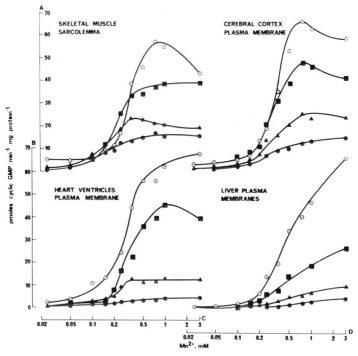

Figure 2. Titration with Mn²⁺ at several fixed GTP concentrations. Skeletal muscle sarco-lemma, 114 μg protein; heart plasma membranes, 59 μg protein; cerebral cortex plasma membranes, 93 μg protein; and liver plasma membranes, 114 μg protein. GTP concentra-tions were 54 μM (●), 102 μM (▲), 251 μM (■) and 490 μM (○). Skeletal muscle sarcolemma, *ordinate A* and *abscissa C;* cerebral cortex plasma membranes, *ordinate A* and *abscissa D;* heart plasma membranes, *ordinate B* and *abscissa C;* liver plasma membranes, *ordinate B* and *abscissa D.*

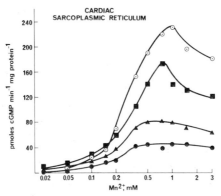

Figure 3. Titration with Mn²⁺ at several fixed concentrations of GTP. Cardiac sarcoplasmic reticulum (42 μg) was incubated under conditions described for Figure 2.

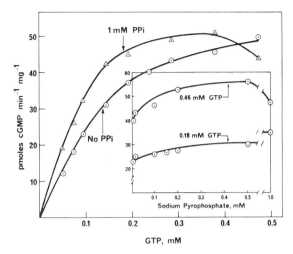

Figure 4. Effect of pyrophosphate. Skeletal muscle sarcolemma (102 μg) was incubated under standard assay conditions containing 2 mM Mn^{2+} and, when added, 1 mM sodium pyrophosphate. GTP concentrations were varied as shown. *Inset*—Sarcolemma were incubated under standard assay conditions containing 2 mM Mn^{2+}, 0.18 mM or 0.46 mM GTP, and variable amounts of sodium pyrophosphate, as shown.

Pyrophosphate (0.02 to 1.0 mM) caused a moderate stimulation of the sarcolemmal enzyme; the action of pyrophosphate was competitive with GTP (Figure 4).

Of interest to note is the finding (Figure 5) that Mg^{2+} stimulates the enzyme activity in the presence of low Mn^{2+} ($Mn^{2+} <$ GTP). However, when Mn^{2+} concentration is equal to or greater than GTP, stimulatory effect of Mg^{2+} was not observed, but instead an inhibition due to Mg^{2+} was seen; Ca^{2+} was also inhibitory (Figure 5*B*).

Regulation of guanylate cyclase in contractile tissues is not understood at present. Stimulation of the cardiac sarcolemmal enzyme by muscarinic cholinergic agonists, which is sensitive to muscarinic blocker, atropine (St. Louis and Sulakhe, 1976), the presence of specific muscarinic receptors in isolated cardiac sarcolemma (Ma, Sulakhe, and Leung, 1977), and influence of cholinergic agonists on the myocardial cGMP level (George *et al.*, 1970) suggest that *in vivo* guanylate cyclase could be regulated by acetyl choline. Although Mn^{2+} ions are most potent in catalyzing the enzyme activity, they are not present in such high amounts in the cell. It is likely that Mg^{2+} regulates the activity of this enzyme, which could exist as a metallo-protein with bound Mn^{2+}, whereas Ca^{2+} and nucleotides other than GTP, especially ATP, could modulate this enzyme activity.

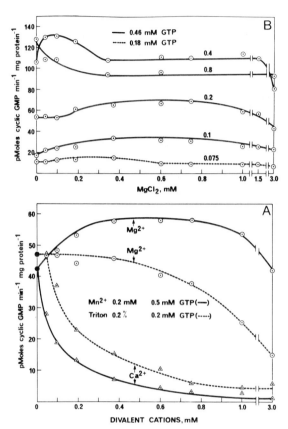

Figure 5. Stimulation of guanylate cyclase by Mg^{2+}. *A,* The solubilized enzyme preparation (80 μg) was incubated under standard assay conditions containing mM Mn^{2+}, shown by the number on each curve, and Mg^{2+}, shown on the abscissa. *B,* The solubilized enzyme (100 μg) was incubated in the standard assay medium containing 0.2 mM $MnCl_2$ and GTP (as shown). Concentrations of Mg^{2+} and Ca^{2+} were as shown on the abscissa.

REFERENCES

GEORGE, W. J., POLSON, J. B., O'TOOLE, A. G., and GOLDBERG, N. D. 1970. Evaluation of guanosine 3′,5′-cyclic phosphate in rat heart after perfusion with acetylcholine. Proc. Natl. Acad. Sci. 66:398–403.

MA, S. K., SULAKHE, P. V., and LEUNG, N. L. 1977. Binding of [³H]-atropine by cardiac plasma membrane-enriched fractions. *In* T. Kobayashi, T. Sano, and N. S. Dhalla (eds.), Recent Advances in Studies on Cardiac Structure and Metabolism, Volume 11. University Park Press, Baltimore.

ST. LOUIS, P. J., and SULAKHE, P. V. 1976. Adenylate cyclase, guanylate cyclase and cyclic nucleotide phosphodiesterases of guinea pig cardiac sarcolemma. Biochem. J. 158:535–541.

SULAKHE, P. V., SULAKHE, S. J., LEUNG, N. L., ST. LOUIS, P. J., and HICKIE, R. A. 1976a. Guanylate cyclase: Subcellular distribution in cardiac muscle, skeletal muscle, cerebral cortex and liver. Biochem. J. 157:705–712.

SULAKHE, P. V., LEUNG, N. L., and ST. LOUIS, P. J. 1976b. Stimulation of calcium accumulation in cardiac sarcolemma by protein kinase. Can. J. Biochem. 54:438–445.

SULAKHE, S. J., LEUNG, N. L., and SULAKHE, P. V. 1976. Properties of particulate, membrane-associated, and soluble guanylate cyclase from cardiac muscle, skeletal muscle, cerebral cortex and liver. Biochem. J. 157:713–719.

Mailing address:
Dr. P. V. Sulakhe,
Department of Physiology,
College of Medicine,
University of Saskatchewan,
Saskatoon, S7N 0W0 (Canada).

Recent Advances in Studies on
Cardiac Structure and Metabolism, Volume 11
Heart Function and Metabolism
Edited by T. Kobayashi, T. Sano, and N. S. Dhalla
Copyright 1978   University Park Press   Baltimore

SIGNIFICANCE OF THE MEMBRANE PROTEIN PHOSPHOLAMBAN IN CYCLIC AMP-MEDIATED REGULATION OF CALCIUM TRANSPORT BY SARCOPLASMIC RETICULUM

M. TADA[1]

The First Department of Medicine, Osaka University Medical School,
Fukushima-ku, Osaka, Japan; and

M. A. KIRCHBERGER[2]

Departments of Medicine, Physiology and Biophysics,
Mount Sinai School of Medicine of the City University of New York,
New York, New York, USA

SUMMARY

Phospholamban (molecular weight = 22,000), which serves as a regulator of Ca transport ATPase (molecular weight = 100,000) of cardiac sarcoplasmic reticulum (SR), becomes resistant to tryptic digestion upon phosphorylation by cAMP-dependent protein kinase (PK). The protective effect of phosphorylation is accompanied by persistence of the PK-induced stimulation of Ca transport. These findings indicate that structural alteration of phospholamban upon phosphorylation is closely associated with changes in the functional properties of cardiac SR.

SR from fast-contracting skeletal muscle of rabbit does not contain a 22,000-dalton substrate for cAMP-dependent PK, nor is Ca transport stimulated by exogenous PK. SR preparation isolated from slow-contracting skeletal muscle of rabbit and dog contains phospholamban, and Ca transport was found to be increased by exogenous cAMP-dependent PK.

In view of the distribution of phospholamban among different types of muscle, a hypothesis is presented to explain the relaxation-promoting effects of catecholamines in cardiac and slow-contracting skeletal muscle in which phospholamban is found. This may also account for the absence of a similar effect of catecholamines in fast-contracting skeletal muscle, which does not contain a similar substrate for PK.

This research was supported by the United States Public Health Service, contract NIH-NHLI-72-2973-M; grants HL-13191 and HL-15764 from the National Heart and Lung Institute; grant AA-00316 from the National Institute on Alcoholic Abuse and Alcoholism; and a Grant-In-Aid from Muscular Dystrophy Associations of America.

[1] Recipient of Japan Heart Foundation Research Grant and a Grant-In-Aid from Muscular Dystrophy Associations of America.

[2] Recipient of a Research Career Development Award from the United States Public Health Service, HL-00053.

INTRODUCTION

Our recent findings suggest that cAMP-dependent protein kinase (PK) produces a two- to threefold increase in the rates of both Ca transport and Ca-activated ATPase of cardiac sarcoplasmic reticulum (SR) through phosphorylation of phospholamban[3], a 22,000-dalton protein of cardiac SR (Kirchberger, Tada, and Katz, 1974, 1975; Tada *et al.,* 1974, 1975a, 1975c; Tada, Kirchberger, and Katz, 1976). Based on these findings, we have proposed a mechanism by which the calcium pump of cardiac SR is regulated through reversible PK-catalyzed phosphorylation of phospholamban (Kirchberger *et al.,* 1975; Tada and Kirchberger, 1975; Tada *et al.,* 1975c, 1976). This hypothesis may explain, on a molecular level, the actions of β-adrenergic agonists, which increase myocardial cAMP levels, on the mechanical properties of heart muscle.

This chapter reports further evidence that phospholamban serves as a regulator of Ca transport by SR of muscles whose contractile response is modulated by catecholamines. A unifying hypothesis to explain the relaxation-promoting effects and other related contractile responses that are produced by catecholamines in various types of muscle is proposed.

INTERACTION BETWEEN
PHOSPHOLAMBAN AND THE CALCIUM PUMP OF CARDIAC SR

Table 1 summarizes the properties of phospholamban and the Ca-activated ATPase of cardiac SR, both of which can exist as phosphoproteins. The ATPase is considered to contain high affinity Ca binding site(s) that are functional in the translocation of Ca from outside to inside the SR membranes when ATPase is phosphorylated to form the reaction intermediate, an acyl-phosphoprotein (MacLennan and Holland, 1975; Tada, Yamamoto, and Tonomura, 1978). The acyl-phosphoprotein intermediate of cardiac SR possesses characteristics essentially similar to those of skeletal muscle SR (Shigekawa *et al.,* 1976). The 22,000-dalton phospholamban can be phosphorylated by cAMP-dependent PK to form a phosphoester (Kirchberger *et al.,* 1974; Tada *et al.,* 1975a) and dephosphorylated by phosphoprotein phosphatase (Tada *et al.,* 1975b; Kirchberger and Raffo, 1977). Phosphorylation and dephosphorylation of phospholamban are accompanied by an increase and decrease, respectively, in the rate of Ca transport (Kirchberger and Chu, 1976; Kirchberger and Raffo, 1977). A protein kinase modulator has recently been found to play a role in the control of phospholamban phosphorylation (Ohmori *et al.,* 1977; Tada *et al.,* 1977).

Brief treatment of unphosphorylated cardiac SR with trypsin in the presence of 1 M sucrose has been found to digest phospholamban while leaving the

---

[3] The term "lamban" derives from $\lambda\alpha\mu\beta\alpha\nu\epsilon\iota\nu$ (=to receive), so that phospholamban may mean "a phosphate receptor."

Table 1. Comparison of the two phosphoproteins formed in the cardiac sarcoplasmic reticulum

	Phospholamban	Ca^{2+}-transport ATPase
1) Physiological function	Substrate for cAMP-dependent protein kinase and Modulator of Ca^{2+}-transport ATPase	Transports Ca^{2+}, which is directly coupled to the contraction-relaxation process
2) Molecular weight	22,000	100,000
3) P-amino acid	Serine	Aspartic acid
4) Nature of phosphoprotein	Phosphoester (stable in hot acid and in hydroxylamine)	Acyl phosphate (labile in hydroxylamine)
5) Amount of phosphorylation	1.0 to 1.4 nmol/mg SR	About 1.2 nmol/mg SR
6) Dependency of phosphorylation on Ca^{2+}	Independent of Ca^{2+}	Dependent on Ca^{2+}
7) Sensitivity to trypsin	Labile to trypsin	Relatively resistant to trypsin

Ca-activated ATPase apparently intact, as determined by its undiminished activity. At the same time, Ca transport by trypsinized cardiac SR, which has lost most of its phospholamban, was not stimulated by PK and cAMP. However, upon phosphorylation, phospholamban becomes resistant to tryptic digestion. This protective effect was accompanied by persistence of the PK-induced stimulation of Ca transport. Under these conditions, phosphorylated phospholamban was not dissociable from the ATPase protein when phosphorylated microsomes were treated with low concentrations of deoxycholate or Triton X-100. These results may indicate that phospholamban is localized at the outer surface of the membrane and that prior phosphorylation of phospholamban prevents attack by the protease, probably due to a phosphorylation-induced alteration in structure or charge distribution (Tada *et al.*, 1975a, 1976).

DISTRIBUTION OF
PHOSPHOLAMBAN IN DIFFERENT TYPES OF MUSCLE

Phosphorylation of cardiac SR by cAMP-dependent PK is seen in SR isolated from muscle from a variety of mammalian species (Kirchberger and Tada, 1976). Treatment of cardiac SR from dog, guinea pig, rabbit, and cat with bovine cardiac PK and cAMP results in increased rates of Ca uptake. In rabbit, guinea pig, and dog cardiac SR, virtually all PK-catalyzed phosphorylation is associated with a component of approximately 22,000 molecular weight. However, in cat cardiac SR, significant additional phosphorylation is associated with a component of approximately 11,000 daltons in some, but not all, preparations of SR. This latter peak of phosphorylation may be similar to a minor peak seen at the same location on electrophoretograms of dog cardiac SR (Figure 1*B*, Peak III) (Tada *et al.*, 1975a).

Treatment of SR from fast-contracting skeletal muscle (fast muscle) of rabbit with cAMP and PK had no effect on the rate of Ca uptake (Kirchberger and Tada, 1976). No radioactivity attributable to PK-catalyzed phosphorylation of fast muscle SR was apparent after it was incubated with cardiac or skeletal muscle PK (Figure 1*A*). The single peak of radioactivity (Peak I) seen in this figure can be attributable to autophosphorylation of the 50,000-dalton cAMP-binding subunit of cardiac PK (Erlichman, Rosenfeld, and Rosen, 1974). These results indicate that a 22,000-dalton protein substrate of cAMP-dependent PK is absent in SR of fast muscle.

Unlike fast muscle SR, SR prepared from dog biceps femoris muscle, which has characteristics typical of slow-contracting skeletal muscle (slow muscle) (Bárány, 1967; Bowman and Nott, 1969), showed a statistically significant increase of about 23% in the initial rate of Ca uptake. A protein of approximately 22,000 daltons was found to be phosphorylated by PK. Similar results

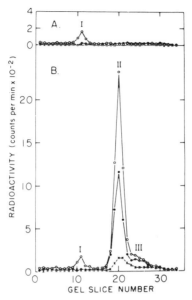

Figure 1. Comparison of effects of different protein kinases and cAMP on SR prepared from (*A*) rabbit fast skeletal muscle and (*B*) dog heart. SR (2.0 mg/ml) were incubated in the presence and absence (X) of bovine cardiac (○) or rabbit skeletal muscle (●) protein kinase (0.45 mg/ml), and 1 μM cAMP, together with 0.5 mM [γ-^{32}P] ATP. Sodium dodecyl sulfate-polyacrylamide gel electrophoresis was carried out as described previously (Tada *et al.*, 1975a; Kirchberger and Tada, 1976). Specific radioactivity of the [γ-^{32}] ATP was 1.83 × 10^7 cpm/μmol. A total of 400 μg of skeletal muscle SR and 415 μg of cardiac SR protein was applied to the gels. The amount of phosphorylation found in the main peak (Peak II) of radioactivity was 0.08 nmol of phosphorus/mg or SR protein for control cardiac SR, 0.45 nmol of phosphorus/mg of SR protein in the presence of skeletal muscle protein kinase, and 0.75 nmol of phosphorus/mg in the presence of bovine cardiac protein kinase. (Reproduced from Kirchberger and Tada (1976) by permission of *Journal of Biological Chemistry.*)

were obtained with SR from rabbit soleus muscle (Kirchberger and Tada, 1976), which is also characterized as slow muscle (Bowman and Nott, 1969).

Recently, essentially similar findings have been reported by Schwartz *et al.* (1976), who showed that Ca uptake by SR from cat soleus muscle could be stimulated by PK, with concomitant phosphorylation of a protein of approximately 20,000 daltons. However, they also reported that PK could stimulate Ca uptake by SR from cat tibialis muscle, which is fast muscle, without phosphorylation of the 20,000-dalton protein. This latter result is not in agreement with our experiments, in which we did not find an effect of cAMP-dependent PK. This discrepancy remains to be resolved.

A HYPOTHESIS FOR THE ROLE OF
PHOSPHOLAMBAN IN CATECHOLAMINE ACTION ON MUSCLE

The present studies suggest that a specific cellular response to hormonally triggered cAMP formation may depend on the presence of specific substrates that can be phosphorylated by cAMP-dependent PK. Thus, the relaxation-promoting effect of catecholamines may be related to the presence in cardiac and slow skeletal muscle of the 22,000-dalton phospholamban whose phosphorylation is catalyzed by PK, while its absence in fast skeletal muscle may be attributed to the absence of an analogous substrate for PK. It is interesting to examine whether an analogous phosphoprotein may mediate the relaxant effects of catecholamines in certain types of smooth muscle by a similar mechanism.

Our previous hypothesis (Kirchberger et al., 1975; Tada and Kirchberger, 1975; Tada et al., 1975, 1976) to explain β-adrenergic control of myocardial contractility may also be applicable to slow skeletal muscle and certain types of smooth muscle. Thus, in cardiac (Tada et al., 1974), slow skeletal (Kirchberger and Tada, 1976; Schwartz et al., 1976), and probably smooth muscle (Andersson et al., 1975), an enhanced rate of Ca uptake into the SR would accelerate the rate of removal of Ca from troponin (Ebashi et al., 1969, 1975) and thereby accelerate relaxation. We must consider why increased intracellular cAMP levels and resulting phosphorylation of phospholamban induce a positive inotropic effect in the heart and in certain types of visceral smooth muscle, but not in slow muscle and other types of smooth muscle, including that of the vascular wall. In the myocardium, which possesses a relatively well-developed network of SR, the increased Ca stores in SR, due to increased rate at which Ca is accumulated during diastole, are considered to increase the amount of Ca available for delivery to the contractile proteins in subsequent contractions, thus producing increased tension development (Fabiato and Fabiato, 1975; Tada and Kirchberger, 1975). A similar mechanism could be considered for visceral smooth muscle, although no direct evidence exists. Conversely, the lack of the inotropic response at increased intracellular cAMP levels in other types of muscle could be attributed to the poorly developed SR, which does not allow Ca to accumulate within SR during the relaxation phase. Justification of such a hypothesis awaits further investigation. Phosphorylation and dephosphorylation of phospholamban in the SR may represent just one means of physiological modulation of the muscular contractility; other regulatory mechanisms, such as phosphorylation of troponin I or the light chain of myosin, are being considered.

Acknowledgments We are greatly indebted to Professor Hiroshi Abe of Osaka University, Osaka, Japan, and Professor Arnold M. Katz of Mount Sinai School of Medicine, New York, USA, for their valuable comments and encouragement during the course of the experiments and preparation of the manuscript.

REFERENCES

ANDERSSON, R., NILSSON, K., WIKBERG, J., JOHANSSON, S., MOHME-LUNDHOLM, M., and LUNDHOLM, L. 1975. Cyclic nucleotides and the contraction of smooth muscle. Adv. Cycl. Nuc. Res. 5:491–518.

BÁRÁNY, M. 1967. ATPase activity of myosin correlated with speed of muscle shortening. J. Gen. Physiol. 50:197–216.

BOWMAN, W. C., and NOTT, M. W. 1969. Actions of sympathomimetic amines and their antagonists on skeletal muscle. Pharmacol. Rev. 21:27–72.

EBASHI, S., ENDO, M., and OHTSUKI, I. 1969. Control of muscle contraction. Quart. Rev. Biophys. 2:351–384.

EBASHI, S., NONOMURA, Y., KITAZAWA, T., and TOYO-OKA, T. 1975. Troponin in tissues other than skeletal muscle. In E. Carafoli et al. (eds.), Calcium Transport in Contraction and Secretion, pp. 405–414. North-Holland Publishing Co., Amsterdam.

ERLICHMAN, J., ROSENFELD, R., and ROSEN, O. M. 1974. Phosphorylation of a cyclic adenosine 3':5'-monophosphate-dependent protein kinase from bovine cardiac muscle. J. Biol. Chem. 249:5000–5003.

FABIATO, A., and FABIATO, F. 1975. Relaxing and inotropic effects of cyclic AMP on skinned cardiac cells. Nature 253:556–558.

KIRCHBERGER, M. A., and CHU, G. 1976. Correlation between protein kinase-mediated stimulation of calcium transport by cardiac sarcoplasmic reticulum and phosphorylation of a 22,000 dalton protein. Biochim. Biophys. Acta 419:559–562.

KIRCHBERGER, M. A., and RAFFO, A. 1977. Phosphoprotein phosphatase-catalyzed dephosphorylation of the 22,000 dalton phosphoprotein of cardiac sarcoplasmic reticulum. In N. S. Dhalla (ed.), Recent Advances in Studies on Cardiac Structure and Metabolism, Volume 11, University Park Press, Baltimore.

KIRCHBERGER, M. A., and TADA, M. 1976. Effects of adenosine 3':5'-monophosphate-dependent protein kinase on sarcoplasmic reticulum isolated from cardiac and slow and fast contracting skeletal muscles. J. Biol. Chem. 251:725–729.

KIRCHBERGER, M. A., TADA, M., and KATZ, A. M. 1974. Adenosine 3':5'-monophosphate-dependent protein kinase-catalyzed phosphorylation reaction and its relationship to calcium transport in cardiac sarcoplasmic reticulum. J. Biol. Chem. 249:6166–6173.

KIRCHBERGER, M. A., TADA, M., and KATZ, A. M. 1975. Phospholamban: A regulatory protein of the cardiac sarcoplasmic reticulum. In A Fleckenstein and N. S. Dhalla (eds.), Recent Advances in Studies on Cardiac Structure and Metabolism, Volume 5, pp. 103–115. University Park Press, Baltimore.

KIRCHBERGER, M. A., TADA, M., REPKE, D. I., and KATZ, A. M. 1972. Cyclic adenosine 3',5'-monophosphate-dependent protein kinase stimulation of calcium uptake by canine cardiac microsomes. J. Mol. Cell. Cardiol. 4:673–680.

MacLENNAN, D. H., and HOLLAND, P. C. 1975. Calcium transport in sarcoplasmic reticulum. Annu. Rev. Biophys. Bioengin. 4:377–404.

OHMORI, F., TADA, M., KINOSHITA, N., MATSUO, H., SAKAKIBARA, H., NIMURA, Y., and ABE, H. 1977. Effect of protein kinase modulator on cAMP-dependent protein kinase-catalyzed phosphorylation of phospholamban and stimulation of calcium transport in cardiac sarcoplasmic reticulum. In N. S. Dhalla (ed.), Recent Advances in Studies on Cardiac Structure and Metabolism, Volume 11, University Park Press, Baltimore.

SCHWARTZ, A., ENTMAN, M. L., KANIIKE, K., LANE, L. K., VAN WINKLE, W. B., and BORNET, E. P. 1976. The rate of calcium uptake into sarcoplasmic reticulum of cardiac muscle and skeletal muscle. Effects of cyclic AMP-dependent protein kinase and phosphorylase b kinase. Biochim. Biophys. Acta 426:57–72.

SHIGEKAWA, M., FINEGAN, J. M., and KATZ, A. M. 1976. Calcium transport ATPase of canine cardiac sarcoplasmic reticulum. A. Comparison with that of rabbit fast skeletal muscle sarcoplasmic reticulum. J. Biol. Chem. 251:6894–6900.

TADA, M., and KIRCHBERGER, M. A. 1975. Regulation of calcium transport by cyclic

AMP. A proposed mechanism for the beta-adrenergic control of myocardial contractility. Acta Cardiologica 30:231–237.

TADA, M., KIRCHBERGER, M. A., and KATZ, A. M. 1975a. Phosphorylation of a 22,000-dalton component of the cardiac sarcoplasmic reticulum by adenosine 3′:5′-monophosphate-dependent protein kinase. J. Biol. Chem. 250:2640–2647.

TADA, M., KIRCHBERGER, M. A., and KATZ, A. M. 1976. Regulation of calcium transport in cardiac sarcoplasmic reticulum by cyclic AMP-dependent protein kinase. *In* P. -E. Roy and N. S. Dhalla (eds.), Recent Advances in Studies on Cardiac Structure and Metabolism, Volume 9, pp. 225–239. University Park Press, Baltimore.

TADA, M., KIRCHBERGER, M. A., and LI, H. -C. 1975b. Phosphoprotein phosphatase-catalyzed dephosphorylation of the 22,000 dalton phosphoprotein of cardiac sarcoplasmic reticulum. J. Cycl. Nuc. Res. 1:329–338.

TADA, M., KIRCHBERGER, M. A., LI, H.-C., and KATZ, A. M. 1975c. Interrelationships between calcium and cyclic AMP in the mammalian heart. *In* Carafoli *et al.* (eds.), Calcium Transport in Contraction and Secretion, pp. 373–381. North-Holland Publishing Co., Amsterdam.

TADA, M., KIRCHBERGER, M. A., REPKE, D. I., and KATZ, A. M. 1974. The stimulation of calcium transport in canine cardiac sarcoplasmic reticulum by adenosine 3′:5′-monophosphate-dependent protein kinase. J. Biol. Chem. 249:6174–6180.

TADA, M., OHMORI, F., NIMURA, Y., and ABE, H. 1977. Effect of myocardial protein kinase modulator on adenosine 3′:5′-monophosphate-dependent protein kinase-induced stimulation of calcium transport by cardiac sarcoplasmic reticulum. J. Biochem. In press.

TADA, M., YAMAMOTO, Y., and TONOMURA, Y. 1978. Molecular mechanism of active calcium transport by sarcoplasmic reticulum. Physiol. Rev. 58. In press.

Mailing address:
Dr. Michihiko Tada,
The First Department of Medicine,
Osaka University Medical School,
Fukushima-ku, Osaka 553 (Japan).

Recent Advances in Studies on
Cardiac Structure and Metabolism, Volume 11
Heart Function and Metabolism
Edited by T. Kobayashi, T. Sano, and N. S. Dhalla
Copyright 1978   University Park Press   Baltimore

AN ADENOSINE 3′:5′-MONOPHOSPHATE-DEPENDENT PROTEIN KINASE FROM HUMAN HEART

S. MATSUSHITA, M. SAKAI, T. KAKU, T. NAKANO, K. KURAMOTO, and M. MURAKAMI

Department of Internal Medicine,
Metropolitan Geriatric Hospital, Tokyo, Japan

SUMMARY

Protein kinase that phosphorylated histone and lesser amounts of protamine was demonstrated in human heart. It was activated three times by 10^{-6} M cyclic adenosine 3′:5′-monophosphate (cAMP) and by 10^{-3} M other cyclic nucleotides. K_m values for cAMP, ATP, Mg^{2+}, and Co^{2+} were about 2×10^{-8} M, 4×10^{-5} M, 2×10^{-3} M, and 1.7×10^{-4} M, respectively. On DEAE cellulose column, the main peak of the enzyme eluted at high NaCl concentration. On Sephadex G-200 gel filtration the majority of the holoenzyme eluted at a peak corresponding to a molecular weight of about 300,000. There was an additional peak corresponding to a molecular weight of about 400,000, with relatively high cAMP binding compared to kinase activity. Right atrium and ventricle showed significantly higher enzyme activities than left atrium and ventricle and interventricular septum. On multivariate analysis of the enzyme activity versus 12 clinical and pathological findings of 122 cases, cardiac hypertrophy and coronary sclerosis were slight but significant negative contributors to the enzyme activity. Multiple correlation coefficient was low, indicating the enzyme activity remained at a relatively stable level, despite different clinical situations. This may be suitable for control of intracellular events through the membrane adenylate cyclase system.

INTRODUCTION

During the past several years, adenosine 3′:5′-monophosphate (cAMP)-dependent protein kinases have been extensively studied, and appear to link the membrane-bound hormone-sensitive adenylate cyclase system and the physiological responses within the cell (Walsh, Perkins, and Krebs, 1968; Kuo and Greengard, 1969). Evidence has been obtained that the mechanism through which cAMP activates the enzyme involves the dissociation of an inactive holoenzyme into a regulatory subunit-cAMP complex and active catalytic subunits. Although animal heart protein kinase has been one of the most intensively studied enzymes (Brostrom *et al.,* 1970; Rubin, Erlichman, and Rosen, 1972; Corbin, Keely, and Park, 1975; Hoffman *et al.,* 1975), that of human heart remained in an obscure form. This chapter is concerned with its enzyme characteristics and its relation to clinical and pathological conditions.

ASSAYS

Protein kinase activity was determined by measuring the incorporation of ^{32}P into histone. The reaction mixture contained, in a final volume of 0.2 ml: 50 mM Na acetate (pH 6.0), 10 mM Mg acetate, 5 mM NaF, 0.1 mM EGTA, 0.1 mM [γ-^{32}P] ATP(20,000 cpm/nmol), 2 mM theophylline, 1 mg/ml calf thymus histone, and enzyme protein. After incubation at 30° C for 15–30 min, the reactions were stopped by the addition of 4 ml of 5% trichloracetic acid and 0.25% Na$_2$WO$_4$ (pH 2.0). Washing of the protein precipitate was done as described by Kuo and Greengard (1970) and was counted in a liquid scintillation counter. The assays were linear for 40 min, and proportional to added enzyme up to 100 μg/ml.

Protein concentration was determined by the method of Lowry *et al.* (1951).

cAMP binding was measured essentially according to the method of Gilman (1970).

RESULTS

Extraction and Partial Purification

Pieces of human left ventricle or whole hearts were obtained at autopsy at our hospital or at Tokyo Metropolitan Medical Examiner's Office and frozen until extraction. Fresh or frozen tissue gave the same enzyme activity. All subsequent operations were carried out at 4° C. Myocardium was homogenized in five volumes (vol/wt) of 5 mM potassium-phosphate buffer and 2 mM EDTA (pH 7.0) in a Waring blender for 2 min. The homogenate was centrifuged at 25,000 × g for 20 min. The protein kinase activity and cAMP binding on the supernatant from 140 left ventricles showed essentially no variation according to hours between death and autopsy.

Protamine sulfate was added to the supernatant (15 mg/dl) and stirred for 10 min and centrifuged.

Solid (NH$_4$)$_2$SO$_4$ was added to the supernatant (32 g/dl) and stirred for 30 min. After centriguation the precipitate was dissolved in about 1/100 volumes of homogenizing buffer, and was dialyzed against the buffer.

The dialyzed fraction was injected into a column, 2.5 × 35 cm, of DEAE cellulose previously equilibrated with the buffer. The column was washed with 200 ml of the buffer. Protein kinase activity was eluted with a linear gradient of 0–0.25 M NaCl and the buffer at a flow rate of 30 ml per hour in 20-ml fractions in a total volume of 1200 ml. After dialysis against the buffer, each fraction was assayed. cAMP-dependent protein kinase activity was resolved into two peaks. The majority of the activity emerged at the higher salt concentration (Type II).

The active fractions were combined and concentrated by precipitation with $(NH_4)_2SO_4$ and dialysis, as described above.

The concentrated protein kinase solution was next injected into a column (2.5 × 90 cm of Sephadex G-200 that had been previously washed with the buffer). Ascending gel filtration was performed at a flow rate of 10 ml per hr in 5-ml fractions. The majority of holoenzyme emerged at a peak corresponding to a molecular weight of about 300,000, according to the method of Andrews (1965) (Figure 1). This is close to the molecular weight (280,000) of bovine heart holoenzyme (Rubin *et al.*, 1972). There was an additional peak corresponding to a molecular weight of about 400,000. Relative to kinase activity, this peak consistently showed higher cAMP binding. If this is not an artifact, this may indicate a different combination of regulatory and catalytic subunits.

PROPERTIES

Most of the kinetic study was performed on first $(NH_4)_2SO_4$ fractionation. cAMP showed stimulation of protein kinase activity at the order of 10^{-9} M and

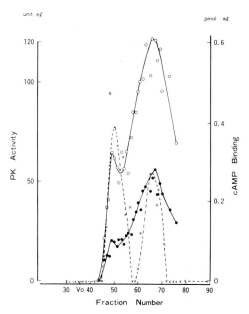

Figure 1. Sephadex G-200 chromatography of human heart protein kinase. *Open circle* and *closed circle* indicate protein kinase activity in the presence and absence of cAMP, respectively. A unit is 1 pmol ^{32}P/min. *Cross* symbol indicates cAMP binding.

up to threefold at 10^{-6} M. Half maximal stimulation occurred at about 2×10^{-8} M. Other cyclic nucleotides also showed stimulation, but at 10^{-6}–10^{-3} M.

The apparent K_m's for ATP, Mg^{2+}, and Co^{2+} were 4×10^{-5} M, 2×10^{-3}M, and 1.7×10^{-4} M, respectively. These values did not change whether or not cAMP was present in incubation medium. Other cold trinucleotides did not depress the labeling, whereas ADP did considerably. Co^{2+} showed slightly higher V_{max} than Mg^{2+}. Mn^{2+} was about one-sixth as effective as Mg^{2+}. Other divalent cations were not good substitutes for Mg^{2+}. Ca^{2+} added to Mg^{2+} inhibited the enzyme activity. Optimum pH was between 6.2 and 7.0 using phosphate buffer.

K_m for histone and protamine was lowered from 0.5 and 0.25 mg/ml to 0.11 mg/ml by cAMP. This is probably due to dissociation of holoenzyme into catalytic and regulatory subunits by the basic substrate. With protamine as substrate, V_{max} was lower and cAMP stimulation was about twofold. Casein was not phosphorylated well.

Enzyme Activity in Atria and Ventricles

Crude extracts from 22 human hearts showed significantly higher protein kinase activities in right side of the heart than in left: right atrium $117 \pm 10, 470 \pm 38$, left atrium $100 \pm 7, 347 \pm 29$, right ventricle $125 \pm 14, 433 \pm 40$, left ventricle $95 \pm 7, 330 \pm 19$, septum $78 \pm 6, 330 \pm 22$ nmol/g wet wt/30 min (mean $\pm$ S.E., without and with cAMP). cAMP-binding showed essentially the same difference.

Correlation Between Enzyme Activity and Clinical or Pathological Findings

Multivariate analysis was performed on enzyme activities of the left ventricles versus available clinical and pathological findings from 122 patients who died in our hospital. Among 12 factors listed in Figure 2, heart weight/height, which is an index of cardiac hypertrophy, and coronary sclerosis were significant contributors in all three categories. Heart failure, sudden death, and antemortem use of digitalis or catecholamine did not show impressive correlation. Multiple correlation coefficients, which mean how much these 12 factors could influence the enzyme activity, were low.

DISCUSSION

The studies described here demonstrate the cAMP-dependent protein kinase system in human heart comparable to that of animal heart. On DEAE cellulose column, human heart showed pattern similar to that of bovine heart, which is mainly Type II (Rubin *et al.*, 1972; Hoffman *et al.*, 1975). In rat heart, on the other hand, protein kinase eluted mainly at low NaCl concentration, which is called Type I (Corbin *et al.*, 1975). Human skeletal muscle showed equal amounts of Type I and II, and human brain mainly Type II (unpublished data).

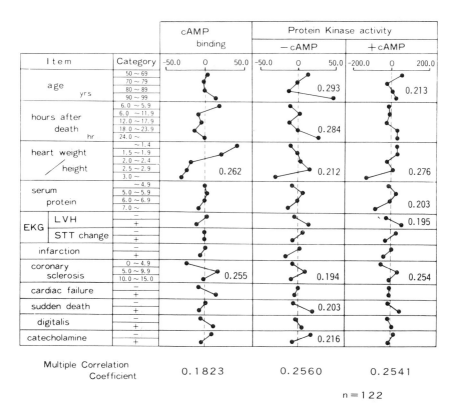

Figure 2. Estimated coefficients and their contributions to enzyme activities. Multivariate analysis was performed on the 12 items listed on the left side versus enzyme activities from 122 cases. The significant correlation coefficients ($p < 0.05$) are written in numbers in the appropriate columns.

Therefore, there is considerable species variation and also organ variation with regard to the type of protein kinase present. The kinetic properties are similar in Type I and II, but Corbin *et al.* (1975) focused attention on the finding that two types of enzyme can be distinguished by the ability of histone or salt to dissociate holoenzyme. Hoffman *et al.* (1975) reported some difference in the kinetics of regulatory subunits.

Right atrium and ventricle showed higher enzyme activity than the left. To our knowledge a comparable study on adenylate cyclase system was not available. The physiological significance of the difference remains to be resolved.

Although cardiac hypertrophy and coronary sclerosis showed significant correlation to the enzyme activity, the overall correlation was low. The relatively stable level of the enzyme is suitable for control of intracellalar events through membrane adenylate cyclase system.

Acknowledgments   We are grateful to Dr. Jushiro Koshinaga of the Tokyo Metropolitan Medical Examiner's Office for human hearts. We thank Miss Michiko Akeda and Yoko Kamiya for their technical assistance. We are indebted to Mr. Takashi Teranishi, Yoshihiro Botan, and Mitsugu Kanba of the Shionogi Computer Center for computer analysis.

REFERENCES

ANDREWS, P. 1965. The gel-filtration behaviour of proteins related to their molecular weights over a wide range. Biochem. J. 96:595–606.

BROSTROM, M. A., REIMAN, E. M., WALSH, D. A., and KREBS, E. G. 1970. A cyclic 3′,5′-AMP-stimulated protein kinase from cardiac muscle. Adv. Enzyme Regul. 8: 191–203.

CORBIN, J. D., KEELY, S. L., and PARK, C. R. 1975. The distribution and dissociation of cyclic adenosine 3′,5′-monophosphate-dependent protein kinases in adipose, cardiac, and other tissues. J. Biol. Chem. 250:218–225.

GILMAN, A. G. 1970. A protein binding assay for adenosine 3′,5′-cyclic monophosphate. Proc. Natl. Acad. Sci. (USA) 67:305–312.

HOFFMAN, F., BEAVO, J. A., BECHTEL, P. J., and KREBS, E. G. 1975. Comparison of adenosine 3′,5′-monophosphate-dependent protein kinases from rabbit skeletal and bovine heart muscle. J. Biol. Chem. 250:7795–7801.

KUO, J. F., and GREENGARD, P. 1969. An adenosine 3′,5′-monophosphate-dependent protein kinase from *Escherichia coli.* J. Biol. Chem. 244:3417–3419.

KUO, J. F., and GREENGARD, P. 1970. Cyclic nucleotide-dependent protein kinases. VIII. An assay method for the measurement of cyclic AMP in various tissues and a study of agents influencing its level in adipose cells. J. Biol. Chem. 245:4067–4073.

LOWRY, O. H., ROSEBROUGH, N. J., FARR, A. L., and RANDALL, R. J. 1951. Protein measurement with the Folin phenol reagent. J. Biol. Chem. 193:265–275.

RUBIN, C. S., ERLICHMAN, J., and ROSEN, O. M. 1972. Molecular forms and subunit composition of a cyclic adenosine 3′,5′-monophosphate-dependent protein kinase purified from bovine heart muscle. J. Biol. Chem. 247:36–42.

WALSH, D. A., PERKINS, J. P., and KREBS, E. G. 1968. A 3′,5′-monophosphate-dependent protein kinase from rabbit skeletal muscle. J. Biol. Chem. 243:3763–3764.

Mailing address:
S. Matsushita, M.D.,
Tokyo Metropolitan Geriatric Hospital,
35-2 Sakae-cho,
Itabashi-ku, Tokyo (Japan).

Recent Advances in Studies on
Cardiac Structure and Metabolism, Volume 11
Heart Function and Metabolism
Edited by T. Kobayashi, T. Sano, and N. S. Dhalla
Copyright 1978   University Park Press   Baltimore

EFFECT OF PROTEIN KINASE MODULATOR ON cAMP-DEPENDENT PROTEIN KINASE-CATALYZED PHOSPHORYLATION OF PHOSPHOLAMBAN AND STIMULATION OF CALCIUM TRANSPORT IN CARDIAC SARCOPLASMIC RETICULUM

F. OHMORI, M. TADA, N. KINOSHITA,
H. MATSUO, H. SAKAKIBARA,
Y. NIMURA, and H. ABE

The First Department of Medicine, Osaka University Medical School,
Fukushima-ku, Osaka, Japan

SUMMARY

The heat-stable protein (protein kinase modulator), partially purified from fresh bovine heart, possessed the ability to inhibit and stimulate adenosine $3':5'$-monophosphate (cAMP)-dependent protein kinase and guanosine $3':5'$-monophosphate (cGMP)-dependent protein kinase activities, respectively. The inhibitory activity of protein kinase modulator on cAMP-dependent protein kinase was abolished almost completely by trypsin treatment, while the ability to stimulate cGMP-dependent protein kinase activity was resistant to trypsin. Fractionation by a linear potassium phosphate gradient on DEAE-cellulose column did not clearly separate both activities. Phosphorylation of cardiac microsomal component, "phospholamban" (molecular weight = 22,000), was inhibited almost completely by the saturating amounts of protein kinase modulator. This inhibition of phospholamban phosphorylation by protein kinase modulator was accompanied by a decreased Ca uptake rate that had been stimulated by cAMP- dependent protein kinase. These findings indicate that protein kinase modulator is functional in controlling the cAMP-dependent protein kinase-catalyzed phosphorylation of phospholamban and the rate of calcium transport, lending further support for the previously proposed mechanism, in which phospholamban is assumed to serve as a regulator of calcium transport in cardiac sarcoplasmic reticulum.

INTRODUCTION

Adenosine $3':5'$-monophosphate-dependent protein kinase (cAMP-PK)-induced stimulation of Ca transport by cardiac sarcoplasmic reticulum has been shown to be mediated by phosphorylation of a 22,000-dalton protein, phospholamban (Kirchberger, Tada, and Katz, 1974; Tada *et al.,* 1974; Tada, Kirchberger, and

This work was supported by the Scientific Research Fund (021512 and 077208) of the Ministry of Education of Japan, a Research Grant 1975 from Japan Heart Foundation, and a Grant-in-Aid from the Muscular Dystrophy Association of America.

Katz, 1975; Kirchberger and Chu, 1976). This protein appears to play a key role in the β-adrenergic control of myocardial contractility (Tada, Kirchberger, and Katz, 1976). To elucidate the mechanism by which sarcoplasmic reticulum Ca transport is regulated by the PK-phospholamban system, we examined effects of a heat-stable and trypsin-labile protein factor from bovine heart (Tada *et al.,* 1977), which possessed characteristics similar to PKM from other tissues (Appleman, Birnbaumer, and Torres, 1966; Walsh *et al.,* 1971; Donnelly *et al.,* 1973a and b; Kuo, 1974, 1975).

METHODS

Cardiac microsomes, which consist mainly of sarcoplasmic reticulum, were prepared from dog heart by the procedures of Harigaya and Schwartz (1969). cAMP-PK from bovine heart (Miyamota, Kuo, and Greengard, 1969) and cGMP-PK from bovine lung (Nakazawa and Sano, 1975) were prepared through DEAE-cellulose chromatography. PKM (protein kinase modulator), partially purified from fresh bovine heart through the ammonium sulfate precipitation (Appleman *et al.,* 1966; Donnelly *et al.,* 1973b), was applied to a column of DEAE cellulose, and eluted with a linear gradient formed by 5 mM and 300 mM potassium phosphate buffer (pH 7.0). Each fraction was dialyzed against 5 mM potassium phosphate buffer, and was subjected to assay for modulation of cAMP-PK and cGMP-PK activities. Standard assay medium for cAMP-PK contained 0.05 mM $[\gamma\text{-}^{32}P]$ ATP (0.1 mCi/μmol), 2.5 mM $MgCl_2$, 1 μM cAMP, 1 mg/ml histone, 120 mM KCl, and 40 mM histidine-HCl buffer (pH 6.8) at 25°. Standard assay medium for cGMP-PK (75 μg/ml) contained 0.01 mM $[\gamma\text{-}^{32}P]$ ATP (0.5 mCi/μmol), 25 mM Mg acetate, 0.1 μM cGMP, 0.5 mg/ml histone, 2.5 mM theophylline, and 100 mM Tris-HCl buffer (pH 7.5) at 25°. Microsomal phosphorylation was measured under essentially similar conditions. Amounts of phosphoprotein were determined by the methods described by Li and Felmly (1973), Kirchberger *et al.* (1974), or Tada *et al.* (1975). Ca uptake was measured by the procedures described previously (Kirchberger *et al.,* 1974; Tada *et al.,* 1974).

RESULTS AND DISCUSSION

When histone phosphorylation by cAMP-PK and cGMP-PK was determined in the presence of PKM, increasing amounts of PKM inhibited cAMP-PK activity, and, at the same time, stimulated cGMP-PK activity. At saturating amounts of PKM, cAMP-PK activity was inhibited more than 95%, and cGMP-PK activity was stimulated about threefold (Table 1). Trypsin treatment of PKM completely abolished the inhibitory activity (Table 1), in accord with the findings by Walsh *et al.* (1971) and Donnelly *et al.* (1973b). Under the same conditions, however,

Table 1. Effects of protein kinase modulator (PKM) on cAMP-dependent and cGMP-dependent protein kinases (PK)*

| | Phosphorylation | |
| | cAMP-PK | cGMP-PK |
	(nmol ^{32}P/mg histone/15 min)	
No PKM	2.09	0.26
PKM	0.07	0.72
Trypsin-treated PKM	2.10	0.63

*PKM was treated by trypsin at 100:1 (PKM:trypsin) ratio for 30 min at 25°C in 40 mM histidine-HCl buffer (pH 6.8). After termination of the incubation with trypsin inhibitor of twofold excess over trypsin, aliquots of the mixture were added to the standard medium for assaying PK activities. The amount of PKM was 90 μl in the reaction mixture.

the stimulatory activity of PKM on cGMP-PK was resistant to trypsin, about 80% of the stimulatory activity being retained (Table 1). Increasing the trypsin: PKM ratio or time of digestion did not appreciably change the stimulatory activity. These differences in trypsin effects may indicate that the abilities of PKM to inhibit and stimulate cAMP-PK and cGMP-PK activities, respectively, are separable. However, fractionation by DEAE-cellulose chromatography did not clearly separate the two activities. A distinct peak of inhibitory activity was found at around 140 mM potassium phosphate, when PKM was fractionated by DEAE-cellulose chromatography. This peak was found to be almost superimposable with a peak of activity to stimulate cGMP-PK.

Effect of PKM on microsomal phosphorylation was examined. cAMP-PK caused marked stimulation of microsomal phosphorylation, amounting to about 1 nmol ^{32}P/mg in 5 min. This phosphorylation was inhibited completely when the saturating amounts of PKM were included in the reaction mixture. Sodium dodecyl sulfate-polyacrylamide gel electrophoresis by the procedures of Tada *et al.* (1975) revealed that PKM completely inhibited phosphorylation of the microsomal component (molecular weight = 22,000). Essentially similar results were obtained by Schwartz *et al.* (1976), who have shown that cAMP-PK-catalyzed phosphorylation of the 20,000-dalton protein of microsomes was inhibited by protein kinase inhibitor from rabbit skeletal muscle.

Since cAMP-PK-catalyzed phosphorylation of the 22,000-dalton phospholamban was found to be closely associated with the stimulation of Ca transport (Kirchberger *et al.*, 1974; Tada *et al.*, 1974, 1975, 1976; Kirchberger and Chu, 1976; Schwartz *et al.*, 1976), we investigated whether PKM, which possesses the ability to inhibit cAMP-PK-catalyzed phosphorylation of phospholamban, could reverse PK-induced stimulation of microsomal Ca uptake. Microsomes were incubated under standard conditions for 5 min, in the presence of various amounts of PKM, and were subjected to assay for Ca uptake by the Millipore method. Preincubation of cardiac microsomes with cAMP-PK resulted in stimulation of the Ca uptake rate from 23 to 63 nmol ^{45}Ca/mg microsomes/min. Increasing amounts of PKM decreased the rate of Ca uptake,

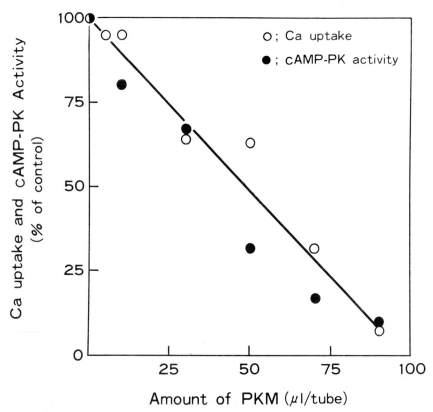

Figure 1. Effects of protein kinase modulator (PKM) on cAMP-dependent protein kinase (cAMP-PK) activity and Ca uptake on cardiac microsomes that had been stimulated by cAMP-PK. cAMP-PK activity (●) was determined under standard conditions (Kirchberger *et al.*, 1974; Tada *et al.*, 1974) in the presence of different amounts of PKM. cAMP-PK activity in the absence of PKM (0.3 nmol ^{32}P/mg histone/min) was taken as control. Microsomes (1 mg/ml) were pretreated with cAMP-PK under conditions essentially similar to those for cAMP-PK activity except that histone and [γ-^{32}P]ATP were substituted for microsomes and cold ATP, respectively, and were subjected to assay for Ca uptake under standard conditions (○) (Kirchberger *et al.*, 1974; Tada *et al.*, 1974). The control value for Ca uptake represents the net stimulation of Ca uptake (40 nmol ^{45}Ca/mg/min) produced by cAMP-PK, that in the absence of cAMP-PK being 22.5 nmol ^{45}Ca/mg/min.

and it was brought back to the basal level of 25 nmol ^{45}Ca/mg microsomes/min in the presence of saturating amounts of PKM. The extent of inhibition of cAMP-PK activity produced by PKM was linearly correlated with the extent of PKM-induced decrease in Ca uptake, which had been stimulated by cAMP-PK (Figure 1). The PKM-induced concomitant decrease in the cAMP-PK activity and PK-stimulated Ca uptake lends further support to the previously proposed control mechanism of Ca transport in cardiac sarcoplasmic reticulum, in which phospholamban is assumed to serve as a regulator of Ca^{2+}-activated ATPase (Tada and Kirchberger, 1975; Tada et al., 1975, 1976).

Acknowledgment We thank Miss Seiko Kako for her expert technical assistance.

REFERENCES

APPLEMAN, M. M., BIRNBAUMER, L., and TORRES, H. N. 1966. Factors affecting the activity of muscle glycogen synthetase. III. The reaction with adenosine triphosphate, Mg^{2+}, and cyclic 3'5'-adenosine monophosphate. Arch. Biochem. Biophys. 116:39–43.

DONNELLY, T. E., JR., KUO, J. F., MIYAMOTO, E., and GREENGARD, P. 1973a. Protein kinase modulator from lobster tail muscle. II. Effects of the modulator on holoenzyme and catalytic subunit of guanosine 3',5'-monophosphate-dependent and adenosine 3',5'-monophosphate-dependent protein kinases. J. Biol. Chem. 248:199–203.

DONNELLY, T. E., JR., KUO, J. F., REYES, P. L., LIU, Y. -P., and GREENGARD, P. 1973b. Protein kinase modulator from lobster tail muscle. I. Stimulatory and inhibitory effects of the modulator on the phosphorylation of substrate proteins by guanosine 3',5'-monophosphate-dependent and adenosine 3',5'-monophosphate-dependent protein kinases. J. Biol. Chem. 248:190–198.

HARIGAYA, S., and SCHWARTZ, A. 1969. Rate of calcium binding and uptake in normal animal and failing human cardiac muscle. Membrane vesicles (relaxing system) and mitochondria. Circ. Res. 25:781–794.

KIRCHBERGER, M. A., and CHU, G. 1976. Correlation between protein kinase mediated stimulation of calcium transport by cardiac sarcoplasmic reticulum and phosphorylation of a 22,000 dalton protein. Biochim. Biophys. Acta 419:559–562.

KIRCHBERGER, M. A., TADA, M., and KATZ, A. M. 1974. Adenosine 3':5'-monophosphate-dependent protein kinase-catalyzed phosphorylation reaction and its relationship to calcium transport in cardiac sarcoplasmic reticulum. J. Biol. Chem. 249:6166–6173.

KUO, J. F. 1974. Guanosine 3':5'-monophosphate-dependent protein kinases in mammalian tissues. Proc. Natl. Acad. Sci. (USA) 71:4037–4041.

KUO, J. F. 1975. Divergent actions of protein kinase modulator in regulating mammalian cyclic GMP-dependent and cyclic AMP-dependent protein kinases. Metabolism 24: 321–329.

LI, H. -C., and FELMLY, D. A. 1973. A rapid paper chromatography assay for protein kinase. Anal. Biochem. 52:300–304.

MIYAMOTA, E., KUO, J. F., and GREENGARD, P. 1969. Cyclic nucleotide-dependent protein kinases. III. Purification and properties of adenosine 3',5'-monophosphate-dependent protein kinase from bovine brain. J. Biol. Chem. 244:6395–6402.

NAKAZAWA, K., and SANO, M. 1975. Partial purification and properties of guanosine 3':5'-monophosphate-dependent protein kinase from pig lung. J. Biol. Chem. 250: 7415–7419.

SCHWARTZ, A., ENTMAN, M. L., KANIIKE, K., LANE, L. K., VAN WINKLE, W. B., and

BORNET, E. P. 1976. The rate of calcium uptake into sarcoplasmic reticulum of cardiac muscle and skeletal muscle. Effects of cyclic AMP-dependent protein kinase and phosphorylase *b* kinase. Biochim. Biophys. Acta 426:57–72.

TADA, M., and KIRCHBERGER, A. M. 1975. Regulation of calcium transport by cyclic AMP. A proposed mechanism for the beta-adrenergic control of myocardial contractility. Acta Cardiol. 30:231–237.

TADA, M., KIRCHBERGER, M. A., and KATZ, A. M. 1975. Phosphorylation of a 22,000-dalton component of the cardiac sarcoplasmic reticulum by adenosine 3′:5′-monophosphate-dependent protein kinase. J. Biol. Chem. 250:2640–2647.

TADA, M., KIRCHBERGER, M. A., and KATZ, A. M. 1976. Regulation of calcium transport in cardiac sarcoplasmic reticulum by cyclic AMP-dependent protein kinase. *In* P. -E. Roy and N. S. Dhalla (eds.), Recent Advances in Studies on Cardiac Structure and Metabolism, Volume 9, pp. 225–239. University Park Press, Baltimore.

TADA, M., KIRCHBERGER, M. A., REPKE, D. I., and KATZ, A. M. 1974. The stimulation of calcium transport in cardiac sarcoplasmic reticulum by adenosine 3′:5′-monophosphate-dependent protein kinase. J. Biol. Chem. 249:6174–6180.

TADA, M., OHMORI, F., NIMURA, Y., and ABE, H. 1977. Effect of myocardial protein kinase modulator on adenosine 3′:5′-monophosphate-dependent protein kinase-induced stimulation of calcium transport by cardiac sarcoplasmic reticulum. J. Biochem. (In press.)

WALSH, D. A., ASHBY, C. D., GONZALEZ, C., CALKINS, D., FISHER, E. H., and KREBS, E. G. 1971. Purification and characterization of a protein inhibitor of adenosine 3′,5′-monophosphate-dependent protein kinases. J. Biol. Chem. 246: 1977–1985.

Mailing address:
Dr. F. Ohmori,
The First Department of Medicine,
Osaka University Medical School,
Fukushima-ku, Osaka 553 (Japan).

Recent Advances in Studies on
Cardiac Structure and Metabolism, Volume 11
Heart Function and Metabolism
Edited by T. Kobayashi, T. Sano, and N. S. Dhalla
Copyright 1978   University Park Press   Baltimore

PHOSPHOPROTEIN
PHOSPHATASE-CATALYZED DEPHOSPHORYLATION
OF THE 22,000-DALTON PHOSPHOPROTEIN OF CARDIAC
SARCOPLASMIC RETICULUM

M. A. KIRCHBERGER[1] and A. RAFFO

Departments of Physiology and Biophysics, and Medicine,
Mount Sinai School of Medicine of the
City University of New York, New York, New York, USA

SUMMARY

Similar time courses were obtained for decreases in the rate of calcium transport by cardiac sarcoplasmic reticulum vesicles previously phosphorylated by cAMP-dependent protein kinase and dephosphorylation of the 22,000-dalton phosphoprotein in these membranes. Dephosphorylation of the 22,000-dalton phosphoprotein can be attributed to a phosphoprotein phosphatase in the sarcoplasmic reticular membranes. This membrane-bound phosphoprotein phosphatase may play a role in the reversal of the relaxation-promoting effect of catecholamines on the heart.

INTRODUCTION

Evidence has previously been presented to indicate that cAMP-dependent protein kinase-catalyzed phosphorylation of a 22,000-dalton protein of the cardiac sarcoplasmic reticulum results in an enhanced rate of calcium transport by these membranes (Kirchberger *et al.,* 1972; Kirchberger, Tada, and Katz, 1974; Tada *et al.,* 1974; Tada, Kirchberger, and Katz, 1975b). A similar phosphoprotein has been found in slow contracting skeletal muscle (Kirchberger and Tada, 1976; Schwartz *et al.,* 1976). These findings suggest a possible role for the 22,000-dalton protein in mediating the relaxation-promoting effects of catecholamines in cardiac and slow skeletal muscle, which are absent in fast skeletal muscle.

Effects of protein kinase-catalyzed phosphorylation reactions can be reversed upon dephosphorylation of the phosphoproteins by phosphoprotein phosphatases (Soderling and Park, 1974). Phosphoprotein phosphatase activity

---

This work was supported by United States Public Health Service Grants HL-15764, HL-18801, and AA-00316.

[1] Recipient of Research Career Development Award HL-00053 from the United States Public Health Service.

has been detected previously in both cytosolic and subcellular membrane fractions of cardiac myocardium (LaRaia and Morkin, 1974; Li, 1975; Tada, Kirchberger, and Li, 1975a). In the present communication, we present evidence to indicate that the dephosphorylation of the 22,000-dalton sarcoplasmic reticular protein is associated with a concomitant decrease in the rate of calcium transport and may be attributed to a phosphoprotein phosphatase that is present in association with the sarcoplasmic reticulum membranes.

METHODS

Canine cardiac microsomes consisting primarily of fragmented sarcoplasmic reticulum were prepared by the method of Harigaya and Schwartz (1969) modified slightly (Kirchberger, Tada, and Katz, 1975).

Rates of calcium transport were compared with the extent of membrane phosphorylation in vesicles (3.0 mg/ml) that were incubated at $25°$ in 40 mM histidine-HCl buffer (pH 6.8), 120 mM KCl, 5 mM $MgCl_2$, 50 mM potassium phosphate, and the following additions: for measuring phosphorylation, 5 mM $[\gamma\text{-}^{32}P]$ATP (specific activity 12 to 14 μCi per μmol), 1 μM cAMP, and 3.0 mg/ml bovine cardiac protein kinase, prepared as described previously (Kirchberger and Tada, 1976); for measuring calcium transport, same as before except that nonradioactive ATP was used. All solutions were adjusted to pH 6.8 prior to addition to the reaction mixture. After 10 min, reaction mixtures were diluted with ice-cold 50 mM potassium phosphate buffer (pH 6.8), and centrifuged for 15 min at 86,000 $\times$ g. Microsomal pellets were resuspended in 80 mM histidine-HCl buffer (pH 6.8), and 240 mM KCl. The resuspended microsomes were then diluted 1:4 by addition to water to start the dephosphorylation reaction; the final microsomal protein concentration was 1.23 mg/ml. At timed intervals, samples were removed and treated as follows: to measure phosphorylation, 200-μl aliquots of ^{32}P-labeled microsomes were added to 2 ml of 10% trichloroacetic acid containing 1 mM KH_2PO_4. Acid-denatured microsomes were then fractionated by sodium dodecyl sulfate-polyacrylamide gel electrophoresis according to Procedure II of Tada et al., 1975b. The extent of microsomal phosphorylation was determined from the number of counts found in the area on the gel corresponding to the 22,000-dalton protein. To measure calcium transport, 75-μl aliquots of phosphorylated microsomes were added to reaction mixtures (final volume 4.0 ml) consisting of 40 mM histidine-HCl (pH 6.8), 120 mM KCl, 5 mM $MgCl_2$, 5 mM ATP, 50 mM potassium phosphate, and a calcium-EGTA [ethylene glycol bis(β-aminoethyl ether)-N,N'-tetraacetic acid] buffer (1 μM Ca^{2+}: 25 μM $CaCl_2$, 63.8 μM EGTA) prepared as described previously (Katz et al., 1970). The final microsome concentration was 23 μg/ml. Samples were taken at timed intervals by the Millipore filtration method.

To measure the effect of ions on microsomal phosphoprotein phosphatase activity, microsomes were phosphorylated with $[\gamma\text{-}^{32}P]$ATP as described above, except that the concentration of protein kinase was 1.5 mg/ml and 25 mM NaF was used instead of 50 mM potassium phosphate. Microsomes were incubated for varying periods of time in the presence and absence of 25 mM NaF, 50 mM potassium phosphate, 5 mM $MgCl_2$, or $MnCl_2$.

RESULTS AND DISCUSSION

When phosphorylated cardiac microsomes labeled with ^{32}P were incubated in buffer at 25°C for varying periods of time, the extent of phosphorylation of the 22,000-dalton phosphoprotein decreased slowly (Figure 1). The time course of the decrease in 22,000-dalton phosphoprotein was similar to a decrease in the rate of calcium transport, the latter measured in microsomes that were phos-

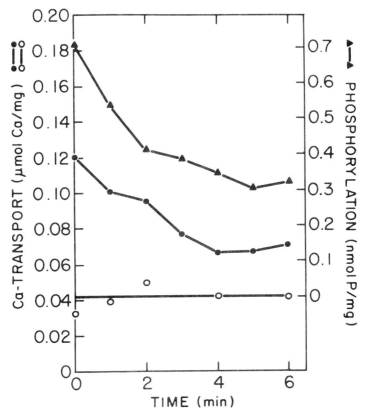

Figure 1. Time course of dephosphorylation of 22,000-dalton phosphoprotein (▲) and decrease in rate of phosphate-facilitated calcium transport (●) by phosphorylated cardiac sarcoplasmic reticulum. Also shown are rates of calcium transport by unphosphorylated microsomes (○) incubated under similar conditions, except that protein kinase and cAMP were omitted from the incubation medium during the 10-min pretreatment.

phorylated and incubated in parallel under identical conditions, except that nonradioactive ATP was used during the phosphorylation reaction. The decrease in the rate of calcium transport could be shown not to be due to aging of microsomes during incubation since no significant loss of activity was found when calcium transport was measured concurrently in unphosphorylated microsomes (Figure 1). In three independent experiments (Figure 2), the decrease in 22,000-dalton phosphoprotein level after incubation correlated significantly with a decreased calcium transport rate (average correlation coefficient = 0.90 ± 0.03, $p < 0.01$). These data suggest that the membranes of the cardiac sarcoplasmic reticulum contain a phosphoprotein phosphatase that catalyzes the dephosphorylation of the 22,000-dalton phosphoprotein also present on these membranes.

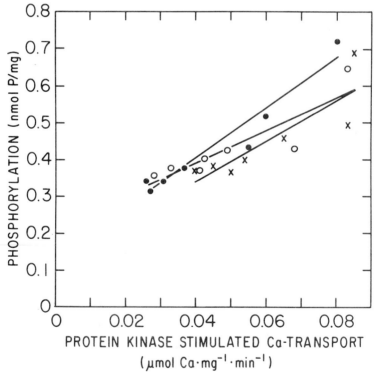

Figure 2. Correlation between amount of 22,000-dalton phosphoprotein and rate of protein kinase-stimulated calcium transport measured after incubating phosphorylated microsomes in buffer solution at 25°C. Protein kinase-stimulated calcium transport represents the rate of calcium transport observed in phosphorylated microsomes minus the rate observed in unphosphorylated microsomes. Shown are three independent experiments (○, ●, x) including the experiment shown in Figure 1 (●).

The rate of decrease in membrane phosphoprotein is sensitive to various ions that are known to affect previously described phosphatases (Kato and Bishop, 1972; Maeno and Greengard, 1972; Soderling and Park, 1974). In the absence of added salts, the amount of phosphoprotein in phosphorylated cardiac sarcoplasmic reticulum decreased from 1.1 nmol P/mg microsomal protein to 0.7 nmol P/mg protein after a 30-min incubation period (Figure 3). Inorganic phosphate (50 mM) and sodium fluoride (25 mM) decreased the extent of

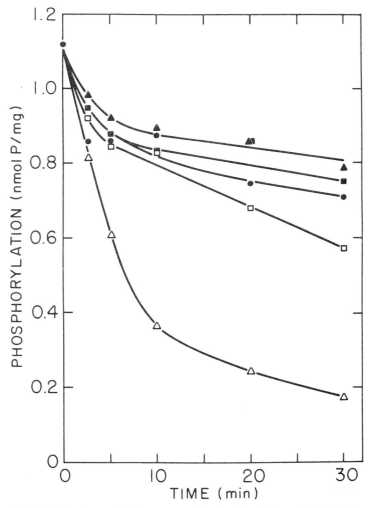

Figure 3. Effect of salts on the time course of dephosphorylation of 22,000-dalton phosphoprotein. Phosphorylated microsomes were incubated in control solution (●), 25 mM NaF (▲), 50 mM potassium phosphate (■), 5 mM MgCl$_2$ (□), or 5 mM MnCl$_2$ (△).

dephosphorylation after 30 min by approximately 10% and 20%, respectively. $MnCl_2$ and $MgCl_2$, each at 5 mM, increased the extent of dephosphorylation by approximately 129% and 32%, respectively, relative to the extent of dephosphorylation observed in the absence of added salts after the 30-min incubation period.

The foregoing data suggest a close functional association of phosphoprotein phosphatase with the membranes of the cardiac sarcoplasmic reticulum. Although the possibility that cytosolic phosphatases become adsorbed onto the membranes during isolation cannot be eliminated, such a cytosolic contaminant is likely to be removed during the preparation of these membranes, which includes one wash in 0.6 M KCl. Treatment of subcellular membranes with solutions of high ionic strength is known to remove loosely associated proteins (Razin, 1972). Furthermore, adsorption of the catalytic subunit of cytosolic cAMP-dependent protein kinase onto membranes derived from bovine cardiac muscle can be prevented when the tissue is homogenized in 0.15 M KCl (Keely, Corbin, and Park, 1975). No differences were detectable with either histone phosphate or phosphorylated cardiac microsomes as substrate for the enzyme found in cardiac sarcoplasmic reticulum isolated in the presence and absence of 0.15 M KCl during initial homogenization.

The phosphoprotein phosphatase associated with cardiac sarcoplasmic reticulum may form part of a complex of enzymes consisting additionally of hormone-sensitive adenylate cyclase (Entman, Levey, and Epstein, 1969; Sulakhe and Dhalla, 1973; Katz et al., 1974) and cAMP-dependent protein kinase (Wray, Gray, and Olsson, 1973; La Raia and Morkin, 1974). This system of enzymes can account for the rapid phosphorylation-dephosphorylation of the 22,000-dalton sarcoplasmic reticular protein that may play a role in the relaxation-promoting effects of catecholamines on the mammalian heart.

REFERENCES

ENTMAN, M. L., LEVEY, G. S., and EPSTEIN, S. E. 1969. Demonstration of adenyl cyclase activity in canine cardiac sarcoplasmic reticulum. Biochem. Biophys. Res. Commun. 35:728–733.

HARIGAYA, S., and SCHWARTZ, A. 1969. Rate of calcium binding and calcium uptake in normal animal and failing human cardiac muscle. Membrane vesicles (relaxing system) and mitochondria. Circ. Res. 25:781–794.

KATO, K., and BISHOP, J. S. 1970. Glycogen synthase-D phosphatase. I. Some new properties of the partially purified enzyme from rabbit skeletal muscle. J. Biol. Chem. 247:7420–7429.

KATZ, A. M., REPKE, D. I., UPSHAW, J., and POLASCIK, M. A. 1970. Characterization of dog cardiac microsomes. Use of zonal centrifugation to fractionate fragmented sarcoplasmic reticulum, $(Na^+ + K^+)$-activated ATPase and mitochondrial fragments. Biochim. Biophys. Acta 204:473–490.

KATZ, A. M., TADA, M., REPKE, D. I., IORIO, J.-M., and KIRCHBERGER, M. A. 1974. Adenylate cyclase: Its probable localization in sarcoplasmic reticulum as well as sarcolemma of the canine heart. J. Mol. Cell. Cardiol. 6:73–78.

KEELY, S. L., JR., CORBIN, J. D., and PARK, C. R. 1975. On the question of translocation of heart cAMP-dependent protein kinase. Proc. Natl. Acad. Sci. (USA) 72:
1501–1504.

KIRCHBERGER, M. A., and TADA, M. 1976. Effects of adenosine 3':5'-monophos-
phate-dependent protein kinase on sarcoplasmic reticulum isolated from cardiac and
slow and fast contracting skeletal muscles. J. Biol. Chem. 251:725–729.

KIRCHBERGER, M. A., TADA, M., and KATZ, A. M. 1974. Adenosine 3':5'-mono-
phosphate-dependent protein kinase-catalyzed phosphorylation reaction and its relationship to calcium transport in cardiac sarcoplasmic reticulum. J. Biol. Chem. 249:
6166–6173.

KIRCHBERGER, M. A., TADA, M., REPKE, D. I., and KATZ, A. M. 1972. Cyclic
adenosine 3',5'-monophosphate-dependent protein kinase stimulation of calcium uptake
by canine cardiac microsomes. J. Mol. Cell. Cardiol. 4:673–680.

LA RAIA, P. J., and MORKIN, E. 1974. Adenosine 3',5'-monophosphate-dependent membrane phosphorylation. A possible mechanism for the control of microsomal calcium
transport in heart muscle. Circ. Res. 35:298–306.

LI, H.-C. 1975. Protein phosphatases from canine heart: Evidence for four different
fractions of this enzyme. FEBS Lett. 55:134–37.

MAENO, H., and GREENGARD, P. 1972. Phosphoprotein phosphatases from rat cerebral
cortex. Subcellular distribution and characterization. J. Biol. Chem. 247:3269–3277.

RAZIN, S. 1972. Reconstitution of biological membranes. Biochim. Biophys. Acta 265:
241–296.

SCHWARTZ, A., ENTMAN, M. L., KANIIKE, K., LANE, L. K., VAN WINKLE, B., and
BORNET, E. P. 1976. The rate of calcium uptake into sarcoplasmic reticulum of cardiac
muscle and skeletal muscle. Effects of cyclic AMP-dependent protein kinase and phosphorylase b kinase. Biochim. Biophys. Acta 426:57–72.

SODERLING, T. R., and PARK, C. R. 1974. Recent advances in glycogen metabolism. Adv.
Cyc. Nucl. Res. 4:283–333.

SULAKHE, P. V., and DHALLA, N. S. 1973. Adenylate cyclase of heart sarcotubular
membranes. Biochim. Biophys. Acta 293:379–396.

TADA, M., KIRCHBERGER, M. A., and LI, H.-C. 1975a. Phosphoprotein phosphatase-
catalyzed dephosphorylation of the 22,000 dalton phosphoprotein of cardiac sarcoplasmic reticulum. J. Cyc. Nucl. Res. 1:329–338.

TADA, M., KIRCHBERGER, M. A., and KATZ, A. M. 1975b. Phosphorylation of a 22,000
dalton component of the cardiac sarcoplasmic reticulum by adenosine 3':5'-monophos-
phate-dependent protein kinase. J. Biol. Chem. 250:2640–2647.

TADA, M., KIRCHBERGER, M. A., REPKE, D. I., and KATZ, A. M. 1974. The stimulation
of calcium transport in canine cardiac sarcoplasmic reticulum by adenosine 3':5'-mono-
phosphate-dependent protein kinase. J. Biol. Chem. 249:6174–6180.

WRAY, H. L., GRAY, R. R., and OLSSON, R. A. 1973. Cyclic adenosine 3':5'-monophos-
phate-stimulated protein kinase and a substrate associated with cardiac sarcoplasmic
reticulum. J. Biol. Chem. 248:1496–1498.

Mailing address:
Dr. M. Kirchberger,
Mount Sinai School of Medicine,
Fifth Avenue and 100th Street,
New York, New York 10029 (USA)

Recent Advances in Studies on
Cardiac Structure and Metabolism, Volume 11
Heart Function and Metabolism
Edited by T. Kobayashi, T. Sano, and N. S. Dhalla
Copyright 1978   University Park Press   Baltimore

EFFECT OF INCREASED cAMP CONTENT ON EXTRACELLULAR DISTRIBUTION OF CALCIUM AND CONTRACTILITY IN RABBIT HEART

Y. ITO, H. MATSUURA, and Y. UEBA

Department of Internal Medicine, Division I,
Kobe University School of Medicine, Kobe, Japan

SUMMARY

Norepinephrine, dexamethasone, and papaverine hydrochloride caused a significant increase in myocardial cAMP level and an alteration of intracellular distribution of Ca, such as the reduction of Ca content on mitochondrial and microsomal fractions, with or without positive inotropic effects, in the rabbit. Positive inotropic effects evoked by norepinephrine were significantly increased under the elevated level of cAMP induced by dexamethasone and papaverine. On the other hand, verapamil showed no effects on cAMP concentration and intracellular Ca distribution of the heart. These results indicate that the accumulation of myocardial cAMP may result in the alteration of intracellular distribution of Ca, and it is suggested that there is an increase in the available Ca for contractile and metabolic mechanisms of the heart.

INTRODUCTION

The role of adenosine $3':1$-monophosphate (cAMP) in mediating certain metabolic effects of catecholamine on heart muscle has been well known and it has been suggested that cAMP induces a positive inotropic effect on the heart as well. However, a principal question in research on myocardial contraction is still whether or not enhancement of myocardial contractility is mediated by cAMP. In order to examine this problem, we have determined myocardial calcium (Ca), which plays a central role in contractile mechanism, and its distribution of intracellular fractions in an elevated cAMP level caused by dexamethasone (Dx), papaverine hydrochloride, and norepinephrine (NE) in the rabbit.

METHODS

The hearts were removed from albino rabbits weighing about 2 kg, were perfused by Langendorff's method with bicarbonate buffered salt solution containing 0.56 mM Ca, and were gassed with 95% oxygen and 5% CO_2 at $37°C$ at a constant pressure of 75 cm in water (Ueba, Ito, and Chidsey, 1971; Ito and Chidsey, 1972).

Calcium determinations were performed on the hearts after the perfusion *in vitro,* and on the tissues rapidly removed from animals (Ueba *et al.,* 1971). The left ventricle with septum was pressed through a stainless steel sieve. A small portion of it was dried for the determination of total Ca content and the remainder was homogenized in a Virtis homogenizer, 45 to 20 vol of 0.25 M sucrose containing 5×10^{-6} M EGTA (ethylene glycol bis(β-aminoethyl ether)-N,N'-tetraacetic acid). A mitochondrial fraction was obtained, sedimenting from 1,000 to 12,000 $\times$ g, and a microsomal fraction was obtained from 12,000 to 37,000 $\times$ g. Protein was measured by the biuret and Lowry's methods. Calcium was extracted with 0.8 M perchloric acid containing 0.4% $LaCl_2$ and measured with a Hitachi 207 atomic absorption spectrophotometer. Myocardial cAMP was extracted and measured by the modified competitive protein binding method of Gilman. Dx, papaverine, and NE were administered to the isolated perfused heart with a Harvard-type infusion pump.

RESULTS AND DISCUSSION

Dx, 3 mg/kg, was intramuscularly injected daily into the rabbit for two days. In the control group, cAMP concentration of the left ventricle was measured 573.4 $\pm$ 29.3 pM/g wet weight ($n = 7$). Twenty-four hours after the injection, cAMP was increased by 40.4%, 804.9 $\pm$ 90.9 pM/g ($p < 0.02$) ($n = 5$), and on the second day by 47.7, 846.9 $\pm$ 35.0 pM/g ($p < 0.001$) ($n = 5$). This finding has not been reported in the literature. Isolated perfused heart from these animals treated with Dx for two days revealed no changes in maximum isometric developed tension.

Myocardial Ca and its distribution of intracellular fractions immediately after removal from the animals pretreated with Dx for two days were determined. No changes in total Ca content of the heart were detected—1.12 $\pm$ 0.07 μM/g in controls ($n = 4$) and 1.02 $\pm$ 0.11 μM/g in Dx-treated hearts ($n = 8$); however, there was a significant decrease of Ca concentration in two intracellular compartments—17.5 $\pm$ 1.0 nM/mg protein in mitochondrial fraction (MT), 16.9 $\pm$ 1.8 nM/mg protein in microsomal fraction (MS) in seven normal rabbits, and 13.5 $\pm$ 0.4 nM/mg protein in MT, and 11.6 $\pm$ 0.7 nM/mg protein in MS in nine Dx-treated rabbits. At that time there was no difference in plasma Ca concentration of two groups, 2.56 $\pm$ 0.13 μM/ml in controls and 2.47 $\pm$ 0.10 μM/ml in Dx-treated animals.

In order to observe the effect of Dx on the heart, Dx was directly infused to the isolated perfused heart at a rate of 0.169 mg/min for 45 min. Dx clearly prohibited the 12.8% of reduction in maximum active tension of control group, and also increased myocardial cAMP concentration by 34.2% at the end of

45-min perfusion of Dx. Ca contents in two intracellular compartments showed a tendency to decrease with Dx infusion, and total Ca of the heart revealed no change.

From these results, it was suggested that intracellular distribution of Ca could be altered under the elevated myocardial cAMP level. In order to answer this question, 1 μg/min of NE was infused to the perfused hearts for 10 min. Maximum active tension was increased by 49.5% as compared to that of controls during its perfusion. Myocardial cAMP concentration was elevated by 48.6% from 460.0 ± 40.2 pM/g in controls ($n = 8$) to 683.4 ± 99.5 pM/g in NE infused hearts ($n = 4$), and Ca contents in MT and MS were decreased by 23.9% from 14.2 ± 0.8 nM/mg protein to 10.8 ± 0.5 nM/mg protein ($p < 0.05$) and 28% from 15.7 ± 1.7 nM&mg protein to 11.3 ± 1.5 nM/mg protein, respectively, but the myocardial total Ca was unchanged.

Papaverine inhibits phosphodiesterase and also increases the intracellular cAMP concentration (Markwardt and Hoffmann, 1970). In the present study, papaverine hydrochloride was infused into the perfused heart at a rate of 0.085 mg/min. Active tension of the heart was decreased by 22% during the 10 min of papaverine infusion, and myocardial concentration of cAMP was increased up to 63%, 751.0 ± 96.3 pM/g ($n = 7$). MT and MS Ca contents ($n = 7$) were decreased

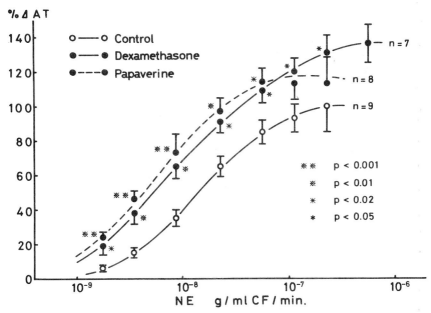

Figure 1. The dose-response curve for norepinephrine in the isolated perfused rabbit hearts. Norepinephrine was cumulatively administered to the heart with the doses ranging from 10^{-9} to 10^{-6} g/ml coronary flow/min. p values: In comparison to controls; AT: Active tension.

by 18.3%, 11.6 ± 0.3 nM/mg protein ($p < 0.01$), and by 16.6%, 13.1 ± 1.0 nM/mg protein, respectively.

Verapamil is structurally related to papaverine and both act as coronary and peripheral vasodilators. In contrast with papaverine, verapamil showed no effects on cAMP concentration of the heart and intracellular distribution of Ca, but a marked reduction of active tension was found with 7.5 μg/min of verapamil.

From these results, it is considered that an elevated cAMP level in myocardial tissue might induce an alteration in the intracellular Ca distribution and thus make available Ca for contraction or metabolism in the heart. For the purpose of examining this consideration, the dose-response curve for NE was determined in the presence of Dx and papaverine in the isolated perfused heart. To avoid the effect of cardiac rate on measurement of myocardial contractile force, the right atrium of the perfused heart was removed and the A-V node was crushed; then the heart was stimulated electrically at a rate of 150/min, at 10% above threshold voltage. NE-induced inotropic effects were markedly increased in the hearts treated with Dx and papaverine, as shown in Figure 1. It is suggested that there is an increase in the available Ca for contractile and metabolic mechanisms under the accumulated cAMP in the heart.

REFERENCES

ITO, Y., and CHIDSEY, C. A. 1972. Intracellular calcium and myocardial contractility IV. Distribution of calcium in the failing heart. J. Mol. Cell. Cardiol. 4:507–517.

MARKWARDT, F., and HOFFMANN, A. 1970. Effects of papaverine derivatives on cyclic AMP phosphodiesterase of human platelets. Biochem. Pharmacol. 19:2519–2520.

UEBA, Y., ITO, Y., and CHIDSEY, C. A. 1971. Intracellular calcium and myocardial contractility I. Influence of extracellular calcium. Amer. J. Physiol. 220:1553–1557.

Mailing address:
Y. Ito,
Department of Internal Medicine, Division I,
Kobe University School of Medicine,
7-chome, Kusunoki-cho, Ikuta-ku,
Kobe, 650 (Japan).

Recent Advances in Studies on
Cardiac Structure and Metabolism, Volume 11
Heart Function and Metabolism
Edited by T. Kobayashi, T. Sano, and N. S. Dhalla
Copyright 1978   University Park Press   Baltimore

INTERACTION OF LANTHANIDES WITH MUSCLE MICROSOMES

N. KRASNOW

Department of Medicine, State University of New York,
Downstate Medical Center, Brooklyn, New York, USA

SUMMARY

The interaction of gadolinium, a lanthanide with calcium-blocking action, with isolated muscle microsomes has been studied. Two classes of binding sites were present, 80 and in excess of 300 nmol/mg in number, respectively. Divalent cation, including Ca, Zn, and Cd, blocked the higher affinity site. Antibiotic ionophores X537A and A23187 enhanced binding, with positive cooperativity. ATP enhanced binding at low concentration (10–20 μM) of nucleotide, and without ATP-hydrolysis. The data suggest a dissociation in the intact membrane between the binding and ATP-hydrolytic portion of the transport site.

INTRODUCTION

The rare earth elements of the lanthanide series—lanthanum, gadolinium, europium, praesodymium, and others—form trivalent cations with a chemistry similar in some respects to calcium. Because they have ionic radii similar to calcium they have been widely used in physiologic studies in both nerve and muscle and are thought to act by blocking calcium movement at the cell membrane. Sanborn and Langer (1970) showed a marked inhibition of contractile activity in perfused heart at 10^{-5} M concentration lanthanum, and suggested that, since electron microscopy did not demonstrate lanthanum intracellularly, it acted on the sarcolemma, perhaps by blocking calcium sites on the mucopolysaccharide coat external to the plasma membrane. Langer and Frank (1972) have also shown an inhibition of calcium flux in cardiac cells.

Despite this interest in a physiologically important tool, there has been little direct study of the interaction of lanthanides with muscle membranes *in vitro*. We (Krasnow, 1972) were able to show an inhibition of *calcium* binding and uptake in cardiac and skeletal muscle microsomes by lanthanum, in concentrations similar to those used by Sanborn and Langer (1970) in their physiologic studies. This effect was only on the inhibition of a calcium influx, since

This work was supported in part by Grant HL 05726, United States Public Health Service, National Heart and Lung Institute, Bethesda, Maryland.

lanthanum has no effect on spontaneous calcium efflux from microsomes. An intriguing aspect of this effect was a time-dependence, which we think accounted for an apparent lack of action by lanthanum in otherwise similar studies by others.

The purpose of the present study was to investigate the *direct* interaction of lanthanides with cardiac and skeletal muscle microsomes.

MATERIALS AND METHODS

Fifty- to one hundred-gram portions of dog heart or rabbit leg muscles were homogenized in a Waring blender, using a sucrose-histidine homogenizing medium buffered with Tris at pH 6.8 in the cold. By differential centrifugation, the fraction of microsomes sedimenting between 9–45,000 g was harvested. In standard assays in our laboratory this preparation usually binds 60–70 nmol/mg calcium from dog heart, and 175–200 nmol/mg from rabbit white skeletal muscle. Assays of lanthanide binding were performed by the Millipore filtration technique in an assay medium containing 100 mM KCl, 4 mM $MgCl_2$, buffered at pH 6.8 by Tris-maleate. In later studies, piperazine-ethane-sulfonate buffer was used to avoid the lanthanide binding of maleic acid. ATP was added as noted. The isotopic lanthanide used was gadolinium-153 (Gd), for its convenience as a fairly long-lived gamma-emitter. The results with heart and skeletal muscle microsomes were similar qualitatively and quantitatively.

RESULTS

Figure 1 shows an experiment in passive binding of Gd to the membranes, that is, no ATP was present. The insert shows the one-phase Lineweaver-Burke plot with a calculated K_m of 3.3×10^{-5} M; on Scatchard plot, a linear two-phase system was usually seen, although in some experiments there was a curvature indicating some negative cooperativity. The two binding sites numbered approximately 80 and in excess of 300 nmol/mg, respectively.

Other cations (Ca, Zn, Al, Cd) block binding competitively, especially the high-affinity site. There was no significant effect on Gd binding by verapamil, ruthenium red, caffeine, or azide. Also, caffeine did not release Gd as it does calcium.

On the other hand, whereas the antibiotic ionophores *release* calcium from microsomes, X537A (20 μM) *increased* gadolinium binding. Figure 2 shows a representative experiment. The Scatchard plot shows an increase in the number of high-affinity binding sites in the presence of X537A, and evidence of positive cooperativity was often seen as well. The effect of another antibiotic ionophore, A23187, more specific for calcium, had a qualitatively similar although lesser effect in 1–2 μM concentration. The enhanced binding was observed whether

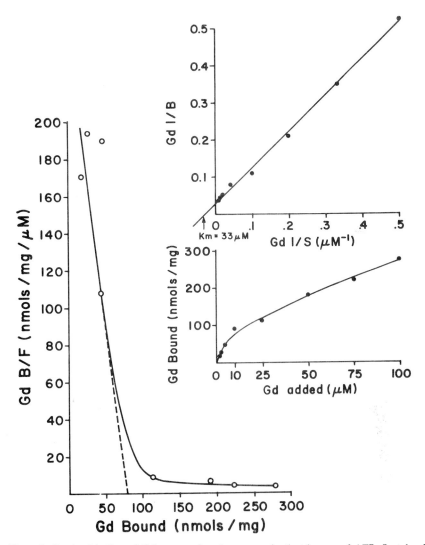

Figure 1. Passive binding of Gd to muscle microsomes, in the absence of ATP. Scatchard plot on *left* indicates two-phase system. Reproduced from Krasnow (1977) with permission.

X537A was present in the medium from the start of the reaction or was added after an initial burst of passive binding. Release of Gd by X537A was not observed.

The binding of lanthanides to muscle microsomes in the presence of ATP is complex. Figure 3 shows the raw data in an experiment in which ATP ($10 \mu M$) is added after completion of the passive binding of Gd to the microsomes. This

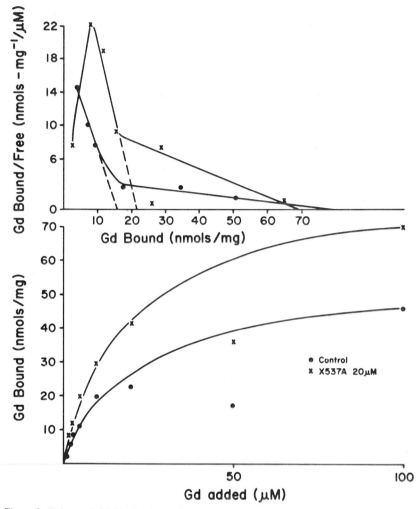

Figure 2. Enhanced Gd binding by X537A. The Scatchard plot (*above*) shows an increase in the number of high-affinity sites.

concentration of ATP produced an additional decrease in Gd concentration in the assay medium of 40 μM, over and above the change produced by passive binding. Note the slow rate of Gd binding when ATP is added, compared to the usual rapid binding of calcium. However, active binding of Gd, that is, binding in the presence by ATP, is complicated by the fact that ATP is a ligand for lanthanides with a binding constant of approximately $10^4 \mathrm{M}^{-1}$, and therefore competes with the vesicles for free lanthanide. In Figure 4, ATP is added at the arrow in *millimolar* concentration, as noted at the right of the graph. On

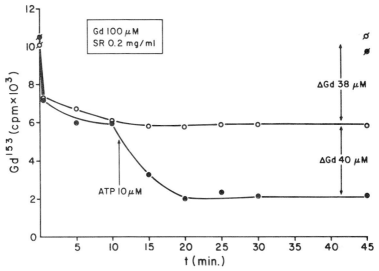

Figure 3. ATP-induced increase in Gd binding. ATP is added at the *arrow* (*solid circles*), inducing a further decline of 40 μM Gd^{153} concentration in the medium compared to the control (*open circles*). *Symbols with diagonal lines* represent samples of unfiltered medium. Reproduced from Krasnow (1977) with permission.

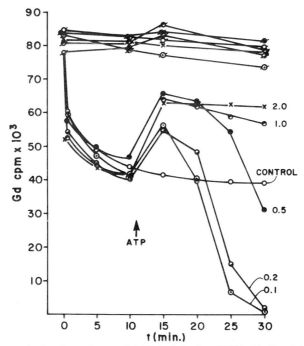

Figure 4. Concentration-dependence of ATP in inducing Gd^{153} binding. The reaction is started at zero time by adding Gd^{153}, and ATP is added at the *arrow. Numbers to the right of each curve* represent ATP concentration (mM); comparable *symbols with diagonal lines* represent unfiltered medium. Reproduced from Krasnow (1977) with permission.

addition of ATP, after passive binding, there is an initial return of Gd counts to the medium, which we interpret as related to a chelation of lanthanide by ATP, which chelate is then soluble and filtrable. When ATP concentration is high, namely millimolar range, the chelation dominates and no vesicle binding of lanthanide occurs. At lower ATP concentrations, however, a slow time-dependent binding of Gd is seen that consumes the isotope in the medium.

We have shown previously that Gd does not activate the magnesium or calcium ATPase present in muscle microsomes, and in high concentrations Gd depresses the calcium ATPase. Nevertheless, it is possible that the apparent increase in Gd binding by low concentrations of ATP could be simply a precipitation of unfiltrable microcrystals of gadolinium phosphate, formed as a result of spontaneous hydrolysis of ATP by the Mg ATPase of the membranes. However, the decrease in concentration of Gd in the medium is greater than can be accounted for even if all of the added ATP were hydrolzed. In Figure 5 the Gd binding in the presence of varying concentrations of ATP is shown by the solid circles, and the corresponding decrease in Gd concentration in the medium shown by crosses. If the decrease in medium concentration of isotope were due to total hydrolysis of ATP with formation of unfiltrable gadolinium phosphate, the curve would be given by the circled crosses, and would be linear with ATP concentration, not curvilinear. The theoretical curve does not fall as low as the observed, and does not therefore account for the lowering of Gd concentration.

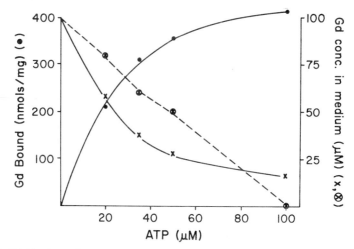

Figure 5. Gd binding (*solid circles*) as a function of ATP concentration. The corresponding decline in Gd concentration in the medium is given by the *cross*. The *circled cross* represents the theoretical change in Gd concentration if unfiltrable Gd PO_4 were produced by spontaneous ATP hydrolysis. For further explanation, see text. Reproduced from Krasnow (1977) with permission.

We also tested whether ATP was completely hydrolyzed by the indirect method of measuring the ability of the system to bind calcium, before and after Gd binding. In Figure 6, right panel, a change of 60 μM Gd in the medium results from the addition of 34 μM ATP. On the left are parallel experiments on calcium binding at three different concentrations of ATP, performed before and then after Gd binding. The ATP concentrations are low enough to be the limiting factors for calcium binding in the system. If ATP had been significantly hydrolyzed to account for the Gd binding, then no subsequent binding of calcium would have been possible. We see here that this is not the case. Allowing for some chelation of ATP by Gd, we see that calcium binding is still supported by ATP despite large amounts of prior gadolinium binding. This indicates that little ATP hydrolysis accompanied the excess Gd binding.

Heating the microsomes for 50 min at 60° C abolished Ca binding but not passive Gd binding. ATP-supported Gd binding was blocked.

DISCUSSION

The present data on passive binding of Gd showing two classes of affinity sites are similar to the study of Lehninger and Carafoli (1971) on mitochondrial membranes, although the affinity of the mitochondrial membrane is more than a full order of magnitude higher than for muscle microsomes.

It is stated, usually on the basis of electron microscopic data, that lanthanides cannot cross membranes. The ionophore data with X537A showing *increased* binding of Gd by the vesicles indicate that, at least under condition of

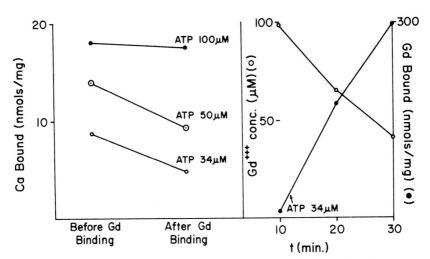

Figure 6. Lack of ATP hydrolysis induced by Gd binding. For further explanation, see text. Reproduced from Krasnow (1977) with permission.

"protection" by the ionophore, Gd *can* cross the membrane to the region of lower concentration in the vesicle interior.

The enhancement of Gd binding by ATP is unusual in that (1) very low concentration of ATP was required, well below the range usually used to demonstrate calcium binding, and (2) the ATP was not hydrolyzed. Whereas calcium transport by muscle microsomes is accompanied by stoichiometric ATP hydrolysis, the enhancement of gadolinium binding by small concentrations of ATP is *not* associated with ATP splitting. The details of this mechanism remain to be worked out, but it may be speculated that Gd binds to one portion of the active transport site, inhibiting calcium movement, but does not affect and is not affected by the ATP hydrolytic site. Shamoo and MacLennan (1975) suggested such a dissociation between an ionophoric site and hydrolytic site on the Ca-ATPase component of muscle microsomes. Ikemoto (1975) also suggested a dissociation in the functional state of transport sites, and it is also possible that Gd in the presence of ATP binds to one component without affecting the other.

We are aware that these actions of lanthanides on muscle microsomes are not necessarily the same as those taking place at the surface membrane of the intact fiber. Microsomes are here used as a model system for lanthanide effects on membranes; any physiologic correspondence remains to be evaluated.

Acknowledgments The interest and encouragement of Professor S. Ebashi and Dr. Y. Ogawa, Department of Pharmacology, University of Tokyo, in whose laboratory some of the early observations of this study were made, are gratefully acknowledged. The technical support of Mrs. L. Shore and Mrs. N. Lazarus and the secretarial assistance of Mrs. Y. Israelite are greatly appreciated.

REFERENCES

IKEMOTO, N. 1975. Transport and inhibitory Ca^{2+} binding sites on the ATPase enzyme isolated from the sarcoplasmic reticulum. J. Biol. Chem. 250:7219–7224.

KRASNOW, N. 1972. Effects of lanthanum and gadolinium ions on cardiac sarcoplasmic reticulum. Biochim. Biophys. Acta 282:187–194.

KRASNOW, N. 1977. Lanthanide binding to cardiac and skeletal muscle microsomes. Effects of adenosine triphosphates, cations and ionophores. Arch. Biochem. Biophys. 181: 322–330.

LANGER, G. A., and FRANK, J. S. 1972. Lanthanum in heart cell culture. J. Cell Biol. 54:441–455.

LEHNINGER, A. L., and CARAFOLI, E. 1971. The interaction of La^{3+} with mitochondria in relation to respiration-coupled Ca^{2+} transport. Arch. Biochem. Biophys. 143: 506–515.

SANBORN, W. G., and LANGER, G. A. 1970. Specific uncoupling of excitation and contraction in mammalian cardiac tissue by lanthanum. J. Gen. Physiol. 56:191–217.

SHAMOO, A. E., and MacLENNAN, D. H. 1975. Separate effects of mercurial compounds on the ionophoric and hydrolytic functions of the $(Ca^{++} + Mg^{++})$ ATPase of sarcoplasmic reticulum. J. Membr. Biol. 25:65–74.

Metabolic Aspect

Recent Advances in Studies on
Cardiac Structure and Metabolism, Volume 11
Heart Function and Metabolism
Edited by T. Kobayashi, T. Sano, and N. S. Dhalla
Copyright 1978   University Park Press   Baltimore

A NEW SPECTROSCOPIC APPROACH TO CARDIAC ENERGY METABOLISM

M. TAMURA[1], N. OSHINO[2], and B. CHANCE

The Johnson Research Foundation, The University of Pennsylvania
School of Medicine, Philadelphia, Pennsylvania, USA

SUMMARY

The optical characteristics of the hemoglobin-free perfused rat heart have been examined in detail. For dual-wavelength spectrophotometry, absorption pairs at 605–620 nm and 587–620 nm are found to be suited for the investigation of the oxidation-reduction changes of cytochrome aa_3 and oxygenation-deoxygenation of myoglobin in cardiac tissue.

Techniques by which the absorption changes of myoglobin and cytochrome aa_3 can be measured during one cycle of contraction-relaxation are presented. The results demonstrate that, in the aerobic state, myoglobin is more oxygenated during the systolic and diastolic periods and deoxygenated in the resting period, whereas cytochrome aa_3 is more reduced in the systole and diastole and oxidized in the resting period.

INTRODUCTION

Two of the main advantages of optical measurements *in vivo* are their non-destructive character and the rapid response to metabolic changes occurring in the organs. Cardiac muscle seems to be well suited for demonstrating the biochemical changes arising from the mechanical work of contraction-relaxation cycle. In this tissue, intracellular oxygen concentration can be monitored optically by oxygenation-deoxygenation of myoglobin, which is determined by the kinetic balance between the oxygen supply from the circulating system and consumption at mitochondria, and respiration can be monitored by the oxidation-reduction state of respiratory components (Chance and Williams, 1965; Oshino *et al.*, 1974; Sugano, Oshino, and Chance, 1974). The measurements, using hemoglobin-free perfused rat heart, are given in this chapter, and the feasibility and usefulness of the method are discussed.

---

[1] Division of Radiation Chemistry on Polymers, The Institute of Scientific and Industrial Research, Osaka University, Suita, Osaka (Japan);

[2] Department of Biodynamics, Nihon Schering, K. K., 6-64, Nishimiyahara, Yodogawa, Osaka (Japan).

RESULTS

The procedures used in the preparation of hemoglobin-free perfused rat heart are described elsewhere (Chance, Salkovitz, and Kovach, 1972). Aerobic and anaerobic conditions were obtained by perfusion with Krebs-Ringer bicarbonate buffer containing 2.5 mM Ca^{2+} and 10 mM glucose, and by equilibration by a gas mixture of 95% O_2 + 5% CO_2, and 95% N_2 + 5% CO_2. The optical absorption spectra were taken by use of a computer-assisted dual-wavelength scanning spectrophotometer (unpublished data), and the time-sharing dual-wavelength spectrophotometer with rotating disc (Theorell *et al.*, 1972) was also used for the absorption measurements of myoglobin and cytochrome aa_3.

The monochromatic light obtained by an interference filter mounted with a rotating disc illuminates the left ventricle uniformly, and the light passed through the left ventricle wall is conducted into the photomultiplier by a thin light-pipe inserted into the left ventricle. The details of the methods will appear elsewhere (Tamura *et al.*).

Optical Characteristics of Perfused Rat Heart

Figure 1A shows the difference spectrum of purified oxymyoglobin minus deoxymyoglobin and carboxymyoglobin, where 540 nm is used as the reference wavelength, and the spectrum of oxymyoglobin is taken as a flat baseline by computer. The difference spectrum of the perfused heart is shown in Figure 1B, where the aerobic steady state is similarly taken as a flat baseline. As is expected from the high content of myoglobin in rat heart ($\sim$ 0.2 μmol/g), the difference spectrum obtained by anaerobiosis is similar to that of purified myoglobin, except for the following: the broad absorption around 600 nm in Figure 1A is shifted to a distinct peak at 605 nm and the relative ratio of absorbance changes at 564 nm and 605 nm is inverted in perfused heart compared to that in purified myoglobin, which arises from the contributions of cytochrome c, aa_3 in this difference spectrum. The CO-inhibited spectrum of the heart (aerobic minus CO-saturated heart) shows more clearly the contribution of the mitochondrial absorption spectra to that of myoglobin.

From the spectra it appears that, in the case of cytochrome aa_3 at 605–620 nm, more than 85% of the absorbance is from cytochrome aa_3 and only 15% is from myoglobin. However, other cytochromes, such as cytochrome c at 550–540 nm and cytochrome b at 564–575 nm, cannot be measured practically by the interference of the absorption of myoglobin.

Behavior of Intracellular
Oxygen Concentration During One Cycle of Contraction-Relaxation

Figure 2 shows the absorption changes of the oxygenation-deoxygenation of myoglobin during the contraction-relaxation cycle together with the left ventric-

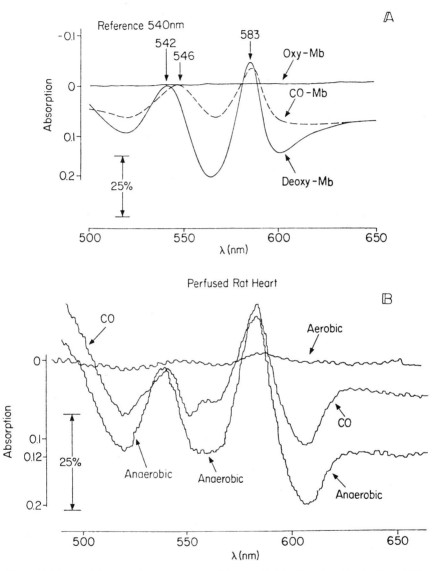

Figure 1. The optical absorption spectra of purified myoglobin (*A*) and perfused rat heart (*B*).

ular pressure changes (LVP) and electrocardiogram (ECG), at an absorption of 581 nm–(587 + 575)/2 nm (Tamura *et al.*). Following the ECG pulse, after contraction starts, the oxygenation of myoglobin occurs with a half-time of approximately 3 msec. The oxygenation is completed within 10 msec when the contraction is halfway to the maximum. The deoxygenation is shown during the

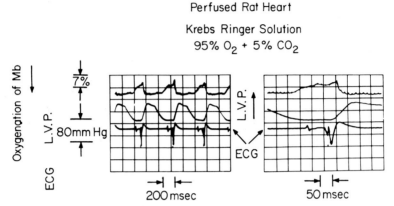

Perfused Rat Heart

Krebs Ringer Solution

95% O_2 + 5% CO_2

Figure 2. The oscilloscope traces of myoglobin absorption changes, left ventricular pressure change (LVP), and electrocardiogram (ECG).

resting state. Thus it can be said that intracellular oxygen concentration is increased during systolic and diastolic periods and decreased in the resting period between concentrations from 10^{-5} M to 10^{-4} M, since approximately 10% of total myoglobin undergoes the periodic cycle of oxygenation-deoxygenation associated with heartbeat under these aerobic conditions.

Periodic Absorption Change of Cytochrome aa₃ During a Single Heartbeat

The periodic absorption changes of cytochrome aa_3 associated with the contraction-relaxation cycle are shown in Figure 3, where cytochrome aa_3 is more reduced in the systolic and diastolic periods and is oxidized in the resting period, having rather moderate oxidation-reduction changes compared with the myoglobin absorption change (Figure 2). Under normal aerobic steady state, similar

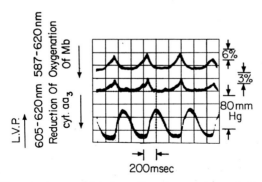

Figure 3. Oscilloscope traces of the absorption changes of myoglobin and cytochrome aa_3 associated with heartbeat. Conditions are aerobic steady state.

to myoglobin, approximately 10–15% of total cytochrome aa$_3$ undergoes the periodic cycle of oxidation-reduction associated with heartbeat.

DISCUSSION

The results of Figure 3 suggest that an increase of respiration rate may occur during systolic and diastolic periods, since the reduction of cytochrome aa$_3$ corresponds to the increase of respiration rate by the state 3–state 4 transition (Chance and Williams, 1965; Oshino *et al.,* 1974). If so, the rapid increase of the oxygenation level of myoglobin during systolic and diastolic periods can be

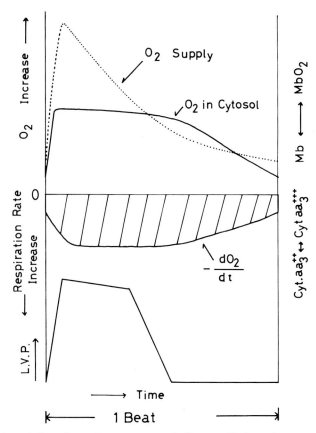

Figure 4. A tentative scheme for oxygen supply from capillaries and consumption during one cycle of contraction-relaxation. *Top: dotted line,* oxygen supply; *solid line,* intracellular oxygen concentration. *Middle:* oxygen consumption rate. The area underneath the curve is the total amount of oxygen utilized by the respiration. The *solid curve* of the *top column* (shown as O$_2$ in Cytosol) is obtained by the difference between the *dotted line* and the *middle curve.*

interpreted by the assumption that oxygen might be supplied from capillaries into tissue in this period, which overcomes the oxygen consumption. In the resting state, on the other hand, the oxygen supply might be stopped, where the oxygen consumption overcomes the supply, causing the decrease of intracellular oxygen concentration. Figure 4 is a tentative illustration of the above, where the intracellular oxygen concentration of the top, as monitored by myoglobin absorption change, is determined by the difference of the oxygen supply (dotted line) and consumption (bottom column). In this figure, we assume the following points: 1) ADP causes the increase of respiration; and 2) ADP might be liberated from muscle during the contraction; however, 3) the buffer system of creatine-phosphate-creatine irons out the fluctuation of ADP, resulting instead in the constant respiration rate over one cycle of contraction-relaxation, as shown in the middle trace.

Although the scheme of Figure 4 must be tested further (Tamura *et al.*), it is clear that the present results open the possibility for studying oxygen metabolism of cardiac tissue during one cycle of contraction-relaxation with millisecond time resolution under nearly physiological conditions.

REFERENCES

CHANCE, B., SALKOVITZ, I. A., and KOVACH, A. G. B. 1972. Kinetics of mitochondrial flavoprotein and pyridine nucleotide in perfused heart. Amer. J. Physiol. 223:207–218.
CHANCE, B., and WILLIAMS, G. R. 1965. The respiratory chain and oxidative phosphorylation. Adv. Enzymol. 17:65–134.
OSHINO, N., SUGANO, T., OSHINO, R., and CHANCE, B. 1974. Mitochondrial function under hypoxic conditions: The steady states of cytochrome aa_3 and their relation to mitochondrial energy states. Biochim. Biophys. Acta 368:198–310.
SUGANO, T., OSHINO, N., and CHANCE, B. 1974. Mitochondrial function under hypoxic conditions. The steady states of cytochrome c reduction and of energy metabolism. Biochim. Biophys. Acta 347:340–358.
TAMURA, M., OSHINO, N., SILVER, I., and CHANCE, B. In preparation.
THEORELL, H., CHANCE, B., YONETANI, T., and OSHINO, N. 1972. The combustion of alcohol and its inhibition by 4-methyl pyrazole in perfused rat liver. Arch. Biochem. Biophys. 151:434–444.

Mailing address:
Dr. M. Tamura
Division of Radiation Chemistry on Polymers,
The Institute of Scientific and Industrial Research,
Osaka University, Suita, Osaka (Japan).

Recent Advances in Studies on
Cardiac Structure and Metabolism, Volume 11
Heart Function and Metabolism
Edited by T. Kobayashi, T. Sano, and N. S. Dhalla
Copyright 1978   University Park Press   Baltimore

SIGNIFICANCE OF HEAT LOSS IN ENERGETICS
OF LEFT VENTRICLE

R. AOYAGI, K. AIZAWA, Y. AIZAWA,
H. MUROOKA, K. TAMURA, and M. MATSUOKA

First Department of Medicine, Niigata University School of Medicine,
Niigata City, Niigata, Japan

SUMMARY

Left ventricular heat loss was examined by measuring the temperatures in the coronary sinus blood, in the aortic blood, and in the left atrial blood by thermistors. The temperature was highest in the coronary sinus blood, in the aortic blood next, and it was the least in the left atrial blood. However, since the aortic blood flow was naturally higher than the coronary sinus blood flow, the heat loss was larger in the left ventricular cavity than in the rest of the chambers. This heat loss was mostly proportional to the magnitude of the changes of both the arterial blood pressure and the aortic blood flow.

INTRODUCTION

Analysis of the complete energy balance of the left ventricle is of great importance in making clear left ventricular pump function. If both the cardiac work and the heat loss were calculated, an evaluation of left ventricular energy efficiency could be approached. However, heat loss of the ventricle has not been examined completely as far as we know (Afonso *et al.,* 1965a,b; Tamura *et al.,* 1976). Therefore, in this preliminary report, we attempted to measure the heat production and the heat loss of the left ventricle in anesthetized dogs, both at rest and during pacing-induced tachycardia.

METHOD

A schematic drawing of the apparatus of the experiment is shown in Figure 1. Heat loss from the left ventricle was measured during the acute experiments of the open-chest mongrel dogs anesthetized with morphine and urethane. A thermistor, Victory Engineering Corporation (U.S.A.), was mounted on the tip of the tube. The time constant of the thermistor was 0.3 sec. Changes in resistance of the matched thermistor induced by blood temperature were recorded on the photorecorder. A special cannula, consisting of the glass tube and

313

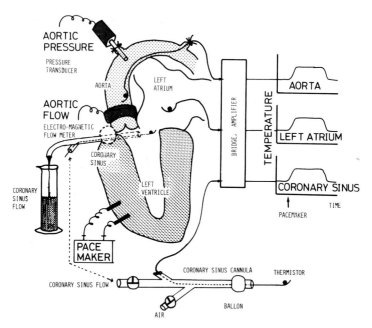

Figure 1. A schematic drawing of the apparatus of the experiment.

a rubber balloon to occlude the flow, was inserted manually into the coronary sinus through the free wall of the right atrium. The special thermistor tubes were inserted into: 1) coronary sinus, 2) root of the aorta, and 3) left atrium. These arrangements were made because the heat dissipation was thought to occur mainly in these three directions. The thermistor tubes were inserted with special care not to touch the inner wall of each cavity. Furthermore, the aortic mean pressure was recorded. The aortic mean flow was measured by electromagnetic flowmeter. The pacemaker wires were connected to the ventricular myocardium, and the heart rate was increased up to twice that of the control period. The chest was closed after surgery and the body was warmed up to normal temperature range by hot pack. Special attention was paid to control of body temperature during the whole period of the experiment. Thus, changes and differences in heat loss were calculated both at rest and during the pacing-induced tachycardia.

RESULTS AND DISCUSSION

The temperature gradient between the coronary sinus blood and the aortic blood was measured by simultaneous measurement of these temperatures. The temperature gradient was plus in all measurements; therefore, the temperature of the coronary sinus blood was always higher than that of the aortic blood. The data clearly indicated that heat was removed while the coronary blood flowed through the coronary vasculature in the left ventricular wall. The magnitude of this temperature gradient was $0.27 \pm 0.05°$ C, expressed as mean and 1 standard deviation. The temperature gradient was also calculated as the differences between the atrial blood and the aortic blood. The temperature gradient was also plus in all measurements. The magnitude of this heat loss into the left ventricular cavity was $0.14 \pm 0.16°$ C. Therefore, the data also clearly indicated that the left atrial blood removed heat from the left ventricular cavity while it was running through this chamber. Moreover, because aortic blood flow is larger than coronary sinus blood flow, the total energy loss in calories should be larger into the left ventricular cavity than into the coronary venous system.

Changes of the temperature gradient were examined by pacing-induced tachycardia (Figure 2). The left panel in the figure shows the temperature gradient between coronary sinus blood and aortic blood. If the aortic blood flow was increased by the pacing, the temperature gradient increased, and the magnitude of this increase was $0.06 \pm 0.11°$ C. If the aortic flow decreased by pacing,

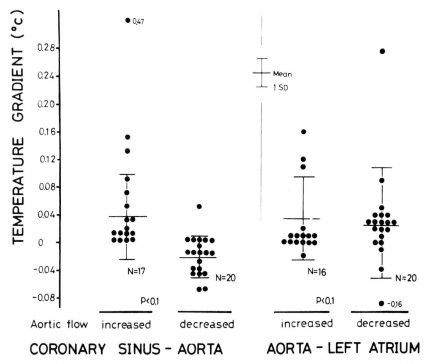

Figure 2. Changes of the temperature gradients during pacing-induced tachycardia. The *left panel* shows the change between the coronary sinus blood and the aortic blood. The *right panel* shows the change between the aortic blood and the left atrial blood.

this gradient decreased, and the magnitude was − 0.02 ± 0.03° C. However, there was no significant difference between the two different gradients. Similarly, as shown in the right panel of Figure 2, the temperature gradient between the aortic blood and the left atrial blood was examined. If the aortic blood flow increased by pacing, the temperature gradient increased, and the magnitude of this gradient was 0.04 ± 0.06° C. On the contrary, however, if the aortic blood flow decreased, the temperature gradient did not change, as is seen in the temperature gradient between the coronary sinus blood and the aortic blood. Therefore, there was no significant difference between these two groups. The magnitude of the changes of these temperature gradients was examined according to the changes of heart rate, aortic blood flow, and aortic pressure. As shown in Figure 3, temperature changes were examined during pacemaker-induced tachycardia. The temperature decreased according to the increase of the heart rate. In dog 1, in Figure 3, the correlation coefficient was 0.72; in dog 2 it was 0.51. The right panel in Figure 3 shows the changes of temperature between the aortic blood and the left atrial blood during pacing-induced tachycardia. Temperature was also decreased according to increase of heart rate by pacing. The correlation coefficient in dog 1 was 0.33; in dog 2 it was 0.68. The data showed that the decrease of heat loss to either the left ventricular cavity or the coronary

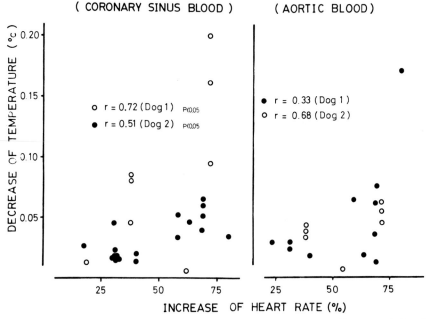

Figure 3. Changes of the temperature gradients according to changes of heart rate induced by pacing.

sinus is dependent on the magnitude of both the arterial pressure and the aortic flow. Changes of temperature in the left atrial blood during the pacing-induced tachycardia were examined, and the results showed that the magnitude of the temperature decreased during pacing-induced tachycardia.

REFERENCES

AFONSO, S., McKENNA, D. H., O'BRIEN, G. S., ROWE, G. G., and CRUMPTON, C. W. 1965a. Left ventricular heat production during induced tachycardia in the intact dog. Amer. J. Physiol. 209:33.

AFONSO, S., ROWE, G. G., LUGO, J. E., and CRUMPTON, C. W. 1965. Left ventricular heat production in intact anesthetized dogs. Amer. J. Physiol. 208:946.

TAMURA, K., AOYAGI, R., MIYANO, S., HIGUMA, N., AIZAWA, Y., AIZAWA, K., and AOKI, T. 1976. The significance and the changes of the heat loss from the left ventricular myocardium. Clin. Physiol. 6:155. (In Japanese.)

Mailing address:
Dr. R. Aoyagi
First Department of Medicine,
Niigata University School of Medicine,
1-Asahinachi, Niigata City, Niigata (Japan).

Recent Advances in Studies on
Cardiac Structure and Metabolism, Volume 11
Heart Function and Metabolism
Edited by T. Kobayashi, T. Sano, and N. S. Dhalla
Copyright 1978 University Park Press Baltimore

MYOCARDIAL ADENINE NUCLEOTIDES AFTER INFUSION OF ADENOSINE

W. ISSELHARD, J. EITENMÜLLER, W. MÄURER, H. WELTER, and H. REINECKE

Institute for Experimental Medicine, University of Köln,
5 Köln 41, Federal Republic of Germany

SUMMARY

In the rabbit heart, continuous infusion (12 ml/hr) of 1% adenosine into the superior caval vein, or of 0.5% adenosine into the left myocardial ventricle, for a period of 3 hr increased the myocardial tissue level of ATP by almost 40% over the control (5.0 μmol/g). Both shorter or longer periods of application and lower or higher concentrations of adenosine, as well as the infusion of adenosine into the left atrium, were less effective. The increase markedly outlasted the period of application of adenosine. It did not result from the adenosine-induced systemic hypotension and decrease in cardiac work, but must be attributed to a direct metabolic effect of the adenosine infusion.

INTRODUCTION

The myocardial tissue levels of adenine nucleotides are fairly constant in physiological situations, despite very large variations in the cardiac workload. However, in certain pathological situations, such as deprivation of oxygen supply, they undergo a rapid reduction. The decrease in the content of energy-rich substances and the simultaneous rapid deterioration of the myocardial function in anaerobiosis prove an insufficient anaerobic energy production. Besides the rapid breakdown of creatine phosphate, the ATP content especially decreases, while ADP, AMP, and adenosine accumulate. Due to a further degradation of these substances, the sum of the adenine nucleotides also diminishes during prolonged periods of anaerobiosis. Upon reoxygenation, the accumulated ADP, AMP, and adenosine are rapidly rephosphorylated, and despite a subnormal content of adenine nucleotides a normal or quasi-normal ATP-ADP-AMP-ratio is achieved. The further restitution of the adenine nucleotides occurs very slowly, at a rate of increase in the myocardial ATP level of 0.06 μmol/g wet tissue/hr (Isselhard *et al.*, 1970b). This second phase of restitution, attributable to a synthesis of new nucleotides, can be markedly accelerated in the myocardium by a postanaerobic continuous application of adenosine (Isselhard *et al.*, 1970a). In the search for further methods of protecting the myocardium during induced anaerobic situations, of improving myocardial anoxic tolerance, or of improving and accelerating postanoxic recovery, it was of interest to investigate whether or not a normal tissue level of ATP can be significantly increased by a continuous administration of adenosine.

METHODS

The experiments were performed on rabbits of 2.5–3.0 kg body weight, anesthetized with Pernocton®, heparinized, and maintained at normal body temperature. Adenosine or saline was administered in three variations: (1) into the left ventricular cavity through a catheter installed via the arteria carotis com., (2) into the vena cava superior cannulated via the vena jugularis superficialis dextra, and (3) into the left atrium after thoractomy in the fifth left ICR. The infusion volume was 12 ml/hr; iso-osmolarity was achieved by the addition of sodium chloride. Phentolamine (Regitin®), xylometazoline-HCl (Otriven®), or noradrenaline was administered intravenously; dosage and volume varied according to the effects to be produced. At the end of the observation period, a broad thoracotomy was performed under artificial ventilation in order to expose the heart, and the metabolic status of the hearts was preserved by the freeze-stop method (Wollenberger, Ristau, and Schoffa, 1960). The technique of the tissue extraction and the biochemical analysis of metabolites by means of enzymatic tests have been previously described (Isselhard and Merguet, 1962; Isselhard, Merguet, and Palm, 1962). Data on the myocardial status are based on the tissue wet weight, consisting of 20.0% tissue dry weight, and refer to left ventricular tissue unless otherwise stated.

RESULTS AND DISCUSSION

A continuous infusion of adenosine resulted in an increase in the myocardial tissue level of ATP, while the tissue levels of ADP and AMP were less changed. The extent of this increase was a function of the mode and duration of application, and of the dose of adenosine (Figure 1). After 3 hr of infusion of 0.5% adenosine solution into the left ventricular cavity, the ATP level had increased from 4.94 μmol/g under control conditions to 6.79 μmol/g, which is an increase of 37.5%. Adenosine solutions of lower and of higher concentrations were less effective. An increase of almost 40% also resulted from the infusion of 1% adenosine into the superior caval vein. The application of adenosine into the left atrium was less effective. The prolongation of adenosine infusion from 3 to 5 hr had no additional effect, except in the group that received 0.5% adenosine in the left atrium.

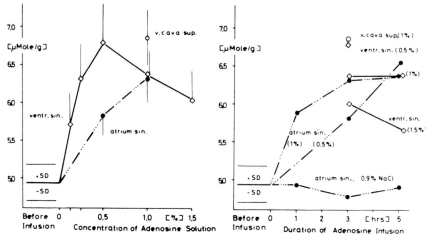

Figure 1. ATP tissue level of left ventricular myocardium of rabbits after infusion of adenosine into the left atrium (•), the left ventrical (◊), and the vena cava sup. (○). *Left:* effect of adenosine concentration after an infusion of 3 hr duration; *Right:* effect of duration of adenosine infusion.

The infusion in control experiments of 12 ml 0.9% NaCl solution per hour did not result in changes in the tissue levels of metabolites investigated in this study.

The increase in ATP, and thus in the sum of adenine nucleotides, is a "metabolic effect" of the adenosine infusion; it does not result from the adenosine-induced, dose-dependent systemic hypotension and decrease in left ventricular work (Figure 2):

1) Hypotension of a similar degree and duration induced by the intravenous application of phentolamine (Regitin® average dose: 1.7 mg/kg/hr) did not alter the normal pattern of adenine nucleotides.

2) The infusion of a 1% adenosine solution into the superior caval vein, together with xylometazoline-HCl (Otriven®, average dose: 600 µg/kg/hr) in doses sufficient to counteract the adenosine-induced hypotension, resulted in an elevated ATP level similar to that after the infusion of adenosine alone. Noradrenaline (average dose: 1300 µg/kg/hr) in combination with adenosine also resulted in a significantly elevated ATP level; the result was slightly less pronounced, apparently due to the massive catecholamine-induced stimulation of the heart.

3) The adenosine-induced rise in myocardial ATP occurred both in the left and the right ventricular tissue. While the systemic blood pressure and the left ventricular work decreased despite an increase in cardiac output, the pulmonary

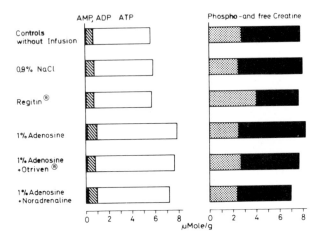

Figure 2. Status of the adenylic acid-creatine phosphate system in the left ventricular myocardium of rabbits at the end of a 3-hr infusion of 1% adenosine and/or various drugs into the vena cava sup.

pressure did not change, and thus the right ventricular work increased. After 3 hr of infusion of 12 ml 0.5% adenosine per hour into the left ventricle, the ATP level in the left ventricular myocardium had increased from 5.09 to 6.79 μmol/g, and in the right ventricular myocardium from 4.23 to 5.78 μmol/g.

Upon discontinuation of the adenosine infusion, the ATP level decreased slowly: a 30% elevated ATP level returned to a normal range after 24 hr.

Adenosine was not detectable in control hearts; it averaged about 0.03 μmol/g in hearts of animals that received an infusion of at least 1% adenosine. The glycogen level was not altered. The tissue level of lactate was not significantly different in animals that received adenosine or saline (4–7 μmol/g) intravenously and intraventricularly. In animals that received adenosine in the left atrium, the lactate level increased continuously (to about 11 μmol/g after 5 hr). The application of adenosine resulted in an increase in the tissue glucose of about 1–2 μmol/g. The administration of adenosine plus noradrenaline caused a massive rise in the tissue level of glucose (20.6 μmol/g) and lactate (17.2 μmol/g), and a 50% reduction of the glycogen level (15.6 μmol/g). In none of the experimental groups did the tissue level of total creatine deviate from the normal range (15.6 $\pm$ 1.9 μmol/g). The myocardial tissue level of creatine phosphate, which increased in accordance with other results during hypotension induced by phentolamine or the infusion of 0.125% and 0.25% adenosine, did not increase, or even decreased, in animals that received adenosine in higher concentrations. A satisfactory interpretation of this finding is difficult. It is unlikely that it results from changes in intracellular metabolic equilibria due to the increased ATP level, because creatine phosphate rapidly returned to normal values with the discontinuation of the adenosine infusion and a consecutive rise in the systematic pressure, but with persisting elevated tissue levels of ATP. It is also unlikely that it is caused by the hypotension-induced underperfusion of myocardial parts: there was neither an overall loss of total creatine or of glycogen nor an increase in the myocardial tissue lactate, and there were no signs of a functional insufficiency during and after the adenosine infusion. Further experiments should investigate whether or not this experimentally induced significant increase in a substantial energy-rich phosphate is of any "biological value," e.g., during or after anaerobiosis.

REFERENCES

ISSELHARD, W., HINZEN, D. H., GEPPERT, E., and MÄURER, W. 1970a. Beeinflussung des post-asphyktischen Wiederaufbaues der Adeninnucleotide in Kaninchenherzen *in-vivo* durch Substratangebot. Pfluegers Arch. 320:195–209.

ISSELHARD, W., MÄURER, W., STREMMEL, W., KREBS, J., SCHMITZ, H., NEUHOF, H., and ESSER, A. 1970b. Stoffwechsel des Kaninchenherzens *in-situ* während Asphyxie und in der post-asphyktischen Erholung. Pfluegers Arch. 316:164–193.

ISSELHARD, W., and MERGUET, H. 1962. Metabolite des Glykolysecyclus und des Adenylsäure-Phosphokreatin-Systems im schlagenden und durchbluteten Warmblüterherzen unter verschiedenen Versuchsbedingungen. Pfluegers Arch. 276:211–235.

ISSELHARD, W., MERGUET, H., and PALM, K. 1962. Bestimmung des Gesamtglykogens neben säurelöslichen Metaboliten in Perchlorsäure-Organhomogenaten. Z. Ges. Exp. Med. 136:174–182.

WOLLENBERGER, A., RISTAU, O., and SCHOFFA, G. 1960. Eine einfache Technik der extrem schnellen Abkühlung Größerer Gewebestücke. Pfluegers Arch. 270:399–412.

Mailing address:
Professor Dr. W. Isselhard,
Institut für Experimentelle Medizin
der Universität zu Köln,
Robert-Koch-Straße 10,
5 Köln 41 (Germany).

Recent Advances in Studies on
Cardiac Structure and Metabolism, Volume 11
Heart Function and Metabolism
Edited by T. Kobayashi, T. Sano, and N. S. Dhalla
Copyright 1978   University Park Press   Baltimore

METABOLIC EFFECT OF pH ON MYOCARDIUM OF HEART-LUNG PREPARATION

S. ANAZAWA, N. SAITO, and M. NAGANO

Department of Internal Medicine, Jikei University,
School of Medicine, Tokyo, Japan

SUMMARY

Cardiac performance and metabolism of heart-lung preparation of rat were studied with acid, normal, and alkali perfusions. Cardiac output, glucose uptake, and myocardial content of lactate, malate, glycerophosphate, and CP were increased in alkali and decreased in acid perfusion of 20 min. On the other hand, when pH of the perfusate was abruptly changed, CP and ATP were decreased independent of the performance. FDP was high and PEP was low in acute acidifying experiments. From these findings it is concluded that cardiac performance and carbohydrate metabolism are accelerated in alkali and depressed in acid perfusion, and that myocardial metabolism could be affected by pH not only secondary to the change of performance but also by itself.

INTRODUCTION

Studies examining the effect of acid-base change of ventricular performance have yielded varying results. Many studies have suggested that acidosis depresses and alkalosis enhances myocardial contractility (Schaer, 1974), whereas others have shown that acidosis per se cannot alter cardiac performance (Beierholm *et al.,* 1975) or only respiratory acid-base disturbance may affect the contractility (Cingolani *et al.,* 1970). Part of this discrepancy could be explained on the basis of differences in the species or preparations used, narcosis, degree of pH shift, oxygen availability, and level of sympathetic tone. The following two series of experiments were performed in an attempt, first, to elucidate the effect of pH on cardiac performance and metabolism, and, second, to clarify which of the two, either performance or metabolism, is more profoundly affected by pH.

MATERIALS AND METHODS

Heart-lung preparations of rats were perfused with Krebs-Ringer bicarbonate buffer containing red blood cells of rat and glucose as substrate. Measurements

325

were made of cardiac output, heart rate, venous pressure, glucose uptake, and myocardial contents of glycolytic intermediates and high-energy phosphates.

In the first series of experiments, perfusion was performed for 20 min with acid (prior to perfusion, 0.25 M HCl was added to adjust the pH of perfusate to 7.0–7.3) and alkali (with 1 M NaHCO$_3$, pH was adjusted to 7.6–8.0) perfusate and compared with normal pH (7.35–7.55) perfusion.

In the second series of experiments, after 15 min of normal pH perfusion, pH of the perfusate was abruptly changed by adding each of 0.125 M HCl, 0.5 M NaHCO$_3$, and 0.2 M Tris separately in 30 sec, and the mean values of pH shift were 7.4–6.73, 7.35–7.50, and 7.38–7.88, respectively. Then, at the 60th sec of infusing these agents, myocardial metabolic compounds were determined.

RESULTS

Cardiac output and glucose uptake were increased stepwise from acid to alkali (Figure 1). Lactate, malate, and glycerophosphate (GP) were high in alkali and low in acid (Figure 2), and creatine phosphate (CP) was significantly high in alkali (Figure 3). The changes of hemodynamics when pH of perfusate was abruptly altered are shown in Figures 4–6. In the HCl and NaHCO$_3$ group, blood flow and heart rate were decreased and venous pressure (VP) was increased, whereas the Tris group revealed slight increases in blood flow and no detectable change in heart rate and VP.

As for the metabolic changes caused by acute acidifying or alkalizing experiments, CP and ATP were decreased in all groups (Figure 7). FDP (fructose

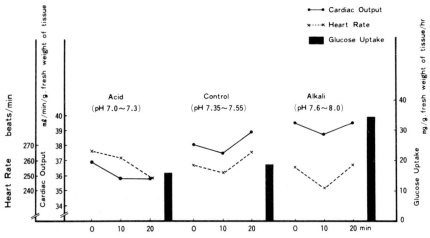

Figure 1. Effect of pH on cardiac hemodynamics and glucose uptake.

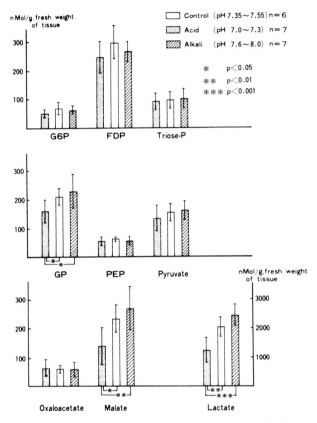

Figure 2. Metabolites in the myocardium after 20-min perfusion.

1:6-diphosphate) was high in the HCl group and low in the Tris group. PEP (phosphoenolpyruvate) was decreased in the HCl group and increased in the Tris and NaHCO₃ groups, but not significantly (Figure 8).

DISCUSSION

The first series of experiments represents overall acceleration of cardiac performance and metabolism in alkali perfusion, and agrees with the results of experiments on isolated rat hearts (Opie, 1965; Scheuer and Berry, 1967). Acceleration of glycolysis may produce more high-energy phosphates than required for increased performance, so excess energy may be stored in the form of CP,

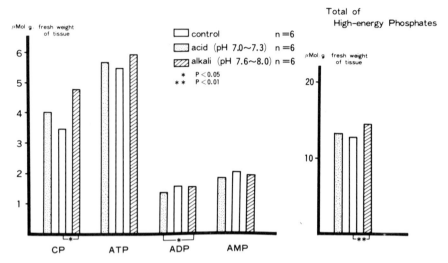

Figure 3. High-energy phosphates in the myocardium after 20-min perfusion.

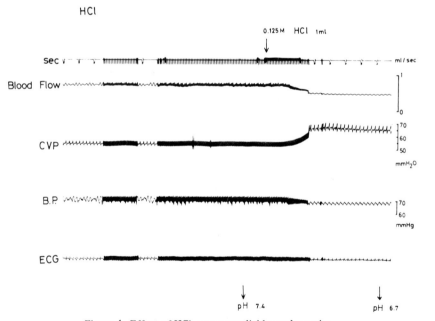

Figure 4. Effect of HCl on myocardial hemodynamics.

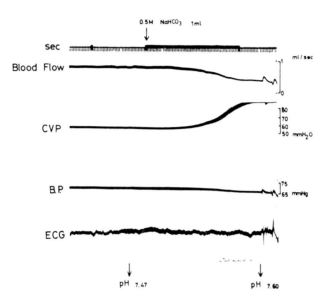

Figure 5. Effect of NaHCO$_3$ on myocardial hemodynamics.

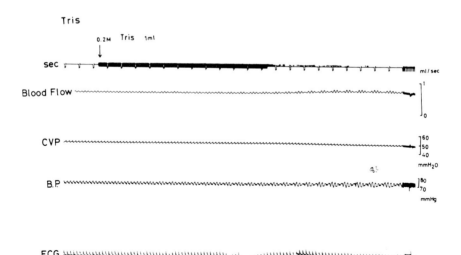

Figure 6. Effect of Tris on myocardial hemodynamics.

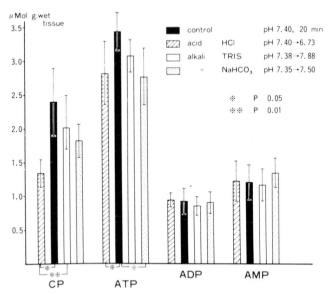

Figure 7. High-energy phosphates in the myocardium when pH of perfusate was changed abruptly.

because Lohman's reaction tends to form CP in high pH. On the other hand, performance and metabolism are depressed in general in acid perfusion; however, ATP is not low and cardiac function is still maintained. From this finding, in acid perfusion it is possible to consider involvement of fatty acid metabolism other than glucose metabolism. There is also the possibility that NADH/NAD ratio might play some role in the metabolism.

In the second series of experiments, in the Tris group, cardiac output slightly increased, whereas in the $NaHCO_3$ group, cardiac performance was found to be decreased, although it was increased in the 20 min of alkali perfusion with $NaHCO_3$ added. It is supposed that within the short duration of 1 min Tris raises intracellular pH but $NaHCO_3$ makes intracellular pH decrease. Concerning the changes of metabolism, experiments alkalized abruptly revealed CP and ATP were decreased, and these findings are different from 20-min perfusion. Could this be considered the result of energy consumption due to increase of cardiac work?

The interrelation of H^+ concentration and myocardial contraction is interesting. It is indicated that Ca^{2+} release from sarcoplasmic reticulum (Nakamaru and Schwartz, 1970) and binding of Ca^{2+} to troponin (Katz and Hecht, 1969) are

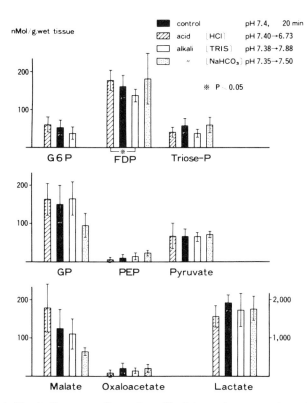

Figure 8. Metabolites in the myocardium when pH of the perfusate was changed abruptly.

increased when pH rises, so it is possible to consider that high pH enhances contraction.

As a view of energy consumption, high-energy phosphate must be saved in acutely acidified experiments, because performance is depressed; but, as a matter of fact, CP and ATP are decreased. From this fact it can be concluded that acute change of pH might affect the metabolism directly. Considering the glycolytic intermediates along the metabolic pathway, a marked difference at the point of FDP and PEP is shown (Figure 9). It is possible to consider that acute pH change affects the glycolytic enzymes leading to disturbance in the metabolic pathway, and, consequently, to depressed energy formation.

Finally, the following speculation was made (Figure 10). Because optimum pH of aldolase is shifted to alkali, acute acidification depresses this enzyme and

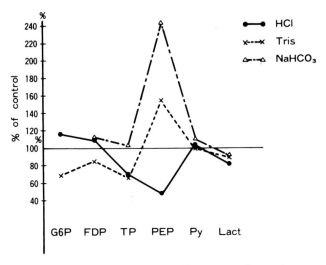

Figure 9. Metabolites represented by percent of control.

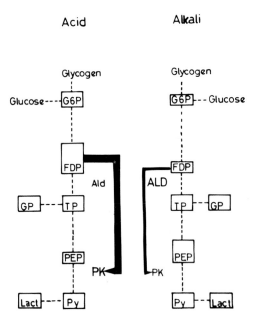

Figure 10. Schematic diagram summarizing the effect of acute change of pH on the metabolic pathway.

FDP will be accumulated. FDP is proved to activate pyruvate kinase (PK), which will result in a low level of PEP. In alkalization, the opposite reaction would occur, that is, active aldolase leads to low FDP and then accumulation of PEP will be mediated by PK. In addition, considering the fact that the FDP level reaches control level with time sequence that we have obtained previously, the disturbed metabolic pathway will be normalized with time; thus, in the steady phase of 20-min perfusion, overall metabolism may be accelerated in alkali perfusion, probably because of activated enzymes such as phosphofructokinase of glyceraldehyde-3-phosphate dehydrogenase.

REFERENCES

BEIERHOLM, E. A., GRANTHAM, R. N., O'KEEFE, D. D., LAVER, M. B., and DAG-GETT, W. M. 1975. Effects of acid-base changes, hypoxia and catecholamine on ventricular performance. Amer. J. Physiol. 228:1555–1561.

CINGOLANI, H. E., MATTIAZZI, A. R., BLESA, E. S., and GONZALEZ, N. C. 1970. Contractility in isolated mammalian heart muscle after acid-base changes. Circ. Res. 26:269–278.

KATZ, A. M., and HECHT, H. H. 1969. The early pump failure of the ischemic heart. Amer. J. Med. 47:497–502.

NAKAMARU, Y., and SCHWARTZ, A. 1970. Possible control of intracellular calcium metabolism by H^+: Sarcoplasmic reticulum of skeletal and cardiac muscle. Biochem. Biophys. Res. Commun. 41:830–836.

OPIE, L. H. 1965. Effect of extracellular pH on function and metabolism of isolated perfused rat heart. Amer. J. Physiol. 209:1075–1080.

SCHAER, H. 1974. Influence of respiratory and metabolic acidosis on epinephrine-inotropic effect in isolated guinea pig atria. Pfluegers Arch. 347:297–307.

SCHEUER, J., and BERRY, M. N. 1967. Effect of alkalosis on glycolysis in the isolated rat heart. Amer. J. Physiol. 213:1143–1148.

Mailing address:
S. Anazawa,
Department of Internal Medicine,
Jikei University, School of Medicine,
Tokyo 105, Minato-ku, Nishishinbashi 3-19-18 (Japan).

Recent Advances in Studies on
Cardiac Structure and Metabolism, Volume 11
Heart Function and Metabolism
Edited by T. Kobayashi, T. Sano, and N. S. Dhalla
Copyright 1978   University Park Press   Baltimore

EFFECTS OF CATECHOLAMINES ON MYOCARDIAL ENERGY METABOLISM AS STUDIED BY AN ORGAN REDOXIMETER

S. IMAI, T. OTORII, K. TAKEDA, Y. KATANO, and Y. NAKAGAWA

Department of Pharmacology,
Niigata University School of Medicine, Niigata City, Japan

SUMMARY

With the use of an organ redoximeter, the effects of noradrenaline, adrenaline, isoproterenol, and phenylephrine on the oxidation-reduction state of the myocardial pyridine nucleotides were studied in the canine heart-lung preparation supported by a donor. Noradrenaline and adrenaline produced an initial, transient improvement, and phenylephrine a sustained improvement, of the redox state, while isoproterenol produced a depression. Pretreatment of the preparation with adrenergic α-blockers resulted in an abolishment of the improvement by noradrenaline, adrenaline, and phenylephrine, while the depression by isoproterenol remained unchanged. Whereas noradrenaline and adrenaline produced a sustained improvement after an adrenergic β-blocker, propranolol, the effect of isoproterenol was abolished. These findings suggest that sympathomimetic amines can produce an improvement of the myocardial energy metabolism through activation of the adrenergic α-receptor. The depression of the myocardial oxidation-reduction state was taken to represent an acceleration of glycolysis.

INTRODUCTION

Although catecholamines are generally believed to induce myocardial hypoxia through augmentation of the myocardial O_2 consumption, an improvement of the myocardial energy metabolism has recently been reported (Williamson and Jamieson, 1966; Ribeilima *et al.,* 1976).

In view of this discrepancy, we have undertaken to study the effects of these substances on the myocardial energy metabolism with the aid of an organ redoximeter.

MATERIALS AND METHODS

Experiments were performed with canine heart-lung preparation supported by a donor. The details of the method were described in a previous publication (Imai *et al.,* 1975). To record the oxidation-reduction state of the pyridine nucleotides within the cell continuously, an organ redoximeter was used (Tateishi Electronics Model HEF-4), constructed on the basic principle developed by Chance and Legallais (1963), but additionally equipped with an analog computer to compensate for an optical artifact derived from variations in tissue blood content (Kobayashi *et al.*, 1971). The practical validity of applying the instrument for monitoring the intracellular oxidation-reduction state of pyridine nucleotides is supported by the experiments of Chance and his collaborators (1965).

Catecholamines were infused continuously into the rubber tubing leading to the venous cannula of the preparation (1–10 µg/ml of noradrenaline and adrenaline and 0.1–1.0 µg/ml of isoproterenol). Phenylephrine (100–300 µg) was injected as a single shot. Blockers were injected into the venous reservoir (1–10 mg of phentolamine mesylate, 10–20 mg of dibenamine hydrochloride, and 0.3–3 mg of propranolol hydrochloride).

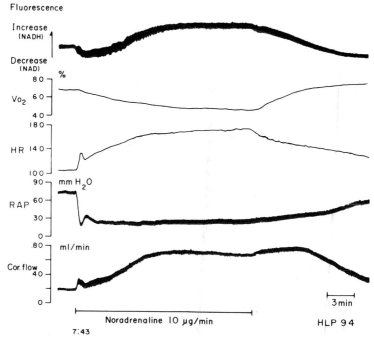

Figure 1. Effects of 10 µg/min of noradrenaline on the oxidation-reduction state of pyridine nucleotides as studied in the canine heart-lung preparation supported by a donor, Fluorescence: Pyridine nucleotides (NADP, NADPH, NAD, and NADH, designated collectively as NADH and NAD) fluorescence recorded by an organ redoximeter. V_{O_2}: Oxygen saturation (%) of the coronary venous blood. HR: Heart rate per minute. RAP: Right atrial pressure. Cor. flow: Coronary sinus outflow. Dog, 11 kg, male. Heart weight: 110 g. Total blood volume at the beginning of the experiment: 1100 ml.

RESULTS

Figure 1 illustrates the effects of 10 μg/min of noradrenaline. A definite decrease in the pyridine nucleotides (PN) fluorescence was observed, followed by an increase, which developed keeping pace with positive inotropic and chronotropic effects, and an increase in the coronary flow. Adrenaline produced qualitatively the same type of response, while isoproterenol produced only an increase in the fluorescence, as shown in Figure 2. Phenylephrine produced much weaker positive inotropic and chronotropic effects as compared with the catecholamines and induced only a decrease in fluorescence (Figure 3).

Pretreatment of the preparation with α-adrenergic blockers, phentolamine or dibenamine, resulted in a dose-dependent inhibition of the fluorescence decrease produced by noradrenaline, adrenaline, and phenylephrine, while the fluores-

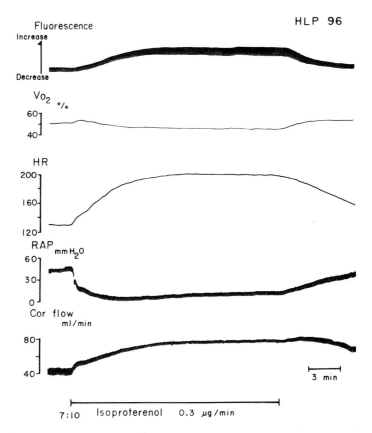

Figure 2. Effects of 0.3 μg/min of isoproterenol on the myocardial oxidation–reduction state. Abbreviations are the same as in Figure 1. Dog, 8 kg, female. Heart weight: 111 g. Total blood volume at the beginning of the experiment: 1000 ml.

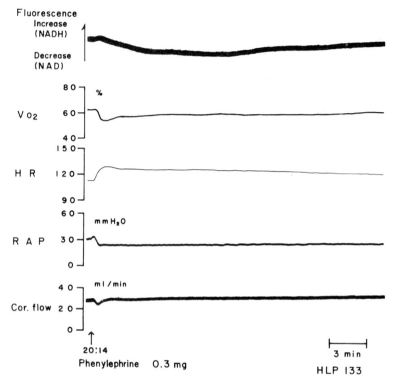

Figure 3. Effects of 0.3 mg of phenylephrine on the myocardial oxidation-reduction state. Abbreviations are as in Figure 1. Total blood volume at the beginning of the experiment: 1500 ml.

cence increase by isoproterenol remained unchanged. Figure 4 depicts the effects of 10 μg/ml of noradrenaline in the presence of 5 mg of phentolamine. Phentolamine itself produced practically no change in the PN fluorescence.

After pretreatment of the preparation with an adrenergic β-blocker, propranolol, which completely abolished the positive inotropic and chronotropic effects of three catecholamines used, noradrenaline and adrenaline produced a dose-dependent decrease in the PN fluorescence, together with a decrease in the coronary flow, which lasted as long as the continuous infusion was maintained. Figure 5 illustrates the effects of 10 μg/ml of noradrenaline. Administration of isoproterenol under this condition resulted in no change in the PN fluorescence.

DISCUSSION

The present results strongly suggest the existence of an adrenergic α-receptor in the myocardium, the direct activation of which by noradrenaline, adrenaline, or

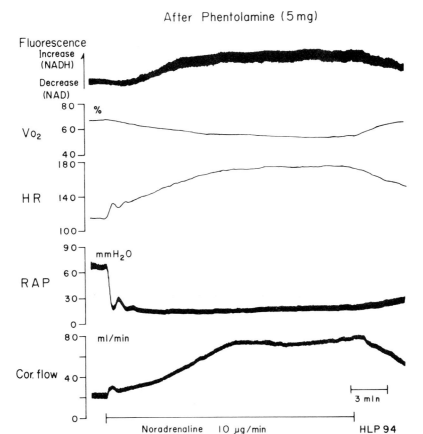

Figure 4. Modification by 5 mg of phentolamine of the effects of 10 μg/min of nor-adrenaline on the myocardial oxidation-reduction state. Abbreviations are as in Figure 1. The preparation is the same as in Figure 1.

phenylephrine results in an acceleration of the myocardial oxidative metabolism. Although the mechanism of this acceleration is not entirely clear at present, the augmentation of the glucose utilization, as demonstrated by Williamson (1964), could be the cause of this acceleration.

The shift of the myocardial oxidation-reduction state to a more reduced state observed with the development of the positive inotropic and chronotropic effects is usually taken to represent a hypoxia of the myocardium consequent to an increased oxygen demand only partially compensated by a simultaneous increase in the coronary blood flow. However, only a minimal reduction of the coronary venous oxygen saturation was observed in the present experiments

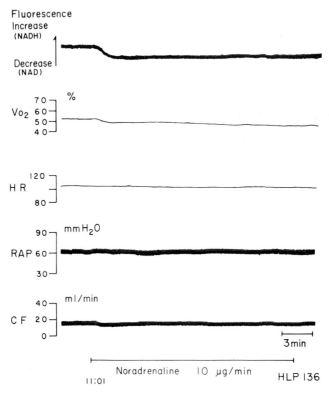

Figure 5. Modification by 1 mg of propranolol of the effects of 10 μg/min of noradrenaline on the myocardial oxidation-reduction state. Dog, 7 kg, female. Heart weight: 80 g. Total blood volume at the beginning of the experiment: 1000 ml.

after administration of isoproterenol. Therefore, a hypoxia of the myocardium is unlikely to be a main factor contributing to the observed fluorescence increase produced by these compounds. An augmentation of the glycolysis and resultant accumulation of lactate within the cytoplasm could be the cause of the increased fluorescence, as postulated by Williamson and Jamieson (1966).

REFERENCES

CHANCE, B., and LEGALLAIS, V. 1963. A spectrofluorometer for recording of intracellular oxidation-reduction state. Trans. Bio-Med. Electron. 10:40–47.

CHANCE, B., WILLIAMSON, J. R., JAMIESON, D., and SCHOENER, B. 1965. Properties and kinetics of reduced pyridine nucleotide fluorescence of the isolated and in vivo rat heart. Biochem. Z. 341:357–377.

IMAI, S., OTORII, T., TAKEDA, K., and KATANO, Y. 1975. Coronary vasodilatation and adrenergic receptors in the dog heart and coronary vasculature. Jpn. J. Pharmacol. 25:423–432.

KOBAYASHI, S., NISHIKI, K., KAEDE, K., and OGATA, E. 1971. Optical consequences of blood substitution on tissue oxidation-reduction state microfluorometry. J. Appl. Physiol. 31:93–96.

RIBEILIMA, J., WENDT, V. E., RAMOS, H., GUDBJARNASON, S., BRUCE, T. A., and BING, R. J. 1964. The effects of norepinephrine on the hemodynamics and myocardial metabolism of normal human subjects. Amer. Heart J. 67:672–678.

WILLIAMSON, J. R. 1964. Metabolic effects of epinephrine in the isolated, perfused rat heart. J. Biol. Chem. 239:2721–2729.

WILLIAMSON, J. R., and JAMIESON, D. 1966. Metabolic effects of epinephrine in the perfused rat heart. 1. Comparison of intracellular redox states, tissue pO_2, and force of contraction. Mol. Pharmacol. 2:191–205.

Mailing address:
Dr. S. Imai,
Department of Pharmacology,
Niigata University School of Medicine,
Niigata City (Japan).

Recent Advances in Studies on
Cardiac Structure and Metabolism, Volume 11
Heart Function and Metabolism
Edited by T. Kobayashi, T. Sano, and N. S. Dhalla
Copyright 1978   University Park Press   Baltimore

CHARACTERISTICS OF ENERGY METABOLISM IN SPECIALIZED MUSCLE OF BOVINE HEART

N. TSUYUGUCHI, K. MATSUMURA, K. MIKAWA, T. NIKI, H. MORI, and K. AKI

The Department of Enzyme Regulation, Institute for Enzyme Research,
School of Medicine, Tokushima University, Tokushima, Japan, and
The Second Department of Internal Medicine, School of Medicine,
Tokushima University, Tokushima, Japan

SUMMARY

Characterization of the energy metabolism pattern of the specialized heart muscle of bovine heart was studied in comparison with that of the ordinary heart muscle. Mitochondrial oxygen consumption of the specialized heart muscle was significantly lower than that of the ordinary heart muscle with succinate as the substrate. On the other hand, there was no significant difference in oxygen consumption between both heart muscles with glutamate + malate as the substrates.

The activity levels of succinate dehydrogenase and lactate dehydrogenase were much lower than those of the ordinary heart muscle. The isozyme pattern of LDH of the specialized heart muscle consisted of one major component of LDH-1 (H4) and that of the ordinary heart muscle consisted of two major components of LDH-1 (H4) and LDH-2 (H3M). The ratio of NADH to NAD of the specialized heart muscle was remarkably lower than that of the ordinary heart muscle. These results indicate that the specialized heart muscle depends not only upon anaerobic metabolism but also upon aerobic metabolism for its energy supply.

INTRODUCTION

It is well known that the cardiac conduction system (specialized heart muscle) is characteristic morphologically and functionally in comparison with the ordinary heart muscle. It has been considered that the specialized heart muscle may be supplied energy predominantly from anaerobic glycolysis because the oxygen consumption and the activity of succinate dehydrogenase are much lower in the specialized heart muscle (Murray, 1954; Schiebler, Stark, and Caesar, 1956; Isaacson and Boucek, 1968; Opie, 1969). It has also been shown that the glycogen concentration is higher (Yamazaki, 1929; Otsuka, Hara, and Okamoto, 1967) and the capacity to survive anoxia is greater (Yamazaki, 1930). In the biochemical study reported here, experiments were focused on characterization of the energy metabolism pattern of the specialized heart muscle in comparison with ordinary heart muscle.

MATERIALS AND METHODS

The specialized heart muscle, composed of atrioventricular node, bundle of His, and right and left bundle branches, was dissected from the bovine heart immediately after sacrifice, with careful avoidance of the ordinary heart muscle. The ordinary heart muscle was dissected from left ventricular wall.

Isolation of mitochondria of bovine heart was performed according to the procedure of Chance and Hagihara (1963). Protein concentrations of mitochondria and postmitochondria fractions were measured according to the method of Lowry *et al.* (1951). Mitochondrial respiration was measured polarographically according to the method of Chance and Williams (1955).

Succinate dehydrogenase activity was measured according to the method of Gutman, Edna, and Singer (1971). Lactate dehydrogenase activity was estimated according to the method of Wroblewski and Ladue (1955). Isozymes of lactate dehydrogenase were separated by disc gel electrophoresis.

The ratio of NADH to NAD was calculated from contents of lactate and pyruvate (Williamson, Lund, and Krebs, 1967). Lactate and pyruvate contents were measured according to the method of Gawehn and Bergmeyer (1974) and Czok and Lamprecht (1974), respectively.

RESULTS

Table 1 presents oxygen consumption and respiratory control index and P/O ratio of heart mitochondria. Oxygen consumption of the specialized heart muscle was significantly lower than that of the ordinary heart muscle with succinate as the substrate. On the other hand, there was no significant difference in oxygen consumption between both heart muscles with glutamate + malate as the substrates. The respiratory control index of the specialized heart muscle was much lower than that of the ordinary heart muscle with succinate as well as glutamate + malate as the substrates. P/O ratios of both heart muscles were almost the same, with values approximated to 2.0 for succinate and 3.0 for glutamate + malate.

Table 2 shows succinate dehydrogenase activity, lactate dehydrogenase activity, lactate and pyruvate contents, and NADH/NAD ratio of both heart muscles. Succinate dehydrogenase activity of the specialized heart muscle was much lower than that of the ordinary heart muscle. Lactate dehydrogenase activity of the specialized heart muscle was also much lower than that of the ordinary heart muscle. Electrophoretic pattern of LDH isozyme revealed that

Table 1. Oxygen consumption, respiratory control index, and P/O ratio of bovine heart mitochondria

Substrate	Heart muscle	O_2 consumption*	RCI	P/O ratio
Succinate	Specialized	126.5 ± 30.4**	2.0 ± 0.3***	1.8 ± 0.2**
	Ordinary	220.2 ± 32.8**	4.7 ± 0.8***	2.2 ± 0.2**
Glutamate + malate	Specialized	138.9 ± 21.8§	3.1 ± 0.9***	2.8 ± 0.2†
	Ordinary	148.6 ± 20.2§	7.9 ± 2.9***	2.9 ± 0.2†

*O_2 Consumption = n atoms 0/mg protein/min.
**$p < 0.001$.
***$p < 0.01$.
†$p < 0.05$.
§Not significant.

the specialized heart muscle had one major component of LDH-1 (H4), and that the ordinary heart muscle had two major components of LDH-1 (H4) and LDH-2 (H3M). Lactate content was much lower, and pyruvate content was much higher, in the specialized heart muscle than in the ordinary heart muscle. Therefore, the ratio of NADH to NAD of the specialized heart muscle was remarkably lower than that of the ordinary heart muscle.

DISCUSSION

The results of mitochondrial respiration suggest that the electron transfer from succinate to respiratory chain in the specialized heart muscle is rate-limiting for

Table 2. Comparison of succinate dehydrogenase activity, lactate dehydrogenase activity, lactate content, pyruvate content, and NADH/NAD ratio between specialized heart muscle and ordinary heart muscle

	Specialized heart muscle	Ordinary heart muscle
Succinate dehydrogenase activity (nmol/mg protein/min)	29.37 ± 8.90*	81.45 ± 20.09*
Lactate dehydrogenase activity (mol/mg protein/min)	0.37 ± 0.07*	2.55 ± 0.30*
Lactate content (μmoi/mg protein/min)	0.85 ± 0.06**	3.15 ± 0.40**
Pyruvate content (nmol/mg protein/min)	117.9 ± 15.4**	27.1 ± 3.2**
NADH/NAD ratio ($\times 10^4$)	8	130

*$p < 0.01$
**$p < 0.001$.

mitochondrial respiration; whereas the electron transfer from NADH-dependent substrates to respiratory chain in the specialized heart muscle is at the same rate as that of the ordinary heart muscle.

Because LDH activity of the specialized heart muscle is very low, the pathway of LDH-catalyzed reaction in the specialized heart muscle is narrower than in the ordinary heart muscle. LDH has five isozymes composed of four subunits of the two parent molecules. H type and M type. H type is found in aerobic tissues, such as cardiac muscles, and M type is found in the more anaerobic tissues, such as voluntary skeletal muscles. From the result of electrophoretic pattern of LDH, LDH isozyme of the specialized heart muscle is considered to be the type found in aerobic tissues.

Furthermore, it appears that LDH in the specialized heart muscle is favorable to production of pyruvate, since the ratio of NADH to NAD of the specialized heart muscle *in vivo* is remarkably lower than that of the ordinary heart muscle.

From these results, it seems that the specialized heart muscle is supplied energy from aerobic metabolism.

REFERENCES

CHANCE, B., and HAGIHARA, B. 1963. Fifth international congress of biochemistry, Vol. 5, p. 3. The Macmillan Company, New York.

CHANCE, B., and WILLIAMS, G. R. 1966. Respiratory enzymes in oxidative phosphorylation. J. Biol. Chem. 217:383–393.

CZOK, R., and LAMPRECHT, W. 1974. Methods of enzymatic analysis, Vol. 3, p. 1446. Academic Press, New York.

GAWEHN, K., and BERGMEYER, H. U. 1974. Methods of enzymatic analysis, Vol. 3, p. 1492. Academic Press, New York.

GUTMAN, M., EDNA, B. K., and SINGER, T. P. 1971. Multiple control mechanisms for succinate dehydrogenase in mitochondria. Biochem. Biophys. Res. Commun. 44: 526–532.

ISAACSON, R., and BOUCEK, R. J. 1968. The atrioventricular conduction tissue of the dog. Histochemical properties; influence of electric shock. Amer. Heart J. 75:206–214.

LOWRY, G. H., ROSENBROUGH, N. J., FARR, A. L., and RANDALL, R. J. 1951. Protein measurement with the Folin phenol reagent. J. Biol. Chem. 193:265–275.

MURRAY, J. B. 1954. Oxygen uptake of atrioventricular conduction tissues of beef heart. Amer. J. Physiol. 177:463–466.

OPIE, L. H. 1969. Metabolism of the heart in health and disease. Part 2. Amer. Heart J. 77:100–122.

OTSUKA, N., HARA, T., and OKAMOTO, H. 1967. Histotopochemische Untersuchungen am Reizleitungssystem des Hundeherzens. Histochemie 10:66–73.

SCHIEBLER, T. H., STARK, M., and CAESAR, R. 1956. Die Stoffwechselsituation des Reizleitungssystems. Klin. Wochenschr. 34:181–183.

WILLIAMSON, D. H., LUND, P., and KREBS, H. A. 1967. The redox state of free nicotinamide-adenine dinucleotide in the cytoplasm and mitochondria of rat liver. Biochem. J. 103:514–527.

WROBLEWSKI, F., and LADUE, J. S. 1955. Lactic dehydrogenase activity in blood. Proc. Soc. Exp. Biol. Med. 90:210–213.

YAMAZAKI, K. 1929. Biochemical studies in the atrioventricular junctional system of heart. 1. The glycogen content. J. Biochem. 10:481–490.

YAMAZAKI, K. 1930. Biochemical studies in the auriculoventricular junctional system of heart. 4. Studies on the anaerobic oxidation of auriculoventricular junctional system. J. Biochem. 12:241–246.

Mailing address:
Dr. N. Tsuyuguchi
The Second Department of Internal Medicine,
School of Medicine, Tokushima University,
Tokushima (Japan).

Recent Advances in Studies on
Cardiac Structure and Metabolism, Volume 11
Heart Function and Metabolism
Edited by T. Kobayashi, T. Sano, and N. S. Dhalla
Copyright 1978   University Park Press   Baltimore

TRANSMURAL MITOCHONDRIAL DIFFERENCES
IN MYOCARDIUM

A. J. WHITTY, M. J. DIMINO, E. A. ELFONT,
G. W. HUGHES, and M. W. REPECK

Department of Research, Sinai Hospital of Detroit,
Detroit, Michigan, USA

SUMMARY

Two functional mitochondrial populations with different sedimentation rates (S) were obtained from homogenates of canine myocardium by rate zonal centrifugation using an iso-osmotic Ficoll gradient. To ascertain the origin of these populations, the left ventricular wall of normal myocardium was divided into subepicardial (outer one-third), intermediate (middle one-third), and subendocardial (inner one-third) layers. The slow S mitochondria comprised 75% of the mitochondrial population of the subepicardial layer. In contrast, the fast S mitochondria contributed 65% of the subendocardial population. Intermediate layer mitochondria resembled those of the subepicardium. Mitochondria isolated from the three layers had approximately the same density, as shown by isopycnic zonal centrifugation. These studies indicate that mitochondria from subepicardial and subendocardial layers of normal myocardium differ in size and shape but not in density. Electron micrographs (EM) of the subepicardium showed many mitochondria as long as 4 to 8 sarcomeres. Mitochondria from the outer and inner layers of normal myocardium had the same oxidative phosphorylation parameters. Acute myocardial infarction, lasting 1 or 2 hr, resulted in the selective loss of the fast S mitochondria. Because the fast S mitochondria are prevalent in the subendocardium, these results may explain the greater vulnerability of this layer to anoxia.

INTRODUCTION

Because mitochondria are the principal sites of oxygen utilization and ATP synthesis, differences in these organelles may have important consequences for the metabolism of the rest of the cell under a stress condition. It is known that in the normal heart there are pO_2 gradients from the epicardium to the endocardium reflecting perfusion differences. In addition, there are gradients in substrates, e.g., glycogen and triglycerides, and there appears to be a greater concentration of myoglobin in the subendocardium. In these studies, mitochondrial differences after myocardial infarction and also in the subepicardial and subendocardial layers of normal myocardium were investigated.

Supported by National Institutes of Health Grants HL 13737 and GRSG-RR 05641 and The Sinai Hospital Guild, Detroit, Michigan.

METHODS

Experimental myocardial ischemia and infarction were produced in dogs by ligating branches of the anterior descending coronary artery. Measurements of intramyocardial pO_2 by means of coaxial oxygen electrodes permitted the demarcation of infarcted, injured, ischemic, and normal areas. Criteria for the identification of the four areas and the recovery of mitochondrial protein following ischemia and infarction are shown in Table 1. Mitochondria, obtained from homogenates of left ventricular myocardium, were separated by differential centrifugation and further resolved by rate zonal centrifugation using an iso-osmotic Ficoll gradient (1% to 30%).

RESULTS

Mitochondria Isolated from Homogenate of Left Ventricular Wall

At an $\omega^2 t = 7.0 \times 10^8$, rate zonal centrifugation permitted not only the separation of two mitochondrial populations but also the isolation of functional mitochondria capable of coupled oxidative phosphorylation (Figure 1). $\omega^2 t$ values below 7.0×10^8 did not yield complete separation of the mitochondrial populations, while values above gave good separation but decreased coupled oxidative phosphorylation. Isopycnic zonal centrifugation demonstrated that the mitochondrial populations had approximately the same densities as evidenced by a single peak. Rate zonal centrifugation yielded two distinct peaks of functional mitochondria in both normal and infarcted areas. While the normal area had approximately the same distribution of slow S mitochondria (found in light end of gradient) and fast S mitochondria (heavy end), there was a progressive loss of fast S mitochondria after 1 and 2 hr infarction (Figure 2, Table 2).

Mitochondria Isolated from
Subepicardial and Subendocardial Layers of Left Ventricular Wall

The left ventricular wall of 15 control dogs was divided into the outer one-third (subepicardial), middle one-third (intermediate), and inner one-third (subendo-

Table 1. Tissue pO_2 criteria used to identify myocardial condition

Condition of myocardium	Tissue pO_2 (mm Hg)	Recoverable mitochondrial protein* (mg/g wet wt)	Recoverable cytochrome oxidase* $(k \times 10^{-3}/g$ wet wt)
Normal	21–35	9.4	1.44
Ischemic	14–20	7.3	1.14
Injured	7–13	4.6	0.78
Infarcted	0–6	3.5	0.65

*Recoverable mitochondrial protein and cytochrome oxidase activity values obtained from a typical heart preparation.

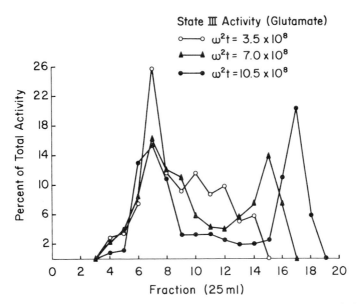

Figure 1. Influence of $\omega^2 t$ on isolation and separation of mitochondrial populations. In these rate zonal centrifugation studies an iso-osmotic Ficoll gradient (1%–30%) was used. Rotor speed was constant (approximately 6000 rpm) with time varied (approximately 15, 30, and 45 min, respectively). Oxidation of glutamate in the presence of ADP (State III) was used as a marker for mitochondria. Coupled oxidative phosphorylation was found with mitochondria separated at 3.5×10^8 and 7.0×10^8, but not at 10.5×10^8. Percent recovery in all runs was approximately 65%.

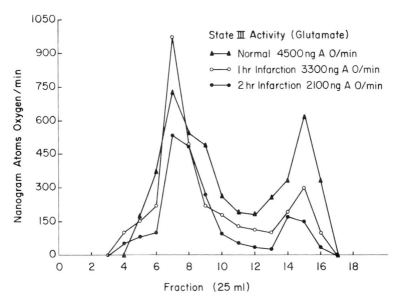

Figure 2. Effect of infarction on distribution of mitochondrial populations. Infarction was induced by coronary ligation of LAD ($\omega^2 t = 7.0 \times 10^8$).

Table 2. Oxidative phosphorylation of heart mitochondrial populations separated by rate zonal centrifugation*

Mitochondrial populations	Recoverable mitochondrial protein infarcted normal	Respiratory control	ADP:O
Normal (4)†			
Slow S		2.3	2.4
Fast S		2.1	2.7
1-hr. infarction (4)†			
Slow S	90%	2.5	2.7
Fast S	50%	2.4	2.9
2-hr. infarction (3)†			
Slow S	40%	2.5	2.1
Fast S	10%	2.0	2.3

*Glutamate used as substrate.
†Number in parentheses indicates dogs per group.

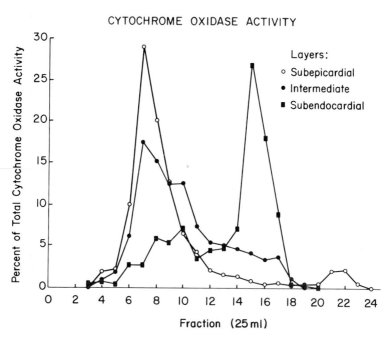

Figure 3. Transmural mitochondrial distribution found in the normal heart. Left ventricular wall divided into equal thirds—subepicardial, intermediate, and subendocardial layers ($\omega^2 t = 7.0 \times 10^8$).

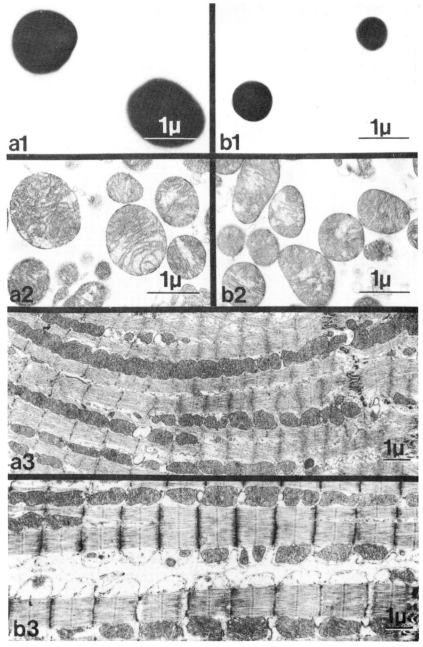

Figure 4. a. Normal subepicardial layer. 1. Isolated, nonsectioned mitochondria fixed in OsO$_4$; diameter range 0.5μ to 1.5μ × 14,100. 2. Isolated, sectioned mitochondria from same sample as above. × 14,000. 3. *In situ* section showing mitochondria extending several sarcomeres. × 7,600. b. Normal subendocardial layer. 1. Isolated, nonsectioned mitochondria fixed in OsO$_4$; diameter range 0.3μ to 1.0μ. × 14,100. 2. Isolated, sectioned mitochondria from same sample as above. × 14,000. 3. *In situ* section showing mitochondria extending usually one sarcomere. × 7,600.

cardial) layers. The subepicardial layer contained a predominance of slow S mitochondria while fast S mitochondria predominated in the subendocardial layer (Figure 3). The intermediate layer resembled the subepicardial layer. There were no significant differences in cytochrome oxidase activity and in oxidative phosphorylation parameters in mitochondria isolated from the layers of normal heart. Electron microscopic studies of both isolated and *in situ* mitochondria confirmed the findings in the separate layers, as seen in Figure 4.

DISCUSSION

These studies demonstrate the existence of two mitochondrial populations that are distributed differently in the subepicardial and the subendocardial layers. While these mitochondrial populations have similar parameters of oxidative phosphorylation, those predominating in the subendocardium were found to be smaller in size, as shown by their faster S and by EM studies. Moreover, it is hypothesized that this vulnerability of the faster migrating mitochondria, which predominate in the subendocardium, may explain why the extent of injury is greater in this layer after myocardial infarction.

Mailing address:
Albert J. Whitty, Ph.D.,
Sinai Hospital of Detroit,
Department of Research,
6767 West Outer Drive,
Detroit, Michigan 48235 (USA).

Recent Advances in Studies on
Cardiac Structure and Metabolism, Volume 11
Heart Function and Metabolism
Edited by T. Kobayashi, T. Sano, and N. S. Dhalla
Copyright 1978   University Park Press   Baltimore

UPTAKE AND RELEASE OF IMMUNOREACTIVE INSULIN IN CORONARY CIRCULATION IN MAN: STUDIES AT REST, DURING EXERCISE, AND DURING GLUCOSE AND INSULIN INFUSIONS

M. L. WAHLQVIST, L. A. CARLSON, L. KAIJSER,
H. LÖW, H. J. PEAK, L. WIDE, and E. G. WILMSHURST

King Gustaf V Research Institute, Karolinska Hospital,
Stockholm; Department of Clinical Chemistry, Uppsala University,
Uppsala, Sweden; and Department of Clinical Science,
John Curtin School of Medical Research,
Australian National University, Canberra, Australia

SUMMARY

Signficant uptake and release of immunoreactive insulin by the heart have been observed in man, and this is related to plasma insulin levels. Exercise and the fed state appear to affect the myocardial handling of insulin. The findings could not be related to myocardial carbohydrate metabolism, but could, during exercise, be related to myocardial lipid metabolism.

INTRODUCTION

When insulin exerts its action on the heart, it is presumably taken up from arterial blood by the myocardium, where it interacts with receptors. Recent work has clarified the nature and control of receptors for insulin (Forgue and Freychet, 1975; Freychet, 1975; Raff, 1976). There remains, however, little information with regard to the peripheral handling of insulin *in vivo* and how this relates to arterial insulin concentrations (Asmal *et al.,* 1971). We have examined the coronary arteriovenous difference in insulin immunoreactivity in man from this point of view and have also assessed its relationship to myocardial substrate utilization.

This work was supported by the Life Insurance Medical Research Fund of Australia and by the Swedish Medical Research Council.

METHODS

Subjects were male volunteers either healthy or with suspected ischemic heart disease. They were examined after an overnight fast. Simultaneous brachial artery and coronary sinus blood samples were obtained (Wahlqvist *et al.*, 1972; Carlson *et al.*, 1973, 1975). Heparin was not administered. Some subjects were examined during prolonged exercise in the supine position on a cycle ergometer (Kaijser *et al.*, 1972) following observations at rest. Four situations were considered: 1) fasting, 2) insulin infusion to raise arterial insulin concentrations, 3) nicotinic acid infusion where arterial free fatty acid (FFA) concentrations were kept low and arterial insulin concentrations tend to be low (Lassers *et al.*, 1972), and 4) a simulated fed state where glucose and a fat emulsion, Intra-lipid®-S, were infused and arterial insulin concentrations elevated (Carlson *et al.*, 1973, 1975; Wahlqvist *et al.*, 1974).

In most categories, subjects were given oral iodine (Lugol's solution) followed by an intravenous injection of about 6μCi of [125] I-albumin as a tracer for plasma albumin two days before the investigation. This enabled estimation of any change in plasma protein concentration as an index of shift of plasma water across the coronary circulation.

Plasma samples for insulin determination were frozen at $-20°$ C until assayed. Insulin was determined using either a radioimmunoassay kit (Radio-chemical Centre, Amersham, England) (Hales and Randle, 1963) or a radioimmunoabsorbent technique (Pharmacia AB, Uppsala) (Wide, Axén, and Porath, 1967). Where insulin was infused, ten replicates of arterial and of coronary sinus plasma were assayed so that the significance of each observation of an arteriovenous difference could be assessed. In the series in which an intravenous fed state was created, each arterial and coronary sinus sample was assessed in three dilutions, each of these in triplicate. In all cases the sample curve was parallel to that of the standard. Other assays were made in duplicate.

Blood samples for determination of glucose, lactate, pyruvate, FFA, triglyceride, "exogenous triglyceride" (plasma triglyceride circulating as Intralipid emulsion), and [125] I-albumin were collected as previously described (Kaijser *et al.*, 1972; Lassers *et al.*, 1972; Wahlqvist *et al.*, 1972; Carlson *et al.*, 1973, 1975).

RESULTS

Uptake

When insulin was infused intravenously in two subjects, each subject had a significant arterial-coronary sinus difference in immunoreactivity (Ia-cs) (Table 1). Ia-cs was also significant and further increased when glucose influsion was combined with insulin infusion.

Table 1. Significance of single observations of extraction of immunoreactive insulin from coronary blood

Subject[§]	Fasting		Insulin infusion		Insulin and glucose infusion	
	Ia[‡]	Ia-cs[‡]	Ia[‡]	Ia-cs[‡]	Ia[‡]	Ia-cs[‡]
FR	3.9	−1.3	28.7	2.4	154.3	37.6
	±0.3	±0.6[ns]	±0.4	±0.6**	±5.6	±9.0***
GR	12.1	0.6	35.9	4.4		
	±0.3	±0.4[ns]	±0.9	±1.1**		

[†]Ia refers to insulin immunoreactivity in arterial blood and Ia-cs to the arterial-coronary sinus difference in insulin immunoreactivity. Significance of Ia-cs is indicated by ns ($p > 0.05$), **($p < 0.01$), ***($p < 0.001$).

[§]Subject FR had a doubtful anginal syndrome and was given an infusion of 2U actrapid insulin in 1% albumin and 0.9% saline per hour. This infusion was then combined with that of 0.4g 20% glucose/min. Subject GR had angina pectoris and the rate of insulin infusion was 4U/hr. Each infusion lasted 1 hr.

[‡]Means ±S.E.M. are shown.

In the intravenous fed state, where infusions of glucose and a fat emulsion were given, resting subjects did not as a group demonstrate a significant myocardial insulin extraction (Ia-cs) (Table 2). When parenterally fed subjects exercised, however, a significant Ia-cs was observed.

Release

There were two circumstances in which a significant release of immunoreactive insulin into coronary venous plasma was observed. One was where fasting subjects exercised for a prolonged period (Table 2). This was associated with a lower arterial insulin immunoreactivity than at rest. This is in contrast to the myocardial handling of insulin during comparable exercise when infusions of glucose and a fat emulsion were given. In that circumstance insulin was taken up.

Insulin release was observed as well during the infusion of nicotinic acid (Table 2). During nicotinate infusion, plasma FFA concentrations were 250 ± 20 μmol/liter, compared with control observations when they were 650 ± 50 μmol/ liter, reflecting the antilipolytic action of nicotinic acid. Although arterial insulin immunoreactivities tended to be lower when nicotinic acid was infused, they were not significantly so.

Water Shifts

Possible water shifts leading to alterations in insulin immunoreactivity across the coronary circulation were assessed by observing the arterial-coronary sinus difference in ^{125}I-albumin. These changes ranged from −1.0 to 0.1% of the arterial levels. The −1.0% change was during the infusion of nicotinic acid when

Table 2. Arterial plasma insulin[†] immunoreactivity (Ia) and arterial-coronary sinus difference in plasma insulin immunoreactivity (Ia-cs)[§] in different experimental categories[‡]

| | Fasting | | Fasting and nicotinic acid[††] | | I.V. fed state[§§] | |
	Rest (12)	Exercise[‡‡] (12)	Rest (9)	Exercise[‡‡] (9)	Rest (36)	Exercise[‡‡] (8)
Ia	17.9	13.8	15.2	11.4	26.8	10.4
	±0.9	±0.8	±1.4	±1.4	±3.2	±2.9
Ia-cs	−1.1	−2.8	−2.3	−1.9	1.2	3.3
	±0.8[ns]	±0.9**	±0.6**	±1.2[ns]	±1.0[ns]	±1.0*

[†] Units are μU/ml.

[§] Significance of Ia-cs is indicated by ns ($p > 0.05$), * ($p < 0.05$), ** ($p < 0.01$).

[‡] Number of observations for each category is shown in parentheses. In each category, mean ±S.E.M. is shown.

[†] Nicotinic acid was infused intravenously at a rate of 200 mg/hr or 400 mg/hr.

[§§] "I.V. Fed State" refers to the infusion of 0.4 g 20% glucose/min, and 0.16–0.17 g triglyceride emulsion as 10% Intralipid®-S/min. Observations were made during infusion lasting 4 hr, the second half of which in some subjects was an exercise period.

[‡‡] Exercise was in the supine position on a cycle ergometer at 50% of the workload, which produced a heart rate of 170/min (W170). It lasted 65–120 min.

subjects exercised and was significant ($p < 0.01$), but in each other experimental category there was a smaller water shift and those shifts were not statistically significant. By contrast, the significant insulin releases were 15–20% of the arterial immunoreactivities. The significant insulin extraction in the fed state exercise group was about 30% of the arterial immunoreactivity.

Relationship Between Ia-cs and Ia

In all experimental categories, significant positive relationships were found between insulin extraction (Ia-cs) and arterial immunoreactivity (Ia) (Table 3). Insulin release was observed below about 20 μU/ml insulin. During exercise in the intravenous fed state, however, extraction was observed at lower Ias.

Relationship Between Ca-cs Substrate and Ia-cs Insulin

Of the carbohydrate and lipid substrates observed, only the extractions of triglyceride and FFA were related to insulin extraction (Table 4). For triglyceride in fasting subjects during exercise, and for FFA in the parenterally fed subjects during exercise, these were negative correlations. The correlations were not dependent on arterial insulin levels. The positive relationships for exogenous triglyceride in the I.V. fed state were no longer evident after partial correlation analysis eliminating the arterial insulin immunoreactivity (rest $r_{1,2,3} = 0.12$; exercise $r_{12.3} = 0.51$).

Table 3. Relationships between arterial-coronary sinus difference in insulin immunoreactivity (Y) and arterial plasma insulin immunoreactivity (X)[†]

	Fasting		I.V. fed state	
	Rest (21)	Exercise (21)	Rest (36)	Exercise (8)
a	−7.2	−8.9	−2.4	0.3
b	0.33	0.51	0.13	0.29
r[§]	0.52*	0.54*	0.44**	0.84**

[†]Regression coefficients for the equation $Y = a + b\,X$ are shown.

[§]r is the correlation coefficient. Significance is indicated by * ($p < 0.05$), ** ($p < 0.01$).

Table 4. Relationships between extraction of substrates (Ca-cs) and extraction of immunoreactive insulin (Ia-cs) from coronary blood[†]

	Fasting		I.V. fed state [§]	
	Rest	Exercise	Rest	Exercise
Glucose	−0.03[ns] (21)	0.05[ns] (21)	0.24[ns] (21)	
Lactate	0.02[ns] (21)	0.02[ns] (21)	0.03[ns] (15)	
Pyruvate	−0.11[ns] (21)	0.08[ns] (21)	0.41[ns] (15)	
FFA	0.05[ns] (21)	−0.04[ns] (21)	0.06[ns] (36)	−0.78* (8)
Triglyceride[‡]	0.08[ns] (21)	−0.45* (21)	0.36* (36)	0.82** (8)
Glycerol	0.02[ns] (21)	0.28[ns] (21)	0.11[ns] (21)	

[†]In each category the correlation coefficient (r) is shown and, beneath it, the number of observations in parentheses. Significance is indicated by ns ($p > 0.05$), * ($p < 0.05$), ** ($p < 0.01$).

[§]"I.V. Fed State" refers to intravenous infusion of glucose and Intralipid®-S.

[‡]In the fasting state, triglyceride refers to total plasma triglyceride and in the "I.V. Fed State" to "exogenous triglyceride."

DISCUSSION

These data provide evidence that there are circumstances in which insulin can be taken up and released by the human heart. The observed changes in plasma insulin immunoreactivity across the coronary circulation cannot be accounted for by water shifts. They are unlikely to depend on movement of insulin between formed elements and plasma (Wahlqvist *et al.,* 1972). They could represent redistribution of insulin between vascular tissue and plasma, but even if this is so, presumably, in turn, movement between cardiac muscle cell membranes and extracellular fluid would occur. That coronary sinus immunoreactive insulin is biologically active has not been tested directly, but is suggested by the radioimmunoassay parallelism between standard, arterial, and coronary sinus insulins. Myocardial cells are thought to degrade insulin to a limited extent, however (Forgue and Freychet, 1975).

The arterial plasma insulin appears to be one, but presumably not the only, determinant of insulin uptake and release by the heart. The indices of determination (r^2) (Table 3) were appreciably less than unity. The Ia-cs/Ia relationship was shifted by exercise. Parenteral feeding with glucose and a fat emulsion appears to prevent the extraction of insulin that occurs when insulin levels are elevated by infusion (Tables 1 and 2).

If coronary plasma flow at rest is taken to be 150 ml/min and myocardial mass about 300 g, at an Ia-cs of -2 μU/ml, the heart could release 1 μU/min/g. This could account for about 10% of the total turnover rate of insulin. The reverse situation could apply at elevated plasma insulin levels or during exercise in the parenterally fed state.

The question remains whether or not the uptake and release of insulin observed affect heart metabolism. No relationship to carbohydrate metabolism was recognized. A negative relationship with triglyceride extraction may be consistent with the reciprocity between lipoprotein lipase in adipose tissue, which is activated by insulin, and in the heart (Borensztajn, Samols, and Rubinstein, 1972). The negative relationship between FFA extraction and insulin extraction was unexpected, considering the antilipolytic action of insulin in adipose tissue, but a different situation may prevail in the heart during exercise and where competition between triglyceride and FFA as substrates may occur (Wahlqvist *et al.,* 1974).

REFERENCES

ASMAL, A. C. I., COX, B. D., BUTTERFIELD, W. J. H., KARAMANOS, B., and WHICHELOW, M. J. 1971. The peripheral uptake of glucose and exogenous insulin. Postgrad. Med. J. (June Suppl.) 407–411.

BORENSZTAJN, J., SAMOLS, D. R., and RUBINSTEIN, A. H. 1972. Effects of insulin on lipoprotein lipase activity in the rat heart and adipose tissue. Amer. J. Physiol. 223: 1271–1275.

CARLSON, L. A., KAIJSER, L., RÖSSNER, S., and WAHLQVIST, M. L. 1973. Myocardial metabolism of exogenous plasma triglyceride in resting man. Acta Med. Scand. 193: 233–245.

CARLSON, L. A., KAIJSER, L., RÖSSNER, S., WAHLQVIST, M. L., and WIDE, L. 1975. Changes in insulin immunoreactivity across the coronary circulation in man during infusions of glucose and a fat emulsion. Eur. J. Clin. Invest. 5:57–61.

FORGUE, M. E., and FREYCHET, P. 1975. Insulin receptors in heart muscle: Demonstration of specific bindings sites and impairment of insulin binding in the plasma membrane of the obese hypoglycemic mouse. Diabetes 24:715–723.

FREYCHET, P. 1975. Recent studies on insulin receptor interactions. Isr. J. Med. Sci. 11:679–686.

GOLDSMITH, S. J. 1975. Radioimmunoassay: Review of basic principles. Sem. Nucl. Med. 5:125–152.

HALES, C. N., and RANDLE, P. J. 1963. Immunoassay of insulin with insulin antibody precipitate. Biochem. J. 88:137–146.

KAIJSER, L., LASSERS, B. W., WAHLQVIST, M. L., and CARLSON, L. A. 1972. Myocardial lipid and carbohydrate metabolism in healthy fasting men during prolonged exercise. J. Appl. Physiol. 32:847–858.

LASSERS, B. W., WAHLQVIST, M. L., KAIJSER, L., and CARLSON, L. A. 1972. Effects of nicotinic acid on myocardial metabolism at rest and during prolonged exercise. J. Appl. Physiol. 33:72–80.

RAFF, M. 1976. Safe regulation of membrane receptors. Nature 259:265–266.

WAHLQVIST, M. L., CARLSON, L. A., EKLUND, B., KAIJSER, L., LASSERS, B. W. LÖW, H., NYE, E. R., and RÖSSNER, S. 1974. Substrate competition in human myocardial metabolism. Adv. Cardiol. 12:94–105.

WAHLQVIST, M. L., KAIJSER, L., LASSERS, B. W., LÖW, H., and CARLSON, L. A. 1972. Release of immunoreactive insulin from the human heart. Eur. J. Clin. Invest. 2: 407–411.

WIDE, L., AXÉN, R., and PORATH, J. 1967. Radioimmunoabsorbent assay for proteins. Chemical coupling of antibodies to insoluble dextran. Immunochemistry 4:381–386.

Mailing address:
Dr. M. L. Wahlqvist
Department of Clinical Science,
John Curtin School of Medical Research,
Australian National University,
Canberra (Australia).

Recent Advances in Studies on
Cardiac Structure and Metabolism, Volume 11
Heart Function and Metabolism
Edited by T. Kobayashi, T. Sano, and N. S. Dhalla
Copyright 1978   University Park Press   Baltimore

INFLUENCE OF CARBOCROMENE ON FREE FATTY ACID METABOLISM OF THE HEART

E. SCHRAVEN

Department of Medical and Biological Research,
Cassella Farbwerke Mainkur AG., Frankfurt (Main), Federal Republic of Germany

SUMMARY

In view of the fact that carbocromene (C) influences the metabolic processes in the heart muscle, its effect on the transport of substrates into the heart tissue was investigated. In rat heart slices C inhibits the uptake of $[1\text{-}^{14}C]$ palmitic acid up to 40%, while $^{14}CO_2$ production is reduced to the same extent. At the same time oxygen consumption diminished by about 20%. Using $3\text{-}O\text{-}[^{14}C]$ methyl-D-glucose as metabolic marker it was shown that the uptake of glucose into the heart tissue increased by 30% under the influence of C. From these results it can be concluded that C inhibits the oxidation of FFA in favor of glucose and diminishes the oxygen-wasting effect of FFA.

INTRODUCTION

Increased plasma concentrations of free fatty acids (FFA) are associated with a rise in myocardial oxygen consumption (Mjøs *et al.*, 1972). This oxygen-wasting effect of FFA can at least partly be explained by reduced glucose utilization. Since the oxidation of substrates in the heart depends on their availability, there are different possibilities for pharmacological interventions. Inhibition of lipolysis, for example by nicotinic acid, leads to a decreased oxygen consumption of about 20%, as was shown by several groups (Mjøs *et al.*, 1976). Mjøs *et al.* (1975) demonstrated that a similar effect could be obtained by enhancing glycolysis with dichloroacetate, an activator of pyruvate dehydrogenase.

Because it is well known that FFA and carbohydrates are interchangeable in heart metabolism, depending on their supply, another way to increase glucose oxidation should be the inhibition of FFA transport into the myocardial cell. The well-documented oxygen-sparing effect of carbocromene, which was introduced into the therapy as a coronary vasodilator, prompted us to study its effect on the transport of substrates into the heart.

METHOD AND RESULTS

Male rats (about 200 g) were anesthetized with ether and the hearts quickly removed. After washing, slices were prepared with a McIlwain chopper. Heart tissue (150 mg) was preincubated for 5 min with and without carbocromene in a Krebs-Ringer albumin buffer. The reaction was started by the addition of [1-^{14} C] palmitate complexed to albumin. Carbocromene in concentrations from 10^{-5} M to 5×10^{-4} M inhibited the uptake of palmitic acid in a dose-dependent manner. With the last-mentioned concentration, the radioactivity in the tissue was reduced by about 30%. The relation between phospholipids, FFA, and triglycerides was mainly unchanged (Figure 1).

This inhibition of FFA uptake leads to a decrease of FFA supply within the cell. In order to maintain the energy metabolism, the diminished supply of FFA has to be overcome by an increase in glucose oxidation. That carbocromene enhances the glucose uptake is shown by the next experiment. Groups of 6 mice were injected with 5 mg of carbocromene/kg intravenously. Ten min later, 1 μCi of 3-O-[^{14} C] methyl-D-glucose was injected, and 5 min after this the animals were killed by decapitation. Under carbocromene the incorporation of radioactivity into the heart was increased by about 30%. Since methylglucose is transported like glucose but not metabolized, this increase of radioactivity means that the uptake of glucose into the heart is enhanced by about 30%.

Both these effects—increased uptake of glucose and decreased incorporation of FFA—should be succeeded by a diminished breakdown of FFA by the citric acid cycle. Therefore, we studied the oxidation of labeled palmitic acid to ^{14} CO$_2$. Rat heart slices prepared as mentioned above were incubated in a

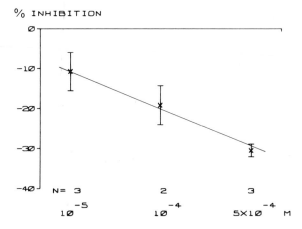

Figure 1. Uptake of [^{14}C] palmitic acid in rat heart slices. Dose-dependent inhibition by carbocromene.

Tyrode solution at 37° C in Warburg flasks. The reaction was started by addition of $[1-{}^{14}C]$ palmitate-albumin complex. The labeled ${}^{14}CO_2$ was absorbed in Hyamine ® and the oxygen consumption was registered after 45 and 90 min of incubation. With increasing concentration of FFA in the incubation medium, carbocromene in a concentration of 5×10^{-4} M inhibited the ${}^{14}CO_2$ production to a maximal amount of about 40%. Parallel to this effect, the oxygen consumption was also diminished by up to 20% (Figure 2).

These effects clearly demonstrate that under the influence of carbocromene the transport and oxidation of FFA in the heart are diminished. The reduction of FFA concentration within the cell is followed by an increase in the oxidation of glucose. The beneficial effect of this switching from FFA to glucose oxidation is theoretically based on an increased ATP production per unit of oxygen consumed, and is practically demonstrated by the decrease in oxygen consumption.

Carbocromene therefore should be of great advantage in hypoxic conditions. This was demonstrated by Salzmann (1967) about 10 years ago. Rabbits were intoxicated with succinylcholine (1.5 mg/kg I.V.). The survival time of the hearts was significantly prolonged under carbocromene (by nearly 50%).

We studied the effect of carbocromene on the tolerance to anoxia of mice exposed to high altitude. Groups of 10 animals—5 controls and 5 drug-treated— were placed in a desiccator that was evacuated to a pressure of 405 mm Hg. This reduced pressure corresponds to an altitude of 5,000 m. Control animals died under this condition within 30 to 50 min. Under the influence of carbocromene the survival time of mice is significantly prolonged.

Hammerl et al. demonstrated in 1969 that 30 min after acute application of carbocromene plasma levels of FFA in patients are increased by about 30%. In

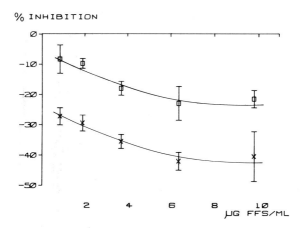

Figure 2. Inhibition of ${}^{14}CO_2$ production from $[{}^{14}C]$ palmitic acid and diminution of O_2 consumption by carbocromene.

contrast, other investigations showed that after long-term treatment with carbo-cromene triglycerides and cholesterol are decreased. The acute effect found by Hammerl can be explained by the diminished consumption of FFA. We there-fore studied the metabolic fate of [^{14}C] palmitic acid under the influence of carbocromene. Rats were anesthetized with chloralose/urethan and the bile duct was cannulated. Two microcuries of palmitic acid bound to albumin were given intravenously, and 60 min later 10 mg carbocromene/kg were injected. As can be seen in Figure 3, carbocromene significantly enhances the excretion of radio-activity after a delay of two hr. Therefore, the lowering of plasma levels of triglycerides and cholesterol after long-term treatment with carbocromene may be explained by an increased excretion of lipids through the bile.

In summary, carbocromene ameliorates the energy metabolism of the heart by inhibition of FFA oxidation and enhancing oxidation of glucose. This was shown by the following arguments:

1. Carbocromene inhibits the uptake of FFA.
2. The uptake of glucose is increased.
3. The oxidation of FFA to $^{14}CO_2$ is inhibited.
4. The consumption of oxygen is simultaneously diminished.
5. G-6-P (glucose-6-phosphate) and F-6-P (fructose-6-phosphate) are slightly but significantly increased.
6. The tolerance to anoxia is enhanced.

The increased oxidation of glucose at the expense of FFA is interpreted as an enhancement of ATP production without an influence on oxygen consumption or as a decrease in oxygen consumption by an unchanged ATP production.

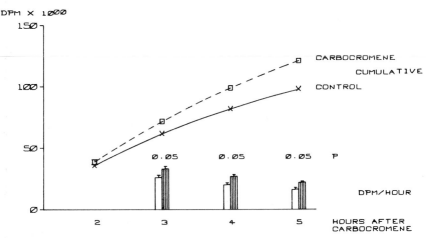

Figure 3. Excretion of radioactivity in the bile after I.V. application of [1-^{14}C] palmitic acid ($n = 7$).

REFERENCES

HAMMERL, H., KRÄNZL, C., NEBOSIS, G., PICHLER, O., and STUDLAR, M. 1969. Über den Einfluss von INTENSAIN auf den Fett- und Kohlenhydratstoffwechsel. Med. Klin. 64:2382.

MJØS, O. D., BUGGE-ASPERHEIM, B., and KIIL, F. 1972. Factors determining myocardial oxygen consumption (MVO_2) during elevation of aortic blood pressure. 2. Relation between MVO_2 and free fatty acids. Cardiovasc. Res. 6:23.

MJØS, O. D., MILLER, N. E., and OLIVER, M. F. 1975. Reduction by sodium dichloroacetate of the severity of acute myocardial ischaemic injury in the dog. Internat. Symp. ISGRCM, Brussels, Abstracts, p. 46.

MJØS, O. D., MILLER, M. B., RIEMERSMA, R. A., and OLIVER, M. D. 1976. Effects of p-chlorophenoxyisobutyrate on myocardial free fatty acid extraction, ventricular blood flow, and epicardial ST-segment elevation during coronary occlusion in dogs. Circulation 53:494.

SALZMANN, G. 1967. Untersuchungen zur Frage der kardialen und cerebralen Überlebenszeit unter Intensain-Wirkung. Dissertation, Frankfurt/Main.

Mailing address:
E. Schraven,
Department of Medical and Biological Research,
Cassella Farbwerke Mainkur AG.,
Frankfurt (Main) (West Germany).

Recent Advances in Studies on
Cardiac Structure and Metabolism, Volume 11
Heart Function and Metabolism
Edited by T. Kobayashi, T. Sano, and N. S. Dhalla
Copyright 1978   University Park Press   Baltimore

METABOLISM OF INDIVIDUAL FATTY ACIDS
IN HEART MUSCLE

K. J. KAKO, S. C. VASDEV, and G. ZAROR-BEHRENS

Department of Physiology, Faculty of Medicine,
University of Ottawa, Ottawa, Ontario, Canada

SUMMARY

We have studied the incorporation of various long chain fatty acids into tissue lipids using various heart preparations. We found that individual fatty acids are incorporated into various lipid fractions at unequal rates. In particular, erucic acid was shown to be a poor acyl donor for various acylation reactions. Labeling of triacylglycerol by exogenous fatty acid was found to be extremely rapid in the perfused rat heart and in the *in vivo* heart.

INTRODUCTION

Heart muscle generates a bulk of energy by oxidizing fatty acids that are taken up from the plasma (Bing *et al.,* 1954). Consequently, mechanisms controlling oxidation of fatty acids have been studied extensively by a number of investigators (see Opie, 1968/69). Some portions of fatty acids taken up by the myocardium are esterified in the cell and transformed to tissue lipids. Therefore, the tissue lipids are not inert substances, but undergo dynamic, relatively active turnover. As a result, under certain pathological conditions triacylglycerol may accumulate in the myocardium (Rona *et al.,* 1959; Opie, 1969; Kikuchi and Kako, 1970). Furthermore, dietary fats contain several major long chain fatty acids, which influence the composition of plasma FFA, and thus secondarily modify the fatty acid composition of cardiac lipids. In an attempt to elucidate factors controlling tissue lipid metabolism, we have examined, using various preparations, the patterns of incorporation of several different fatty acids into cardiac lipids. In addition, we have studied the metabolism of erucic acid. This fatty acid, being a major component of some species of rapeseed oil, is known to accumulate preferentially in the myocardium and ultimately produce necrotic changes in the heart (see Engfelt, 1976).

This work was supported by grants from the Medical Research Council of Canada and the Ontario Heart Foundation.

Figure 1 illustrates schematically the metabolic fate of fatty acids in the cardiac cell. Fatty acids, after their passage through the cell membrane, are activated to form CoA esters, and then are either oxidized in the mitochondria, or acylated into complex lipids. Phosphatidic acid serves as a precursor of neutral glycerides as well as of phospholipids, which are mostly formed in the sarcoplasmic reticulum. Therefore, when ^{14}C-labeled fatty acid is administered to the intact animal, to a heart perfusion system, or to a tissue slice preparation, various tissue lipids become radioactive.

Figure 2 illustrates the results of an experiment in which we injected albumin-bound [1-[14] C] oleic acid through the jugular veins of anesthetized rats at time 0. At various times after injection, hearts were excised, and cardiac lipids were extracted and isolated by thin-layer chromatography. Figure 2 clearly demonstrates that the radioactivity of the triacylglycerol increased very rapidly following the injection of the fatty acid. The activity in the phospholipid fraction formed a relatively large fraction of the total tissue labeling in the first 100 sec or so, but it decreased thereafter. Thus, this graph resembles a precursor-produced relationship between these two lipids.

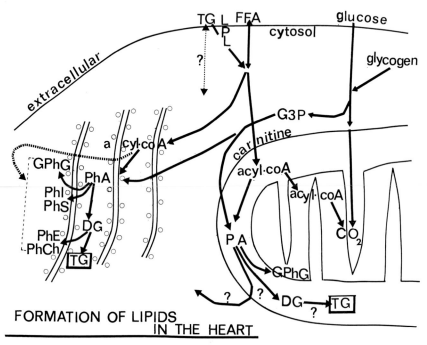

FORMATION OF LIPIDS IN THE HEART

Figure 1. Pathway of lipid formation in the heart. Abbreviations are: TG (triacyglycerol), DG (diacylglycerol), LPL (lipoprotein lipase), PHA and PA (phosphatidic acid), GPhG (glycerophosphoryl-glycerol), PhI (phosphatidylinositol), PhS (phosphatidylserine), PhE (phosphatidylethanolamine), PhCh (phosphatidylcholine) and G3P (glycerol 3-phosphate).

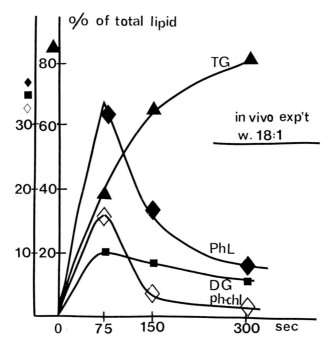

Figure 2. Relative distribution of radioactivity of oleic acid in the *in situ* heart. [1-^{14}C] oleic acid (5 μCi) was injected through the jugular veins of anesthetized rats. The animals were sacrificed after 75, 150, or 300 sec. Abbreviations are: TG (triacylglycerol), PhL (phospholipids), DG (diacylglycerol), and Ph.chl (phosphatidylcholine).

The distribution of the fatty acid carbon in tissue lipids observed at 300 sec after injection in intact rats was compared with the distribution found in the perfused heart preparation (Figure 3). In the latter experiment, the heart was perfused for 30 min (Dhalla *et al.,* 1973) in a recirculating apparatus in the presence of 0.5 mM albumin-bound fatty acid. The results obtained with heart perfusion were found to be quite similar to those with the *in vivo* experiments described above (Vasdev and Kako, 1977). Thus, some 60% of the total radioactivity of tissue lipids was found in the triacylglycerol fraction in both preparations (Figure 3). There was very little labeling (less than 10%) in the fatty acid and diacylglycerol fractions. This was in contrast to the results obtained with heart tissue slices, in which more than 70% of the total activity was found in the tissue fatty acid fraction (Figure 3). Despite this difference in the relative magnitude of ^{14}C incorporation into tissue lipids, labeling patterns of individual phospholipids were somewhat more reproducible among the three preparations studied (Figure 4). Phosphatidylcholine was labeled to the greatest extent with all three preparations (39-59%), whereas phosphatidic acid was labeled to the least extent (3-10%); phosphatidylethanolamine (approx. 10%) and phospha-

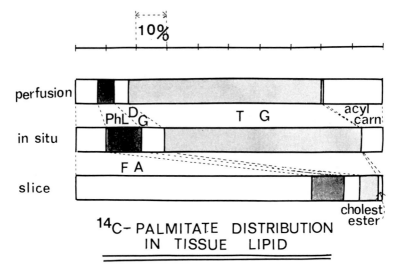

Figure 3. Comparison of the relative distribution of [¹⁴C] palmitate in tissue lipids in the three heart preparations. Procedures for heart perfusion and the *in situ* experiment are described in the text. The experiment with rat heart tissue slices was carried out by incubating tissue slices in a Krebs phosphate buffer containing 5 mM glucose and 0.5 mM fatty acid for 30 min at 37°C. Abbreviations are: PhL (phospholipids), DG (diacylglycerol), TG (triacyglycerol), FA (fatty acid), acyl carn (acylcarnitine) and cholest ester (cholesterol ester).

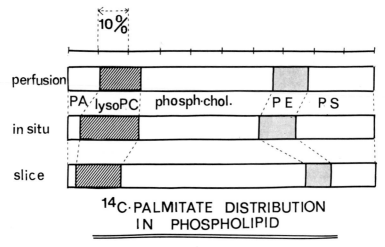

Figure 4. Comparison of the relative distribution of [¹⁴C] palmitate in tissue phospholipids in the three heart preparations. Abbreviations are: PA (phosphatidic acid), phosph·chol (phosphatidylcholine), lyso PC (lysophosphatidylcholine), PE (phosphatidylethanolamine), and PS (phosphatidylserine).

tidylserine (approx. 20%) were also labeled. These experiments were carried out with palmitate as the labeled precursor. It was further found that the distribution of different fatty acids, such as palmitic, oleic, linoleic, and erucic acids, in the tissue lipid fraction differed, but the patterns of incorporation of individual fatty acids were similar among the three different preparations.

The metabolic patterns of different fatty acids in the myocardium were then studied in more detail by using the rat heart perfusion system. Our study revealed that palmitic, oleic, linoleic, and erucic acids were taken up by the heart at similar rates. However, the magnitude of incorporation of individual fatty acids into various cardiac lipids varied. Oleic acid was incorporated preferentially into triacylglycerol, whereas erucic acid accumulated greatly in tissue fatty acids (Figure 5). More linoleic acid was found in the phospholipid fraction. The pattern of labeling of tissue phospholipids varied also, depending upon the kind of precursor fatty acids. Erucic acid was relatively rapidly incorporated into phosphatidic acid, whereas linoleic acid was rapidly incorporated into phosphatidylcholine (Figure 5). The radioactivity in the phosphatidylserine was highest with oleic acid as compared with other fatty acids, whereas phosphatidylethanolamine was labeled equally well irrespective of fatty acid precursors.

The distinctive pattern of cellular metabolism of erucic acid was further revealed upon examination of the kinetics of changes in the radioactivities of

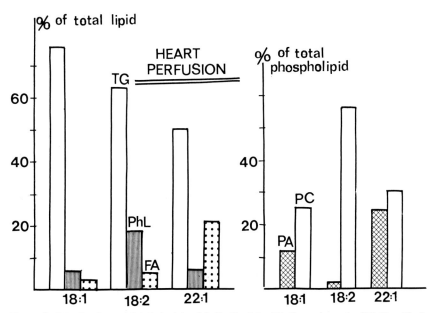

Figure 5. Distribution of labeled oleic (18:1), linoleic (18:2), and erucic (22:1) acids in tissue lipids of perfused rat hearts. For abbreviations, see legends to Figures 1 and 2.

tissue lipids (Figure 6). In this experiment, 2.5 μCi of [1-^{14}C] palmitic acid was added at time 0 and the heart perfusion was continued for various durations of time. The results demonstrated that the label in triacylglycerol was extremely rapidly increased, whereas the radioactivity in fatty acid and diacylglycerol increased slowly over the time period of 300 sec. It is therefore evident that the tissue lipids can be acylated relatively rapidly with exogenous fatty acyl molecules. In contrast, Figure 7 illustrates the results obtained with erucic acid as the radioactive precursor. In this experiment, the rapidly increasing activity was not that of triacylglycerol but that of tissue erucic acid; tissue diacylglycerol labeling was also rapidly increased, but the radioactivity in triacylglycerol and phospholipids was not as rapid during the initial 300-sec period. Therefore, under these experimental conditions erucic acid accumulated in the heart tissue mainly in

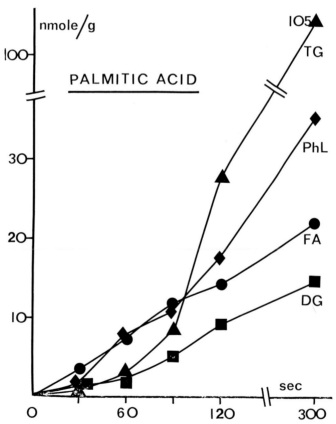

Figure 6. Time course of changes in radioactivities of individual lipid fractions of perfused hearts after the addition of [1-^{14}C] palmitic acid. (Reproduced by permission of *Biochimica et Biophysica Acta.*)

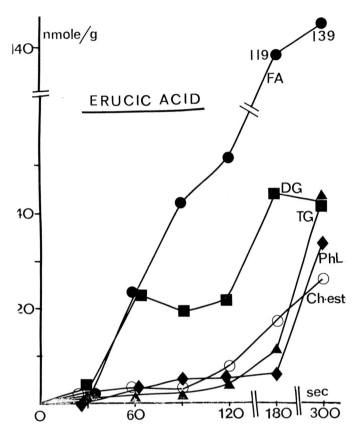

Figure 7. Time course of changes in radioactivities of individual lipid fractions of perfused hearts after the addition of [14-¹⁴C] erucic acid. (Reproduced by permission of *Biochimica et Biophysica Acta.*)

the form of fatty acid. Our study, in addition, suggests that acylation of diacylglycerol containing erucoyl moieties is slow.

The results of these studies demonstrated that individual fatty acids are not utilized at equal rates in esterification reactions leading to the formation of cardiac lipids. In particular, erucic acid, a component of rapeseed oil, does not appear to be a substrate that can be readily acylated to cardiac glycerides. This postulate was tested by studying the selectivity of one of the lipid-forming reactions, namely, that of acyl-CoA:1-palmitoylglycerol 3-phosphate acyltransferase (Figure 8). We assayed activities of this enzymatic reaction in rabbit heart microsomes by measuring the formation of diacylglycerol 3-phosphate using various acyl-CoA esters as acyl donors (Zaror-Behrens and Kako, 1976). The maximal reaction rate of the acyl transfer reaction was approximately equal

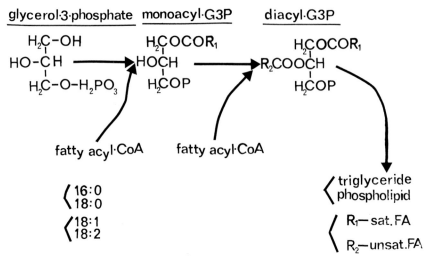

Figure 8. Schematic presentation of glycerol 3-phosphate acylation reactions leading to the formation of diacylglycerol 3-phosphate (phosphatidic acid).

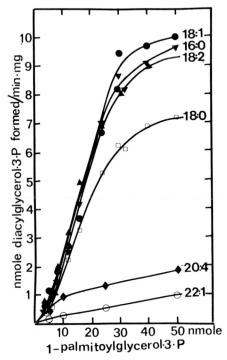

Figure 9. Initial velocity of the acyl-CoA:1-acylglycerol 3-phosphate acyltransferase reaction of rabbit heart microsomes. The rate of acylation was measured at various concentrations of 1-palmitoylglycerol 3-phosphate in the presence of different acyl donors, i.e., 18:1 (oleic), 16:0 (palmitic), 18:2 (linoleic), 18:0 (stearic), 20:4 (arachidonic), and 22:1 (erucic). (Reproduced by permission of *Biochimica et Biophysica Acta.*)

when oleic, palmitic, or linoleic acid served as the acyl donor (Figure 9). Stearic acid was acylated to a slightly lesser extent, and arachidonic and erucic acids were utilized to a very small extent. Thus, the latter two fatty acids are not favorable substrates for this, and perhaps for some other, acylation reactions in rabbit heart microsomes.

REFERENCES

BING, R. J., SIEGEL, A., UNGAR, I., and GILBERT, M. 1954. Metabolism of the human heart. II. Studies of fat, ketone and amino acid metabolism. Amer. J. Med. 16:504–515.

DHALLA, N. S., MATOUSHEK, R. F., SUN, C. N., and OLSON, R. E. 1973. Metabolic, ultrastructural and mechanical changes in the isolated rat heart perfused with aerobic medium in the absence or presence of glucose. Can. J. Physiol. Pharmacol. 51:590–603.

ENGFELT, B. (ed.). 1976. Morphological and biochemical effects of orally administered rapeseed oil in rat myocardium. Acta Med. Scand. Suppl. 585.

KIKUCHI, T., and KAKO, K. J. 1970. Metabolic effects of ethanol on the rabbit heart. Circ. Res. 26:625–634.

OPIE, L. H. 1968/69. Metabolism of the heart in health and disease. Parts I, II, and III. Amer. Heart J. 76:685–698; 77:100–122 and 383–410.

RONA, G., CHAPPEL, C. I., BALAZS, T., and GAUDRY, R. 1959. An infarct-like myocardial lesion and other toxic manifestations produced by isoproterenol in the rat. Arch. Pathol. 67:443–455.

VASDEV, S. C., and KAKO, K. J. 1977. Incorporation of fatty acids into rat heart lipids: In vivo and in vitro studies. J. Mol. Cell. Cardiol. In press.

ZAROR-BEHRENS, G., and KAKO, K. J. 1976. Positional and fatty acid specificity of monoacyl- and diacylglycerol 3-phosphate formations by rabbit heart microsomes. Biochim. Biophys. Acta. In press.

Mailing address:
K. J. Kako, M.D.,
Department of Physiology, Faculty of Medicine,
University of Ottawa, Nicholas Street,
Ottawa, Ontario, KIN 9A9 (Canada).

Recent Advances in Studies on
Cardiac Structure and Metabolism, Volume 11
Heart Function and Metabolism
Edited by T. Kobayashi, T. Sano, and N. S. Dhalla
Copyright 1978   University Park Press   Baltimore

MYOCARDIAL FATTY ACID AND CARDIAC PERFORMANCE

F. TAKENAKA and S. TAKEO

Department of Pharmacology, Kumamoto University Medical School,
Kumamoto, Japan

SUMMARY

Isoproterenol enhanced myocardial triglyceride utilization and incorporation of exogenous fatty acid into triglyceride fraction in the perfused rat heart in the presence of glucose. However, in the absence of glucose, cardiac performance was considerably aggravated by isoproterenol. This suggests that glucose might be an essential fuel in the heart stimulated by isoproterenol.

INTRODUCTION

It has been reported that epinephrine enhanced fatty acid utilization in the perfused heart (Kreisberg, 1966; Gartner and Vahouny, 1972; Crass, Shipp, and Piper, 1976). In the present study, effects of isoproterenol and exogenous substrates on myocardial triglyceride utilization and cardiac performance were investigated in isolated, perfused rat hearts.

METHODS

Male albino Wistar rat hearts were perfused with a modified Locke-Ringer solution by Langendorff technique without recirculation. Exogenous substrates added to the perfusing solution were 5.5 mM glucose and 0.4 mM sodium myristirate bound to 0.5% albumin. Sodium myristirate was employed as an exogenous fatty acid tracer, since myristiric acid content in the rat heart was very low. Isoproterenol was applied to the heart at a concentration of 4×10^{-6} M in the absence of myristirate and 4×10^{-7} M in its presence. Isometric tension development of the heart was monitored by a force-displacement transducer, and heart rate by a cardiotachometer. Total myocardial lipids were extracted from the myocardial homogenate by using chloroform-methanol. Methylesters of fatty acid moieties in triglyceride (TG) fraction separated by thin-layer chromatography were prepared and analyzed by means of gas chromatography.

Lipolytic activity was measured according to the method of Risack in adipose tissue and that of Mosinger (Risack, 1961; Mosinger, 1965).

RESULTS

In the heart perfused for 30 min in the absence of isoproterenol, changes in cardiac performance and myocardial triglyceride fatty acid (TGFA) content are shown in Figure 1.

Cardiac contraction and myocardial TGFA content at 30-min perfusion significantly decreased in the heart without substrates, when compared with those in the presence of glucose. When hearts were perfused with a solution containing myristirate, cardiac contractions in the hearts both with and without glucose were initially depressed, and followed by a gradual improvement. Triglyceride fatty acid content at 30-min perfusion was as high as the initial level in the presence of glucose and reduced to 64% in its absence. Both values were significantly higher than those in the hearts without myristirate.

Effects of Isoproterenol in the Presence of Glucose

When isoproterenol was applied to the heart perfused with a solution containing glucose (Figure 2), cardiac performance was augmented during 30-min perfusion and TGFA content at 30-min perfusion was 27% of the initial value, which was significantly different from that of the heart without isoproterenol.

When isoproterenol was applied to the heart perfused with a solution containing glucose and myristirate (Figure 2), cardiac performance was augmented without any initial depression. Triglyceride fatty acid content at 30-min perfusion was 84% of the initial level, which was significantly lower than that of the heart without isoproterenol. Initial content of myristiric acid was 0.187 ± 0.026, while its values in the heart perfused for 30 min with and without isoproterenol were 3.653 ± 0.335 and 2.895 ± 0.244 μmol/g dry weight, respectively. This indicates that myristirate incorporation into TG fraction was significantly increased by isoproterenol.

Myocardial lipolytic activity was 0.327 ± 0.015 μeq/mg protein in *in vitro* experiments and declined to 0.230 ± 0.016 μeq/mg protein after incubating for 1 hr. The lipolytic activities incubated with 4×10^{-6} M and 4×10^{-4} M isoproterenol for 1 hr were 0.269 ± 0.015 ($0.1 > p > 0.05$) and 0.258 ± 0.016 μeq/mg protein ($0.3 > p > 0.2$), respectively.

Effects of Isoproterenol in the Absence of Glucose

When isoproterenol was applied to the heart perfused without substrates, cardiac performance was initially augmented and followed by a gradual depression. Triglyceride fatty acid content at 30-min perfusion was 36% of the initial value,

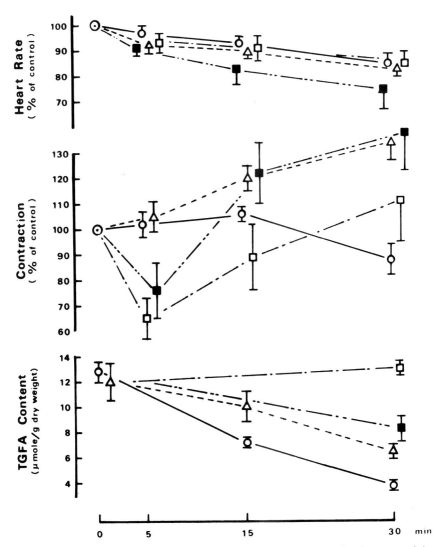

Figure 1. Changes in cardiac performance and triglyceride fatty acid(TGFA) content of the heart perfused with a modified Locke-Ringer solution containing or without substrates. *n* = 7–15. o——; heart in the absence of substrates. △————; heart in the presence of glucose. ■ ————; heart in the presence of myristirate. □ —————; heart in the presence of glucose and myristirate.

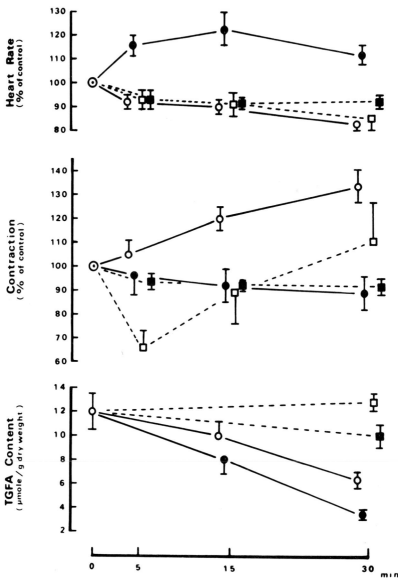

Figure 2. Changes in cardiac performance and triglyceride fatty acid(TGFA) content of the heart perfused with a modified Locke-Ringer solution in the presence of glucose. *n* = 7–15. ○———; heart in the presence of glucose. □————; heart in the presence of glucose and myristirate. ●———; heart in the presence of isoproterenol and glucose. ■————; heart in the presence of isoproterenol, glucose and myristirate.

which was not significantly different from that without isoproterenol. When isoproterenol was applied to the heart perfused with a solution containing myristirate, marked bradycardia or ventricular arrest occurred within 10 min of perfusion.

DISCUSSION

The present experiments demonstrated an enhanced utilization of myocardial TG by isoproterenol as reported by epinephrine (Kreisberg, 1966; Gartner *et al.,* 1972; Crass *et al.,* 1976). In addition, enhanced myocardial turnover of TG content was indicated by applying exogenous myristirate to the heart. The effect on myocardial lipolytic activity suggests that hydrolysis of myocardial TG may not accompany an increase in myocardial lipase activity or it may not occur solely due to the direct effect of isoproterenol. The fact that enhanced decrease in TG content by isoproterenol was not observed in the perfused heart without substrates may be explained by "TG mobilization-resistant pools," the value of which was suggested as about 30% of the initial content (Olson, 1967; Crass *et al.,* 1976). Triglyceride content at 30-min perfusion in the heart perfused without exogenous substrates was 29% of the initial value in the present study. In the heart receiving isoproterenol, TGFA content 15 min after the start of the perfusion was not different from that of the heart without isoproterenol, indicating that myocardial TG utilization did not appear as promptly as glucose utilization by catecholamines (Williamson, 1964). The slow activation of TG utilization might result in a lack of energy supply sufficient to meet the increase in energy demand of the heart by isoproterenol, leading to an irregular contraction of the heart perfused with exogenous myristirate in the absence of glucose. Such an assumption may be supported by the finding that isoproterenol did not significantly increase the lipolytic activity of the myocardium. It is concluded that glucose might be an essential fuel in the heart stimulated by catecholamines.

REFERENCES

CRASS, M. F., III, SHIPP, J. C., and PIPER, G. M. 1976. Effects of catecholamines on myocardial endogenous substrates and contractility. Amer. J. Physiol. 228:618–627.

GARTNER, S. L., and VAHOUNY, G. M. 1972. Effects of epinephrine and cyclic 3', 5'-AMP in the perfused rat hearts. Amer. J. Physiol. 222:1121–1124.

KREISBERG, R. A. 1966. Effect of epinephrine on myocardial triglyceride and free fatty acid utilization. Amer. J. Physiol. 210:385–389.

MOSINGER, F. 1965. Photometric adaptation of Dole's microdetermination of free fatty acids. J. Lipid Res. 6:157–159.

OLSON, R. E. 1967. Utilization of exogenous and endogenous lipids by isolated perfused rat heart. *In* G. Marchetti and B. Taccardi (eds.), Coronary Circulation and Energetics of the Myocardium, pp. 162–185.

RISACK, M. F. 1961. An epinephrine-sensitive lipolytic activity in adipose tissue. J. Biol. Chem. 236:657–662.

WILLIAMSON, J. R. 1964. Metabolic effects of epinephrine in the isolated, perfused rat heart. J. Biol. Chem. 239:2721–2729.

Mailing address:
F. Takenaka, M.D.,
Professor of Pharmacology,
Department of Pharmacology,
Kumamoto University Medical School,
Honjo 2-2-1, Kumamoto City, Kumamoto (Japan).

Recent Advances in Studies on
Cardiac Structure and Metabolism, Volume 11
Heart Function and Metabolism
Edited by T. Kobayashi, T. Sano, and N. S. Dhalla
Copyright 1978   University Park Press   Baltimore

FREE FATTY ACID CONTENT OF MYOCARDIAL
INTERSTITIAL SPACES OF DOG

P. JULIEN, G. R. DAGENAIS, L. GAILIS, and P. -E. ROY

Department of Pathology and Institut de Cardiologie de Québec,
Université Laval, Québec, Canada

SUMMARY

Morphological and biochemical observations from our laboratory have shown the presence
of lipids in the cardiac interstitial spaces of the dog. The present study was designed to
assess the importance of free fatty acids (FFA) in these lipids using FFA or sucrose tracers
in 14 anesthetized fasting open-chest mongrel dogs. Endogenous FFA and labeled tracers
were measured in arterial and coronary sinus plasma; they were also determined in lymph
collected from cardiac efferent lymphatic trunks.

[^{14}C] sucrose was infused at a constant rate in the femoral vein of 5 dogs. The
concentration of the tracer in the lymph was 90% of the arterial concentration after 60 min
of infusion. On the other hand, when [1-^{14}C] palmitate was infused at the same rate in 7
dogs, the ratio of lymph to arterial tracer concentration was only 20% (60 min) and 25%
(120 min), even though the myocardial extraction and oxidation of the tracer were stable.
This ratio tended to reach a plateau ($\geqslant$ 90%) only 24 hr after a bolus injection of the tracer.
This tracer study shows the presence of a pool of myocardial fatty acids with a relatively
slow turnover rate that may constitute an important reservoir of FFA.

INTRODUCTION

Morphological observations from our laboratory (Roy, 1975) have shown the
presence of lipid droplets in the interstitial spaces of human and canine hearts.
Moreover, biochemical findings from Stokke *et al.* (1974) and Julien and Roy
(1975) have also revealed the presence of different lipid components, such as
phospholipids, cholesterol, triglycerides and free fatty acids, in the cardiac
lymph which is representative of the interstitial fluid (Schultze and Heremans,
1966). These morphological and biochemical observations led us to consider the
possibility of cardiac interstitial spaces serving as a reservoir of fatty acids. The
present study was undertaken to verify this hypothesis by attempting to saturate
the myocardial interstitial spaces with labeled free fatty acid (FFA).

This work was supported by grants from the Canadian Heart Foundation and the
Medical Research Council of Canada. A fellowship from the Canadian Heart Foundation is
gratefully acknowledged.

METHODS

Procedure

Fourteen mongrel dogs, weighing about 20 Kg, and after fasting for a period of at least 18 hr, were anesthetized with sodium pentobarbital (30 mg/kg body weight, supplemented as required). Cardiac lymph was obtained from efferent lymphatic trunks cannulated near the cardiac lymphatic ganglion according to the method described by Kluge and Ullal (1971) and Julien *et al.* (1974). A femoral artery was cannulated for blood sampling and pressure monitoring. A catheter was introduced into a jugular vein and advanced to the coronary sinus. Normal saline solution was infused intravenously to replace the total loss of fluid. The electrocardiogram, heart rate, systolic and left ventricular end-diastolic pressures, and ventricular dp/dt were monitored while arterial and coronary sinus pO_2, O_2 saturation, pCO_2, pH, total and individual FFA, labeled FFA $^{14}CO_2$, and lactate were being determined. No glucose or heparin was used during these experiments.

Biochemical Analysis

Plasma and lymph palmitate were extracted by the method of Dole (1956) and measured using a gas chromatographic method (Dagenais, Marquis, and Gailis, 1975). [^{14}C] sucrose (specific activity: 4.9 mCi/mmol) or [1-^{14}C] palmitate (specific activity: 44.2 mCi/mmol) was infused at a constant rate in femoral vein. Labeled carbon dioxide was measured as reported by Dagenais *et al.* (1975).

Calculations

1. Percent myocardial extraction of [1-^{14} C] palmitate was measured as:

$$\frac{A^* - CS^*}{A^*} \times 100$$

where A^* and CS^* represent the arterial and coronary sinus concentration of the tracer.

2. Percent myocardial palmitate oxidation, based on $C^{14}O_2$ released, was calculated as:

$$\frac{(^{14}CO_2 \; \overline{cs} - {}^{14}CO_2 \, \overline{a})}{(A^* - CS^*)} \times 100$$

where $\overline{cs}$ and $\overline{a}$ designate the $^{14}CO_2$ concentrations in coronary sinus and arterial plasma, respectively.

RESULTS

During these metabolic studies, no evidence of myocardial ischemia was observed. Figure 1 illustrates an example from one of the experiments. During a constant infusion of $[1\text{-}^{14}C]$ palmitate, the myocardial extraction of palmitate remained nearly constant—about 50% throughout the experiment. The myocardial oxidation of the extracted palmitate also remained constant—about 60% of the amount extracted. Furthermore, the arterial, coronary sinus, and lymph palmitate-specific activities remained stable. The lymph-specific activity represented 25% of the arterial-specific activity.

Figure 2 shows that during the infusion of $[1\text{-}^{14}C]$ palmitate in 7 dogs the ratio of lymph to arterial tracer concentrations was only 20% at 60 min and 25% at 120 min, even though the myocardial extraction and oxidation of the tracer were stable. On the other hand, when $[^{14}C]$ sucrose was infused at the same rate, in 5 dogs, the concentration of the tracer in the lymph was 90% of the arterial concentration after 60 min of infusion. A ratio of 90% was obtained with $[^3H]$ palmitate only 24 hr after a bolus injection in 2 dogs.

The lymph flow varied between 4 and 12 ml/hr while the coronary blood flow could reach 6,000 ml/hr. The small loss of free fatty acids in the lymph represented only 0.3% of the myocardial extraction.

DISCUSSION

It has been shown that the mean arterial concentration and lymphatic concentration of total FFA are not different (Julien, Gailis, and Roy, 1977). However, the percentage of oleic acid in the plasma is higher than in the lymph, while

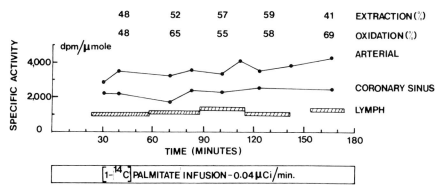

Figure 1. Data from one of the experiments showing myocardial extraction and oxidation of extracted $[1\text{-}^{14}C]$ palmitate and myocardial balance of palmitate-specific activity during a continuous infusion of $[1\text{-}^{14}C]$ palmitate.

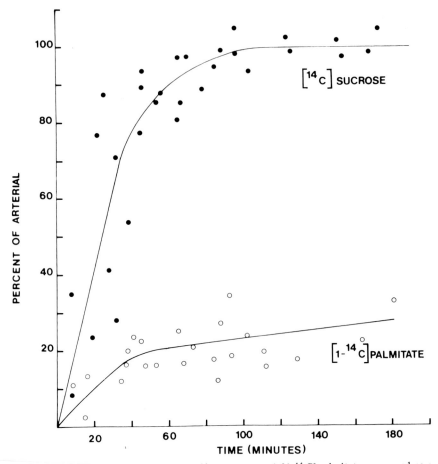

Figure 2. Cardiac lymph saturation of [^{14}C] sucrose and [1-^{14}C] palmitate, expressed as a percentage of their arterial concentration, in relation to time. Values were obtained with a continuous infusion of arterial tracers in 12 dogs.

stearic and myristic acids are significantly lower in plasma (Julien *et al.*, 1977).

In order to test the possibility that different FFA in the interstitial spaces are not in immediate equilibrium with those in plasma, the specific activity of palmitate was measured. This study showed that after two hr of infusion the lymphatic palmitate specific activity was only 25% of the arterial value. The lower specific activity did not result from lower endogenous palmitate concentration in the interstitial fluid since its concentrations in both lymph and plasma were similar.

In order to appreciate the time course of saturation of the lymph space, [^{14}C] sucrose infusion demonstrated that its low specific activity in the cardiac lymph was not due to a slow transit time through the interstitial spaces because the myocardial interstitial fluid was saturated to 90% or more after 60 min of infusion. The low specific activity obtained after $[1\text{-}^{14}C]$ palmitate infusion shows that there was a fatty acid reservoir with a relatively slow turnover rate not yet saturated after 180 min of infusion. The only way that we were able to achieve a specific activity of palmitate in the cardiac lymph of 90% of the arterial value was by waiting 24 hr after a bolus injection of labeled palmitate.

These findings confirm that the heart has a lipid pool (Opie, 1969) with a slow turnover. Furthermore, they indicate that the cardiac interstitial spaces can be considered one possible location of this pool.

REFERENCES

DAGENAIS, G. R., MARQUIS, Y., and GAILIS, L. 1975. Assessment of myocardial free fatty acid metabolism in humans during heparin infusion. *In* P.-E. Roy and G. Rona (eds.), Recent Advances in Studies on Cardiac Structure and Metabolism, Vol. 10, The Metabolism of Contraction, pp. 3—16. University Park Press, Baltimore.

DOLE, V. P. 1956. A relationship between non-esterified fatty acids in plasma and the metabolism of glucose. J. Clin. Invest. 35:150—154.

JULIEN, P., GAILIS, L., and ROY, P.-E. 1977. Evidence for lipids in the cardiac interstitial spaces. In press.

JULIEN, P., GAILIS, L., BLOUIN, A., and ROY, P. -E. 1974. Technique de canulation des vaisseaux lymphatiques cardiaques. Union Méd. Can. 103:1941—1943.

JULIEN, P., and ROY, P. -E. 1975. Lipid composition of cardiac lymph. *In* P. -E. Roy and G. Rona (eds.), Recent Advances in Studies on Cardiac Structure and Metabolism, Vol. 10, The Metabolism of Contraction, pp. 37—46. University Park Press, Baltimore.

KLUGE, T., and ULLAL, S. R. 1971. A standardized technique for drainage and collection of cardiac lymph. Acta Physiol. Scan. 83:433—436.

OPIE, L. H. 1969. Metabolism of the heart in health and disease. Part II. Amer. Heart J. 77:100—122.

ROY, P.-E. 1975. Lipid droplets in the heart interstitium: Concentration and distribution. *In* P. -E. Roy and G. Rona (eds.), Recent Advances in Studies on Cardiac Structure and Metabolism, Vol. 10, The Metabolism of Contraction, pp. 17—27. University Park Press, Baltimore.

SCHULTZE, H. E., and HEREMANS, J. -F. 1966. *In* Molecular Biology of Human Proteins, pp. 587—669. Elsevier Publ. Co., Amsterdam.

STOKKE, K. T., FJELD, N. B., KLUGE, T. H., and SKREDE, S. 1974. Lipid composition and cholesterol esterification in lymph. Scan. J. Clin. Lab. Invest. 33:199—206.

Mailing address:
Pierre Julien,
Centre de Recherches,
Hôpital Laval,
2725 Chemin Ste-Foy,
Ste-Foy, Québec, G1V-4G5 (Canada).

Pharmacological Aspect

Recent Advances in Studies on
Cardiac Structure and Metabolism, Volume 11
Heart Function and Metabolism
Edited by T. Kobayashi, T. Sano, and N. S. Dhalla
Copyright 1978 University Park Press Baltimore

ELECTROLYTE-DEPENDENCE OF CARDIAC GLYCOSIDE ACTIONS AT THE CELLULAR AND SUBCELLULAR LEVEL

W. KLAUS and U. FRICKE

Institute of Pharmacology, University of Cologne,
Federal Republic of Germany

SUMMARY

On the basis of studies on cardiac glycoside (CG) electrolyte interactions with myocardial function, (Na^+,K^+)-ATPase activity, CG uptake and microsomal binding, a model for the mode of action of CG at the subcellar level is presented.

INTRODUCTION

Clinical experience has shown that the extracellular concentration of certain electrolytes is able to modulate both the onset and the intensity of the positive inotropic and toxic actions of cardiac glycosides (CG). Although the theoretical implications of this behavior have been studied extensively in the past (Lee and Klaus, 1971), some aspects remained controversial. Therefore, the influence of the determinant electrolytes, K^+, Na^+, and Ca^{2+}, was studied at different levels of CG actions: myocardial function, activity of membrane ATPase, cardiac uptake, and microsomal binding.

METHODS

The pharmacological actions were tested on papillary muscles or isovolumically perfused guinea pig hearts. The latter preparation was also used in the uptake studies (Fricke and Klaus, 1975). The activity of the myocardial membrane ATPase was determined as previously described (Fricke and Klaus, 1974). The binding of CG to this preparation was studied using the sedimentation technique; the degree of phosphorylation was measured according to Neufeld and Levy (1970).

These studies were supported by grants from the Deutsche Forschungsgemeinschaft.

RESULTS AND DISCUSSION

K^+-Dependence

The clinically well-known antagonism between the action of CG and $[K^+]_e$ on myocardial function can easily be demonstrated in pharmacological experiments (Fricke and Klaus, 1971). An analysis of the absolute changes in contractile force induced by CG at different $[K^+]_e$ indicates a reduction of the inotropic maximum by increasing the $[K^+]_e$ due to an "earlier" manifestation of toxicity in the course of the dose-response relationship. This behavior may reflect a different sensitivity of these two functional parameters to changes in $[K^+]_e$. The antagonistic influence of $[K^+]$ has also been shown repeatedly on the CG-induced inhibition of the (Na^+,K^+)-ATPase (Lee and Klaus, 1971). These actions of high $[K^+]_e$ on myocardial function and on ATPase activity obviously are based on an antagonistic influence of $[K^+]$ on the interaction of CG with the heart muscle cell, i.e., the (Na^+,K^+)-ATPase as shown by Dutta and Marks (1969) and Lindenmayer (1970). The reduced binding of CG observed under these conditions is accompanied by a corresponding reduction in the ATP-induced phosphorylation of the enzyme (Hegyvary and Post, 1971). Because the phosphorylated ATPase intermediate is generally accepted as the specific binding site of CG, the antagonistic effect of high $[K^+]$ can easily be explained.

Ca^{2+}-Dependence

The interaction between CG and Ca^{2+} actions is well known as a functional synergism. Regarding the absolute changes in contractile force induced by CG at different $[Ca^{2+}]_e$, however, a lack of dependence (digoxin) or even a reduction in effectiveness (ouabain) could be demonstrated Alken, Fricke, and Klaus, 1974). The inhibitory action of CG on the (Na^+,K^+)-ATPase was not altered by variation of the $[Ca^{2+}]$ (unpublished data). On the other hand, the myocardial uptake of CG was reduced by high $[Ca^{2+}]_e$ (Fricke and Klaus, 1975). This is paralleled with a diminished microsomal binding of CG that most probably is due to a concomitant effect of $[Ca^{2+}]$ on the degree of phosphorylation of the ATPase system (Figure 1).

Na^+ Dependence

Both the inotropic and the toxic response of the myocardium to CG are dependent on $[Na^+]_e$; the higher $[Na^+]_e$, the more pronounced are the positive inotropic as well as the toxic effects (Figure 2). It is obvious, however, that at low $[Na^+]_e$ the toxicity (as indicated by the breaking-off of the curves) appears "earlier" (i.e., at a lower inotropic level) in the course of the dose-response relationship than at high $[Na^+]_e$. This again may indicate a certain dissociation between the inotropic and toxic actions of CG, as observed already in the CG-K^+ interrelationships. Similar to the CG influence on the functional parameters, the

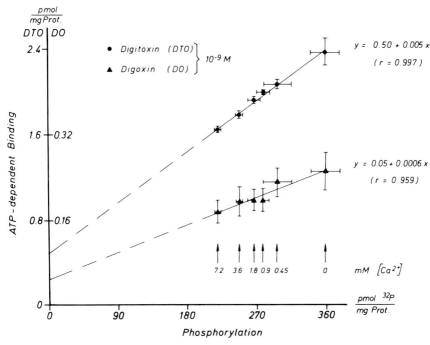

Figure 1. Correlation between the extent of phosphorylation of the (Na^+,K^+)-ATPase and the binding of digitoxin or digoxin at different $[Ca^{2+}]$.

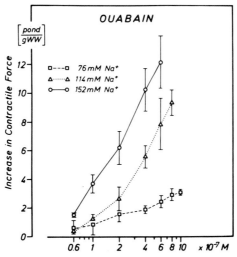

Figure 2. Dose-response curves for the inotropic action of ouabain at different $[Na^+]_e$, determined on isolated perfused guinea pig hearts.

ouabain-induced inhibition of the (Na^+,K^+)-ATPase is more pronounced at high $[Na^+]$ (Lindenmayer, 1970). In good agreement with this behavior, an increased uptake of CG into the myocardium has been observed by increasing the $[Na^+]_e$ (Dutta and Marks, 1969). A more detailed analysis of the influence of $[Na^+]$ on the microsomal binding of ouabain, however, revealed two distinct processes involved in this relationship (Figure 3A): one binding site activated at low $[Na^+]$ and a second site of interaction was predominant at high $[Na^+]$. The first type of ouabain binding is strongly correlated to the degree of phosphorylation of the ATPase system under the same conditions (Figure 3B). On the basis of the

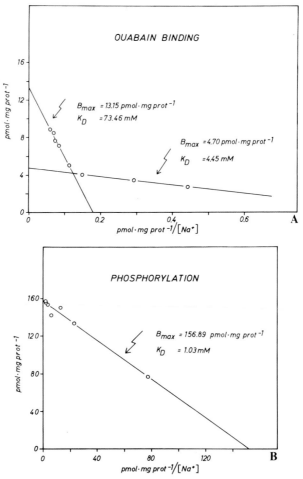

Figure 3. $[Na^+]$-dependence of ouabain binding to (3A), and phosphorylation of (3B), a microsomal (Na^+,K^+)-ATPase preparation. Analysis according to Hofstee (1952). B_{max} = maximum binding capacity. K_D = $[Na^+]$ for half maximum effect.

commonly accepted CG-ATPase reaction sequence (Post *et al.*, 1969) it is tempting to assume that the maximum binding of CG to the phosphorylated enzyme intermediate is induced at rather low $[Na^+]$, whereas the total amount of CG interacting with this system is determined by a different activating influence of high $[Na^+]$. This behavior may best be explained on the basis of a Na^+-dependent translocation process similar to the uptake mechanism of CG by the intestinal mucosa (Lauterbach, 1975).

CONCLUSION

Considering the outlined influences of the different electrolytes on the above-mentioned CG actions, a model of these interrelationships (Figure 4) may be developed on the basis of the reaction scheme originally proposed by Post *et al.* (1969).

CG are known to interfere with this system by forming a complex with the phosphorylated intermediate $E_2 \sim P$. The above-mentioned differences in the electrolyte-dependence of CG actions may be understood if we assume:

a) that this complex may act as a carrier (additional conformation change $E_2 \rightarrow E'_2$) providing a Na^+-induced translocation of CG from an outer to an inner compartment (which may well be located within the surface membrane),

b) that the concentration of the CG-enzyme complex determines the toxic actions of CG (by reducing the energy transfer for the cation transport below a critical level), and

c) that the concentration of CG in the inner compartment determines the inotropic action (by interfering with the state of calcium binding).

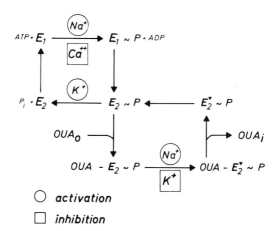

Figure 4. Proposed interaction scheme of CG and electrolytes at the level of the membrane ATPase. For details, see text.

A decrease in [Na$^+$] will cause a diminution of the phosphorylated intermediate, thereby reducing the number of specific binding sites, and, furthermore, will impair the translocation reaction of the carrier system. This type of interaction explains that the inotropic response to CG is more dependent on [Na$^+$] than the toxic action.

A similar reduction of the number of binding sites will be obtained by an increase in [K$^+$] resulting in a diminished toxicity. The relatively more pronounced influence of [K$^+$] on the inotropic action may tentatively be explained by an additional inhibitory effect on the translocation. An increase in [Ca^{2+}] inhibits the first step of phosphorylation by competition with [Na$^+$] (Portius and Repke, 1967). The resulting decrease in phosphorylated intermediate is responsible both for the increase in toxicity (due to an impairment of the energy transfer utilized for the cation transport) and the diminished inotropic activity of CG (due to a reduction of the number of binding sites thereby affecting the translocation).

REFERENCES

ALKEN, R. G., FRICKE, U., and KLAUS, W. 1974. Divergent influences of Ca^{2+} on the action of several cardiotonic steroids in isolated heart muscle preparations. Eur. J. Pharmacol. 26:331–337.

DUTTA, S., and MARKS, B. H. 1969. Factors that regulate ouabain-H3 accumulation by the isolated guinea pig heart. J. Pharmacol. Exp. Ther. 170:318–325.

FRICKE, U., and KLAUS, W. 1971. Comparative studies of the influence of various K$^+$-concentrations on the action of k-strophanthidin, digitoxin and strophanthidin-3-bromoacetate on papillary muscle and on membrane ATPase of guinea pig hearts. Eur. J. Pharmacol. 15:1–7.

FRICKE, U., and KLAUS, W. 1974. A simple preparation technique for a microsomal Na$^+$-K$^+$-activated ATPase from cardiac tissues of different species. Prep. Biochem. 4:13–29.

FRICKE, U., and KLAUS, W. 1975. Dependence of the cardiac uptake of digitalis glycosides on the extracellular calcium concentration in isolated guinea pig hearts. Eur. J. Pharmacol. 30:182–187.

HEGYVARY, C., and POST, R. L. 1971. Binding of adenosine triphosphatase to sodium and potassium ion-stimulated adenosine trisphosphatase. J. Biol. Chem. 246:5234–5240.

HOFSTEE, B. H. J. 1952. On the evaluation of the constants V_m and K_M in enzyme reactions. Science 116:329–331.

LAUTERBACH, F. 1975. Resorption und Sekretion von Arzneistoffen durch die Mukosaepithelien des Gastrointestinaltraktes. Arzneim.-Forsch. 25:479–488.

LEE, K. S., and KLAUS, W. 1971. The subcellular basis for the mechanism of inotropic action of cardiac glycosides. Pharmacol. Rev. 23:193–261.

LINDENMAYER, G. A. 1970. Biochemical responses of the cardiac cell to various stresses, a molecular mechanism for cardiac glycoside-induced compensation. Thesis, Houston, Texas.

NEUFELD, A. H., and LEVY, H. M. 1970. The steady state level of phosphorylated intermediate in relation to the two sodium-dependent adenosine triphosphatases of calf brain microsomes. J. Biol. Chem. 245:4962–4967.

PORTIUS, H. J., and REPKE, K. R. H. 1967. Eigenschaften und Funktion des Na$^+$-K$^+$-

aktivierten, Mg^{2+}-abhängigen Adenosintriphosphat-Phosphohydrolase-Systems des Herz-muskels. Acta Biol. Med. Germ. 19:907–938.

POST, R. L., KUME, S., TOBIN, T., ORCUTT, B., and SEN, A. K. 1969. Flexibility of an active center in sodium-plus-potassium adenosine triphosphatase. J. Gen. Physiol. 54: 306S–326S.

Mailing address:
Dr. W. Klaus
Institute of Pharmacology,
University of Cologne, Cologne
(Federal Republic of Germany).

Recent Advances in Studies on
Cardiac Structure and Metabolism, Volume 11
Heart Function and Metabolism
Edited by T. Kobayashi, T. Sano, and N. S. Dhalla
Copyright 1978   University Park Press   Baltimore

EFFECT OF OUABAIN ON SODIUM MOVEMENT IN CARDIAC CELLS

T. AKERA, M. K. OLGAARD, and T. M. BRODY

Department of Pharmacology, Michigan State University,
East Lansing, Michigan 48824, USA

SUMMARY

A computer simulation indicates that intracellular sodium concentration within a space near the inner surface of sarcolemma fluctuates during a cycle of myocardial function. The sodium transient (a transient increase in sodium ion concentration associated with membrane excitation) is enhanced by the inhibition of (Na^+,K^+)-ATPase by ouabain, but an accumulation of myocardial sodium does not occur until the inhibition exceeds a critical point. The critical magnitude of sodium pump inhibition that causes a progressive sodium accumulation is dependent on the heart rate.

INTRODUCTION

A 20 to 40% inhibition of cardiac (Na^+,K^+)-ATPase, an enzyme system responsible for the active transport of Na^+ and K^+ across the cell membrane, has been found at the time when the positive inotropic effect of digitalis is observed (Akera, Larsen, and Brody, 1970; Besch *et al.*, 1970; Ku *et al.*, 1974; Schwartz *et al.*, 1974). Nevertheless, the majority of studies (Lee and Klaus, 1971) failed to yield data consistent with sodium pump inhibition, i.e., an accumulation of sodium in these hearts. Since the magnitude of positive inotropic response to digitalis appears to be related to the magnitude of sodium pump inhibition during the onset and also the offset of drug action (Ku *et al.*, 1974), we attempted to examine the possible relationship between the inhibition of sodium pump activity and the intracellular sodium concentration. The specific question asked was whether we should expect an accumulation of myocardial sodium at the time when the sodium pump is inhibited by 40%.

In order to understand drug-induced changes in intracellular sodium concentrations, it is first necessary to describe the sodium concentration profile across the myocardial cell during a cycle of myocardial function. The intracellular

Supported by United States Public Health Service Research Grants HL-16052 and HL-16055.

sodium concentration in the mammalian myocardium is maintained at a level substantially lower than that of the extracellular space. On membrane excitation, sodium flows down a concentration and electrical gradient into the cell (Figure 1). The initial rapid sodium influx during phase 0 of action potential is followed by an additional sodium influx during phase 2 (Langer, 1974). Thus, the rate of sodium influx during the early phase of each cycle is significantly greater than that during the resting state or the later phase of the cycle. Therefore, the concentration of sodium ion in a space close to the inner aspect of the cell membrane fluctuates during a cycle of myocardial function, increasing during membrane excitation and returning to resting levels prior to the next membrane excitation. Diffusion exchange of sodium may occur between the intracellular space close to the sarcolemma and that deeper within the cell. Thus, the profile of sodium concentration across the cell should be such that the average sodium concentration is uniform throughout the cell, at approximately 30 mM, but the fluctuation of intracellular sodium concentration associated with myocardial function is greatest in a space closer to the sarcolemma and becomes smaller as the distance from the sarcolemma increases.

Because it is not possible to monitor sodium concentration in a small intracellular space with a time resolution fast enough to follow its changes during a cycle of myocardial function, a computer simulation was performed using the published data for sodium influx rates (Langer, 1974) and the (Na^+, K^+)-ATPase activity of partially purified dog heart enzyme preparations assayed in the presence and absence of ouabain at varying sodium concentrations as an estimate of sodium pump activity (for details, see Akera et al., 1976).

The change in intracellular sodium concentration with respect to time was calculated by subtracting the rate of efflux from the rate of influx at each

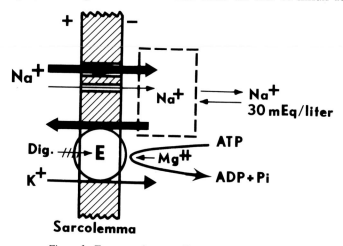

Figure 1. Transmembrane sodium movements.

half-millisecond time point in the cardiac cycle for a total of 500 msec (Figure 2). This time period corresponds to a heart rate of 120 beats per min. The figure shows that there is a rapid increase in intracellular sodium concentration during the first millisecond, that there is a sharp break in the curve at the 1-msec point corresponding to the closing of the fast sodium channel, and that, due to relatively large sodium influx during an early phase 2 period, intracellular sodium concentration increases further and reaches a peak at about 70 msec, a time when the efflux rate equals the influx rate. Following the peak the intracellular sodium concentration declines, since sodium pump activity is still high due to a high intracellular sodium concentration, but the rate of sodium influx is now decreased. It has been shown previously that the material to be pumped, i.e., intracellular sodium, regulates the activity of the pumping system (Post, 1968; Thomas, 1972; Langer, 1974). As the intracellular sodium concen-

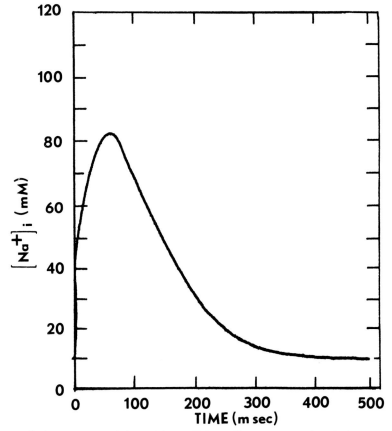

Figure 2. Computer simulation of intracellular sodium concentration during a cycle of myocardial function.

tration declines, so does pump activity. Prior to the next excitation, the intracellular sodium concentration has returned to its resting level of about 10 mM. The average concentration during the cycle is equal to the average intracellular sodium ion concentration of 30 mM.

Moderate inotropic, maximal inotropic, and arrhythmic doses of ouabain cause 20, 40, and 60% inhibition of cardiac (Na^+,K^+)-ATPase activity, respectively (Akera *et al.,* 1970). A 20% inhibition of sodium pump activity elevates the peak of the sodium transient (a transient increase in intracellular sodium concentration associated with membrane excitation), but the intracellular sodium concentration returns to control resting levels at the end of the cycle. Thus, a 20% inhibition of sodium pump activity will cause an enhancement of the sodium transient but will not cause a myocardial sodium accumulation. Similarly, the computer simulation indicates that a 40% inhibition of sodium pump activity fails to cause a progressive accumulation of myocardial sodium. However, a 60% inhibition of sodium pump activity causes a progressive accumulation of myocardial sodium with each cardiac cycle, since intracellular sodium concentration does not return to the resting level before the next membrane excitation when the cycle time is 500 msec.

These data indicate that inotropic concentrations of ouabain will produce a minimal myocardial sodium accumulation at relatively slow heart rates (below 120 beats per min) but will result in a progressive sodium accumulation at higher rates. In order to test the predictability of the computer simulation, electrically driven Langendorff preparations of guinea pig hearts were perfused with Krebs-Henseleit solution (6 ml/min) at 34° C. After a 45-min equilibration period, 0.4 μM ouabain, which has been shown to produce approximately 20% inhibition of cardiac (Na^+,K^+)-ATPase in this species (Ku *et al.,* 1976), was perfused. Under these conditions, ouabain produced a 32.9 ± 3.4% increase in contractile force (mean ± S.E.M. of sixteen experiments) at 20 min. At this time, the stimulation rate was increased to 240 per min for an additional 5-min period in half of the ouabain-treated and half of the control preparations. No cardiac arrhythmias were observed. In controls, there was no significant change in intracellular sodium content following the change in stimulation rate from 120 to 240 beats per min. With the ouabain-treated hearts, there was also no increase in sodium concentration at a perfusion rate of 120 per min when compared with control. When the rate was changed to 240 per min for a 5-min period in the ouabain-treated hearts, however, there was a significant (34.7%) increase in myocardial sodium content. Thus, the results predicted by the computer simulation were obtained.

These studies indicate that the inhibition of $(Na^+ K^+)$-ATPase by ouabain enhances the sodium transient, but does not cause a progressive accumulation of myocardial sodium until the inhibition exceeds a critical point. These results also indicate that the failure of positive inotropic concentrations of cardiac glycosides to cause myocardial sodium accumulation is not incompatible with the hypothesis that the (Na^+,K^+)-ATPase inhibition is the mechanism for the inotropic action of cardiac glycosides.

REFERENCES

AKERA, T., BENNETT, R. T., OLGAARD, M. K., and BRODY, T. M. 1976. Cardiac Na^+,K^+-ATPase inhibition by ouabain and myocardial sodium: A computer simulation. J. Pharmacol. Exp. Ther. 199:287–297.

AKERA, T., LARSEN, F. S., and BRODY, T. M. 1970. Correlation of cardiac sodium- and potassium-activated adenosine triphosphatase activity with ouabain-induced inotropic stimulation. J. Pharmacol. Exp. Ther. 173:145–151.

BESCH, H. R., JR., ALLEN, J. C., GLICK, G., and SCHWARTZ, A. 1970. Correlation between the inotropic action of ouabain and its effects on subcellular enzyme systems from canine myocardium. J. Pharmacol. Exp. Ther. 171:1–12.

KU, D., AKERA, T., PEW, C. L., and BRODY, T. M. 1974. Cardiac glycosides: Correlation among Na^+,K^+-ATPase, sodium pump and contractility in the guinea pig heart. Naunyn Schmiedebergs Arch. Pharmacol. 285:185–200.

KU, D. D., AKERA, T., TOBIN, T., and BRODY, T. M. 1976. Comparative species studies on the effect of monovalent cations and ouabain on cardiac Na^+,K^+-ATPase and contractile force. J. Pharmacol. Exp. Ther. 197:458–469.

LANGER, G. A. 1974. Ionic movements and the control of contraction. *In* G. A. Langer and A. J. Brady (eds.), The Mammalian Myocardium, pp. 193–217. John Wiley and Sons, New York.

LEE, K. S., and KLAUS, W. 1971. The subcellular basis for the mechanism of inotropic action of cardiac glycosides. Pharmacol. Rev. 23:193–261.

POST, R. L. 1968. The salt pump of animal cell membranes. *In* J. Järnefelt (ed.), Regulatory functions of Biological Membranes, pp. 163–176. Elsevier Publishing Co., Amsterdam.

SCHWARTZ, A., ALLEN, J. C., VAN WINKLE, W. B., and MUNSON, R. 1974. Further studies on the correlation between the inotropic action of ouabain and its interaction with the Na^+,K^+-adenosine triphosphatase: Isolated perfused rabbit and cat hearts. J. Pharmacol. Exp. Ther. 191:119–127.

THOMAS, R. C. 1972. Intracellular sodium activity and the sodium pump in snail neurons. J. Physiol. (Lond.) 220:51–71.

Mailing address:
Tai Akera,
Department of Pharmacology,
Michigan State University,
East Lansing, Michigan 48824 (USA)

Recent Advances in Studies on
Cardiac Structure and Metabolism, Volume 11
Heart Function and Metabolism
Edited by T. Kobayashi, T. Sano, and N. S. Dhalla
Copyright 1978   University Park Press   Baltimore

EFFECTS OF HYPOXIA AND DIGITALIS GLYCOSIDES ON MYOCARDIAL STIFFNESS

K. TAUBERT, J. T. WILLERSON, W. SHAPIRO,
and G. H. TEMPLETON

Departments of Physiology and Internal Medicine,
University of Texas Health Science Center and Dallas V. A. Hospital,
Dallas, Texas, USA

SUMMARY

The influences of hypoxia and of the interactions of hypoxia with digoxin and ouabain on myocardial stiffness were studied at two extracellular calcium concentrations (2.5 mM and 4.0 mM) in isolated, isometrically contracting cat papillary muscles. Stiffness ($\Delta T/\Delta L$), defined as a change in tension (ΔT) in response to an imposed length change (ΔL), was measured during contraction and during rest by use of a sinusoidal forcing function. Neither digoxin, ouabain, nor increased extracellular calcium altered contraction or resting stiffness in the well-oxygenated environment. Resting stiffness was increased at the end of hypoxia only in the presence of digoxin in both 2.5 mM and 4.0 mM Ca. Contraction stiffness was increased in 2.5 mM Ca by hypoxia alone and by hypoxia in the presence of digoxin or ouabain, but was not increased in experiments carried out in 4.0 mM Ca. Thus it appears that hypoxia *per se* increases contraction stiffness, but increasing extracellular calcium from 2.5 mM to 4.0 mM prevents the increase elicited by hypoxia; resting stiffness, however, is increased by hypoxia only in the presence of digoxin, and this occurs in both 2.5 mM and 4.0 mM Ca.

INTRODUCTION

Several previous experimental and clinical studies have been directed toward the measurement of myocardial stiffness, or its reciprocal, compliance, but few have evaluated the effects of periods of hypoxia, either alone or in combination with digitalis, on stiffness. In isolated cardiac muscle, Tyberg *et al.* (1970) found that hypoxia *per se* did not alter series elastic stiffness, whereas Greene and Weisfeldt (1974) found that the combination of hypoxia and digoxin increased resting tension during the recovery phase after hypoxia.

Because the combined effects of digitalis and hypoxia on myocardial stiffness have not been evaluated during contraction and their effects on resting

This research was supported by National Institutes of Health Ischemic Heart Disease Specialized Center of Research (SCOR) Grant HL-17669 and by a grant from the Veterans Administration (5750-03).

stiffness have only been measured indirectly, we felt it was important to examine their influences on resting and contraction stiffness of isolated cardiac muscle utilizing the sinusoidal forcing function. This technique, developed in our laboratory (Templeton *et al.*, 1973), provides a sensitive measure of dynamic stiffness, which includes elastic and viscous components.

METHODS

Thirty-seven papillary muscles were removed from the right ventricles of adult cats of either sex, previously anesthesized with sodium pentobarbital (40 mg/kg, I.P.). The muscles were suspended between a tension transducer and a lever and lowered into a muscle bath containing a Krebs-Ringer bicarbonate buffer with 2.5 mM extracellular calcium (Ca). Muscles were oxygenated with 95% O_2, 5% CO_2 at a temperature of 30° C and a stimulation rate of 12/min. Voltage used for stimulation was threshold + 20%, which equaled about 90 V. The muscles contracted isometrically with the exception of a small sinusoidal stretch applied to the lever. The amplitude of the stretch was held constant at 0.5% L_{max} and the frequency was 20 Hz. This sinusoidal stretch was sufficient to induce a sinusoidal tension response during contraction as well as during rest. The sinusoidal tension response was filtered from the waveform by Fourier analysis for the purpose of measuring the amplitude of each sinusoidal tension cycle during contraction and rest. Approximately 40 stiffness values were then determined for each data collection period by dividing the amplitude of the sinusoidal tension cycle by the constant amplitude of the applied sinusoidal stretch. Data collected during both contraction and rest were analyzed by dividing each stiffness value by the simultaneously measured muscle tension, thus giving a stiffness: tension (ST:T) ratio, which represented stiffness per unit tension. Since stiffness is linearly related to tension (Nilsson, 1972; Templeton *et al.*, 1973), an intervention's ability to alter stiffness for a given tension could be analyzed by the ST:T ratio. Drugs utilized in these studies included digoxin (2×10^{-6} M; Burroughs-Wellcome) and ouabain (8.7×10^{-7} M; Lilly).

RESULTS

Contraction and resting stiffness were unaltered by digoxin in the well-oxygenated environment in 11 muscles in 2.5 mM Ca. In 9 other muscles, extracellular calcium was raised from 2.5 to 4.0 mM 30 min before digoxin was added to the muscle bath. Neither 4.0 mM Ca nor the combination of 4.0 mM Ca and digoxin altered contraction or resting stiffness under these circumstances. Similar experiments were carried out with ouabain in 2.5 and 4.0 mM Ca, and ouabain also did not alter contraction or resting stiffness in the well-oxygenated environment.

Figure 1 shows the results of comparisons of measurements of resting ST:T ratios before and after a 25-min period of hypoxia for three groups of muscles in 2.5 mM Ca and three groups in 4.0 mM Ca. All muscles were made hypoxic by changing the gas mixture to 95% N_2, 5% CO_2. Within either extracellular calcium concentration, muscles were either made hypoxic after control measurements had been made and thus had no glycoside present, or they were made hypoxic at the peak inotropic effect of ouabain or digoxin. In 2.5 mM Ca, the mean ST:T ratios before hypoxia were 0.20 for the 7 control muscles, 0.22 for the 4 muscles in the ouabain group, and 0.18 for the 7 muscles in the digoxin group. There was a modest increase in the absolute ST:T ratio in all three of these groups, but only the group of muscles made hypoxic at peak digoxin effect had a significant increase in resting ST:T ratios at the end of hypoxia ($p < 0.02$). In 4.0 mM Ca, ST:T ratios before hypoxia were 0.25 for the 4 control muscles, 0.21 for the 6 muscles in the ouabain group, and 0.28 for the 6 muscles in the digoxin group. For those muscles in the control group and the ouabain group, the ST:T ratios were unaltered by hypoxia; in the digoxin group, however, there was a tendency for the ST:T ratio to increase at the end of hypoxia (14%, $p = 0.05$). In none of the 6 groups shown in Figure 1 was there a significant change in resting tension during hypoxia. Thus, within either extracellular calcium

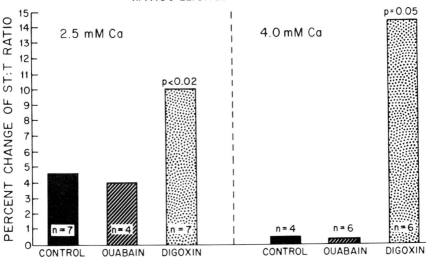

Figure 1. Each *bar* represents percent change in the resting ST:T ratio at the end of hypoxia as compared to the measurement obtained immediately prior to hypoxia. *p* values are for paired comparisons of ST:T ratios before and at the end of hypoxia.

concentration resting stiffness for any given resting tension was increased at the end of hypoxia only in the presence of digoxin.

Figure 2 illustrates the changes in contraction stiffness for 5 of the 6 previous groups. In 2.5 mM Ca the contraction ST:T ratio was 0.11 in all three groups of muscles prior to hypoxia. This value was significantly increased by 20% in the 5 control muscles ($p < 0.05$), by 36% in the 4 muscles in the ouabain group ($p < 0.02$), and by 35% in the 9 muscles in the digoxin group ($p < 0.005$). In 4.0 mM Ca the contraction ST:T ratio was 0.13 in both the ouabain and digoxin groups before hypoxia and the change at the end of hypoxia was not significant in either of the two groups.

DISCUSSION

The present study analyzed the effects of cardiac glycosides and increased extracellular calcium on resting and contraction stiffness of isolated cardiac muscle in the well-oxygenated environment and during hypoxic depression. The findings from these studies indicate that neither digoxin, ouabain, nor modestly increased extracellular calcium concentration alters resting or contraction stiffness in the well-oxygenated environment. During hypoxia, resting stiffness for any given resting tension was increased only in the presence of digoxin, and

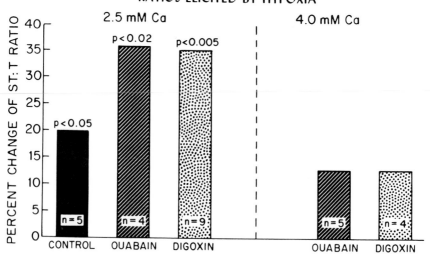

Figure 2. Each *bar* represents percent change in the contraction ST:T ratio at the end of hypoxia as compared to the measurement obtained immediately prior to hypoxia. *p* values are for paired comparisons of the ST:T ratios before and at the end of hypoxia.

this occurred in both 2.5 and 4.0 mM Ca, although in neither case was the increase greater than 15%. One other group of investigators (Greene and Weisfeldt, 1974) evaluated changes in resting tension as an indicator of resting stiffness and found no changes in resting tension during hypoxia in the presence or absence of digoxin, although resting tension did increase during reoxygenation in the digoxin group. An important point, as indicated by the present study, is that changes in resting tension do not necessarily reflect changes in resting stiffness, for the normal direct relationship between stiffness and tension may be altered under certain circumstances.

Measurements of contraction stiffness showed that it was increased by hypoxia per se, and the increases were greater when digoxin or ouabain were present. When the level of extracellular calcium was increased from 2.5 to 4.0 mM, the increase in contraction stiffness at the end of hypoxia was no longer significant. Tyberg and associates (1970) performed quick-release experiments during hypoxia and found no changes in contraction stiffness, whereas Templeton, Adcock, and Willerson (1973), utilizing the sinusoidal forcing function, found increased contraction stiffness for any given tension during hypoxia. The quick-release technique, however, has been considered to measure elastic stiffness, whereas the sinusoidal forcing function measures both elastic and viscous stiffness (Templeton *et al.,* 1973).

The clinical significance of these results remains uncertain. Similar studies need to be done in the intact animal and in humans so that the physiologic, metabolic, and hemodynamic correlates to the changes in stiffness can be determined.

REFERENCES

GREENE, H. L., and WEISFELDT, M. L. 1974. Combined effects of digitalis and hypoxia on myocardial diastolic stiffness. J. Clin. Invest. 53:30A (Abstract).

NILSSON, E. 1972. Influence of muscle length on mechanical parameters of myocardial contraction. Acta Physiol. Scand. 85:1–23.

TEMPLETON, G. H., ADCOCK, R. C., and WILLERSON, J. T. 1973. Influence of hypoxia on isolated papillary muscle stiffness and its elastic and viscous components. Circulation 48:262 (Abstract).

TEMPLETON, G. H., DONALD, T. C., MITCHELL, J. H., and HEFNER, L. L. 1973. Dynamic stiffness of papillary muscle during contraction and relaxation. Amer. J. Physiol. 224:692–698.

TYBERG, J. V., YEATMAN, L. A., PARMLEY, W. W., URSCHEL, C. W., and SONNENBLICK, E. H. 1970. Effects of hypoxia on mechanics of cardiac contraction. Amer. J. Physiol. 218:1780–1788.

Mailing address:
Dr. Kathryn Taubert,
Biomedical Sciences Program
University of California, Riverside,
Riverside, California 92502 (USA).

Recent Advances in Studies on
Cardiac Structure and Metabolism, Volume 11
Heart Function and Metabolism
Edited by T. Kobayashi, T. Sano, and N. S. Dhalla
Copyright 1978   University Park Press   Baltimore

THYROID HORMONE-INDUCED SUPERSENSITIVITY TO THE CARDIAC PHOSPHORYLASE-ACTIVATING EFFECT OF ADRENERGIC AMINES

J. H. McNEILL

Division of Pharmacology and Toxicology, Faculty of Pharmaceutical Sciences,
University of British Columbia, Vancouver, British Columbia, Canada

SUMMARY

Previous reports from this and other laboratories have clearly demonstrated that thyroid hormone pretreatment of rats produces a supersensitivity in the heart to the phosphorylase-activating effect of the adrenergic amines. The enhancement of the amine response is not due to changes in amine metabolism or inactivation. In addition we have reported that both the synthesis and breakdown of cardiac cyclic AMP is unaffected by pretreatment of animals with thyroid hormone. Calcium is also involved in the activation of phosphorylase and it was considered possible that the enhancement of the adrenergic amine response could take place at the calcium activation step. In order to test this possibility hearts were removed from euthyroid and hyperthyroid rats and perfused by the Langendorff technique. Injections of $CaCl_2$ or norepinephrine were made by means of a side arm cannula, and dose-response and time-response studies were carried out in which contractile force, heart rate and phosphorylase activation were determined. Both agonists increased all three parameters in a dose-dependent manner. Hearts from hyperthyroid animals responded to norepinephrine with greater increases in phosphorylase a than did those from euthyroid animals. However, no marked difference was noted between the two groups when $CaCl_2$ was injected and phosphorylase or contractile force was monitored. Hearts from hyperthyroid animals were, however, supersensitive to the chronotropic effect of calcium. It is concluded that hearts from hyperthyroid animals do not exhibit supersensitivity to the phosphorylase activating effect of $CaCl_2$. We are presently investigating the effect of dibutyryl cyclic AMP on phosphorylase activation in the heart in order to determine if hyperthyroid hearts are more sensitive to the actions of this agent.

INTRODUCTION

Thyroid hormone pretreatment does not enhance the inotropic or chronotropic effects of the adrenergic amines (Benfey and Varma, 1963; Margolius and Gaffney, 1965; Van der Schoot and Moran, 1965), but it does sensitize the heart and other tissues to the lipolytic and glycogenolytic effects of the catecholamines (Hornbrook *et al.,* 1965; McNeill and Brody, 1968; Krishna, Hynie,

Supported by grants from the British Columbia Heart Foundation and the Medical Research Council of Canada.

and Brodie, 1968; McNeill, Muschek, and Brody, 1969; Young and McNeill, 1974). The activation of the enzyme glycogen phosphorylase by adrenergic amines has been extensively studied in the hearts of several species. Enzyme sensitivity is greatly enhanced by production of the hyperthyroid state, but the mechanism involved is, as yet, unknown. It is not attributable to blockade of amine uptake, to a reserpine-like supersensitivity, or to an alteration in the synthesis or breakdown of cyclic AMP (McNeill and Brody, 1968; McNeill, 1969; McNeill *et al.,* 1969; Young and McNeill, 1974).

In addition to the catecholamines, it is known that calcium can activate phosphorylase in the heart (Friesen, Allen, and Valadares, 1967). Because it has been reported that thyroid hormone can alter some aspects of calcium metabolism in the heart, notably to increase the accumulation and exchange of calcium in the sarcoplasmic reticulum (Nayler *et al.,* 1971; Suko, 1971), it seemed possible that an increased release of bound calcium by, for example, norepinephrine could account for the thyroid hormone supersensitivity. Therefore, in the present study the effect of calcium on phosphorylase activation in hearts obtained from euthyroid and hyperthyroid rats was studied. Some preliminary data on the effect of dibutyryl cyclic AMP on phosphorylase activation are also presented.

MATERIALS AND METHODS

Wistar female rats (200–250 g) were used throughout the study. Animals were injected with heparin sodium (2.8 mg/kg subcutaneously (s.c.)) 60 min before sacrifice. The animals were stunned by a blow to the head and the heart was rapidly removed and perfused by the Langendorff technique using Chenoweth-Koelle solution (Chenoweth and Koelle, 1946) at a flow rate of 2.8 ml/min at 37°C as described by McNeill and Muschek (1972). Flow rate was maintained by means of a Holter micro-infusion roller pump (Extracorporeal Medical Specialties, King of Prussia, Pa., model RL175). Contractility was monitored by means of a Palmer clip placed in the apex of the heart and connected to a Grass force displacement transducer and recorded on a Grass model 7 polygraph.

Diastolic tension was adjusted to 2 g. The hearts were allowed to equilibrate for 8 min before calcium chloride dissolved in buffer solution was injected in a volume of 0.5 ml via a sidearm cannula over a 30-sec period. Noradrenaline injections were made in the same manner in a volume of 0.2 ml injected rapidly. At various times following injection, the hearts were frozen using a pair of tongs (Wollenberger, Ristan, and Schoffa, 1960) previously chilled in a mixture of alcohol-Dry Ice. The hearts were then stored at −80°C until assayed. In a few experiments dibutyryl cyclic AMP was injected over a 15-sec period via sidearm cannula and hearts were frozen 5 min later.

Phosphorylase was measured in the direction of glycogen synthesis as previously described by McNeill and Brody (1966). Since total phosphorylase did not change, all results are presented as percentage phosphorylase *a* which is: (phosphorylase activity in the absence of AMP/phosphorylase activity in the presence of AMP) $\times$ 100. The hearts were assayed for cyclic AMP using a modification of the protein-binding assay of Gilman (1970) with a cyclic AMP kit (TRK, 432 Amersham/Searle, Oakville, Ontario).

Animals were made hyperthyroid by the subcutaneous injection of 500 μg/kg of 3,3',5'-triiodo-L-thyronine in alkaline saline administered daily for 3 days. This treatment has previously been shown to make rats hyperthyroid (McNeill *et al.,* 1969).

Statistical analysis was done by the Student *t*-test for unpaired data for phosphorylase *a* and cyclic AMP, and for paired data for the positive inotropic effect (Lewis, 1966). A probability of < 0.05 was chosen as the criterion of significance.

Drugs used were the following: l-Arterenol HC1, heparin sodium, 3,3',5'-triiodo-L-thyronine, and dibutyryl cyclic AMP (all from Sigma Chem. Corp.) and calcium chloride dihydrate (MC and B, Norwood, Ohio).

RESULTS

Initial experiments were carried out in which norepinephrine (0.05 and 0.10 μg) was injected into the perfused hearts and phosphorylase measured. In hearts from euthyroid animals the percent of phosphorylase *a* increased from approximately 5% in buffer solution-injected preparations to 13.4 ± 1.6 and $33.8 \pm 6.5\%$ phosphorylase *a* with the two doses of norepinephrine. In hearts from hyperthyroid animals the phosphorylase *a* values were 37.9 ± 3.7 and $49.3 \pm 3.0\%$, a highly significant increase over control. Thus the thyroid hormone pretreatment did enhance the phosphorylase-activating effect of norepinephrine.

Injections of calcium chloride into the perfused hearts also produced dose-dependent increases in phosphorylase *a*. The data are presented in Table 1 and indicate that there was no significant difference between the two groups of hearts over a dose range of 0.5–8.0 mg of $CaCl_2$. In other experiments not shown, propranolol (10^{-6} M) did not affect the calcium response but did block the response to norepinephrine. Changes in contractile force produced by both norepinephrine and calcium chloride were also monitored. While both agonists produced an inotropic effect, there was no difference between the hearts obtained from euthyroid and hyperthyroid animals.

The chronotropic effect of $CaCl_2$ was also investigated, and the results are shown in Table 2. Pretreatment with triiodothyronine markedly affected the rate-increasing effect of $CaCl_2$ over a dose range of 1.0–8.0 mg. In another set of

Table 1. The effect of various doses of $CaCl_2$ on the percent of phosphorylase *a* in hearts* from euthyroid and hyperthyroid animals

Treatment**	Dose of $CaCl_2$ (mg)	Percent phosphorylase *a*
Euthyroid (7)	0.5	12.6 ± 1.5
Hyperthyroid (6)		12.2 ± 0.4
Euthyroid (8)	1.0	17.3 ± 3.7
Hyperthyroid (8)		14.3 ± 2.1
Euthyroid (32)	2.0	20.9 ± 1.4
Hyperthyroid (18)		20.0 ± 2.0
Euthyroid (7)	4.0	29.6 ± 1.4
Hyperthyroid (5)		34.0 ± 5.0
Euthyroid (6)	8.0	31.4 ± 3.0
Hyperthyroid (5)		39.9 ± 4.7

*Hearts were frozen at a time when phosphorylase activation was at its peak as determined by a time-response study.
**Numbers in parentheses indicate the number of animals.

experiments, injections of 2.0 mg calcium chloride were made into hearts obtained from both groups, and cyclic AMP was determined at 15 sec prior to the peak of the contractile response, at the peak of the contractile response, and at 4 10-sec intervals thereafter. Control values were 0.25 ± 0.05 nm/g for the hyperthyroid hearts and 0.27 ± 0.03 nm/g for the euthyroid hearts. These values did not change significantly at any time interval tested following the injection of calcium.

In the preliminary experiments with dibutyryl cyclic AMP it was found that hearts from hyperthyroid animals were more sensitive to this agent with regard

Table 2. The effect of increasing doses of calcium on heart rate in hearts from hyperthyroid and euthyroid rats ($N = 4$)

Treatment	Dose of $CaCl_2$ (mg)	Increase in rate over rate prior to injection (beats/min)
Euthyroid	1.0	24 ± 0
Hyperthyroid		30 ± 3[a]
Euthyroid	2.0	36 ± 4.9
Hyperthyroid		54 ± 11.4*
Euthyroid	4.0	36 ± 12.9
Hyperthyroid		139 ± 20.9*
Euthyroid	8.0	56 ± 14.1
Hyperthyroid		160 ± 28.1*

*Significantly greater than euthyroid.

Table 3. The effect of time on the phosphorylase-activating response to 100 μmol of dibutyryl cyclic AMP in the perfused rat heart*

Time	Percent phosphorylase a	
	Euthyroid	Hyperthyroid
30″	15.5 ± 1.12 (3)	17.3 ± 1.34 (3)
2′	22.2 (2)	20.5 (2)
5′	45.8 ± 2.87 (5)	65.0 ± 0.8 (5)**

*Numbers in parentheses indicate the number of animals.
**Significantly greater than euthyroid; $p < 0.01$.

to the activation of phosphorylase. In these experiments (Table 3) 100 μmol of dibutyryl cyclic AMP were injected into the heart and phosphorylase analyzed at various times thereafter. The difference between the two groups is apparent, particularly at the 5-min time interval.

DISCUSSION

The data presented confirm that thyroid hormone pretreatment will enhance the phosphorylase-activating effect of norepinephrine. The data also confirm the work of Friesen et al. (1967) that calcium can activate phosphorylase directly without releasing catecholamines. There were no differences between euthyroid and hyperthyroid animals with regard to the inotropic or phosphorylase-activating response. Hearts from hyperthyroid animals were more sensitive to calcium when the chronotropic response was monitored. This may indicate a change in membrane permeability in the nodal tissue of the heart as a result of the thyroid hormone pretreatment. Calcium injections did not elevate cyclic AMP in the rat heart. It is apparent from these data that thyroid hormone-induced supersensitivity to the phosphorylase-activating effects of norepinephrine is not due to a supersensitivity to calcium. From the preliminary data obtained with dibutyryl cyclic AMP it is concluded that hearts obtained from hyperthyroid animals are more sensitive to the phosphorylase-activating effect of this agonist. Thus, a supersensitivity to cyclic AMP, perhaps at the level of protein kinase, may exist in the heart in the hyperthyroid state.

REFERENCES

BENFEY, B. G., and VARMA, D. R. 1963. Cardiac and vascular effects of sympathomimetic drugs after administration of tri-iodothyronine and reserpine. Br. J. Pharmacol. 21:174–181.
CHENOWETH, M. B., and KOELLE, E. S. 1946. An isolated heart perfusion system

adapted to the determination of non-gaseous metabolites. J. Lab. Clin. Med. 31: 600–608.

FRIESEN, A. J. D., ALLEN, G., and VALADARES, J. R. E. 1967. Calcium-induced activation of phosphorylase in rat hearts. Science 155:1108–1109.

GILMAN, A. G. 1970. A protein binding assay for adenosine 3′,5′-cyclic monophosphate. Proc. Natl. Acad. Sci. USA 67:305–312.

HORNBROOK, K. R., QUINN, P. V., SIEGEL, J. H., and BRODY, T. M. 1965. Thyroid hormone regulation of cardiac glycogen metabolism. Biochem. Pharmacol. 14:925–936.

KRISHNA, G., HYNIE, S., and BRODIE, B. B. 1968. Effects of thyroid hormone on adenylate cyclase in adipose tissue and on free fatty acid mobilization. Proc. Natl. Acad. Sci. 59:884–889.

LEWIS, A. E. 1966. Biostatistics. Reinhold Publishing Corporation, New York, N.Y.

MARGOLIUS, H. S., and GAFFNEY, T. E. 1965. The effects of injected norepinephrine and sympathetic nerve stimulation in hypothyroid and hyperthyroid dogs. J. Pharmacol. Exp. Ther. 149:32–35.

McNEILL, J. H. 1969. Amine-induced cardiac phosphorylase *a* after reserpine triiodothyronine pretreatment. Eur. J. Pharmacol. 7:235–238.

McNEILL, J. H., and BRODY, T. M. 1966. The effect of antihistamines, cocaine and reserpine on amine-induced rat cardiac phosphorylase activation. J. Pharmacol. Exp. Ther. 152:478–486.

McNEILL, J. H., and BRODY, T. M. 1968. The effect of triiodothyronine pretreatment on amine-induced rat cardiac phosphorylase activation. J. Pharmacol. Exp. Ther. 161: 40–46.

McNEILL, J. H., and MUSCHEK, L. D. 1972. Histamine effects on cardiac contractility, phosphorylase and adenyl cyclase. J. Mol. Cell. Cardiol. 4:611–624.

McNEILL, J. H., MUSCHEK, L. D., and BRODY, T. M. 1969. The effect of triiodothyronine on cyclic AMP, phosphorylase and adenyl cyclase in rat heart. Can. J. Physiol. Pharmacol. 47:913–916.

NAYLER, W. G., MERRILLEES, N. C. R., CHIPPERFIELD, D., and KURTZ, J. B. 1971. Influence of hyperthyroidism on the uptake and binding of calcium by cardiac microsomal fractions and on mitochrondrial structure. Cardiovasc. Res. 4:469–482.

SUKO, J. 1971. Alterations of calcium uptake and calcium activated ATPase of cardiac sarcoplasmic reticulum in hyper- and hypothyroidism. Biochim. Biophys. Acta. 252: 324–327.

VAN DER SCHOOT, J. B., and MORAN, N. C. 1965. An experimental evaluation of the reported influence of thyroxine on the cardiovascular effects of catecholamines. J. Pharmacol. Exp. Ther. 149:336–345.

WOLLENBERGER, A., RISTAN, O., and SCHOFFA, G. 1960. Eine einfache Technik der extremen schnellen Abkulung grosserer Gewebstucke. Arch. Ges. Physiol. 27:399–412.

YOUNG, B. A., and McNEILL, J. H. 1974. The effect of noradrenaline and tyramine on cardiac contractility, cyclic AMP and phosphorylase *a* in normal and hyperthyroid rats. Can. J. Physiol. Pharmacol. 52:373–383.

Mailing address:
John H. McNeill
Division of Pharmacology and Toxicology
Faculty of Pharmaceutical Sciences
University of British Columbia
Vancouver, B.C. V6T 1W5 (Canada).

Recent Advances in Studies on
Cardiac Structure and Metabolism, Volume 11
Heart Function and Metabolism
Edited by T. Kobayashi, T. Sano, and N. S. Dhalla
Copyright 1978   University Park Press   Baltimore

EVIDENCE FOR OPPOSING INFLUENCES OF CYCLIC GMP AND CYCLIC AMP ON FORCE OF CONTRACTION IN MAMMALIAN MYOCARDIUM

H. NAWRATH

Pharmakologisches Institut der Universität Mainz,
6500 Mainz, Federal Republic of Germany

SUMMARY

The inotropic effects of the 8-Br-derivatives of cyclic GMP and cyclic AMP were investigated in guinea pig or rat auricles and papillary muscles from cats. In guinea pig auricles, 8-Br-cyclic GMP had a concentration-dependent negative inotropic effect, whereas 8-Br-cyclic AMP had a concentration-dependent positive inotropic effect. A negative inotropic effect of 8-Br-cyclic GMP in rat auricles was obtained with 30 times lower doses than in guinea pig auricles; the pacemaker activity of spontaneously beating rat right auricles did not change in response to 8-Br-cyclic GMP. In cat papillary muscles, 8-Br-cyclic GMP (3×10^{-4} M) also produced a negative inotropic effect. In contrast, 8-Br-cyclic AMP (3×10^{-4} M) did not affect force of contraction; however, after pretreatment with the strong phosphodiesterase inhibitor papaverine (2×10^{-5} M) 8-Br-cyclic AMP (3×10^{-4} M) had a strong positive inotropic effect also in cat papillary muscles. The results suggest opposite influences of cyclic GMP and cyclic AMP on force of contraction in mammalian myocardium.

INTRODUCTION

Several studies appear to confirm the general concept that the stimulation of cardiac contractility by adrenergic influences is associated with increased myocardial cAMP concentrations, and depression of contractility by cholinergic influences with increased cyclic GMP levels (for review, see Goldberg *et al.,* 1975). Whereas experimental evidence has accumulated that cyclic AMP or dibutyryl cyclic AMP exerts positive inotropic effects similar to that of adrenaline (Kukovetz and Pöch, 1970; Skelton, Levey, and Epstein, 1970; Fabiato and Fabiato, 1975) no direct action of cyclic GMP or its derivatives on force of contraction of isolated mammalian myocardium is described.

This research was supported by a grant from the Deutsche Forschungsgemeinschaft (Na 105/1).

the influence of the 8-Br-derivatives of cyclic GMP and cyclic AMP on force of contraction of isolated mammalian myocardium are described.

METHODS

The experiments were performed on isolated heart muscle preparations from guinea pigs, rats, and cats of either sex. Guinea pigs were killed by a blow on the head, rats and cats were anesthetized with ether, and the hearts were quickly removed and transferred to a dissection chamber with warmed, oxygenated Tyrode solution. Left or right auricles from guinea pigs and rats and papillary muscles from cats were dissected from the heart and attached to a muscle holder with a bipolar platinum stimulating electrode and mounted vertically in a muscle chamber containing 5 ml Tyrode solution that was continuously gassed with 95% O_2–5% CO_2 and heated to $35°C$. The composition of the Tyrode solution was (mM): NaCl, 136.9; KCl, 5.4; $MgCl_2$, 1.05; $CaCl_2$, 1.8; NaH_2PO_4, 0.42; $NaHCO_3$, 11.9; glucose, 5.6. The muscles were connected to an inductive force displacement transducer by means of a stainless steel wire. The preparations were driven electrically (left auricles at 2/sec and papillary muscles at 0.2/sec) with rectangular pulses of 2-msec duration; intensity of voltage was 10–15% above threshold. Contractions were monitored under isometric conditions at the apex of the preload-active tension curve and recorded on a Hellige paper recorder.

8-Br-cyclic AMP, 8-Br-cyclic GMP, and cyclic GMP were purchased from Boehringer/Mannheim. Papaverine-HCl and atropine sulfate were purchased from Boehringer/Ingelheim. All drugs were freshly dissolved in distilled water, and 0.1 ml of the corresponding stock solutions were injected into the muscle chamber. Each concentration of the drug was tested in individual preparations.

RESULTS AND DISCUSSION

Figure 1 shows the influence of 8-Br-cyclic GMP and 8-Br-cyclic AMP on force of contraction in guinea pig left auricles 30 min after drug addition. 8-Br-cyclic GMP exerted a concentration-dependent negative inotropic effect at concentrations above 10^{-4} M, whereas 8-Br-cyclic AMP had a concentration-dependent positive inotropic effect at concentrations above 3×10^{-5} M. A strong negative inotropic effect of 8-Br-cyclic GMP was also seen in rat left auricles; in this preparation the same effects were found with 30 times lower concentrations than in guinea pig left auricles. Therefore, all control experiments were done in rat left auricles:

1. 10^{-3} cyclic GMP itself did not affect force of contraction.
2. 10^{-3} M NaBr also did not affect force of contraction.

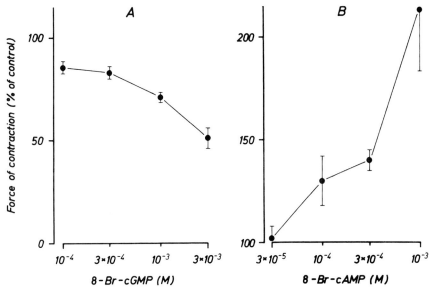

Figure 1. Influence of 8-Br-cyclic GMP and 8-Br-cyclic AMP on force of contraction in guinea pig left auricles. Values are means ± S.E. of 4–8 preparations each. 8-Br-cyclic GMP had a concentration-dependent negative inotropic effect (*A*), and 8-Br-cyclic AMP had a concentration-dependent positive inotropic effect (*B*).

3. Pretreatment with 5×10^{-6} M atropine did not change the response to 10^{-4} M 8-Br-cyclic GMP.

In contrast to the negative inotropic effect of 8-Br-cyclic GMP, the frequency of spontaneously beating rat right auricles did not change under the influence of the drug. In papillary muscles from cats, 8-Br-cyclic GMP (3×10^{-4} M) also had a negative inotropic effect, whereas 8-Br-cyclic AMP (3×10^{-4} M) did not affect force of contraction; however, after pretreatment with the strong phosphodiesterase inhibitor papaverine (2×10^{-5} M), a distinct positive inotropic effect was seen with 8-Br-cyclic AMP (3×10^{-4} M) also in cat papillary muscles. Therefore, the evidence suggests an opposite influence of cyclic GMP and cyclic AMP on force of contraction in atrial as well as in ventricular myocardium. This would be another example for the validity of the yin-yang hypothesis of the opposing roles of cyclic GMP and cyclic AMP in physiologic regulation.

    In contrast to the negative inotropic effects of 8-Br-cyclic GMP, the frequency of spontaneously beating rat right auricles was not changed by the drug. This points to a difference in the action of acetylcholine on rat atrial muscle. It has been shown in voltage-clamp experiments that the negative inotropic effect of acetylcholine in mammalian atrial muscle can be explained by an increase in potassium conductance at lower doses, and, additionally, by a decrease in calcium conductance at higher doses (Ten Eick *et al.,* 1976). It remains to be elucidated whether similar membrane conductance changes are brought about by the action of cyclic GMP and can be related to the corresponding changes in force of contraction.

REFERENCES

FABIATO, A., and FABIATO, F. 1975. Relaxing and inotropic effects of cyclic AMP on skinned cardiac cells. Nature 253:556–558.

GOLDBERG, N. D., HADDOX, M. K., NICOL, S. E., GLASS, D. B., SANFORD, C. H., KUEHL, F. A., and ESTENSEN, R. 1975. Biologic regulation through opposing influences of cyclic GMP and cyclic AMP: the yin yang hypothesis. *In* G. I. Drummond, P. Greengard, and G. A. Robison (eds.), Advances in Cyclic Nucleotide Research Vol. 5, pp. 307–330. Raven Press, New York.

KUKOVETZ, W. R., and PÖCH, G. 1970. Cardiostimulatory effects of cyclic 3′,5′-adenosine monophosphate and its acylated derivatives. Naunyn-Schmiedebergs Arch. Pharmak. 266:236–254.

SKELTON, C. L., LEVEY, G. S., and EPSTEIN, S. E. 1970. Positive inotropic effects of dibutyryl cyclic adenosine 3′,5′-monophosphate. Circ. Res. 26:35–43.

TEN EICK, R., NAWRATH, H., McDONALD, T. F., and TRAUTWEIN, W. 1976. On the mechanism of the negative inotropic effect of acetylcholine. Pfluegers Arch. 361: 207–213.

Mailing address:
Dr. Med. Hermann Newrath,
Pharmakologisches Institut der Universität Mainz,
Obere Zahlbacher Strasse 67,
D-6500 Mainz (Federal Republic of Germany).

Recent Advances in Studies on
Cardiac Structure and Metabolism, Volume 11
Heart Function and Metabolism
Edited by T. Kobayashi, T. Sano, and N. S. Dhalla
Copyright 1978   University Park Press   Baltimore

MECHANISM OF CHOLINERGIC ANTAGONISM
OF THE EFFECTS OF ISOPROTERENOL ON HEARTS
FROM HYPERTHYROID RATS

A. M. WATANABE, D. R. HATHAWAY, and H. R. BESCH, JR.

Departments of Medicine and Pharmacology, and the Krannert Institute of Cardiology,
Indiana University School of Medicine, Indianapolis, Indiana, USA

SUMMARY

The purpose of this study was to examine the mechanism by which acetylcholine antagonizes the contractile and metabolic effects of catecholamines on hearts from hyperthyroid rats. Experiments were performed on isolated perfused hearts obtained from male euthyroid and age-matched male hyperthyroid (T_3 for 3 days) rats. All hearts were perfused with buffer ($37°C$) containing 1.25 mM Ca^{2+} and paced at a rate of 210 stimuli/min. Contractility, assessed as the first derivative of tension development, increased more in hyperthyroid rats in response to 10^{-9} and 3×10^{-9} M isoproterenol (Iso) than in euthyroid animals (10^{-9} M Iso: + 24% in hyperthyroid hearts versus +13% in euthyroid hearts). Similarly, phosphorylase activation by Iso was greater in hearts from hyperthyroid rats. Whereas 10^{-8} M Iso activated phosphorylase from 10% to only 20% in euthyroid hearts, 10^{-9}, 3×10^{-9} M Iso activated phosphorylase from 10% to 21%, and 35% to 42%, respectively, in hyperthyroid hearts. Acetylcholine (ACh) antagonized both the positive inotropic and phosphorylase-activating effects of Iso. For example, Iso-induced increases in dT/dt and phosphorylase activation were reduced from +29% to +8% and from 42% to 35%, respectively, by 3×10^{-7} M ACh. These effects of ACh were accompanied by an attenuation of the amount of cyclic adenosine monophosphate (cAMP) generated by Iso. Dibutyryl cyclic guanosine monophosphate (dbcGMP) in concentrations of 10^{-6} and 10^{-5} M mimicked these effects of ACh. 10^{-6} M dbcGMP attenuated Iso induced dT/dt from +29% to +12% and phosphorylase activation from 42% to 32%. These effects of dbcGMP occurred without a change in the amount of cAMP generated by Iso. These results suggest that ACh may antagonize the effects of Iso on hyperthyroid rat hearts by acting at more than one level. ACh may attenuate the generation of cAMP by Iso. Furthermore, perhaps by means of cyclic guanosine monophosphate, ACh may antagonize the effects of cAMP formed by Iso stimulation.

INTRODUCTION

Several lines of evidence suggest that hearts taken from hyperthyroid animals are more sensitive to catecholamines than are hearts from euthyroid animals, al-

---

This work was supported by Grants HL 06308, HL 14159, HL 05363, and HL 05749 from the National Heart and Lung Institute; by the American Heart Association, Indiana Affiliate; and by the Herman C. Krannert Fund. Dr. Besch is supported by the Showalter Research Trust Fund.

though controversies persist on this point (Levey, 1971). Furthermore, data suggest that hyperthyroid animals have less vagal tone regulating the cardio-vascular system than do euthyroid animals (Cairoli and Crout, 1967). Our previous investigations have shown that the cholinergic system antagonizes the effects of catecholamines on normal hearts and may serve as a modulator of the effects of the adrenergic system on the heart (Watanabe and Besch, 1975). The purpose of this study was to examine the interaction between the adrenergic and cholinergic limbs of the autonomic nervous system in hyperthyroid hearts.

METHODS

Adult male Cox-Wistar rats (250–300 g) were treated for three days with triiodothyronine at a dose of 500 μg/kg/day. On the fourth day the animals were heparinized, sacrificed by cervical dislocation and the herats removed and perfused by the Langendorff method. The atria were excised and the hearts were paced at a rate of 210 beats/min. At specified times, hearts were frozen with Wollenberger clamps precooled in liquid nitrogen. The resulting tissue was pulverized in liquid nitrogen and the powder stored under liquid nitrogen until assayed for cyclic AMP and percent phosphorylase a levels. Cyclic AMP was assayed according to the competitive protein binding method of Brown *et al.* (1971) as previously described (Watanabe and Besch, 1974). Phosphorylase was determined by a modification of the method of Gilboe, Larson, and Nuttall (1972) and measured as the ratio of incorporation of D-[α-^{14}C]glu-cose-1-phosphate into glycogen in the absence and presence of 3 mM 5'-AMP.

RESULTS AND DISCUSSION

Hearts from hyperthyroid rats responded with a greater increase in contractility than did hearts from euthyroid rats when low concentrations of isoproterenol were used. For example, with 10^{-9} M isoproterenol, contractility of hyperthy-roid hearts was increased 25% over control levels, whereas that of euthyroid hearts was increased only 12% above control levels. The response of hearts from euthyroid rats and hyperthyroid rats was similar at higher concentrations of isoproterenol. Hyperthyroid hearts also seemed to generate more cyclic AMP in response to isoproterenol than did euthyroid hearts at the lower concentrations of isoproterenol. Again, the differences were seen only at the lowest concentra-tion of isoproterenol, i.e., 10^{-9} M . These differences were, however, quite small. At 3×10^{-9} M and higher the amount of cyclic AMP generated was similar in the two groups of hearts.

Hyperthyroid hearts showed a marked increase in the percent phosphorylase a formed in response to isoproterenol at all concentrations of isoproterenol studied (Figure 1). Although the basal percent phosphorylase a was similar in

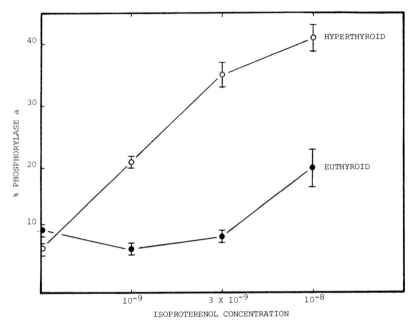

Figure 1. Effect of isoproterenol on percent phosphorylase *a* in euthyroid and hyperthyroid rat hearts. Each *point* is the mean ± S.E.M. of 6 to 8 hearts.

hyperthyroid and euthyroid hearts, hyperthyroid hearts responded to 10^{-9} M isoproterenol with a 20% conversion to phosphorylase *a* and a 34% conversion to phosphorylase *a* at 3×10^{-9} M. The euthyroid hearts did not respond to isoproterenol with conversion of phosphorylase *b* to *a* until a concentration of 10^{-8} M isoproterenol was used. Thus, hyperthyroid hearts appeared to be more responsive to isoproterenol whether the response was assessed by biochemical means (cyclic AMP levels and percent phosphorylase *a*) or by physiological means (rate of development of contractile force).

The next phase of our studies was designed to assess the anti-adrenergic effects of acetylcholine in hyperthyroid hearts. The cholinergic agent was given simultaneously with a fixed concentration of isoproterenol. Acetylcholine produced a complex biphasic effect on the contractile action of isoproterenol (Figure 2). When given alone, isoproterenol produced a rapid increase in contractility that peaked at about 30 sec and stabilized thereafter. At a low dose, 3×10^{-8} M, acetylcholine produced some attenuation of the positive inotropic effect of isoproterenol. The maximal attenuation by acetylcholine was seen at a dose of 10^{-7} M. With a higher concentration, 3×10^{-7} M, acetylcholine did not attenuate the inotropic effect of isoproterenol but rather actually seemed to potentiate the positive inotropic effects of the catecholamine. In the same

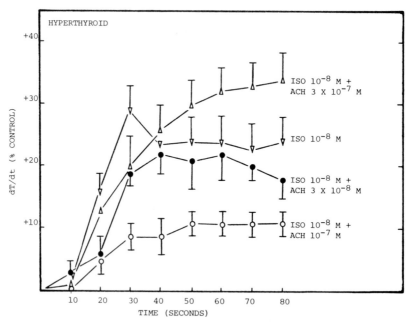

Figure 2. Effect of acetylcholine on the positive inotropic action of isoproterenol (10^{-8} M) in hyperthyroid hearts. Each *point* represents the mean ± S.E.M. of 6 to 8 hearts.

hearts the percent phosphorylase *a* activity was also attenuated by acetylcholine. This seemed to occur without any marked reduction in the amount of cyclic AMP generated (Figure 3). As with the physiological effect of acetylcholine, this latter metabolic effect was biphasic, with the maximal attenuation occurring at a concentration of 10^{-7} M.

The effects of acetylcholine were mimicked by dibutyryl cyclic GMP. As in the case with acetylcholine, dibutyryl cyclic GMP appeared to produce a complex biphasic effect, depending on the concentration of the nucleotide analog used (Figure 4). With 10^{-6} M dibutyryl cyclic GMP there was a substantial blunting of the positive inotropic effect of isoproterenol. With higher concentrations of dibutyryl cyclic GMP (10^{-5} M), the initial positive inotropic effect of isoproterenol was blunted, but the later contractile effect of isoproterenol (at 60 to 80 sec) was not attenuated. Dibutyryl cyclic GMP, just as acetylcholine, also attenuated the percent phosphorylase a formed in response to isoproterenol (Figure 5). This attenuation occurred even though the amount of cyclic AMP generated in response to isoproterenol was not reduced, but rather actually seemed to be slightly potentiated (Figure 5).

These results confirm the enhanced responsiveness of hyperthyroid hearts to adrenergic agents. Furthermore, we have shown that acetylcholine antagonizes

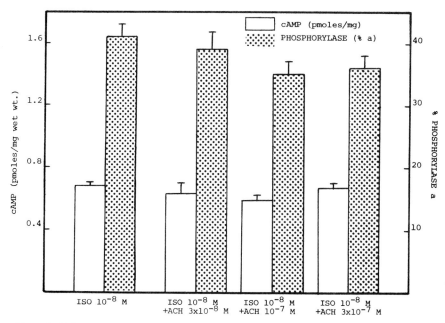

Figure 3. Effect of isoproterenol, when given alone and when given with varying concentrations of acetylcholine, on cyclic AMP levels and percent phosphorylase *a* in hyperthyroid hearts. Values are means ± S.E.M. of 6 to 8 hearts.

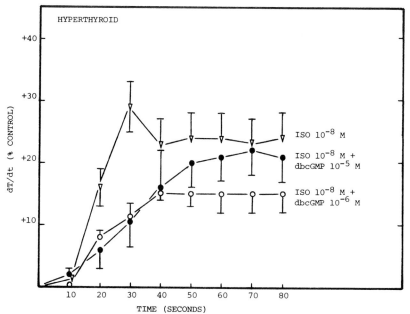

Figure 4. Effect of dibutyryl cyclic GMP on the positive inotropic action of isoproterenol. Each *point* represents the mean ± S.E.M. of 6 to 8 hearts.

427

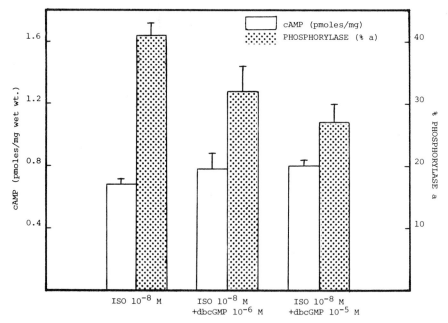

Figure 5. Effect of isoproterenol, alone and combined with dibutyryl cyclic GMP (dbcGMP), on cyclic AMP levels and percent phosphorylase *a* in hyperthyroid hearts. Values represent mean ± S.E.M. of 4 to 6 hearts.

both the inotropic and metabolic actions of isoproterenol and this antagonism can be mimicked by dibutyryl cyclic GMP, a lipid-soluble analog of cyclic GMP. It appears that acetylcholine may attenuate the effects of isoproterenol on hyperthyroid hearts by antagonizing the effects of cyclic AMP within the cell without substantially altering the steady-state levels of cyclic AMP. This effect of acetylcholine may be mediated by cyclic GMP.

Acknowledgments We gratefully acknowledge the expert technical assistance of Mr. Bruce Henry and the secretarial assistance of Ms. Carol Holliday.

REFERENCES

BROWN, B. L., ALBANO, J. D. M., EKINS, R. P., and SCHERZI, A. M. 1971. Simple and sensitive assay method for the measurement of adenosine 3':5'-cyclic monophosphate. Biochem. J. 121:561–562.

CAIROLI, V. J., and CROUT, J. R. 1967. Role of the autonomic nervous system in the resting teachycardia of experimental hyperthyroidism. J. Pharmacol. Exp. Ther. 158: 55–65.

GILBOE, D. P., LARSON, K. L., and NUTTALL, F. Q. 1972. Radioactive method for the assay of glycogen phosphorylase. Anal. Biochem. 17:20–27.

LEVEY, G. S. 1971. Catecholamine sensitivity, thyroid hormone and the heart. Amer. J. Med. 50:413–420.

WATANABE, A. M., and BESCH, H. R., JR. 1975. Interaction between cyclic adenosine monophosphate and cyclic guanosine monophosphate in guinea pig ventricular myocardium. Circ. Res. 37:309–317.

Mailing address:
August M. Watanabe, M.D.,
Department of Medicine,
Indiana University School of Medicine,
1100 West Michigan Street,
Indianapolis, Indiana 46202 (USA).

Recent Advances in Studies on
Cardiac Structure and Metabolism, Volume 11
Heart Function and Metabolism
Edited by T. Kobayashi, T. Sano, and N. S. Dhalla
Copyright 1978 University Park Press Baltimore

ALPHA-ADRENERGIC REDUCTION OF CYCLIC ADENOSINE MONOPHOSPHATE LEVELS IN RAT VENTRICULAR MYOCARDIAL CELLS

A. M. WATANABE, H. R. BESCH, JR., D. R. HATHAWAY, R. A. HARRIS, and B. B. FARMER

Departments of Medicine and Pharmacology, and the Krannert Institute of Cardiology, Indiana University School of Medicine, Indianapolis, Indiana, USA

SUMMARY

The purpose of this study was to examine the effects of alpha-adrenergic receptor (α) stimulation on cyclic adenosine monophosphate (cAMP) levels in myocardium. Experiments were performed on isolated myocardial cells obtained by perfusing hearts from adult rats with collagenase and hyaluronidase. Alpha-stimulation with phenylephrine (Pe) or with epinephrine (Epi) plus propranolol (10^{-6} M) reduced cAMP levels below that of control cells, the threshold of effect for Pe occurring at 10^{-8} M and for Epi occurring at 10^{-9} M. Cyclic AMP levels were significantly reduced from control values of 3.9 ± 0.2 ($\overline{X} \pm$ S.E.M.) pmol/mg dry wt to 3.2 ± 0.6 pmol/mg dry wt by Pe. Similarly, α-stimulation produced by Epi (10^{-6} M) plus propranolol (10^{-6} M) resulted in a reduction of cAMP levels to 2.8 ± 0.4 pmol/mg dry wt. Alpha-agonists also attenuated the stimulation of cAMP levels induced by isoproterenol (Iso), glucagon, and theophylline. For example, cAMP levels rose to 10.3 ± 0.2 pmol/mg dry wt following administration of 10^{-5} M Iso alone but rose to only 72% of this value when Pe (10^{-5} M) was added to 10^{-5} M Iso. Similarly, 10^{-6} M Pe reduced maximal glucagon-stimulated cAMP levels from 7.0 ± 0.5 to 5.0 ± 0.5 pmol/mg dry wt. Both Pe (10^{-7} M) and Epi (10^{-7} M) plus propranolol (10^{-6} M) reduced theophylline-stimulated cAMP levels from 10.4 ± 1.5 to about 7.5 pmol/mg dry wt. All of these α-reducing effects on cAMP levels were attenuated or abolished by phentolamine. Iso or Epi alone increased cAMP levels, the threshold for the former occurring at 10^{-9} M and for the latter occurring at 10^{-7} M. These results suggest that adrenergic agents can either increase or decrease cAMP levels of myocardium, increases being mediated by β-adrenergic receptors, whereas decreases appear to be mediated by α-adrenergic receptors. Furthermore, α-agonists can attenuate cAMP generation occurring in response to two different hormones or to theophylline.

INTRODUCTION

Although many studies have shown that activation of alpha (α)-adrenergic receptors results in changes in both the mechanical (Govier, 1967) and electrophysiological (Govier *et al.*, 1966) properties of the heart, no intracellular

This work was supported by grants HL 06308, HL 14159, HL 05363, and HL 05749 from the National Heart and Lung Institute; by the American Heart Association, Indiana Affiliate; and by the Herman C. Krannert Fund. Dr. Besch is supported by the Showalter Research Trust Fund.

messenger or biochemical basis for these changes has been identified. The purpose of this study was to examine the effects of α-adrenergic receptor stimulation on cyclic adenosine-3':5' monophosphate (cyclic AMP) levels in rat myocardium in an attempt to determine whether or not this messenger may be involved in mediating some of the effects of α-receptor stimulation.

METHODS

Experiments were performed on isolated myocardial cells obtained by perfusing hearts from adult rats with collagenase and hyaluronidase (Farmer *et al.*, 1976). Isolated cells were incubated in buffer with and without varying concentrations of α-adrenergic and β-adrenergic receptor agonists and antagonists. After appropriate periods of exposure to drugs, experiments were terminated by addition of trichloroacetic acid to the reaction mixture followed by disruption of the cells with a polytron homogenizer. Cyclic AMP was measured with a competitive protein binding assay (Gilman, 1970; Brown *et al.*, 1971) as previously described (Watanabe and Besch, 1974).

RESULTS AND DISCUSSION

Activation of β-adrenergic receptors resulted in stimulation of adenylate cyclase and an increase in the intracellular concentration of cyclic AMP, as expected (Figure 1). The classical order of β-adrenergic receptor potency for catecholamines was observed, isoproterenol being about one and one-half orders of magnitude more potent than epinephrine and norepinephrine in inducing increases in cyclic AMP levels. The threshold concentration for stimulation by isoproterenol was between 10^{-9} M and 10^{-8} M, and 10^{-5} M produced a 250% increase in cyclic AMP concentrations.

In contrast to these effects of β-adrenergic receptor agonists, α-adrenergic stimulation lowered myocyte cyclic AMP levels (Figure 2). Phenylephrine in concentrations of 10^{-8} to 10^{-6} M lowered cyclic AMP levels, and this reduction was abolished by the α-adrenergic antagonist phentolamine (10^{-6} M). Higher concentrations of phenylephrine increased cyclic AMP levels, reflecting the weak β-adrenergic agonist properties of this amine. This latter effect of phenylephrine was not altered by phentolamine.

The mixed adrenergic receptor agonist epinephrine, when given with the β-adrenergic receptor blocker propranolol, also lowered cyclic AMP levels in myocytes (Figure 3). The maximal effect of epinephrine plus propranolol occurred with 10^{-6} M epinephrine when the cyclic AMP level was reduced 28% below basal values.

When α-receptors were stimulated in previously basal or "resting" cardiac cells, the fall in cyclic AMP levels was very small. However, when cyclic AMP

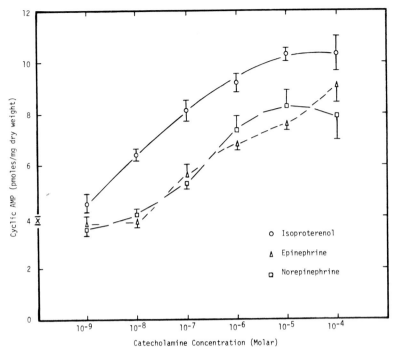

Figure 1. Effect of catecholamines on cyclic AMP concentrations in isolated heart cells. Values represent means ± standard error of the mean (S.E.M.) of 4 to 16 preparations of cells for each point. Basal value: 3.9 ± .01 pmol/mg dry weight; $n = 45$.

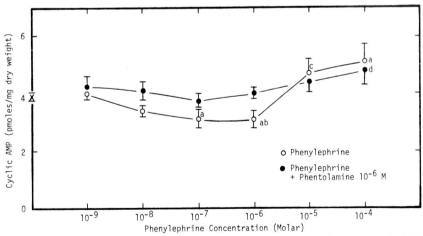

Figure 2. Effect of phenylephrine alone and with phentolamine (10^{-6} M) on cyclic AMP concentrations in isolated heart cells. Each point is the mean ± S.E.M. of 4 to 7 preparations. Basal value: 3.9 ± .01 pmol/mg dry weight; $n = 45$. *a* $p < 0.001$ compared to basal; *b*, $p < 0.001$ compared to phenylephrine plus phentolamine; *c*, $p < 0.05$ compared to basal; *d*, $p < 0.01$ compared to basal.

433

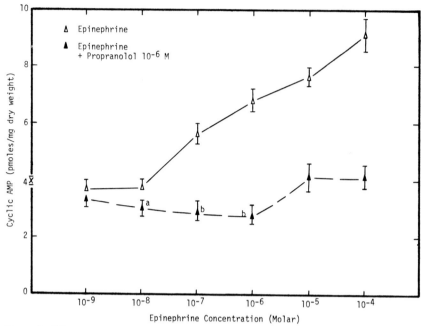

Figure 3. Effect of epinephrine alone and with propranolol (10^{-6} M) on cyclic AMP levels in isolated heart cells. Each *point* is the mean ± S.E.M. of 4 to 16 different preparations. Basal value: 3.9 ± .01 pmol/mg dry weight; $n = 45$. *a*, $p < 0.01$ compared to basal; *b*, $p < 0.001$ compared to basal.

levels were increased, the α-adrenergic reduction of cyclic AMP levels was magnified. The effect of α-adrenergic stimulation with phenylephrine during activation of adenylate cyclase by glucagon is presented in Table 1. Phenylephrine significantly attenuated the amount of cyclic AMP generated in response to glucagon. Phentolamine abolished this effect of phenylephrine. Similar results were observed when cyclic AMP levels were increased by the phosphodiesterase inhibitor theophylline (Table 2). Both phenylephrine and epinephrine plus propranolol appeared to attenuate the amount of cyclic AMP generated in the presence of theophylline. These effects of the α-adrenergic agonists tended to be attenuated by phentolamine.

During the past decade it has been demonstrated that activation of α-adrenergic receptors can lead to a reduction in cyclic AMP levels in several different tissues derived from a variety of species, including frog skin (Abe *et al.*, 1969), human blood platelets (Robison, Langley, and Burns, 1972), rat pancreatic islets (Turtle and Kipnis, 1967), toad bladder (Handler, Bensinger, and Orloff, 1968), and human lung (Austen, 1974). Moreover, in several of these

Table 1. Effect of glucagon alone and with phenylephrine on cyclic AMP levels in heart cells

Additions	Cyclic AMP (pmol/mg dry wt)
(−) Glucagon	3.9 ± 0.1
(+) Glucagon (10^{-7} M)	7.0 ± 0.5
(+) Phenylephrine (10^{-7} M)	5.3 ± 0.3*
(+) Phenylephrine (10^{-6} M)	5.0 ± 0.5*
(+) Phenylephrine (10^{-7} M)	
(+) Phentolamine (10^{-6} M)	7.1 ± 0.5†

*$p < 0.05$ compared to glucagon alone.
†$p < 0.05$ compared to phenylephrine alone.

studies the functional response associated with the fall in cyclic AMP level was opposite that associated with a rise in cyclic AMP concentration.

The present study indicates that in the rat myocardium, under the conditions of our study, α-adrenergic stimulation can result in a reduction of cyclic AMP levels. The physiological significance of our findings is not clear at the present. However, other investigators have demonstrated a cardiodepressant effect of α-adrenergic receptor stimulation (Imai, Shigei, and Hashimoto, 1961; James *et al.,* 1968). If an increase in cyclic AMP levels mediates the positive inotropic effect of catecholamines, a reduction in cyclic AMP levels could logically be expected to produce the opposite effect. It thus appears possible that activation of α-adrenergic receptors, under certain conditions, produces cardiodepressant effects by reducing tissue cyclic AMP levels.

Table 2. Effect of theophylline alone and with the α-adrenergic agonists phenylephrine and epinephrine plus propranolol on cyclic AMP levels in isolated myocytes

Additions	Cyclic AMP (pmol/mg dry wt)
(−) Theophylline	3.9 ± 0.1
(+) Theophylline (10^{-3} M)	10.4 ± 1.5
(+) Phenylephrine (10^{-7} M)	7.7 ± 0.3*
(+) Phenylephrine (10^{-7} M)	
(+) Phentolamine (10^{-6} M)	9.4 ± 0.4
(+) Epi (10^{-7} M) + Prop (10^{-6} M)	7.6 ± 0.6
(+) Epi (10^{-7} M) + Prop (10^{-6} M)	
(+) Phentolamine (10^{-6} M)	8.6 ± 0.4

*$p < 0.05$ compared to theophylline alone.

Acknowledgments We gratefully acknowledge the technical assistance of Mr. Bruce Henry and Miss Carolyn Hicks and the secretarial assistance of Ms. Carol Holliday.

REFERENCES

ABE, K., ROBISON, G. A., LIDDLE, G. W., BUTCHER, R. W., NICHOLSON, W. E., and BAIRD, C. E. 1969. Role of cyclic AMP in mediating the effects of MSH, norepinephrine, and melatonin on frog skin color. Endocrinology 85:674–682.

AUSTEN, K. F. 1974. Reaction mechanisms in the release of mediators of immediate hypersensitivity from human lung tissue. Fed. Proc. 33:2256–2262.

BROWN, B. L., ALBANO, J. D. M., EKINS, R. P., and SGHERZI, A. M. 1971. Simple and sensitive assay method for the measurement of adenosine 3':5' cyclic monophosphate. Biochem. J. 121:561–562.

FARMER, B. B., HARRIS, R. A., JOLLY, W. W., HATHAWAY, D. R., KATZBERG, A., WATANABE, A. M., BESCH, H. R., JR., and WHITLOW, A. L. 1977. Isolation and characterization of adult rat heart cells. Arch. Biochem. Biophys. 179:545–558.

GILMAN, A. G. 1970. Protein binding assay for adenosine 3',5'-cyclic monophosphate. Proc. Natl. Acad. Sci. USA 67:305–312.

GOVIER, W. C. 1967. A positive inotropic effect of phenylephrine mediated through alpha adrenergic receptors. Life Sciences 6:1361–1365.

GOVIER, W. C., MOSAL, N. C., WHITTINGTON, P., and BROOM, A. H. 1966. Myocardial alpha and beta adrenergic receptors as demonstrated by atrial functional refractory-period changes. J. Pharmacol. Exp. Ther. 154:255–263.

HANDLER, J. S., BENSINGER, R., and ORLOFF, J. 1968. Effect of adrenergic agents on toad bladder response to ADH, 3',-5' AMP, and theophiline. Amer. J. Physiol. 215:1024–1031.

IMAI, S., SHIGEI, T., and HASHIMOTO, K. 1961. Antiaccelerator action of methoxamine. Nature 189:493–494.

JAMES, T. N., BEAR, E. S., LANG, R. F., and GREEN, E. W., 1968. Evidence for adrenergic alpha receptor depressant activity in the heart. Amer. J. Physiol. 215:1366–1375.

ROBISON, A. G., LANGLEY, P. E., and BURNS, T. W. 1972. Adrenergic receptors in human adipocytes–Divergent effects on adenosine 3', 5'-monophosphate and lipolysis. Biochem. Pharmacol. 21:589–592.

TURTLE, J. R., and KIPNIS, D. M. 1967. An adrenergic receptor mechanism for the control of cyclic 3',5'-adenosine monophosphate synthesis in tissues. Biochem. Biophys. Res. Comm. 28:797.

WATANABE, A. M., and BESCH, H. R., JR. 1974. Cyclic adenosine monophosphate modulation of slow calcium influx channels in guinea pig hearts. Circ. Res. 35:316–324.

Mailing address:
August M. Watanabe, M.D.,
Department of Medicine,
Indiana University School of Medicine,
Indianapolis, Indiana 46202 (USA).

Recent Advances in Studies on
Cardiac Structure and Metabolism, Volume 11
Heart Function and Metabolism
Edited by T. Kobayashi, T. Sano, and N. S. Dhalla
Copyright 1978 University Park Press Baltimore

EFFECT OF DILTIAZEM ON CALCIUM- AND NORADRENALINE-INDUCED CONTRACTIONS IN ISOLATED RABBIT AORTA

T. NAGAO, T. IKEO, M. SATO,
H. NAKAJIMA, and A. KIYOMOTO

Pharmacological Research Laboratory,
Tanabe Seiyaku Co. Ltd., Saitama, Japan

SUMMARY

The effect of diltiazem on calcium- and noradrenaline-induced contractions was investigated in the K-depolarized aortic strip of the rabbit. Diltiazem inhibited the contraction induced by calcium ions dose-dependently. A lower concentration of diltiazem produced no significant influence on the contraction induced by noradrenaline, while a higher concentration suppressed it. It is assumed that in the rabbit aorta diltiazem effectively inhibits the contraction mediated by the influx of calcium ions but it is less effective with the contraction induced by the release of sequestered calcium.

INTRODUCTION AND METHOD

Diltiazem, a new 1,5-benzothiazepine derivative, is a potent coronary vasodilator with a calcium-antagonistic property (Sato *et al.*, 1971; Nakajima *et al.*, 1975). This chapter investigates the calcium-antagonistic mechanism of the compound in the vascular smooth muscle by examining its effect on the contractions induced by $CaCl_2$ and noradrenaline (NA). Isolated strips of the rabbit aorta were used and the experiments were carried out in K-depolarizing solution (KCl, 160 mM; glucose, 5.5 mM; tris-HCl buffer, 12.5 mM; pH, 7.4).

RESULTS

As shown in Figure 1, diltiazem shifted the dose-response curve for Ca^{2+} in a parallel fashion to the right, suggesting that the compound competitively antagonizes Ca^{2+} under K-depolarized condition.

NA could evoke the contraction of the preparation even in Ca^{2+}-free K-depolarizing solution (Devine, Somlyo, and Somlyo, 1972). This contraction was

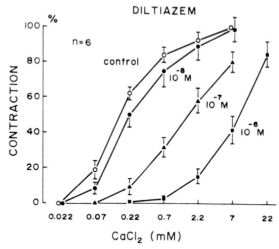

Figure 1. Antagonistic action of diltiazem on Ca^{2+}-induced contraction in K-depolarized rabbit aortic strip. The *points* and *vertical bars* indicate the mean value and S.E.M.

blocked by phentolamine and thus is assumed to be mediated by α-adreno-ceptor.

Lanthanium ion is assumed to inhibit the influx of Ca^{2+} (van Breemen, 1969). In the presence of La^{3+} (0.5 mM), the development of the contraction caused by 2.2 mM Ca^{2+} was completely abolished, while the initial phasic response evoked by NA (1 μM) was not inhibited. These results suggest that the initial phasic response induced by NA is ascribed to the release of sequestered calcium, while the contraction induced by Ca^{2+} is due to the influx of Ca^{2+}.

Procaine at the concentration of 0.1 mM caused no effect on Ca^{2+}-induced contraction, whereas it depressed NA-induced contraction by approximately 30% of the control.

As shown in Figure 2, diltiazem inhibited Ca^{2+}-induced contraction more strongly than NA-induced contraction. The inhibitory effect of diltiazem $(10^{-8}-10^{-4} M)$ on Ca^{2+}-induced contraction was found to be dose-dependent, while NA-induced contraction was not affected significantly by a lower concentration of the compound $(10^{-7}-10^{-6} M)$. Diltiazem at 2 higher concentration $(10^{-5}-10^{-4} M)$ suppressed NA-induced contraction significantly.

Figure 3 shows the effects of prolonged exposure of preparation to diltiazem and phentolamine on the contraction induced by Ca^{2+} or NA. When the preparation was treated with diltiazem, Ca^{2+}-induced contraction was rapidly reduced and maximum effect could be obtained after treatment for a short period. On the other hand, the inhibitory effect of diltiazem on NA-induced contraction became remarkable as the exposure period was prolonged. In con-

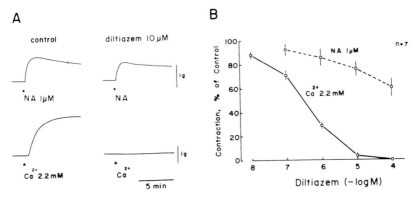

Figure 2. Effects of diltiazem on the noradrenaline (NA)- and Ca^{2+}-induced contractions in K-depolarized aortic strip. *A,* an example of experimental records. *B,* dose-response curve for the effect of diltiazem. The *points* and *vertical bars* indicate the mean value and S.E.M.

trast to the effect of diltiazem, phentolamine considerably inhibited NA-induced contraction immediately after the addition of the compound.

From these results, it is inferred that, in K-depolarized aortic strip of rabbits, diltiazem readily inhibits the contraction induced by influx of Ca^{2+}, while the compound is less effective with the contraction caused by release of sequestered Ca^{2+}.

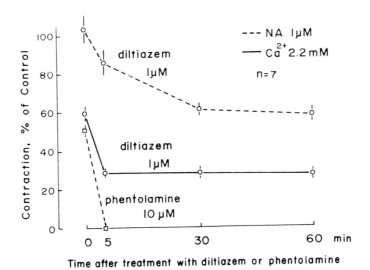

Figure 3. Effects of prolonged exposure to diltiazem and phentolamine on the noradrenaline (NA)- or Ca^{2+}-induced contractions in K-depolarized rabbit aortic strip. The *points* and *vertical bars* indicate the mean value and S.E.M.

REFERENCES

DEVINE, C. E., SOMLYO, A. V., and SOMLYO, A. P. 1972. Sarcoplasmic reticulum and excitation-contraction coupling in mammalian smooth muscles. J. Cell. Biol. 52: 690–718.

NAKAJIMA, H., HOSHIYAMA, M., YAMASHITA, K., and KIYOMOTO, A. 1975. Effect of diltiazem on electrical and mechanical activity of isolated cardiac ventricular muscle of guinea pig. Jpn. J. Pharmacol. 25:383–392.

SATO, M., NAGAO, T., YAMAGUCHI, I., NAKAJIMA, H., and KIYOMOTO, A. 1971. Pharmacological studies on a new 1,5-benzothiazepine derivative (CRD-401). I. Cardiovascular actions. Arzneim. Forsch. 21:1338–1343.

VAN BREEMEN, C. 1969. Blockade of membrane calcium fluxes by lanthanum in relation to vascular smooth muscle contractility. Arch. Int. Physiol. Biochim. 77:710–716.

Mailing address:
T. Nagao,
Pharmacological Research Laboratory,
Tanabe Seiyaku Co., Ltd.,
2-2-50 Todashi, Saitama (Japan).

Recent Advances in Studies on
Cardiac Structure and Metabolism, Volume 11
Heart Function and Metabolism
Edited by T. Kobayashi, T. Sano, and N. S. Dhalla
Copyright 1978   University Park Press   Baltimore

EFFECTS OF INSULIN ON MAMMALIAN CARDIAC MUSCLE

I. IMANAGA

Second Department of Physiology, Kanazawa Medical University,
Uchinada, Ishikawaken 920-02, Japan

SUMMARY

Insulin increases the contractile force of myocardium with hyperpolarization and a faster rate of fall of the action-potential plateau. This phenomenon is augmented in the reduced-K^+ or ouabain solution. It is suggested that the insulin-induced positive inotropism can be explained by facilitation of inward movement of Ca^{2+}, which possibly is associated with an increase in outward movement of K^+.

INTRODUCTION

A recent review by Taylor and Majid (1971) implies that insulin is playing an important role in maintenance and regulation of the myocardial function.

This author reported previously (Imanaga, 1973) that extracellularly applied insulin (glucagon-free) had a positive inotropic action on the isolated ventricular papillary muscle.

Since development of contraction is ultimately dependent on the concentration of Ca^{2+} supplied to myofilaments, insulin may modify a mobilization of Ca^{2+} across the cell membrane. It is interesting to observe how insulin acts on Ca^{2+} transport.

MATERIALS AND METHODS

Papillary muscle isolated from canine right ventricle was used in this experiment. The preparation was 0.9–1.0 mm thick and 5–6 mm long. The muscle was mounted in the three-compartment chamber (Wood, Heppner, and Weidmann, 1969), perfused with well-oxygenated Tyrode and test solutions at constant temperature ($37°$ C) in the compartment for electrical and mechanical measurements and driven rhythmically (0.5 Hz) with electrical stimulation. Transmembrane potentials were measured by conventional glass-microelectrode technique and mechanical contractions (isometric twitch contraction) were picked up by RCA-5734. They were displayed on a dual-beam oscilloscope simultaneously and were photographed. Measurements of input resistance and membrane resistance were based on the theory of Weidmann (1951), Kamiyama and Matsuda (1966), and Fozzard and Sleator (1967).

Glucagon-free bovine crystalline insulin (26.7 U/mg, Lot No. 0665GF, Shimizu Seiyaku Co., Ltd., Japan) was applied, final concentration to be 0.3 to 0.5 IU/ml.

RESULTS

Effects on Electrical Activities

The resting membrane potential (RP) begins to increase progressively just after an application of insulin and becomes almost steady in 10 to 15 min. The hyperpolarization is remarkable in lower $[K^+]_o$ and not significant in higher $[K^+]_o$ (Table 1).

The input resistance is reduced by insulin (Figure 1A). Generally, the membrane resistance increases as the membrane is depolarized and it is maximal at the plateau phase of action potential (Weidmann, 1951; Fozzard and Sleator, 1967). Insulin reduces the increase in the membrane resistance, above all at the plateau phase (Figure 1B).

Maximum rate of rise and overshoot of action potential are not affected by insulin. Action potential duration at the 30% level of repolarization [APD(30%)] is shortened by about 20%, and APD at the 70% level [APD(70%)], is prolonged by about 30% in 20 min (Figures 2 and 3).

Effects on Mechanical Activities

An increase in contractile force appears 1 min after insulin, develops steeply in a few minutes, reaches to almost maximum (about 200% of control) in 15 to 20 min, and is kept steady during the presence of the hormone (Figure 3). Time to peak contraction is not changed and relaxation is slightly prolonged (Figures 2 and 3). The positive inotropic action of insulin lasts about an hour after removal of the hormone (not shown). This increase in contractile force is brought about together with changes of RP and APDs (Figures 2 and 3).

Table 1. Effect of insulin on resting membrane potential

$[K^+]_o$ mM	Control ($-$mV)	Insulin ($-$mV)	Difference
0	107.8 ± 2.6	114.0 ± 4.8	8.3 ± 2.3*
2.7	93.9 ± 1.7	98.2 ± 4.2	5.8 ± 1.9*
13.5	71.0 ± 2.0	68.8 ± 3.2	-3.3 ± 2.5**
27.0	51.7 ± 3.9	49.5 ± 2.6	-3.0 ± 2.4**

*$p < 0.01$, significant.
**$p > 0.01$, not significant.

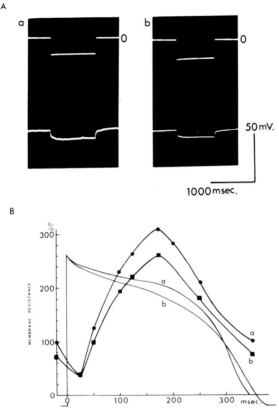

Figure 1. Effects of insulin on membrane resistance. *A:* For measurement of input membrane resistance, electrotonic potential produced by anodal current of 1000 msec at resting membrane. *a,* control; *b,* 5 min after insulin (0.3 IU/ml). The *upper trace* shows 0 mV and strength of current; the *lower,* resting potential and deflection of voltage. *B:* Resistance of active membrane calculated from potential deflection produced by weak anodal current (30 msec, 10 Hz). Traces of action potentials are superimposed. *a* and *b* are the same as those in *A.*

Effects on Action of Reduced-K⁺ and Ouabain Solution

The reduced-K⁺ solution raises the force of contraction, accompanied by short-ening of APD(30%), prolongation of APD(70%), and hyperpolarization of the membrane (Figure 4*A*). These observations are consistent with those obtained by Prasad and Callaghan (1969) and Graham, Bennett, and Ware (1969). Insulin accelerates the action of the reduced-K⁺ solution on electrical and mechanical properties. That is, RP is more negative, APD(30%) more shortened, APD(70%) more prolonged, and force of contraction augmented (Figure 4*A*).

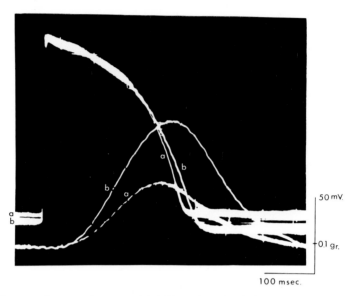

Figure 2. Transmembrane action potential (AP) and mechanical contraction are photographed simultaneously. Two APs and contractions are superimposed. *a* and *b* are the same as those in Figure 1.

Ouabain of 1×10^{-7} g/ml depolarizes the membrane by about 10 mV (from 86.5 ± 2.3 to $77.6 \pm 5.4(-mV)^*$), shortens APD(30%) ($86.3 \pm 2.5\%^*$) and APD(70%) ($81.2 \pm 3\%^*$) and increases contractile force ($286 \pm 55\%^*$). Insulin makes RP more negative (to $85.1 + 3.1(-mV^*)$), APD(30%) shorter (to $72.9 + 4.0\%^*$), APD(70%) longer (to $95.9 \pm 3.5\%^*$), and peak contraction greater ($403 \pm 55\%^*$) (100% means control value, mean $\pm$ S.E.;* means significant ($p < 0.01$)) (Figure 4*B*).

Effects on Mechanical Properties in Variation of $[Ca^{2+}]_o$ and Stimulating Frequency

The S-curve relationship between $[Ca^{2+}]_o$ and peak contraction is shifted upward. The augmentation is smaller in higher values of $[Ca^{2+}]_o$ (6–8 mM) and remarkable in 3–4 mM (Figure 5).

When muscle is stimulated in higher frequency, peak contraction becomes greater (frequency potentiation) (Koch-Weser and Blinks, 1963; Edman and Johannsson, 1976). Insulin potentiates this phenomenon more at each frequency (from 0.1 to 1.0 Hz) (Figure 6).

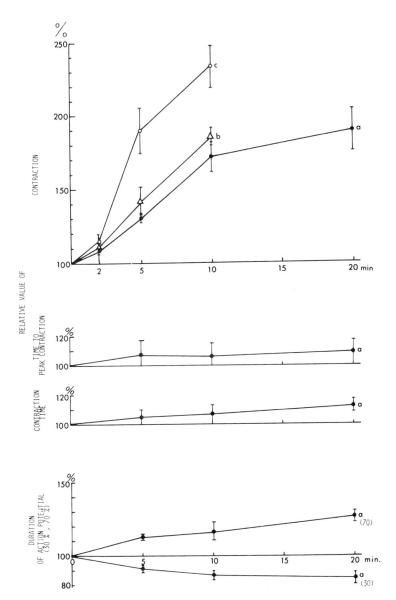

Figure 3. Time course of effects of insulin (0.5 IU/ml) on mechanical contraction and AP. *a,* in control solution ($[K^+]_o$ = 2.7 mM); *b,* in reduced K^+ solution ($[K^+]_o$ = 0.5 mM); *c,* in K^+-free solution. 100% means value before insulin. *Vertical bars* mean S.E.

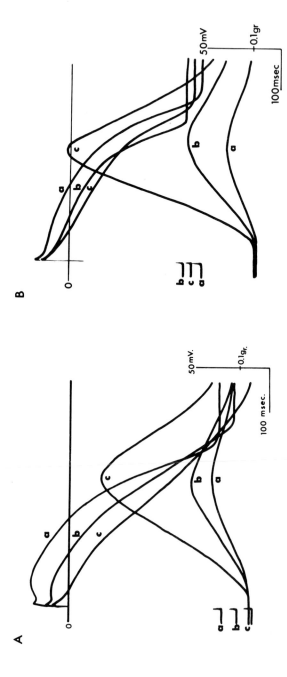

Figure 4. Effects of insulin on mechanical contraction and AP in K⁺-free and ouabain solution. Three contractions and APs traced from films. *A:* *a,* in control solution; *b,* 10 min after in K⁺-free solution; *c,* 10 min after insulin (0.5 IU/ml) in the K⁺-free solution. *B:* *a,* in control solution; *b,* 10 min after ouabain (1 × 10⁻⁷ g/ml) solution; *c,* 10 min after insulin (0.5 IU/ml) in the ouabain solution.

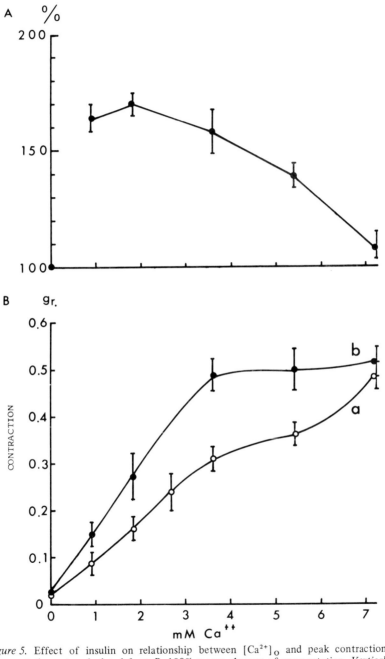

Figure 5. Effect of insulin on relationship between $[Ca^{2+}]_O$ and peak contraction. *A:* Augmentation rate calculated from *B.* 100% means absence of augmentation. *Vertical bars* mean S.E. *B: a,* control; *b,* 10 min after insulin (0.3 IU/ml).

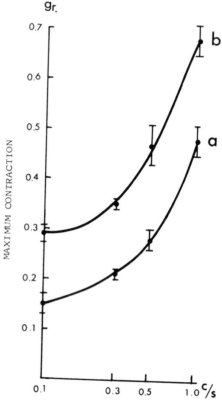

Figure 6. Effect of insulin on frequency potentiation. *a,* control; *b,* 10 min after insulin (0.3 IU/ml). *Vertical bars* mean S.E.

DISCUSSION

Changes of RP and input resistance suggest that in myocardial cell as well as in skeletal muscle (Zierler, 1959) and liver (Williams *et al.,* 1971) insulin increases the permeability of the membrane to K^+ and uptake of K^+ in the cell. The shortening of APD(30%) by insulin, due to the faster rate of fall of the plateau phase, may be caused by an acceleration of outward movement of K^+ or inward movement of Ca^{2+}, since the plateau phase is related to K^+ outflow (Hoffman and Cranefield, 1960; Noble and Tsien, 1969) and Ca^{2+} inflow (Reuter, 1967; Beeler and Reuter, 1970; New and Trautwein, 1972). The movement of K^+ is over that of Ca^{2+}. The increase in the membrane conductance at the plateau phase supports the above possibility.

It is interesting that insulin augments the action of the reduced-K^+ or ouabain solution on both electrical and mechanical properties.

Prasad and Callaghan (1969) and Prasad (1972) reported that in K^+-free solution, the shortening of the plateau phase of action potential and the rise in contractile force resulted from inhibition of (Na^+, K^+)-ATPase, and they concluded that this positive inotropism was due to increased Ca^{2+} influx associated with K efflux (Langer and Brady, 1966).

On the other hand, ouabain-induced positive inotropism is considered to be increased Ca^{2+} inflow in relation to the Na^+-Ca^{2+} exchange mechanism, coming after inhibition of the Na^+ pump (Glitsch, Reuter, and Scholz, 1970).

However, it is doubtful that insulin inhibits (Na^+, K^+)-ATPase, since the enzyme is rather stimulated when the enzyme is inhibited (Gavryck, Moore, and Thompson, 1975). If more Ca^{2+} is accumulated in the intracellular Ca^{2+} store by Na^+-Ca^{2+} exchange in K^+-free or ouabain solution, Ca^{2+} inflow raised by insulin may release more Ca^{2+} from the store to myoplasm.

Ca^{2+} influx rises rapidly as $[Ca^{2+}]_o$ is varied from 0 to 4 mM, but it rises more slowly at higher $[Ca^{2+}]_o$ (Langer, 1971). Moreover, a rise in contracting frequency accumulates more Ca^{2+} in the intracellular Ca^{2+} store (Langer, 1965; Sands and Winegrad, 1970; Edman and Johannsson, 1976). These two findings come from analysis of the data.

Results in this experiment suggest that insulin facilitates Ca^{2+} influx. Therefore, more Ca^{2+} may act directly on myofilaments or be released from the store to myoplasm by the facilitated Ca^{2+} inflow. If the Na-pump system is in the plateau phase, this increase in Ca^{2+} inflow may be associated with an increase in K^+ outflow.

REFERENCES

BEELER, G. W., JR. and REUTER, H. 1970. Membrane calcium current in ventricular myocardial fibres. J. Physiol. 207:191–209.

EDMAN, K. A. P., and JOHANNSSON, M. 1976. The contractile state of rabbit papillary muscle in relation to stimulation frequency. J. Physiol. 254:565–581.

FOZZARD, H. A., and SLEATOR, W. 1967. Membrane ionic conductances during rest and activity in guinea pig atrial muscle. Amer. J. Physiol. 212:945–952.

GAVRYCK, W. A., MOORE, R. D., and THOMPSON, R. C. 1975. Effect of insulin upon membrane-bound $(Na^+ + K^+)$-ATPase extracted from frog skeletal muscle. J. Physiol. 252:43–58.

GLITSCH, H. G., REUTER, H., and SCHOLZ, H. 1970. The internal sodium concentration on Ca fluxes in isolated guinea pig auricle. J. Physiol. 209:25–43.

GRAHAM, G. D., BENNETT, R. B., and WARE, F. 1969. Potassium effects on transmembrane potentials in frog ventricle. Amer. J. Physiol. 216:1360–1366.

HOFFMAN, B. F. and CRANEFIELD, P. F. 1960. Electrophysiology of the Heart, pp. 285–290. McGraw-Hill Book Company, New York.

IMANAGA, I. 1973. Effects of insulin on mammalian cardiac muscle. Jpn. Circ. J. 37:909.

KAMIYAMA, A., and MATSUDA, K. 1966. Electrophysiological properties of the canine ventricular fiber. Jpn. J. Physiol. 16:407–420.

KOCH-WESER, J., and BLINKS, J. R. 1963. The influence of the interval between beats on myocardial contractility. Pharmacol. Rev. 15: 601–652.

LANGER, G. A. 1965. Calcium exchange in dog ventricular muscle: Relation to frequency of contraction and maintenance of contractility. Circ. Res. 17:78–89.

LANGER, G. A. 1971. The intrinsic control of myocardial contraction-ionic factors. New Engl. J. Med. 285:1065–1071.

LANGER, G. A., and BRADY, A. J. 1966. Potassium in dog ventricular muscle: Kinetic studies of distribution and effects of varying frequency of contraction and potassium concentration of perfusate. Circ. Res. 18:164–177.

NEW, W., and TRAUTWEIN, W. 1972. The ionic nature of slow inward current and its relation to contraction. Pflüegers Arch. 334:24–38.

NOBLE, D., and TSIEN, R. W. 1969. Outward membrane currents activated in the plateau range of potentials in cardiac Purkinje fibres. J. Physiol. 200:205–231.

PRASAD, K. 1972. Membrane Na^+-K^+-ATPase and electromechanics of human heart. *In* N. S. Dhalla (ed.), Myocardial Biology: Recent Advances in Studies on Cardiac Structure and Metabolism, Vol. 4, pp. 91–105. University Park Press, Baltimore.

PRASAD, K., and CALLAGHAN, J. C. 1969. Effect of replacement of potassium by rubidium on the transmembrane action potential and contractility of human papillary muscle. Circ. Res. 24:157–166.

REUTER, H. 1967. The dependence of slow inward current in Purkinje fibres on the extracellular calcium concentration. J. Physiol. 192:479–492.

SANDS, S. D., and WINEGRAD, S. 1970. Treppe and total calcium content of the frog ventricle. Amer. J. Physiol. 218:908–910.

TAYLOR, S. H., and MAJID, P. A. 1971. Insulin and the heart. J. Mol. Cell. Cardiol. 2:293–317.

WEIDMANN, S. 1951. Effect of current flow on the membrane potential of cardiac muscle. J. Physiol. 115:227–236.

WILLIAMS, T. F., EXTON, J. H., FRIEDMANN, N., and PARK, C. R., 1971. Effects of insulin and adenosine 3'-5'-monophosphate on K^+ flux and glucose output in perfused rat liver. Amer. J. Physiol. 221:1645–1651.

WOOD, E. H., HEPPNER, R. L., and WEIDMANN, S. 1969. Inotropic effects of electrical currents. Circ. Res. 24:409–445.

ZIERLER, K. L. 1959. Effect of insulin on membrane potential and potassium content of rat muscle. Amer. J. Physiol. 197:515–523.

Mailing address:
Dr. I. Imanaga,
Second Department of Physiology,
Kanazawa Medical University,
Uchinada, Ishikawaken 920-02 (Japan).

Recent Advances in Studies on
Cardiac Structure and Metabolism, Volume 11
Heart Function and Metabolism
Edited by T. Kobayashi, T. Sano, and N. S. Dhalla
Copyright 1978   University Park Press   Baltimore

INOTROPIC AND CHRONOTROPIC EFFECTS
OF ANTIARRHYTHMIC AGENTS ON ISOLATED
BLOOD-PERFUSED CANINE VENTRICULAR TISSUE

K. HASHIMOTO, T. TSUKADA, and H. MATSUDA

Department of Pharmacology, Niigata University,
School of Medicine, Niigata, Japan

SUMMARY

In the isolated blood-perfused canine ventricular tissue, antiarrhythmic agents could be classified as having: 1) positive chronotropic and inotropic effects (procainamide), 2) negative chronotropic but positive inotropic effects (quinidine), and 3) negative chronotropic and inotropic effects (lidocaine, ajmaline, diphenylhydantoin, and propranolol).

INTRODUCTION

Blood-perfused isolated canine ventricular preparation has been demonstrated to be suitable for physiological and pharmacological studies of cardiac contraction and automaticity (Endoh and Hashimoto, 1970; Hashimoto *et al.*, 1975). The present experiment was performed to investigate the effects of antiarrhythmic agents using this preparation.

METHODS

The ventricular septum with the right anterior papillary muscle was isolated from 12 dogs (6–10 kg), and perfused at a constant pressure of 100 mm Hg via the anterior septal artery with arterial blood from a donor dog, as previously described (Endoh and Hashimoto, 1970; Hashimoto *et al.*, 1975). The preparation was stimulated with an electronic stimulator, when necessary, at 2 Hz, 3-msec duration, and twice threshold voltage.

Drugs were injected intra-arterially through a rubber tube close to the preparation. Drugs used were quinidine HCl, procainamide HCl, lidocaine HCl, diphenylhydantoin Na, ajmaline HCl, and *dl*-propranolol HCl.

Statistical analysis was performed using paired *t*-test.

This study was supported by a grant from the Ministry of Education of Japan (077036-1975).

RESULTS

Spontaneously Beating Preparation

Ventricular preparation fibrillated soon after the blood perfusion was started; but usually within an hour fibrillation suddenly ceased, and regular spontaneous contraction started. The average values of the automaticity and the contractile force were 30 ± 4 beats/min and 1.5 ± 0.3 g, respectively (mean ± S.E., n = 11). Intra-arterial injection of antiarrhythmic agents produced effects within 10 sec that lasted 3 to 5 min. Typical records are illustrated in Figure 1. Quinidine depressed ventricular automaticity; however, it had no effect on contractile force. Procainamide differed from other drugs and increased automaticity and contractile force. Lidocaine, diphenylhydantoin, and ajmaline had negative chronotropic and inotropic effects, but the latter two had more potent and longer actions. Propranolol also had negative chronotropic and inotropic effects, but the curves in Figures 2 and 3 were not dose-dependent. This is due to the variation in the sensitivity of the preparations, and also to longer action (often over 30 min) and incomplete recovery to the control values. The summarized dose-response relationships are shown in Figure 2.

Electrically Driven Preparation

Cardiac contractility is very dependent on the rate of contraction; therefore, the inotropic effects of the agents were examined in the electrically driven condition at 2 Hz. The average developed tension was 2.9 ± 0.6 g (n = 9). The dose-response relationships of the inotropic effects are illustrated in Figure 3. Quinidine and procainamide had positive inotropic effects, but higher doses had weaker effects, resulting in depression of the dose-response curves. These positive inotropic effects were not modified by pretreatment with propranolol (10–30 μg). Other drugs had dose-related negative inotropic effects, even though the influence of negative chronotropic effects was eliminated.

DISCUSSION

Among antiarrhythmic agents studied, procainamide increased spontaneous ventricular automaticity, while other agents decreased it. In order to examine whether or not this positive effect of procainamide was therapeutic, 40 mg/kg procainamide was injected intravenously to the donor dog. This dose of procainamide, sufficient to suppress ventricular arrhythmia caused by two-stage coronary ligation (Matsubara *et al.,* 1976), also increased the rate and contractile force of the isolated preparation (Hashimoto, Tsukada, and Matsuda, unpublished data). These effects of procainamide differ from those reported by Rosen, Gelband, and Hoffman (1972), who used isolated canine Purkinje fiber superfused with arterial blood from the donor dog.

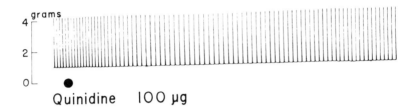

Quinidine   100 µg

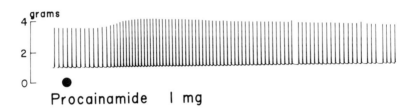

Procainamide   1 mg

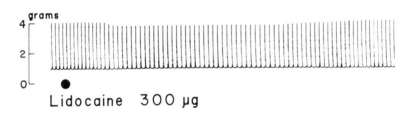

Lidocaine   300 µg

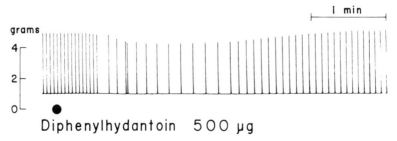

Diphenylhydantoin   500 µg

Figure 1. Effects of antiarrhythmic agents on the contractile force and rate of spontaneously beating ventricular preparation.

Spontaneous automaticity

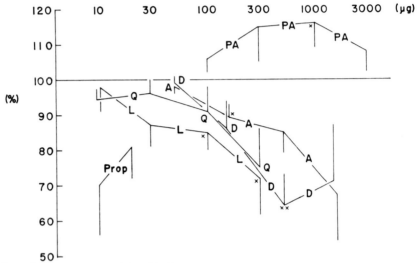

Figure 2. Dose-response relationship for spontaneous automaticity. *Abscissa:* doses in μg. *Ordinate:* average percent values as compared to the control values of 100%. PA, procainamide ($n = 5–9$); Q, quinidine ($n = 5–8$); D, diphenylhydantoin ($n = 3–8$); A, ajmaline ($n = 4–6$); L, lidocaine ($n = 5–8$); Prop, propranolol ($n = 4$); x, $p < 0.05$; xx, $p < 0.01$. *Vertical bars* represent S.E.

Contractile force (Electrically driven preparation, 2 Hz)

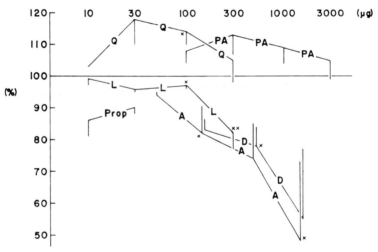

Figure 3. Dose-response relationship for contractile force of electrically driven (2 Hz) preparation. PA, procainamide ($n = 5–9$); Q, quinidine ($n = 5–8$); D, diphenylhydantoin ($n = 3–8$); A, ajmaline ($n = 4–6$); L, lidocaine ($n = 5–8$); Prop, propranolol ($n = 4$); x, $p < 0.05$; xx, $p < 0.01$. *Vertical bars* represent S. E.

Contractile force of the electrically drive preparation was increased by both quinidine and procainamide. The direct positive inotropic effect of quinidine has been reported by Himori and Taira (1976). Procainamide also showed similar effects. Nahas, Lachapelle, and Tremblay (1969) reported that in the rat heart procainamide produced a transient positive inotropic effect followed by a negative one, but in this experiment only the positive inotropic effect was observed. These two drugs may be used safely under myocardial depression produced by other antiarrhythmic agents.

In conclusion, antiarrhythmic agents can be classified according to their effects on ventricular tissue as having: 1) positive chronotropic and inotropic effects (procainamide), 2) positive inotropic but negative chronotropic effects (quinidine), and 3) negative chromotropic and inotropic effects (ajmaline, diphenylhydantoin, lidocaine, and propranolol).

REFERENCES

ENDOH, M., and HASHIMOTO, K. 1970. Frequency-force relationship in the blood-perfused canine papillary muscle preparation. Jpn. J. Physiol. 20:320–331.

HASHIMOTO, K., ENDOH, M., KIMURA, T., and HASHIMOTO, K. 1975. Effects of halothane on automaticity and contractile force of isolated blood-perfused canine ventricular tissue. Anesthesiology 42:15–25.

HIMORI, N., and TAIRA, N. 1976. Effects of quinidine on blood flow rate and developed tension in blood-perfused canine papillary muscle. Clin. Exp. Pharmacol. Physiol. 3:1–7.

MATSUBARA, I., HASHIMOTO, K., KATANO, Y., TSUKADA, T., NABATA, H., and IMAI, S. 1976. Antiarrhythmic effects of dl-1-(tert. butylamino)-3-[(2-propinyloxy) phenoxy]-2-propanol hydrochloride (Kö 1400-Cl), a new adrenergic β-blocking agent. Folia Pharmacol. Jpn. In press. (In Japanese.)

NAHAS, J., LACHAPELLE, J., and TREMBLAY, G. M. 1969. Comparative effect of procainamide and lidocaine on myocardial contractility. Can. J. Physiol. Pharmacol. 47:1038–1042.

ROSEN, M. R., GELBAND, H., and HOFFMAN, B. F. 1972. Canine electrocardiographic and cardiac electrophysiologic changes induced by procainamide. Circulation 46: 528–536.

Mailing address:
Dr. K. Hashimoto
Department of Pharmacology
Niigata University School of Medicine,
Niigata (Japan).

Recent Advances in Studies on
Cardiac Structure and Metabolism, Volume 11
Heart Function and Metabolism
Edited by T. Kobayashi, T. Sano, and N. S. Dhalla
Copyright 1978 University Park Press Baltimore

INFLUENCE OF QUINIDINE ON
ATP-LINKED CALCIUM BINDING
BY HEART MITOCHONDRIA AND MICROSOMES

J. A. C. HARROW and N. S. DHALLA

Pathophysiology Laboratory, Department of Physiology,
Faculty of Medicine, University of Manitoba, Winnipeg, Canada

SUMMARY

The action of quinidine on heart microsomal and mitochondrial calcium binding in the presence of MgATP was studied under different experimental conditions and compared with other antiarrhythmic agents such as procaine amide and lidocaine. Quinidine stimulated microsomal calcium binding but depressed mitochondrial calcium binding. Although procaine amide stimulated microsomal calcium binding, it did not affect mitochondrial calcium binding. On the other hand, lidocaine depressed calcium binding by mitochondria without affecting calcium binding by the microsomal fraction. The stimulation of microsomal calcium binding by quinidine was not apparent at high concentrations of Mg^{2+}, low concentrations of ATP, or low concentrations of Ca^{2+}. The depressant action of quinidine on mitochondrial calcium binding was not observed at low concentrations of Mg^{2+} or ATP but was more pronounced at low concentrations of Ca^{2+}. These results suggest that the action of quinidine on mitochondria may play a major role in eliciting cardiodepressant effect.

INTRODUCTION

The cardiodepressant action of high concentrations of quinidine has been explained on the basis of its inhibitory effect on microsomal calcium uptake (Fuchs, Gertz, and Briggs, 1968; Shinebourne, White, and Hamer, 1969). However, recent studies from our laboratory (Harrow and Dhalla, 1975, 1976) have indicated that quinidine inhibited mitochondrial calcium uptake also and the sensitivity of mitochondrial calcium uptake to quinidine was comparable to that for the microsomal calcium uptake. Furthermore, it was shown that microsomal calcium binding, when studied under optimal conditions (10 mM Mg^{2+} and 4 mM ATP) for calcium uptake was not affected by quinidine, whereas mitochondrial calcium binding was depressed (Harrow and Dhalla, 1976). It should be noted that the terms calcium binding and calcium uptake by microsomes and mitochondria are used to describe ATP-dependent calcium accumulation in the

---

This work was supported by a grant from the Medical Research Council of Canada.

absence and presence of calcium precipitating agents, oxalate and phosphate, respectively. Although the exact significance of these *in vitro* processes is not clear with respect to functional changes in the heart, some investigators believe that calcium binding is a better physiological measure of contractility than calcium uptake. In this chapter, therefore, we report the effects of quinidine on calcium binding by heart subcellular fractions under different experimental conditions. Other antiarrhythmic agents such as procaine amide and lidocaine, which like quinidine decrease myocardial contractile force in high doses (Szekeres and Papp, 1971; Harrow and Dhalla, 1975), were also used for the purpose of comparison with quinidine.

METHODS

Both mitochondrial and heavy microsomal fractions from the rabbit heart ventricles were isolated and purified according to procedures described elsewhere (Harrow and Dhalla, 1976). The protein concentrations of these fractions were measured by the method of Lowry *et al.* (1951). For calcium binding determination, both mitochondrial and microsomal fractions were preincubated for 3 min in 2 ml of a medium containing 100 mM KCl, 20 mM Tris-HCl, pH 6.8 to 7.0, 2 mM $Mg Cl_2$ at $25°C$ in the absence or presence of drugs. The mitochondrial and microsomal protein concentrations in the incubation medium were 0.3 to 0.7 mg/ml. The reaction was started by the addition of 2 mM ATP and 0.1 mM $^{45}Ca Cl_2$ and stopped by millipore filtration (millipore size 0.45 μm) after 4 min of incubation. The radioactivities in the protein-free filtrate and protein precipitate on the filter were analyzed in a Packard Tri-Carb scintillation spectrometer and the amount of calcium bound to the subcellular particles was calculated. The drugs used in this study were quinidine gluconate, procaine amide hydrochloride, and lidocaine hydrochloride. All the determinations were made in duplicate and all changes in the experimental conditions are described in the text. The results were analyzed statistically by Student t test.

RESULTS

Before studying the effects of drugs on ATP-dependent calcium binding by the rabbit heart mitochondrial and microsomal fractions, it was felt necessary to examine some of its characteristics. By using 10 mM $Mg Cl_2$ and 2–4 mM ATP in the incubation medium, both microsomes and mitochondria were found to bind 34 to 48 nmol Ca^{2+}/mg protein in 10 min in the presence of 0.1 mM $^{45}Ca Cl_2$ at $25°$ C. Under these conditions calcium binding with microsomal fraction reached maximum within 2 min, whereas 75 to 80% of the mitochondrial calcium binding occurred within 5 min. On the other hand, the values for calcium binding by microsomes and mitochondria varied from 66 to 75 nmol Ca^{2+}/mg protein/10 min when 2 mM Mg ATP was used in the incubation medium; about 80 to 95% of this calcium binding took place within 5 min by microsomes and mitochondria, respectively. On varying the concentrations of Mg^{2+} and ATP over a wide range, it was found that maximal calcium binding by subcellular fractions was obtained when 2 mM Mg ATP was used in the incubation medium. It should be mentioned that some of the apparent calcium binding reported here is due to calcium accumulation in the lumen of mitochondria or microsomal vesicles. Calcium binding by the mitochondrial fraction employed in this study was inhibited by 75 to 80% of the control values by 4 mM sodium azide or 3 μg/ml of oligomycin, whereas microsomal calcium binding was not affected by these agents. Furthermore, the endogenous calcium in the microsomal and mitochondrial fractions as measured by atomic absorption spectrophotometry (Sulakhe and Dhalla, 1971) was 8–11 and 13–17 nmol/ mg protein, respectively.

The actions of quinidine, procaine amide, and lidocaine (10^{-7} to 5×10^{-3}M) on calcium binding in the presence of 2 mM Mg ATP were studied at different intervals of incubation. The time courses of calcium binding by microsomal or mitochondrial fractions in the absence or presence of 1 mM guinidine, procaine amide, and lidocaine are shown in Table 1. None of these agents in concentrations from 10^{-7} to 10^{-4} M showed any effect on microsomal or mitochondrial calcium binding. Quinidine and procaine amide at concentrations of 10^{-3} M or higher produced a significant ($p < 0.05$) stimulatory action at the earlier time intervals of incubation, whereas lidocaine had no significant effect on microsomal calcium binding. On the other hand, quinidine and lidocaine, unlike

Table 1. Time course of calcium binding by rabbit heart heavy microsomes or mitochondria in the presence of 1 mM quinidine, procaine amide, and lidocaine†

| Incubation time | Calcium binding (nmol/mg protein) | | | |
	Control	Quinidine	Procaine amide	Lidocaine
A. Heavy microsomes:				
30 sec	37 ± 3	61 ± 3*	49 ± 2*	41 ± 2
1 min	47 ± 3	64 ± 1*	66 ± 4*	54 ± 3
2 min	53 ± 2	63 ± 3*	66 ± 3*	60 ± 4
5 min	60 ± 3	71 ± 2*	76 ± 2*	70 ± 4
10 min	72 ± 2	72 ± 4	74 ± 4	75 ± 3
B. Mitochondria:				
30 sec	39 ± 3	37 ± 4	42 ± 4	36 ± 3
1 min	45 ± 3	46 ± 3	56 ± 4	55 ± 2
2 min	64 ± 2	48 ± 2*	59 ± 3	53 ± 3*
5 min	69 ± 4	54 ± 3*	76 ± 4	53 ± 2*
10 min	73 ± 3	58 ± 4*	79 ± 4	54 ± 4*

†Results are the means ± standard errors of 6 experiments.
*Significantly different from the control ($p < 0.05$).

procaine amide, at concentrations of 10^{-3} M or higher produced a significant (p < 0.05) depressant effect on mitochondrial calcium binding at the later time intervals of incubation.

In order to gain further information concerning stimulation of microsomal calcium binding and depression of mitochondrial calcium binding by quinidine, the actions of 1 mM quinidine were studied at different concentrations of Ca^{2+}, ATP, or Mg^{2+} in the incubation medium. The results shown in Table 2 reveal that quinidine did not increase (p> 0.05) calcium binding by microsomal fraction when 5 to 50 μM calcium was added in the incubation medium. Although quinidine significantly (p < 0.05) decreased mitochondrial calcium binding at all concentrations of calcium used in this study, its depressant effect in terms of percent decrease from the control value was greater at low concentrations of calcium. Lowering the concentration of ATP in the incubation medium abolished the microsomal stimulation and mitochondrial depression produced by quinidine (Table 3). Although quinidine stimulated (p < 0.05) microsomal calcium binding in the presence of 0.2 to 2.0 mM Mg^{2+}, the magnitude of stimulation was greater at low concentrations in comparison to the high concentrations of Mg^{2+} (Figure 1). On the other hand, no depressant effect of quinidine on mitochondria was apparent at low concentrations (0.1 to 1.5 mM) of Mg^{2+}. When 4 to 10 mM Mg^{2+} was used in the incubation medium, quinidine (1 mM) decreased mitochondrial calcium binding by about 30% of the control value but did not increase microsomal calcium binding when estimated at 0.5, 1, 3, and 5 min after starting the reaction.

In order to demonstrate the specificity of drug action on the ATP-dependent calcium binding, the effects of quinidine, procaine amide, and lidocaine were examined on the Mg ATP-independent calcium binding by heart microsomal and mitochondrial preparations. The results in Figure 2 indicate that lidocaine in concentrations from 10^{-7} to 10^{-4} M, but not quinidine or procaine amide,

Table 2. Influence of Ca^{2+} on the effect of quinidine on calcium binding by rabbit heart heavy microsomes and mitochondria†

	Calcium binding (nmol/mg protein)			
	Heavy microsomes		Mitochondria	
Ca^{2+} (μM)	Control	Quinidine	Control	Quinidine
5	7.0 ± 0.6	7.1 ± 0.7	2.9 ± 0.3	0.8 ± 0.2*
10	11.2 ± 0.7	10.4 ± 0.5	5.2 ± 0.5	1.5 ± 0.4*
25	16.4 ± 1.8	19.3 ± 1.3	15.5 ± 1.5	6.2 ± 0.7*
50	32.3 ± 2.5	34.7 ± 2.7	38.9 ± 2.9	20.5 ± 2.4*
100	62.1 ± 2.1	75.1 ± 3.0*	70.2 ± 3.2	52.6 ± 2.6*

†Results are the means ± standard errors of 3 experiments. Incubation time was 5 min.
*Significantly different from the control (p < 0.05).

Table 3. Influence of ATP on the effect of 1 mM quinidine on calcium binding by rabbit heart heavy microsomes and mitochondria†

| ATP (mM) | Calcium binding (nmol/mg protein) | | | |
| | Heavy microsomes | | Mitochondria | |
	Control	Quinidine	Control	Quinidine
0.05	38 ± 3	30 ± 2	35 ± 2	39 ± 3
0.10	47 ± 2	53 ± 4	40 ± 2	48 ± 2
0.50	53 ± 3	57 ± 4	57 ± 3	53 ± 3
1.00	59 ± 3	65 ± 3	60 ± 3	45 ± 4*
2.00	61 ± 4	75 ± 2*	68 ± 4	50 ± 2*

†Results are the means ± standard errors of 5 experiments. The incubation time was 5 min.

*Significantly different from the control ($p < 0.05$).

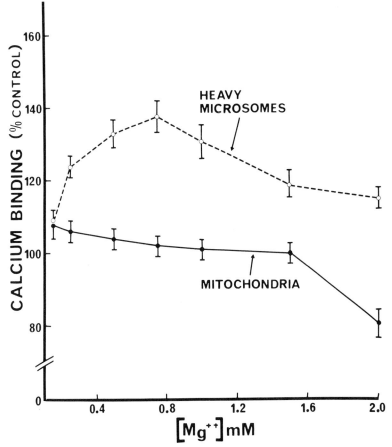

Figure 1. Influence of Mg^{2+} on the effect of 1 mM quinidine on ATP-dependent calcium binding by rabbit heart heavy microsomes and mitochondria. The time of incubation was 5 min. Results are the means ± standard error of 5 experiments.

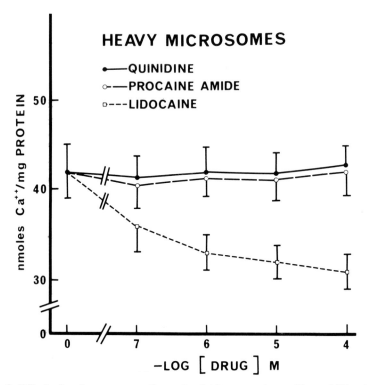

Figure 2. Effect of various concentrations of quinidine, procaine amide, and lidocaine on Mg ATP-independent calcium binding by rabbit heart microsomal fraction. Each value is a mean ± standard error of 4 experiments.

decreased ATP-independent calcium binding by the rabbit heart microsomes significantly ($p < 0.05$). On the other hand, both procaine amide ($10^{-7} - 10^{-4}$ M) and lidocaine ($10^{-6} - 10^{-4}$ M), but not quinidine, depressed ($p < 0.05$) ATP-independent calcium binding by the rabbit heart mitochondria (Figure 3). It should be mentioned that the significance of the ATP-independent calcium binding by subcellular organelles is not clear at present. The possibility that this action of procaine amide and lidocaine may contribute to stabilizing the cardiac muscle seems intriguing, and in this regard these agents may differ from quinidine in their mechanism of action.

DISCUSSION

In this study we have demonstrated that quinidine stimulated cardiac microsomal calcium binding, and under similar experimental conditions we were also able to demonstrate depression in calcium uptake by quinidine (Harrow and

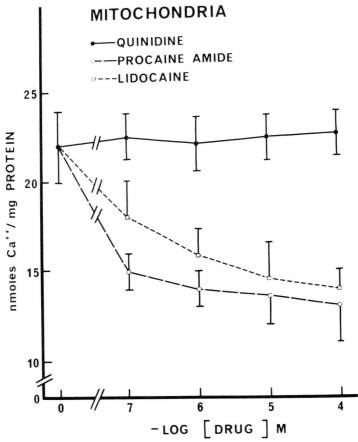

Figure 3. Effect of various concentrations of quinidine, procaine amide, and lidocaine on Mg ATP-independent calcium binding by rabbit heart mitochondrial fraction. Each value is a mean ± standard error of 4 experiments.

Dhalla, 1976). Depression of calcium uptake and stimulation of calcium binding by quinidine have also been shown to occur in skeletal muscle microsomes (Fuchs *et al.*, 1968; Scales and McIntosh, 1968; Balzer, 1972). Such experiments on the interaction of quinidine with microsomal membranes provide pharmacologic evidence in support of the concept that calcium binding and uptake are two different processes. In this regard it has been shown that the microsomal calcium uptake, but not calcium binding, was increased by cyclic AMP-protein kinase (Katz and Repke, 1973; Dhalla, Varley, and Harrow, 1974). Furthermore, different agents, such as antibiotic ionophore, X537A, and arsenate, were also reported to be more potent inhibitors of calcium uptake than calcium binding by heart microsomes (Entman *et al.*, 1973). Calcium binding by the fragments of sarcoplasmic reticulum from different types of failing hearts was observed to be depressed under experimental conditions showing no alteration in calcium uptake (Nayler et al., 1971; Muir et al., 1970; Sulakhe and Dhalla, 1971; Varley and Dhalla, 1973).

In contrast to microsomal calcium binding, heart mitochondrial calcium binding was decreased by quinidine. The depressant action of quinidine on mitochondrial calcium binding was of greater magnitude at low concentrations than at high concentrations of calcium in the incubation medium. However, decreasing the concentration of Mg^{2+} and decreasing the concentration of ATP or Ca^{2+} in the incubation medium were observed to abolish the depressant effect of quinidine on mitochondrial calcium binding. On the other hand, increasing the concentration of MG^{2+} and decreasing the concentration of ATP or Ca^{2+} in the incubation medium were observed to abolish the stimulation of microsomal calcium binding by quinidine. It is unlikely that the opposite effects of quinidine on mitochondrial and microsomal calcium binding are due to its chelating action. These observations concerning opposite responses of mitochondrial calcium binding and microsomal calcium binding to quinidine may be due to some fundamental differences between mitochondrial and microsomal membranes. In this regard it should be noted that mitochondrial calcium binding, unlike microsomal calcium binding, is known to be sensitive to sodium azide and oligomycin (Sulakhe and Dhalla, 1971; Varley and Dhalla, 1973).

Although quinidine, procaine amide, and lidocaine are known to produce cardiodepressant effect in high doses (Harrow and Dhalla, 1975; Szekeres and Papp, 1971), these antiarrhythmic drugs are found to possess some differences with respect to their actions on mitochondrial and microsomal calcium binding. For example, microsomal calcium binding was stimulated by both quinidine and procaine amide whereas lidocaine was ineffective. On the other hand, mitochondrial calcium binding was depressed by quinidine and lidocaine but not by procaine amide. This can be interpreted to mean that the subcellular sites of action of quinidine may be different from those for procaine amide and lidocaine. In this regard it should be noted that quinidine, unlike procaine amide and lidocaine has been shown to decrease calcium uptake by heart microsomes and mitochondria (Harrow and Dhalla, 1976). In view of the fact that quinidine decreased microsomal calcium uptake and increased microsomal calcium binding, it is difficult to readily explain its cardiodepressant effect on the basis of its action on the sarcotubular system. On the other hand, quinidine not only decreased mitochondrial calcium uptake but calcium binding also. Furthermore, the inhibitory effect of quinidine on mitochondrial calcium binding was quite pronounced at low concentrations of calcium in the incubation medium. These observations suggest that the mitochondrial action of quinidine may contribute greatly in eliciting the cardiodepressant effect.

REFERENCES

BALZER, H. 1972. The effect of quinidine and drugs with quinidine-like action (propranolol, verapamil and tetracaine) on the calcium transport system of isolated sarcoplasmic reticulum vesicles of rabbit skeletal muscle. Naunyn Schmiedebergs Arch. Pharmacol. 274:256–272.

DHALLA, N. S., VARLEY, K. G., and HARROW, J. A. C. 1974. Effect of epinephrine and adenosine cyclic 3', 5'-monophosphate on heart mitochondrial and microsomal calcium uptake. Res. Commun. Chem. Pathol. Pharmacol. 9:489–500.

ENTMAN, M. L., SNOW, T. R., FREED, D., and SCHWARTZ, A. 1973. Analysis of calcium binding and release by canine cardiac relaxing system (sarcoplasmic reticulum). J. Biol. Chem. 248:7762–7772.

FUCHS, F., GERTZ, E. W., and BRIGGS, F. N. 1968. The effect of quinidine on calcium accumulation by isolated sarcoplasmic reticulum of skeletal and cardiac muscle. J. Gen. Physiol. 52:955–968.

HARROW, J. A. C., and DHALLA, N. S. 1975. Subcellular and functional effects of quinidine, procaine amide and lidocaine on rat myocardium. Can. J. Physiol. Pharmacol. 53:1058–1064.

HARROW, J. A. C., and DHALLA, N. S. 1976. Effect of quinidine on calcium transport activities of the rabbit heart mitochondria and sarcotubular vesicles. Biochem. Pharmacol. 25:897–902.

KATZ, A. M., and REPKE, D. I. 1973. Calcium-membrane interactions in the myocardium: Effects of ouabain, epinephrine and 3', 5'-cyclic adenosine monophosphate. Amer. J. Cardiol. 31:193–201.

LOWRY, D. H., ROSEBROUGH, N. J., FARR, A. L., and RANDALL, R. J. 1951. Protein measurement with folin phenol reagent. J. Biol. Chem. 193:265–275.

MUIR, J. R., DHALLA, N. S., ORTEZA, J. M., and OLSON, R. E. 1970. Energy-linked calcium transport in subcellular fractions of the failing rat heart. Circ. Res. 26:429–438.

NAYLER, W. G., STONE, J., CARSON, V., and CHIPPERFIELD, D. 1971. Effect of ischemia on cardiac contractility and calcium exchange ability. J. Mol. Cell. Cardiol. 2:125–143.

SCALES, B., and McINTOSH, D. A. D. 1968. Studies on the radiocalcium uptake and the adenosinetriphosphatase of skeletal and cardiac sarcoplasmic reticulum fractions. J. Pharmacol. Exp. Ther. 160:249–260.

SHINEBOURNE, E. L., WHITE, R., and HAMER, J. 1969. A qualitative distinction between the beta-receptor blocking and local anesthetic actions of antiarrhythmic agents. Circ. Res. 24:835–841.

SULAKHE, P. V., and DHALLA, N. S. 1971. Excitation-contraction coupling in heart. VII. Calcium accumulation in subcellular particles in congestive heart failure. J. Clin. Invest. 50:1019–1027.

SZEKERES, L., and PAPP, G. J. 1971. Experimental Cardiac Arrhythmias and Antiarrhythmic Drugs. Akademiai Kiado, Budapest.

VARLEY, K. G., and DHALLA, N. S. 1973. Excitation-contraction coupling in heart. XII. Subcellular calcium transport in isoproterenol-induced myocardial necrosis. Exp. Mol. Pathol. 19:94–105.

Mailing address:
Dr. Naranjan S. Dhalla,
Professor of Physiology,
Faculty of Medicine,
University of Manitoba,
Winnipeg, R3E OW3 (Canada).

Recent Advances in Studies on
Cardiac Structure and Metabolism, Volume 11
Heart Function and Metabolism
Edited by T. Kobayashi, T. Sano, and N. S. Dhalla
Copyright 1978   University Park Press   Baltimore

EFFECTS OF HALOTHANE ANESTHESIA ON MYOCARDIAL CONTRACTILITY, CORONARY AS WELL AS SYSTEMIC HEMODYNAMICS, AND MYOCARDIAL METABOLISM IN DOGS

T. SAITO, K. OKAZAKI, N. OHTA,
S. SAKATA, Y. TANAKA, R. TONOGAI,
T. TOMINO, and Y. TOMINO

Department of Anesthesiology,
Tokushima University School of Medicine, Tokushima, Japan

SUMMARY

Halothane depressed coronary and other systemic circulations as arterial halothane concentration rose in dogs. Myocardial oxygen consumption decreased as the cardiac action, especially "myocardial contractility," was depressed, while the whole-body oxygen usage remained steady.

Lactate and pyruvate levels in arterial, mixed venous, and coronary venous blood did not show any signs of tissue hypoxia or development of anaerobic metabolism even in very deep halothane anesthesia. Coronary blood flow seemed well maintained for the demand, and changed almost in parallel with the myocardial oxygen consumption during the observation.

INTRODUCTION

Although there are several papers (Kettler, 1973; Merin, 1973; Rowe, 1974; Vance *et al.*, 1975; Fahmy and Laver, 1976) dealing with the effects of anesthesia on hemodynamics and myocardial metabolism published in the recent years, precise observations on the "dose-response relation" seem still lacking.

The purpose of our study was to observe the influences of halothane on depth of anesthesia, with special reference to coronary hemodynamics, myocardial performance, and metabolism of the heart.

METHOD

Fifteen adult mongrel dogs were used in the study. Anesthesia was induced with thiamylal I.V. and succinylcholine I.M. injections, and an endotracheal catheter was implanted. Respiration was controlled by Harvard pump.

P_aO_2 and P_aCO_2 were maintained around 100 and 40 torr, respectively, by regulating either the O_2/N_2 ratio in the inhaled gas mixture or the performance of the respirator throughout the study.

After completion of the preparatory surgery and application of transducers to appropriate positions under halothane anesthesia, the animals were allowed to wake up to the lightest possible level of anesthesia. Control data and samples were obtained thereafter.

RESULTS

The animals inhaled 1% halothane for 1 hr, 1.5% for 1 hr, and 2% for 2 hr, successively. Arterial halothane concentration rose as the inhaled halothane concentration increased. Mean aortic pressure declined significantly as anesthesia deepened, while heart rate decreased slightly, and only at a very deep plane of anesthesia did the reduction become statistically significant. Both cardiac index and the left coronary arterial blood flow decreased profoundly and significantly as the arterial halothane concentration rose, as shown in Figure 1. The left coronary blood flow/cardiac output ratio decreased slightly in the mean values during the course of anesthesia, although the changes were not significant. Calculated left ventricular work decreased significantly as anesthesia deepened.

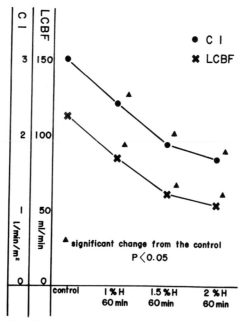

Figure 1. Effects of halothane anesthesia on the cardiac index (CI) and the left coronary arterial blood flow (LCBF).

Left ventricular dp/dt_{max} was depressed significantly by the halothane inhalation, in spite of rather mild depression of so-called V_{max} calculated from the left ventricular pressure pulse. Only at a very deep plane of anesthesia was the reduction of V_{max} statistically significant. Figure 2 shows the changes. Oxygen consumption of the whole body remained essentially unchanged, while the myocardial oxygen consumption sharply decreased as the halothane anesthesia deepened.

Lactate levels in arterial, mixed venous, and coronary venous blood were maintained virtually unchanged, except for a significant decrease in the mixed venous blood noted at the end of the first hour, as shown in Figure 3. The pyruvate level was raised by the halothane inhalation and the L/P ratio decreased significantly as a result. Interpretation of the change is difficult so far and should be studied further. At the least, there seemed to be very little possibility of myocardial hypoxia and increase in anaerobic metabolism caused by the anesthetic, even in very deep level of anesthesia.

The correlation between principal circulatory parameters and myocardial VO_2 was investigated. The results are summarized in Table 1.

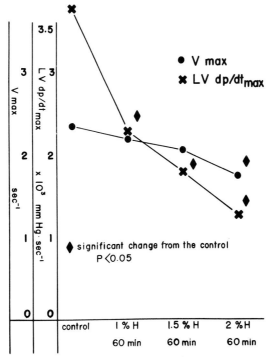

Figure 2. Changes in the left ventricular dp/dt_{max} (LV dp/dt_{max}) and V_{max}.

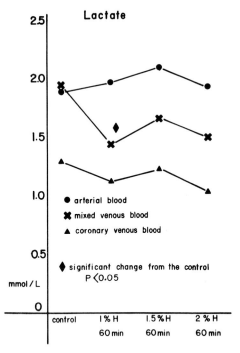

Figure 3. Blood lactate levels during the halothane inhalation.

Table 1. Correlations between two principal parameters during the experiment

Parameters		$r_{x \cdot y}$	Significance
Myocardial $\dot{V}o_2$	X	−0.33	$0.05 < p < 0.1$
Body $\dot{V}o_2$	Y		
Heart rate	X	0.40	$0.01 < p < 0.02$
Myocardial $\dot{V}o_2$	Y		
Mean aortic pressure	X	0.60	$p < 0.001$
Myocardial $\dot{V}o_2$	Y		
Cardiac index	X	0.50	$0.001 < p < 0.01$
Myocardial $\dot{V}o_2$	Y		
Left ventricular work	X	0.63	$p < 0.001$
Myocardial $\dot{V}o_2$	Y		
V_{max}	X	0.64	$p < 0.001$
Myocardial $\dot{V}o_2$	Y		
LV dp/dt$_{max}$	X	0.80	$p < 0.001$
Myocardial $\dot{V}o_2$	Y		
dF/dt$_{max}$ (aorta)	X	0.76	$p < 0.001$
Myocardial $\dot{V}o_2$	Y		
Myocardial $\dot{V}o_2$	X	0.89	$p < 0.001$
Left coronary blood flow	Y		
Total peripheral resistance	X	0.51	$0.001 < p < 0.01$
Left coronary vascular resistance	Y		

Myocardial VO_2 and whole-body VO_2 did not show a significant correlation during the course of the experiment. The left ventricular dp/dt_{max} and myocardial VO_2 have shown the closest correlation in the study. Heart rate and mean aortic pressure seemed less important determinants of myocardial oxygen consumption.

The left coronary blood flow and the VO_2 of the myocardium perfused by the left coronary artery revealed a very close and significant correlation. So-called myocardial contractility, represented particularly by the left ventricular dp/dt_{max}, seemed to be playing a major role in determining myocardial oxygen consumption in the halothane anesthesia. The changes in LV dp/dt_{max} and the maximum acceleration of aortic blood flow were almost identical, and depressed sharply as anesthesia deepened. Very close correlation was observed between the two. The maximum acceleration also correlated very well with the myocardial oxygen consumption.

REFERENCES

FAHMY, N. R., and LAVER, M. B. 1976. Hemodynamic response to ganglionic blockade with pentolinium during N_2O-halothane anesthesia in man. Anesthesiology 44:6.

KETTLER, D. 1973. Sauerstoffbedarf und Sauerstoffversorgung des Herzens in Narkose. Springer-Verlag, Berlin.

MERIN, R. G. 1973. Inhalation anesthetics and myocardial metabolism: Possible mechanisms of functional effects. Anesthesiology 39:216.

ROWE, G. G. 1974. Responses of the coronary circulation to physiologic changes and pharmacologic agents. Anesthesiology 41:182.

VANCE, J. P., SMITH, G., THORBURN, J., and BROWN, D. M. 1975. The combined effect of halothane-induced hypotension and hypocapnia on canine myocardial blood flow and oxygen consumption. Br. J. Anaesth. 47:825.

Mailing address:
Takao Saito, M.D., Professor,
Department of Anesthesiology,
Tokushima University School of Medicine,
Kuramoto-cho, Tokushima 770 (Japan).

Recent Advances in Studies on
Cardiac Structure and Metabolism, Volume 11
Heart Function and Metabolism
Edited by T. Kobayashi, T. Sano, and N. S. Dhalla
Copyright 1978   University Park Press   Baltimore

DOSE-DEPENDENT DEPRESSION OF CARDIAC FUNCTION AND METABOLISM BY INHALATION ANESTHETICS IN CHRONICALLY INSTRUMENTED DOGS

R. G. MERIN,
T. KUMAZAWA, and
N. L. LUKA

University of Rochester School of Medicine,
Department of Anesthesiology,
Rochester, New York, USA

SUMMARY

Halothane, methoxyflurane, and enflurane produce dose-dependent depression in ventricular function in the dog. Myocardial blood flow and oxygen consumption are decreased accordingly without evidence of myocardial tissue hypoxia. Low-dose fluroxene does not depress the heart, while there is less depression with high-dose fluroxene than with the other anesthetics. In spite of this depression, myocardial blood flow was unchanged, and the decreased oxygen consumption during high-dose fluroxene was a result of decreased oxygen extraction by the heart. Sympathetic nervous system stimulation produced by fluroxene anesthesia is probably responsible for these effects, but further work is necessary for confirmation of this hypothesis.

INTRODUCTION

We have previously shown that high-dose halothane, methoxyflurane, and fluroxene depress left ventricular function and metabolism when compared to low doses of the same anesthetics in acutely prepared dogs (Kumazawa and Merin, 1975). In isolated muscle, low-dose anesthesia produces significant depression as well (Kemmotsu, Hashimoto, and Shimosato, 1974). This study was designed to evaluate the effects of low and high concentrations of four halogenated inhalation anesthetics in trained chronically instrumented dogs.

METHODS

The details of our method have been published (Merin, Kumazawa, and Luka, 1976a). In brief, catheters were surgically implanted in the thoracic aorta (TA),

This research was supported by United States Public Health Service Grant HL 13257. Dr. Merin was supported throughout the period of this investigation by United States Public Health Service Grant HL 31752 (Research Career Development Award).

left atrium (LA), great cardiac vein (GCV), left anterior descending coronary artery (LADCA), and main pulmonary artery (MPA). A pressure transducer was sewn in the left ventricular (LV) apex, and atrial pacing wires were placed (Figure 1). Between 2 and 22 weeks after the surgery, the animals were studied awake and during low (MAC, minimum alveolar anesthetic concentration; Eger, Saidman, and Brandstater, 1965) and high concentrations of the anesthetics. Ventilation and F_iO_2 were adjusted during anesthesia so that P_aCO_2 and P_aO_2 approximated the awake values. The results from 5 animals are reported for halothane and enflurane, and from 3 dogs with methoxyflurane and fluroxene. Paired t-tests were used to evaluate the former, and changes were considered significant in the 3 dog groups if all animals reacted in the same direction. Cardiovascular pressures were transduced through Statham gauges (LA and TA) or through a high fidelity amplifier recording system (LV). Cardiac output was measured by dye dilution. Coronary (myocardial) blood flow was estimated from the washout curve of ^{133}Xe in the gCV (Merin *et al.*, 1976a). Oxygen and lactate in aortic and GCV blood were measured by conventional techniques (Merin *et al.*, 1976a).

RESULTS AND DISCUSSION

Controlled variables were unchanged with halothane, enflurane (Merin, Kumazawa, and Luka, 1976b), and methoxyflurane (Table 1), but there was metabolic

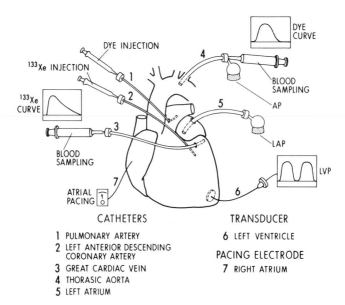

Figure 1. Schematic depiction of instrumentation. LVP, left ventricular pressure; LAP, left atrial pressure; AP, aortic pressure.

Table 1. Controlled variables*

Variable	Awake	Methoxyflurane		Awake	Fluroxene	
% Anesthesia (ET)	0	0.34	0.75	0	6.36	12.7
P_aCO_2 (torr)	30	27	30	33	32	34
pHa	7.45	7.47	7.41	7.46	7.36[+]	7.29[+]
P_aO_2 (torr)	80	101	89	197	184	190
Hgb (g/dl)	10.9	11.0	11.7	11.9	14.2	12.7
Temp (°C)	36.5–38.5	38.2	37.9	36.5 –38.5	38.3	38.2

*ET = end tidal; Hgb = hemoglobin.
[+] = different from awake.

acidosis with both doses of fluroxene (Table 1). The changes in hemodynamics produced by halothane, enflurane, and methoxyflurane were remarkably similar (Figures 2 and 3). High doses unquestionably depressed ventricular function, since cardiac output and ventricular pressure derivatives were all markedly reduced in spite of increased heart rate and filling pressures (LAP). Low-dose anesthesia also increased heart rate, but depressed pressure and output derivatives considerably less without changing filling pressures, so that the interpreta-

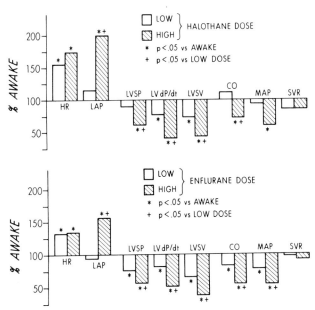

Figure 2. Cardiodynamic effects of halothane and enflurane. HR, heart rate; LAP, left atrial pressure; LVSP, left ventricular systolic pressure; LV$dP/dt$, rate of rise of LVSP; LVSV, left ventricular stroke volume; CO, cardiac output; MAP, mean aortic pressure; SVR, systemic vascular resistance.

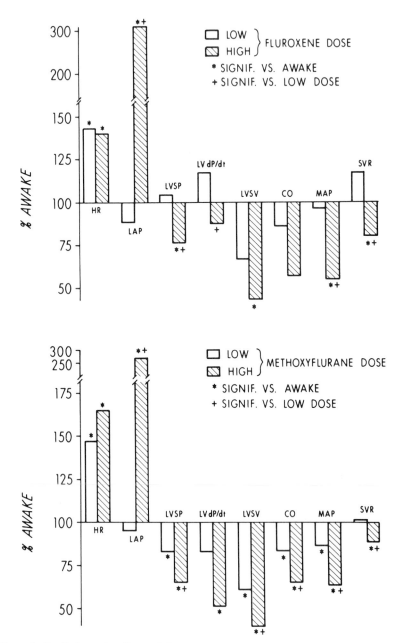

Figure 3. Cardiodynamic effects of fluroxene and methoxyflurene. MBF, myocardial blood flow; $\dot{V}O_2$, myocardial O_2 uptake.

tion is somewhat less clear. However, if the effects of pacing tachycardia are compared with the effects of the low-dose anesthetics, it is apparent that there was appreciable depression, for the heart rate increase alone *increased* LV dP/dt and aortic pressure and decreased LAP (Table 2). During halothane, methoxyflurane, and enflurane, appropriate changes in myocardial blood flow and oxygen consumption accompanied the hemodynamic changes (Figures 4 and 5). The decrease in oxygen extraction and increase in lactate extraction suggest that myocardial oxygen delivery was adequate for the demand (Scheuer, 1967).

As in the acute experiments, fluroxene behaved differently (Kumazawa and Merin, 1975). Again, the dose-related metabolic acidosis was seen. At the low concentration there was no evidence for ventricular depression (Figure 3), although the number of experiments is too small for definitive conclusions. However, as noted previously (Kumazawa and Merin, 1975), high-dose fluroxene depressed ventricular function, although to a lesser degree than the other anesthetics (Figures 2 and 3). The metabolic effects are particularly interesting. Myocardial oxygen consumption mirrored the hemodynamic effects in that it did not change during low-dose anesthesia and decreased during high dose (Figure 5). However, the latter effect was a result of decreased oxygen extraction, because myocardial blood flow did not drop in spite of markedly decreased aortic pressures. Lactate extraction was also puzzling. It decreased slightly during low-dose anesthesia but, unlike the acute experiments, increased markedly during high-dose anesthesia. With all the anesthetics, arterial lactate concentrations increased (Merin *et al.,* 1976 a and b) but only with fluroxene was there a dose-related increase. It seems likely that fluroxene is stimulating the sym-

Table 2. Effect of atrial pacing†

	Control		Paced	
HR	80.3 ±	3.6	129.1 ±	3.6*
LAP (torr)	4.4 ±	0.7	2.2 ±	0.7*
LV dP/dt (% awake)	100		109.6 ±	2.6*
LVSV (ml)	40.5 ±	1.8	29.3 ±	1.5*
LVSW (Gm.m.)	49.7 ±	3.3	39.6 ±	2.7*
CO (ml/min)	3230 ±	170	3760 ± 180	*
MAP (torr)	94.1 ±	2.8	108.5 ±	2.4*
SVR (prn)	1.70 ±	0.05	1.63 ±	0.6
MBF (ml/100g/min)	56.5 ±	2.8	63.5 ±	2.8*
$\dot{V}O_2$ (ml/100g/min)	6.0 ±	0.4	6.8 ±	0.4*
O_2 extraction (%)	76.6 ±	1.3	76.8 ±	1.6
Lactate extraction (%)	15.2 ±	8.5	15.3 ±	6.4

†HR = heart rate; LAP = left ventricular pressure; LV dP/dt = rate of rise of left ventricular pressure; LVSV = left ventricular stroke volume; LVSW = left ventricular stroke work; CO = cardiac output; MAP = mean aortic pressure; SVR = systemic vascular resistance; MBF = myocardial blood flow; $\dot{V}O_2$ = myocardial oxygen uptake.

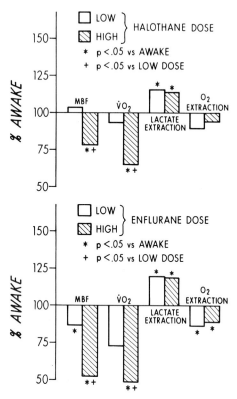

Figure 4. Myocardial oxygenation with halothane and enflurane. Abbreviations as in Figure 2.

pathetic nervous system in the dog, as was previously suggested in man (Cullen *et al.,* 1970) and reported in the cat (Skovsted and Price, 1970). This would explain the lack of depression of myocardial blood flow at the low dose and the maintenance at the high dose. It is puzzling that this sympathetic nervous stimulation was unable to overcome the negative inotropic effect of high-dose fluroxene in the dog, as had been seen in man (Cullen *et al.,* 1970). However, the sympathoadrenal response of the dog has been noted to be different from adult man, but similar to that seen in infants (Price, 1960). Although the data are scant, it is possible that the difference may relate to a different proportion of norepinephrine and epinephrine being secreted by the adrenal medulla in the dog and man. Alternatively, there may be some difference in adrenergic receptor response. However, this hypothesis cannot be established from these investigations and must be confirmed by further experimentation.

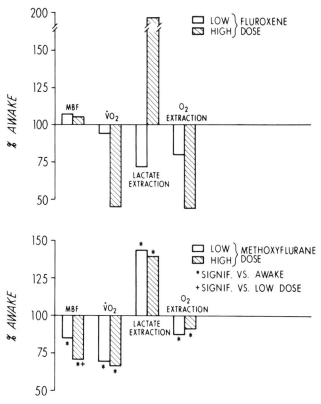

Figure 5. Myocardial oxygenation with methoxyflurane and fluroxene. Abbreviations as in Figure 2.

Acknowledgments The conscientious technical assistance of Ms. Sally Basch was crucial to the conduct of this experiment. In addition, we are grateful for the technical assistance provided by Adrienne Barton, Ruth Howard, and John Young. Veterinary support was supplied by Drs. Robert Garman and Allan L. Kraus. Drs. William Simon and David Goldstein designed the on-line myocardial blood flow apparatus for this experiment.

REFERENCES

CULLEN, D. J., EGER, E. I., SMITH, N. T., SAWYER, D. C., GREGORY, G. A., and JOAS, T. C. 1970. Cardiovascular effects of fluroxene in man. Anesthesiology 32: 218–226.

EGER, E. I., II, SAIDMAN, L. J., and BRANDSTATER, B. 1965. Minimum alveolar anesthetic concentration, a standard of anesthetic potency. Anesthesiology 26:756–763.

KEMMOTSU, O., HASHIMOTO, Y., and SHIMOSATO, S. 1974. Effects of fluroxene and enflurane on contractile performance of isolated papillary muscles from failing hearts. Anesthesiology 40:252–260.

KUMAZAWA, T., and MERIN, R. G. 1975. Effects of inhalation anesthetics on cardiac function and metabolism in the intact dog. *In* P.-E. Roy and G. Rona (eds.), Recent Advances in Studies on Cardiac Structure and Metabolism, Vol. 10, The Metabolism of Contraction, pp. 71–79. University Park Press, Baltimore.

MERIN, R. G., KUMAZAWA, T., and LUKA, N. L. 1976a. Myocardial function and metabolism in the conscious dog and during halothane anesthesia. Anesthesiology 44:402–415.

MERIN, R. G., KUMAZAWA, T., and LUKA, N. L. 1976b. Enflurane depresses myocardial function, perfusion, and metabolism in the dog. Anesthesiology. 45:501–507.

PRICE, H. L. 1960. General anesthesia and circulatory homeostasis. Physiol. Rev. 40: 187–218.

SCHEUER, J. 1967. Myocardial metabolism in cardiac hypoxia. Amer. J. Cardiol. 19: 385–392.

SKOVSTED, P., and PRICE, H. L. 1970. Central sympathetic excitation caused by fluroxene. Anesthesiology 32:210–217.

Mailing address:
Robert G. Merin, M.D.,
Department of Anesthesiology,
University of Rochester Medical Center,
601 Elmwood Avenue,
Rochester, New York 14642 (USA).

Recent Advances in Studies on
Cardiac Structure and Metabolism, Volume 11
Heart Function and Metabolism
Edited by T. Kobayashi, T. Sano, and N. S. Dhalla
Copyright 1978   University Park Press   Baltimore

EFFECTS OF MORPHINE AND HALOTHANE
ON CANINE CARDIAC FUNCTION
BEFORE AND AFTER CARDIOPULMONARY BYPASS

T. KUMAZAWA, M. NAKAGAWA, E. IKEZONO,
M. SUNAMORI, R. HATANO, N. YAMAMOTO, and T. SUZUKI

Department of Anesthesiology and Department of Surgery,
Tokyo Medical and Dental University, Tokyo, Japan

SUMMARY

In an effort to compare the effects of anesthetics on cardiac functions and metabolism, mongrel dogs were anesthetized with morphine (3 mg/kg, N_2O 50% in oxygen) or halothane (0.7%, N_2O 50% in oxygen). Hb, Ht, pO_2, pCO_2, pH, O_2 content, lactate, and pyruvate in the arterial and coronary sinus blood were measured and ECG, LVP, CVP, AP, and CO were recorded. Aorta was cross-clamped for 30 min under cardiopulmonary bypass (CPB). Hemodynamic and metabolic survey were continued until 120 min of recovery period. Results were as follows: Hemodynamics, such as LVP, AP, and CO, were depressed after CPB, then gradually returned to control level. Subendocardial ischemia observed through ST depression and QRS widening on ECG, as well as DPTI/TTI ratio under 1.0, disappeared in the recovery period. Lactate was produced by the heart after anoxic arrest and was extracted at 120 min after CPB. Halothane and morphine did not show any significant differences of effects on cardiac function and metabolism in this study.

INTRODUCTION

Halothane has frequently been used in the anesthetic management of patients undergoing open heart operations. Recently, large doses of morphine (0.5 ~ 3.0 mg/kg) are more commonly used for cardiovascular stability with minimal cardiac depression. In an effort to investigate the differences between the effect of halothane and morphine on cardiac function, we undertook the study described in this chapter.

METHODS

Twenty-three mongrel dogs were anesthetized with 15 mg/kg secobarbital intravenously and were intubated orotracheally. Eleven dogs were ventilated with 50% N_2O, 0.7% halothane, and O_2. The other twelve dogs were ventilated with 50% N_2O and O_2 and received 3 mg/kg morphine intravenously over 20 min.

Through a left thoracotomy, coronary sinus and left ventricle were cannulated and an electromagnetic flowmeter was placed around the ascending aorta. Femoral arteries and veins were cannulated for blood sampling, pressure measurement, infusion, and blood return from cardiopulmonary bypass (CPB). After 20 min of cardiovascular hemodynamic stabilization, control measurements were taken. Aorta was cross-clamped for 30 min under CPB. The survey was continued for 120 min after aorta clamp-off. Rectal temperature was maintained at the control value by external heating and/or heat exchanger in bypass. Prime solution contained Ringer's lactate without blood.

RESULTS

Hemodynamics at Control Condition

There were no significant differences between the effects of morphine and halothane on heart rate, cardiac index, stroke index, mean aortic pressure, and systemic vascular resistance at the control state (Figure 1). Left ventricular pressure, left ventricular work index, left ventricular stroke work index, and left ventricular end-diastolic pressure did not show any significant differences between the anesthetics (Figure 2). Although we saw very similar effects of the anesthetics, a different response to changes of after-load by binding of descending aorta was shown. Increasing left ventricular after-load induced increase in left ventricular peak pressure with both anesthetics. However, aortic flow maximum was significantly decreased on halothane and was not depressed on morphine (Figure 3).

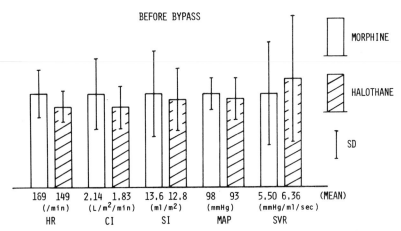

Figure 1. Hemodynamics at the control state. HR, heart rate; CI, cardiac index; SI, stroke index; MAP, mean aortic pressure; SVR, systemic vascular resistance.

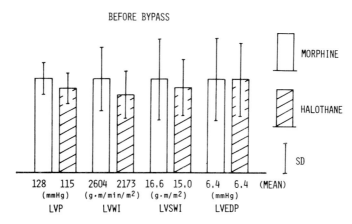

Figure 2. Hemodynamics at the control state. LVP, left ventricular pressure; LVWI, left ventricular work index; LVSWI, left ventricular stroke work index; LVEDP, left ventricular end-diastolic pressure.

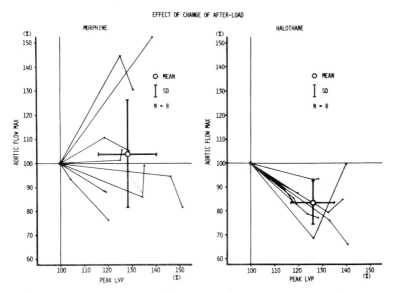

Figure 3. Relationship between peak left ventricular pressure and aortic flow maximum after elevating of left ventricular after-load.

Hemodynamics after Cardiopulmonary Bypass

Figures 4 and 5 show hemodynamic changes after CPB. Morphine and halothane did not show any significant hemodynamic difference at any time. Mean aortic pressure, left ventricular pressure, and left ventricular work index were depressed after CPB compared with control. DPTI/TTI ratio (Buckberg *et al.*, 1972) decreased significantly at 30 and 60 min after clamp-off, but gradually increased and recovered to control value at 120 min.

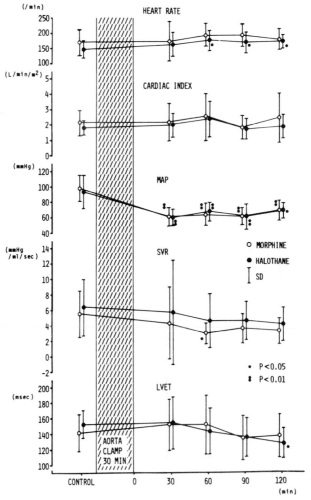

Figure 4. Change in hemodynamics after cardiopulmonary bypass. MAP, mean aortic pressure; SVR, systemic vascular resistance; LVET, left ventricular ejection time.

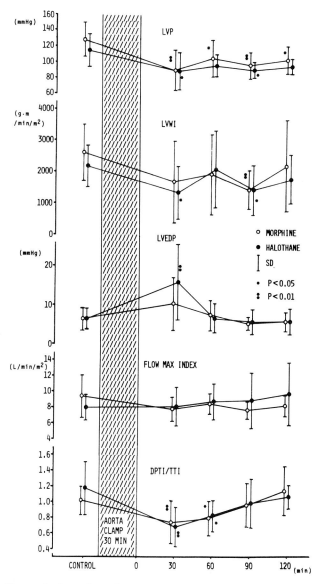

Figure 5. Change in hemodynamics after cardiopulmonary bypass. LVP, left ventricular pressure; LVWI, left ventricular work index; LVEDP, left ventricular end-diastolic pressure; Flow Max Index, aortic flow maximum/body surface; DPTI/TTI, diastolic pressure time index/tension time index.

Mortality Rates

After aortic clamp-off, some dogs could not recover from depressed hemo-dynamic state and died. Mortality rates after CPB were 3/12 in the morphine group and 4/11 in the halothane group. There seem to be no differences between the anesthetics, but the Hb value after CPB was well correlated with mortality rates. Twelve dogs showed very low Hb, less than 5 g/dl, after CPB, and 5 of them died. In the other eleven dogs, with Hb higher than 5 g/dl, only 2 died.

Metabolic changes

We could not find any significant differences between the anesthetics in effects on blood gas, acid-base balance, and extraction of oxygen and lactate by the heart. The mean value of lactate extraction by the heart showed lactate production only at the time just after clamp-off.

DISCUSSION

Since Lowenstein recommended large doses of morphine as a safe anesthetic for patients with minimal circulatory reserve (Lowenstein *et al.,* 1969), morphine has being used for open heart operations more widely than halothane. Although the advantages of using morphine are thought to be the strong analgesia induced, the ease of after-care of ventilation, and the hemodynamic stability, hemo-dynamic and metabolic differences between the agents are not well shown. A prospective comparison of the agents for 128 open heart operations did not show any marked differences in effects on hemodynamics and mortality rates (Conahan *et al.,* 1973). It was suggested that morphine increased total vascular capacitance more than halothane by comparison of blood requirements during open heart surgery (Stanley *et al.,* 1974). Our study did not show any significant hemodynamic differences between the agents except for the response to elevating after-load. This difference indicates that halothane decreases cardiac functional reserve, but morphine does not, at least not as much as halothane. This may be the cause of hemodynamic stability during morphine anesthesia exhibited in patients with heart diseases.

Acknowledgment The conscientious and able technical assistance of Mr. Keiichi Iizuka made this work possible.

REFERENCES

BUCKBERG, G. D., TOWERS, B., PAGLIA, D. E., MULDER, D. G., and MALONEY, J. V. 1972. Subendocardial ischemia after cardiopulmonary bypass. J. Thorac. Cardiovasc. Surg. 64:669–684.

CONAHAN, T. J., OMINSKI, A. J., WOLLMAN, H., and STROTH, R. A. 1973. A prospective random comparison of halothane and morphine for open-heart anesthesia: One year's experience. Anesthesiology 38:528–535.

LOWENSTEIN, E., HOLLOWEL, P., LEVINE, F. H., DAGGETT, W. M., AUSTEN, W. G., and LAVER, M. B. 1969. Cardiovascular response to large doses of intravenous morphine in man. New Engl. J. Med. 281(25):1389–1393.

STANLEY, T. H., GRAY, N. H., ISERN-AMARAL, J. H., and PATTON, C. 1974. Comparison of blood requirements during morphine and halothane anesthesia for open-heart surgery. Anesthesiology 41:34–38.

Mailing address:
Dr. Teruo Kumazawa,
Department of Anesthesiology,
Tokyo Medical and Dental University,
5-45, Yushima 1-chome, Bunkyo-ku,
Tokyo (Japan).

Recent Advances in Studies on
Cardiac Structure and Metabolism, Volume 11
Heart Function and Metabolism
Edited by T. Kobayashi, T. Sano, and N. S. Dhalla
Copyright 1978   University Park Press   Baltimore

EFFECT OF ACETALDEHYDE ON FUNCTIONING OF CARDIAC MUSCLE AT THE ULTRASTRUCTURAL LEVEL

W. G. NAYLER and E. FASSOLD

Department of Medicine, Cardiothoracic Institute,
University of London, London, England

SUMMARY

The effect of acetaldehyde, the hepatic metabolite of alcohol, on the functioning of cardiac muscle was investigated at the subcellular level. Concentrations of acetaldehyde that occur in plasma failed to alter either the microsomal Ca^{2+}-accumulating and ATPase activity or the Ca^{2+}-accumulating activity of the mitochondria. These same concentrations of acetaldehyde inhibited the Ca^{2+}-dependent myofibrillar ATPase.

INTRODUCTION

An association between chronic alcoholism and ventricular pump dysfunction is now firmly established (Brigden, 1972). Several investigators have shown that this dysfunction cannot be explained in terms of malnutrition or vitamin deficiency. Others have attempted to establish the basis for this alcohol-induced dysfunction by adding alcohol directly to subcellular fractions of heart muscle (Swartz *et al.*, 1974), but high concentrations of alcohol have had to be used before a significant response can be obtained. Recently, several investigators (James and Bear, 1967; Gailis and Verdy, 1971; Schreiber *et al.*, 1974) suggested that some of the deleterious effects of ingested alcohol may be due to its hepatic metabolite, acetaldehyde. The experiments described in this chapter were undertaken to investigate whether concentrations of acetaldehyde (0.02–0.3 M) that occur in plasma have a deleterious effect at the subcellular level.

METHODS

Mitochondrial, myofibrillar, and sarcoplasmic reticulum-rich (SR-rich) microsomal fractions were prepared from ventricular muscle freshly excised from

Supported by grants from the Medical Research Council and The British Heart Foundation.

adult male guinea pigs (Dunken-Hartley strain). The details of the homogenization and differential centrifugation techniques that were used have been described in detail elsewhere (Nayler et al., 1975a, b). The subcellular fractions were characterized in terms of their ultrastructure (m $\times$ 48,000), their Ca^{2+}-accumulating activity, and their enzymic profiles (Nayler et al., 1976), which included: cytochrome oxidase; succinic dehydrogenase; $(Na^+ + K^+)$-activated, ouabain-sensitive ATPase, and oligomycin-insensitive and azide-sensitive ATPase activities. To establish whether acetaldehyde has an effect on the functioning of these various organelles they were pre-incubated with acetaldehyde for 30 min at either 25 or 37° C before the various Ca^{2+}-accumulation and ATPase assays were performed. The assays were performed on a paired basis, acetaldehyde being added to the test and omitted from the control preparations. Because acetaldehyde evaporates rapidly, the reaction tubes (test and control) had to be layered with 0.5 ml mineral oil.

Ca^{2+}-Accumulating and ATPase Activity
of Sarcoplasmic Reticulum-rich Microsomal Fractions

Ca^{2+}-accumulation was measured in the absence ("Ca^{2+}-binding") and presence ("calcium uptake") of oxalate, as previously described (Nayler et al., 1976). The "binding" reaction mixture contained 100.0 mM KCl; 5.0 mM $MgCl_2$; 40.0 mM histidine buffer of pH 7.0; 5.0 mM ATP; 50 μM $^{45}Ca^{2+}$ and 30 μg protein/ml. The reaction was started by adding ATP. The "uptake" reaction mixture was similar to that used for the binding studies except that its $^{45}Ca^{2+}$ concentration was increased to 100 μM, its protein concentration was reduced to 15 μg/ml and 5.0 mM K oxalate was added. ATPase activity was monitored as previously described using an ATP regenerating system (Nayler et al., 1975a, 1976).

Ca^{2+}-Accumulating Activity of Mitochondria

The mitochondria were incubated in a reaction mixture containing 5.0 mM Tris-succinate; 100.0 mM KCl; 10.0 mM $MgCl_2$; 5.0 mM NaN_3; 0.01–1.0 mM Ca^{2+}, with and without 4.0 mM $KH_2 PO_4$; 4.0 mM Na_2 ATP; 2.0 mM Tris-maleate buffer, pH 6.8, and 0.1 M EDTA. The uptake reaction was started by adding 100 μM Ca^{2+} labeled with $^{45}Ca^{2+}$.

Myofibrillar ATPase Activity

The ATPase activity of the myofibrils was assayed in a reaction mixture containing 70.0 mM KCl; 20 mM imidazole, pH 7.0; 6.0 mM $MgCl_2$; 5 mM NaN_3; 0.01–1.0 mM Ca^{2+}, with and without EGTA. The reaction was started by adding ATP Na_2.

RESULTS

Concentrations of acetaldehyde (0.02–0.3 M) that occur in the plasma of humans failed to cause any significant change in the Ca^{2+}-accumulating activity of cardiac SR-rich microsomal preparations, irrespective of whether the reaction was performed in the presence of a precipitating anion. Concentrations of acetaldehyde in excess of 20 mM did, however, reduce the Ca^{2+}-accumulating activity of these preparations.

Figure 1 shows that although plasma concentrations (0.02–0.3 mM) of acetaldehyde had no effect on the activity of the Ca^{2+}-activated ATPase in these SR-rich preparations, higher concentrations (> 20 mM) were inhibitory.

Similarly (Figure 2), relatively high concentrations of acetaldehyde were required before any change in the Ca^{2+}-accumulating activity of the mitochondria could be detected.

Figure 3 shows that cardiac myofibrils that have been preincubated together with relatively small concentrations of acetaldehyde (0.02–0.2 mM) exhibit an altered myofibrillar ATPase activity, the activity of the Ca^{2+}-dependent ATPase being significantly reduced. Halving the duration of preincubation with the acetaldehyde failed to alter the amount of inhibition that occurred. Kinetic studies showed this inhibition to be of a competitive nature, V_{max} remaining constant and the K_m increasing (with respect to ATP). Higher concentrations of acetaldehyde, e.g., 20 and 100 mM, had an even greater inhibitory effect, but only on the Ca^{2+}-dependent ATPase.

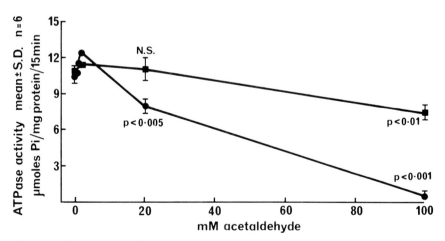

Figure 1. Effect of 0.02–100 mM acetaldehyde on the activity of the Ca^{2+}-independent and Ca^{2+}-dependent ATPases in guinea pig cardiac microsomes. The microsomes were preincubated with the acetaldehyde for 60 min. N.S., not significant at $p = 0.05$ (paired t-test). ■, Ca^{2+}-independent ATPase; ●, Ca^{2+}-activated ATPase.

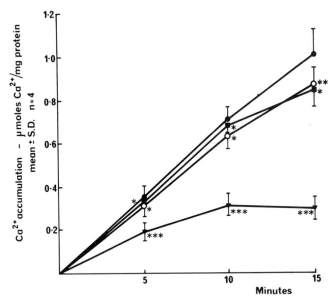

Figure 2. Effect of acetaldehyde on the Ca^{2+}-accumulating activity of guinea pig cardiac mitochondria. The mitochondria were preincubated with the acetaldehyde for 60 min at $25°C$ before the Ca^{2+}-accumulation studies were started. N.S., not significant at $p = 0.05$. •, control; ■, 10mM A; ○, 20 mM A; ▼, 100 mM A; * N.S.; ** $p < 0.01$; *** $p < 0.001$.

DISCUSSION

These results show that although concentrations of acetaldehyde that occur in plasma do not interfere with the Ca^{2+}-accumulating activity of either the mitochondria or the SR-rich microsomal fractions, they inhibit the activity of the Ca^{2+}-dependent myofibrillar ATPase enzyme. This inhibition cannot be a nonspecific phenomenon, because the Ca^{2+}-dependent ATPase activity of the microsomes was not affected, unless excessively high concentrations of acetaldehyde were used. Nor was the Ca^{2+}-independent ATPase affected.

The importance of the myofibrillar ATPase enzyme is now firmly established, and there seems little reason to doubt that its inhibition would lead to pump dysfunction similar to that caused by alcohol. This does not mean, however, that alcohol per se may not also have a direct effect on the functioning of cardiac muscle at a subcellular level. It does seem probable, however, that the effect of alcohol's hepatic metabolite must also be considered when attempts are made to explain the pump dysfunction that is associated with the consumption of alcohol (Burch and Walsh, 1960). Presumably the change in the Ca^{2+}-accumulating activity of the SR-rich microsomal fractions that Bing et al. (1974)

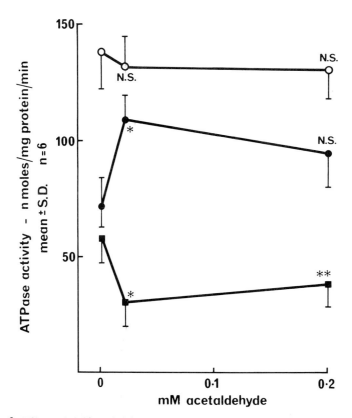

Figure 3. Effect of 0.02 and 0.2 mM acetaldehyde on the activity of the myofibrillar ATPase enzyme. Note that it is the activity of the Ca^{2+}-dependent ATPase that is inhibited. ●, Ca^{2+}-independent ATPase; ■, Ca^{2+}-dependent ATPase; ○, total ATPase; * $p < 0.05$; ** $p < 0.025$; N.S., $p = 0.05$.

detected in their alcohol-fed dogs reflects a direct effect of alcohol and not an effect of the metabolite acetaldehyde.

REFERENCES

BING, R. J. TILLMANNS, H., FAUVEL, J. M., SELLER, K., and MAO, J. C. 1974. Effects of prolonged alcohol administration on calcium transport in heart muscle in the dog. Circ. Res. 35:33–38.

BRIGDEN, W. 1972. Alcoholic cardiomyopathy. *In* G. E. Burch (ed.), Cardiomyopathy. F. A. Davis Company, Philadelphia.

BURCH, G. E., and WALSH, J. J. 1960. Cardiac insufficiency in chronic alcoholism. Amer. J. Cardiol. 6:864–874.

GAILIS, L., and VERDY, M. 1971. The effect of ethanol and acetaldehyde on the metabolism and vascular resistance of the perfused heart. Can. J. Biochem. 49:227–233.

JAMES, T. N., and BEAR, E. S. 1967. Effects of ethanol and acetaldehyde on the heart. Amer. Heart J. 74:243–255.

NAYLER, W. G., DUNNETT, J., and BERRY, D. 1975a. The calcium accumulating activity of subcellular fractions isolated from rat and guinea pig heart muscle. J. Mol. Cell. Cardiol. 7:275–288.

NAYLER, W. G., DUNNETT, J., and BURIAN, W. 1975b. Further observations on species-determined differences in the calcium-accumulating activity of cardiac microsomal fractions. J. Mol. Cell. Cardiol. 7:663–676.

NAYLER, W. G., SULLIVAN, A. T., DUNNETT, J., SLADE, A. M., and TRETHEWIE, E. R. 1976. The effect of a cardiotoxic component of the venom of the Indian Cobra (*Naja nigrieollis*) on the subcellular structure and function of heart muscle. J. Mol. Cell. Cardiol. 8:541–560.

SCHREIBER, S. S., ORATZ, M., ROTHSCHILD, M. A., REFF, F., and EVANS, C. 1974. Alcoholic cardiomyopathy. II. The inhibition of cardiac muscle protein synthesis by acetaldehyde. J. Mol. Cell. Cardiol. 6:207–213.

SWARTZ, M. H., REPKE, D. I., KATZ, A. M., and RUBIN, E. 1974. Effects of ethanol on calcium binding and calcium uptake by cardiac microsomes. Biochem. Pharmacol. 23:2369–2378.

Mailing address:
Dr. W. G. Nayler,
Cardiothoracic Institute,
2 Beaumont Street,
London, W1N 2DX (England).

Recent Advances in Studies on
Cardiac Structure and Metabolism, Volume 11
Heart Function and Metabolism
Edited by T. Kobayashi, T. Sano, and N. S. Dhalla
Copyright 1978   University Park Press   Baltimore

POSSIBLE MODE OF ACTION OF NITROGLYCERIN ON HEART MITOCHONDRIA

L. SZEKERES, P. VÁGHY, P. BOR, and K. CSETE

Department of Pharmacology,
University Medical School of Szeged,
6701 Szeged, P.O.B. 115, Hungary

SUMMARY

Nitroglycerin has no effect on the electron transport and oxidative phosphorylation of isolated rabbit heart mitochondria at 5×10^{-4} M and lower concentrations. However, it diminished the phosphate-induced energy-dependent potassium fluxes through the mitochondrial membrane in both directions; thus it was able to prevent the impairment of the efficiency of oxidative phosphorylation produced by increased ion transport.

INTRODUCTION

In spite of extensive research, the mechanism of the beneficial effect of nitroglycerin (GTN) in angina pectoris is still not fully understood. According to the present view, this action is partly due to the diminution of the preload and the afterload (Brachfeld, Bozer, and Gorlin, 1959; Gorlin *et al.,* 1959) and partly to the redistribution of the myocardial blood flow in favor of the ischemic area (Winbury, 1971). However, the possibility of a direct metabolic action of the drug reducing O_2 demand of the myocardial tissue should also be considered. There are some data in favor of this assumption, based on experiments made on dog heart homogenates (Bachand, Somani, and Hardman, 1969; Somani *et al.,* 1969), on sliced atrial tissue of rabbits (Levy, 1970), as well as on our earlier findings concerning GTN action on myocardial pO_2 values of the intact rabbit atria at constant O_2 supply and work load (Vághy *et al.,* 1973).

Because the precise mechanism of the O_2-sparing action of GTN is not known, our present experiments were devoted to the analysis of this question. Furthermore, because GTN is assumed to penetrate the cell (Gailis and Nguyen, 1975), its action on the mitochondrial function deserves special interest. We have studied the influence of GTN on oxidative phosphorylation as well as on the mitochondrial ion transport.

METHODS

Mitochondria were isolated from the rabbit heart according to Lindenmayer, Sordahl, and Schwartz (1968). The mitochondrial O_2 consumption was determined polarographically using an oscillating platinum oxygen electrode and a silver reference electrode, both immersed in a thermostabilized cuvette. Energy-linked ion transport was determined in the same sample simultaneously by measuring the osmotic swelling-shrinkage cycles of the mitochondria by their light absorbence at 520 nm. The ADP/O ratio was calculated according to Estabrook (1967).

RESULTS AND DISCUSSION

The left panel of Figure 1 shows optimal values for the RCI and the ADP/O ratio in sucrose medium containing appropriate concentrations of alcohol, the solvent of GTN. It also shows that neither O_2 uptake nor oxidative phosphorylation is affected by 5×10^{-4} M GTN. Accordingly, in this relatively low concentration the drug has neither uncoupling effect nor direct inhibiting action on the electron transport chain. The small ADP-induced mitochondrial shrinking is not affected either.

The finding that, in a medium providing optimal function of the mitochondria, GTN proved to be ineffective is not surprising, if we take into consideration that the beneficial action of this drug appears in the more or less hypoxic myocardium.

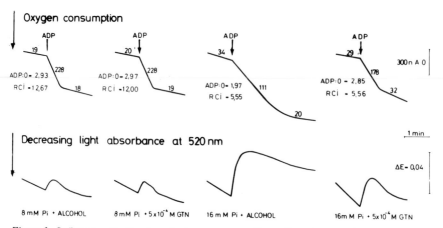

Figure 1. Influence of nitroglycerin in sucrose medium. Experimental conditions were: sucrose, 250 mM; Tris HCl, 10 mM; pyruvate, 0.125 mM; pH, 7.40; 37° C. Cuvette volume was 5 ml. The reaction was started by the addition of 6.15 mg mitochondrial protein (Mw). ADP (2072 nmol) was added where indicated.

Since elevated myocardial inorganic phosphate (Pi) concentration is one of the earliest and most sensitive indicators of impaired aerobic energy production, the right panel of Figure 1 shows the influence of increased Pi concentration on oxidative phosphorylation and on the mitochondrial ion transport.

A Pi concentration of 16 mM markedly inhibited the rate and efficiency of oxidative phosphorylation, simultaneously augmenting the ADP-induced mitochondrial shrinkage. This latter effect is probably due to potassium loss from the intramitochondrial space (Kimmich and Rasmussen, 1967; Safer and Schwartz, 1967).

Under these circumstances the same concentration of GTN that is ineffective in the presence of low Pi concentrations proved to be highly effective in preventing the phosphate-induced decrease of the rate and efficiency of oxidative phosphorylation as well as the shrinkage of mitochondria, probably by decreasing the potassium loss from the mitochondria.

It is well known that efficiency of the oxidative phosphorylation is impaired at very early stages of hypoxia. On the other hand, not shrinking, but swelling, of the mitochondria was shown to be the earliest hypoxic morphological alteration (Jennings, 1969).

The discrepancy is probably attributable to the fact that sucrose, representing a nonphysiological constituent of the medium, was used. Therefore, in the following experiments it was replaced by KCl, since potassium is the dominant cation of the intracellular space. RCI values were much lower in this latter medium, which is mainly the consequence of an increased state 4 respiration. Also, sensitivity to Pi was considerably increased. This is shown in Figure 2,

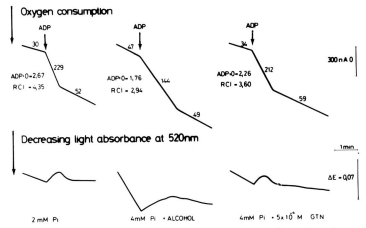

Figure 2. Influence of nitroglycrein in potassium chloride medium. Experimental conditions were: potassium chloride, 150 mM; pyruvate, 1 mM; pH, 7.40; 37° C. Cuvette volume was 5 ml. The reaction was started by the addition of 5.55 mg mitochondrial protein (Mw). ADP (2072 nmol) was added where indicated.

where elevation of the Pi concentration from 2 to 4 mM markedly increased swelling and considerably reduced the ADP/O ratio and the RCI.

Swelling is an osmotic process due to intramitochondrial accumulation of ions (Rottenberg and Solomon, 1969; Brierley *et al.*, 1971), mainly of potassium in this case. We have shown that it does not occur in the absence of the easily penetrating phosphate anion. This ion accumulation represents an energy-requiring process, since rotenon or antimycin A, inhibitors of the electron transport chain, prevented the swelling-inducing effect of Pi. Uncoupling concentrations of DNP similarly inhibited swelling; therefore, in order to produce swelling, not only the normal function of the electron transport chain is needed, but also the energy produced by it.

The fact that addition of ADP to the medium prevented or abolished further swelling is indicative of a competition for available energy (Safer and Schwartz, 1967) between ion accumulation and oxidative phosphorylation. Conversely, separate inhibition of the oxidative phosphorylation, even from endogenous ADP, by oligomycin promoted swelling because more energy became available for ion accumulation.

GTN (5×10^{-4} M) considerably reduced swelling of the mitochondria and simultaneously increased RCI, and ADP/O ratio if higher, 4 mM; Pi concentration was present in the medium.

On the strength of these data the sequence of early hypoxic changes could be imagined as follows: As a consequence of impaired aerobic energy production, intracellular Pi concentration increases, promoting energy-linked potassium accumulation in the mitochondria. This may cause mitochondrial swelling, and,

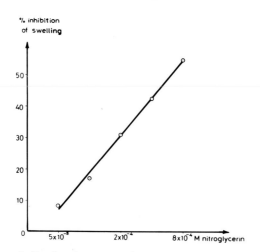

Figure 3. Influence of nitroglycerin on phosphate-induced swelling in the presence of 2 mg oligomycin/mg mitochondrial protein. Medium: KCl, 150 mM; pyruvate, 1 mM; potassium phosphate buffer, 10 mM; pH, 7.20; 37° C.

by diverting available energy from oxidative phosphorylation to ion transport, reduce efficiency of oxidative phosphorylation. This in turn further increases intracellular Pi and results in the development of a vicious circle. GTN may act predominantly on the first process, inhibiting or at least reducing phosphate-induced increased inward and outward ion transport in the mitochondria. It exerts a mitochondrial membrane-stabilizing action.

This is supported also by our observation, shown in Figure 3, that GTN exerts a dose-dependent inhibition of swelling in the presence of oligomycin; even a 5×10^{-5} M concentration proved to be effective.

Acknowledgment The authors gratefully acknowledge the excellent technical assistance of Authné Fehér Mária.

REFERENCES

BACHAND, R. T., JR., SOMANI, P., and HARDMAN, H. F. 1969. Inhibition of oxygen utilisation (QO_2) by nitroglycerin in the myocardial homogenate preparation. Fed. Proc. 28:671.

BRACHFELD, N., BOZER, J., and GORLIN, R. 1959. Action of nitroglycerin on the coronary circulation in normal and in mild cardiac subjects. Circulation 19:697–704.

BRIERLEY, G. P., JURKOWITZ, M., SCOTT, K. M., and MEROLA, A. J. 1971. Ion transport by heart mitochondria XXII. Spontaneous, energy-linked accumulation of acetate and phosphate salts of monovalent cations. Arch. Biochem. Biophys. 147: 545–556.

ESTABROOK, R. W. 1967. Mitochondrial respiratory control and the polarographic measurement of ADP:O ratios. *In* R. W. Estabrook and M. E. Pullman (eds.), Methods in Enzymology 10, p. 41. Academic Press, New York.

GAILIS, L., and NGUYEN, M. -H. 1975. The effect of sulfhydryl reagents on the heart rate and coronary flow of the isolated perfused guinea-pig heart. Arch. Int. Pharmacodyn. 218:19–28.

GORLIN, R., BRACHFELD, N., MacLEOD, C., and BOPP, P. 1959. Effect of nitroglycerin on the coronary circulation in patients with coronary artery disease or increased left ventricular work. Circulation 19:705–718.

JENNINGS, R. B. 1969. Early phase of myocardial ischemic injury and infarction. Amer. J. Cardiol. 24:753–765.

KIMMICH, G. A., and RASMUSSEN, H. 1967. Inhibition of mitochondrial respiration by loss of intramitochondrial K^+. Biochim. Biophys. Acta 131:413–420.

LEVY, J. V. 1970. Effect of organic nitrates on myocardial oxygen consumption in vitro. Brit. J. Pharmacol. 38:743–748.

LINDENMAYER, G. E., SORDAHL, L. A., and SCHWARTZ, A. 1968. Reevaluation of oxidative phosphorylation in cardiac mitochondria from normal animals and animals in heart failure. Circ. Res. 23:439–450.

ROTTENBERG, H., and SOLOMON, A. K. 1969. The osmotic nature of the ion-induced swelling of rat-liver mitochondria. Biochim. Biophys. Acta 193:48–57.

SAFER, B., and SCHWARTZ, A. 1967. Active transport of potassium ion in heart mitochondria. Circ. Res. 21:25–31.

SOMANI, P., BACHAND, R. T., JR., HARDMAN, H. F., and LADDU, A. R. 1969. Nutritional circulation in the heart II. A reappraisal of the effect of nitroglycerin on myocardial hemodynamics, oxygen consumption and nutritional blood flow in the isolated supported heart preparation. Eur. J. Pharmacol. 8:1–13.

VÁGHY, P., BOR, P., CSETE, K., and SZEKERES, L. 1973. On the possibility of a direct action of nitroglycerin on myocardial metabolism. Symposium on Pharmacodynamics of Circulation, Smolenice.

WINBURY, M. M. 1971. Redistribution of left ventricular blood flow produced by nitroglycerin. Circ. Res. 28–29: Suppl. I-140–I-147.

Mailing address:
Dr. L. Szekeres
Department of Pharmacology,
University Medical School of Szeged,
6701 Szeged, F.O.B. 115 (Hungary).

Recent Advances in Studies on
Cardiac Structure and Metabolism, Volume 11
Heart Function and Metabolism
Edited by T. Kobayashi, T. Sano, and N. S. Dhalla
Copyright 1978   University Park Press   Baltimore

ALTERATIONS OF LEFT VENTRICULAR FUNCTION AND REGIONAL MYOCARDIAL BLOOD FLOW INDUCED BY NITRATES IN PATIENTS WITH CORONARY ARTERY DISEASE

W. RUDOLPH, E. FLECK, J. DIRSCHINGER,
C. LORACHER, R. BRANDT, A. REDL, and D. HALL

German Heart Center, Lothstrasse 11, 8000 Munich 2,
Federal Republic of Germany

SUMMARY

In patients with coronary artery disease and left ventricular asynergy, an improved regional wall motion can frequently be seen after the administration of nitrates. These agents produce an increase in regional myocardial blood flow only in those regions found to have reversible wall motion impairment, even though comparable reductions of preload and afterload occur in the presence of irreversible asynergy. This increase in flow is most probably the result of a decreased extravascular component of the coronary vascular resistance. In contrast, due to the nitrate-induced reduction in oxygen requirements mediated by decreased wall tension, regional flow in healthy myocardium decreases. This results in a more homogeneous distribution in flow between healthy and diseased myocardial regions. Irreversibly damaged zones show no changes in regional blood flow. It is assumed that reversible asynergy represents chronic, ischemic myocardium, while irreversible asynergy represents myocardial scar. The nitrate-induced improvement in contraction in asynergic zones yielded by the reduction in afterload and increased regional blood flow is hemodynamically reflected in an increase in ejection fraction, mean normalized systolic ejection rate, and velocity of mean circumferential fiber shortening, as well as in an unchanged or increased stroke volume, depending on the extent of preload reduction. Concurrent with unchanged values of ejection-phase contractility indices, irreversibly damaged myocardium consistently displays a reduction in stroke volume after nitrate administration. A significant difference in the effects of glyceryl trinitrate, isosorbide dinitrate, and sodium nitroprusside was not observed.

INTRODUCTION

Characteristic findings in coronary artery disease (CAD) are regional perfusion disturbances and compromised left ventricular wall motion (Rudolph *et al.,* 1976). The present study was proposed to determine the influence of nitrates on regional myocardial blood flow (RMBF) and left ventricular function.

MATERIAL AND METHODS

In a total of 129 patients with CAD end-systolic (ESV) and end-diastolic volumes (EDV), mean normalized systolic ejection rate (MNSER), velocity of mean circumferential fiber shortening (VCF), ejection fraction (EF), regional ventricular wall motion (RVWM), and regional myocardial blood flow (RMBF) were determined before and after the administration of either 2.4 mg glyceryl trinitrate (GTN) s.1., 15 mg isosorbide dinitrate (ISDN) s.1., or sodium nitroprusside (NP) in an average dosage of 100 μg i.v. In addition, systolic (LVSP) and end-diastolic left ventricular pressure (LVEDP) as well as heart rate and ejection time were recorded.

ESV and EDV (n = 53) were calculated from the left ventriculogram (RAO 30° projection) according to the area-length method (Kennedy, Trenholme, and Kasser, 1970). RVWM (n = 129) was quantitatively analyzed from superimposed images of end-diastolic and end-systolic ventricular contours by calculating the percent systolic shortening of the longitudinal and 6 hemi-axes in RAO projection and of 11 radially ordered axes in the LAO projection. Healthy controls demonstrate a characteristic contraction profile (Loracher, Dacian, and Rudolph, 1975). Measurements of RMBF in the region of distribution of the left coronary artery were performed with the Xenon[133] wash-out technique by means of a computerized gamma-camera system (Cannon, Bell, and Dwyer, 1972; Rudolph *et al.*, 1976).

RESULTS

One hundred and four asynergic zones were found in the 129 CAD patients. Fifty-nine of the 104 (57%) asynergic zones showed improved contraction after the administration of nitrates, and thus could be designated as being reversibly asynergic. The remaining 45 asynergic zones studied showed no change (Figure 1). The quantitative evaluation of left ventricular wall motion demonstrated that the administration of nitrates yielded improved contraction in 83% of all hypokinetic zones, while only 15% of akinetic regions showed improvement. An increase in RVWM in dyskinetic areas was not observed. The extent of the improvement in wall motion resulting from either GTN, ISDN, or NP did not significantly differ.

GTN, ISDN, and NP uniformly reduce LVSP and LVEDP and decrease ventricular volumes. Patients with irreversible wall damage consistently show increased volumes. The nitrate-induced decrease in end-diastolic volume in reversibly as well as in irreversibly damaged myocardium is of approximately the same magnitude. A more marked reduction in systolic volume can be demonstrated in the presence of reversible impairment. Corresponding to a varying degree of end-systolic volume reduction, nitrates exert a varying influence on the

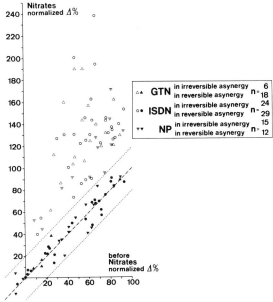

Figure 1. Alterations in regional ventricular wall motion after administration of isosorbide dinitrate (ISDN), glyceryl trinitrate (GTN), and sodium nitroprusside (NP). Patients with reversible asynergy *(open symbols)* display improved ventricular wall motion. Irreversibly asynergic regions *(closed symbols)* show no change. The magnitude of changes in wall motion induced by glyceryl trinitrate, isosorbide dinitrate, and nitroprusside does not differ significantly. Normalized Δ% represents the quotient of the actual percent systolic shortening and the least normal percent systolic shortening of the hemi-axis. 100% represents the lowest limit of normal. Values exceeding 100% result from improvement in contraction extending to the upper limit of normal.

stroke volume. The stroke volume in patients with reversible asynergy remains constant, while that of patients with irreversible disease decreases significantly. Furthermore, the ejection-phase contractility indices, EF, MNSER, and VCF, only show significant increases in the presence of improved RVWM.

Left ventricular filling pressure is an additional determinant of stroke volume changes after nitrate administration. In the presence of an elevated end-diastolic pressure, an increase in stroke volume can only be attained in patients with reversible disease. The stroke volume of patients with irreversible wall motion impairment remains unchanged or decreases slightly. In the presence of normal end-diastolic pressure, patients with irreversible disease uniformly show a significant decrease in stroke volume.

Hypoperfusion was documented in 92% of asynergic regions by defective uptake in the Xenon [133] scintigram, and, in 87% of the asynergic regions, by delayed Xenon wash-out characteristics. NP and ISDN lead to increased RMBF in hypoperfused zones in the presence of reversible wall motion impairment. At the same time, nitrates were seen to induce a marked decrease in flow in areas of normal myocardium (Figure 2).

DISCUSSION

The decrease in RMBF in normal myocardium and the increase in RMBF in hypoperfused zones induced by nitrates result in a more homogeneous distribution of flow between healthy and diseased myocardial regions. The decrease in flow through healthy myocardium is most probably the result of reduced oxygen requirements subsequent to decreased ventricular wall tension. In contrast, the increased flow through hypoperfused regions appears to represent a decreased extravascular component of the coronary vascular resistance, which, in turn, is the result of reduced left ventricular volume and filling pressure due to the venous pooling effect of nitrates (Becker and Pitt, 1971; da Luz *et al.*, 1975; Rudolph *et al.*, 1976).

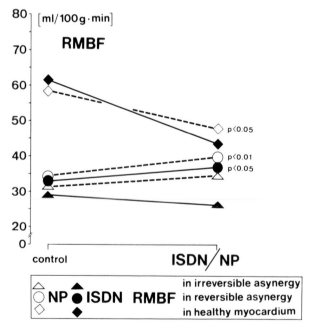

Figure 2. Influence of nitrates on regional myocardial blood flow in patients with coronary artery disease. As compared with normally perfused regions (*squares*), the myocardial blood flow in post-stenotic, asynergic regions (*circles* and *triangles*) is significantly diminished ($p < 0.001$). Regional flow decrease after the administration of isosorbide dinitrate and sodium nitroprusside in healthy zones (*squares*) increases in reversibly asynergic zones (*circles*), and shows no change in irreversibly asynergic regions (*triangles*).

Generally, the nitrate-induced increase in RMBF is accompanied by improved ventricular wall motion. The finding of reversibility in asynergic myocardium can be construed as evidence for the presence of chronic ischemia (Loracher *et al.*, 1975; Rudolph *et al.*, 1976). In addition to increased perfusion, the reduction of impedance to ventricular ejection accounts for the wall-motion improvement (Miller *et al.*, 1975).

Unchanged values of RMBF are found to be consistent with irreversibly impaired ventricular wall motion, probably indicating the presence of myocardial scar (Rudolph *et al.*, 1976). The increase in EF, MNSER, and VCF and the greater reduction of end-systolic volume associated with an unchanged or increased stroke volume can be explained on the basis of the nitrate-induced recruitment of previously poorly contracting myocardium. The varying response of the stroke volume can be viewed as being a function of the left ventricular filling pressure or preload.

In the presence of irreversibly damaged myocardium, reduction of the filling pressure below optimal level renders the Starling mechanism inadequate and results uniformly in a decrease in stroke volume. In the dosages used, no significant difference in the effect of GTN, ISDN, and NP could be ascertained.

REFERENCES

BECKER, L., and PITT, B. 1971. Regional myocardial blood flow, ischemia, and antianginal drugs. Ann. Clin. Res. 3:353.

CANNON, P. J., DELL, R. B., and DWYER, E. M. 1972. Measurement of regional myocardial perfusion in man with 133-Xenon and a scintillation camera. J. Clin. Invest. 51:964.

DA LUZ, P., FORRESTER, J., WYATT, H. L., TYBERG, J. V., CHAGRASULIS, R., PARMLEY, W. W., and SWAN, H. J. C. 1975. Hemodynamic and metabolic effects of sodium nitroprusside on the performance and metabolism of regional ischemic myocardium. Circulation 52:400.

KENNEDY, J. W., TRENHOLME, S. E., and KASSER, I. S. 1970. Left ventricular volume and mass from single-plane cineaniocardiogram. Amer. Heart J. 80:343.

LORACHER, C., DACIAN, S., and RUDOLPH, W. 1975. Erkennung reversibel-asynerger Myokardbezirke durch quantitative Analyse des linksventrikulären Cineangiogramms vor und nach Gabe von Nitraten. Verh. Dtsch. Ges. Kreislaufforschg. 41:166.

MILLER, R. R., VISMARA, L. A., ZELIS, R., AMSTERDAM, E. A., and MASON, D. T. 1975. Clinical use of sodium nitroprusside in chronic ischemic heart disease. Circulation 51:328.

RUDOLPH, W., DACIAN, S., DIRSCHINGER, J., FLECK, E., LORACHER, C., and REDL, A. 1976. Der Einfluss von Nitraten auf regionale Myokarddurchblutung und regionale Ventrikelwandbewegung. Med. Klin. 71:687.

Mailing address:
Professor W. Rudolph,
German Heart Center,
Lothstrasse 11,
8000 Munich 2 (Federal Republic of Germany).

Pathophysiological Aspect

Recent Advances in Studies on
Cardiac Structure and Metabolism, Volume 11
Heart Function and Metabolism
Edited by T. Kobayashi, T. Sano, and N. S. Dhalla
Copyright 1978   University Park Press   Baltimore

GLYCOLYTIC ATP AND ITS PRODUCTION DURING ISCHEMIA IN ISOLATED LANGENDORFF-PERFUSED RAT HEARTS

O. L. BRICKNELL
and
L. H. OPIE

MRC Ischaemic Heart Disease Research Unit, Department of Medicine,
Groote Schuur Hospital and University of Cape Town, South Africa

SUMMARY

The perfused rat heart was used to assess the possible contribution of glycolytically produced ATP to the maintenance of the action potential in the normoxic heart, and to the maintenance of membrane integrity in the underperfused, ischemic heart. During normoxia, pyruvate (10 mM) was nearly as able as glucose (10 mM) to maintain the normal action potential. During ischemia (reduction of perfusion pressure of Langendorff heart from 100 to 20 cm H_2O), total tissue values of ATP and creatine phosphate were similar in pyruvate and in glucose hearts. However, pyruvate-perfused hearts had higher tissue levels of cyclic AMP during the ischemic period, and during the reperfusion period they had an increased release of lactate dehydrogenase and an increased incidence of arrhythmias when compared with glucose hearts. It is proposed that these differences can be related to a higher rate of production of glycolytic ATP. The anatomical, biochemical, and pharmacological evidence favoring a cytoplasmic compartment of ATP located in relation to the cell membrane is reviewed.

INTRODUCTION

As already well established by Bing and subsequent workers (Bing, 1965; Opie, 1969), the major fuels of the human heart are glucose, lactate, and free fatty acids, but the uptake of glucose is usually low. Of these fuels, only glucose is able to produce ATP extramitochondrially, i.e., in the cytoplasm; in all other cases, ATP must be produced intramitochondrially to be exported to the cytoplasm by the atractyloside-sensitive ATP-ADP translocase system described by Klingenberg and Pfaff (1966).

Most studies on man show a small but definite positive arteriovenous difference of glucose during basal conditions (Opie, 1969) and the approximate rates of generation of glycolytic ATP can be calculated assuming that glycogen is not a major fate of the glucose extracted. Values for glycolytic ATP production are very low when compared with total ATP production. Nevertheless, it has been suggested that glycolytic ATP may have a special role in the maintenance of membrane activity and in the generation of the action potential (Figure 1). The major evidence for this is electrophysiological and is discussed later. This paper examines the projected role of glycolytically produced ATP in the heart with special reference to normal or ischemic Langendorff-perfused rat hearts.

METHODS

The action potential of the normoxic, isolated, perfused rat heart was studied by inserting floating micro-electrodes into Langendorff hearts perfused horizontally

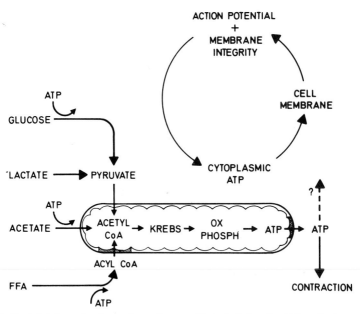

Figure 1. Postulated mechanisms of nonglucose effects in ischemia. Although glucose uses cytoplasmic ATP in its activation, there is a net gain of cytoplasmic ATP during glycolysis and it is *hypothetically* suggested that such ATP may be compartmented and available in relation to the cell membrane to help maintain the action potential and membrane integrity. Pyruvate (or lactate) neither produces nor uses cytoplasmic ATP, but by oxidative phosphorylation (ox phosph) produces mitochondrial ATP that passes through the Klingenberg-translocase to reach the cytoplasm and chiefly to be used for contraction. In normoxia, such ATP can also be used to maintain the action potential (see text). In ischemia, glycolytic ATP production from glucose may become important (see text). Acetate, which uses up cytoplasmic ATP and has a low P/O ratio (see Opie, 1973), and free fatty acids (FFA), which also use extramitochondrial ATP in their activation, should be harmful to the cell membrane (see text). Accumulation of acyl-CoA in ischemic hearts may depend on FFA uptake (see Opie, 1975).

but at 65 cm H_2O pressure. The perfusate was a Krebs-Henseleit (1932) bicarbonate buffer, pH 7.4, 30° C, equilibrated with 95% O_2, 5% CO_2 and containing either glucose (10 mM) or pyruvate (10 mM), but keeping the perfusate (Na^+) at 140 mEq/liter.

To study the possible role of glycolytic ATP in ischemic rat hearts, isolated

To study the possible role of glycolytic ATP in ischemic rat hearts, isolated perfused rat hearts were again perfused according to the technique of Langendorff (1895) by a Krebs-Henseleit bicarbonate buffer, pH 7.4, equilibrated with 95% O_2, 5% CO_2, but the temperature was 37° C. An initial control perfusion period at 100 cm H_2O perfusion pressure lasted for 10 min, followed by an "ischemic" period of 30 min with a perfusion pressure of 20 cm H_2O, and then a reperfusion period of 100 cm H_2O for 30 min. Exogenous substrates were: glucose, 11 mM; pyruvate, 5 mM; acetate, 4 mM, or palmitate, 0.5 mM, bound to 0.1 mM albumin (Figure 2). Release of lactate dehydrogenase (LDH) and the

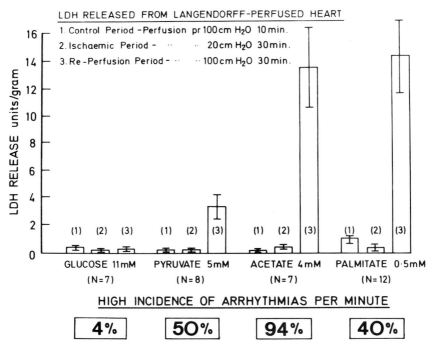

Figure 2. Effect of substrates on lactate dehydrogenase (LDH) release and on arrhythmias in ischemic rat heart. The various substrates used were: glucose, 11 mM; pyruvate, 5 mM; acetate, 4 mM, and palmitate, 0.5 mM (bound to albumin, 0.1 mM). The rationale for the choice of substrates is shown in Figure 1. Note that LDH release is not increased in the ischemic period, but rises during the reperfusion period in pyruvate and especially in acetate and palmitate hearts. The peak incidence of arrhythmias (per minute) in the reperfusion period is shown below; the major differences lie between the very low incidence with glucose and the much higher incidence with nonglucose fuels.

incidence of reperfusion arrhythmias were followed as indices of membrane integrity. Some hearts were freeze-clamped at the end of the ischemic period for measurements of high-energy phosphate compounds, cyclic AMP, glycogen, and lactate. Pooled glycogen values were compared with pooled values from another series of hearts at the end of the perfusion period. Oxygen uptake, glucose uptake, and lactate output were measured by conventional means and glycolytic flux determined by the net glycogen breakdown (and the glucose uptake, where appropriate).

RESULTS AND DISCUSSION

Normoxic hearts

In normally oxygen-perfused hearts, we found that the general shape of the action potential during perfusion with pyruvate was very similar to perfusion with glucose; these studies were done at perfusion temperatures of $30°$ C to achieve a slower heart rate and easier manipulation of the micro-electrode. The duration of the action potential in pyruvate hearts was 92% of that of glucose hearts. In the perfused rat heart, however, pyruvate is well established as an inhibitor of glycolysis (Williamson, 1965). At $37°$ C, glycolytic flux during pyruvate perfusions was almost entirely eliminated, probably due to very high citrate values (Bricknell and Opie, 1977), with resultant inhibition of the key enzyme, phosphofructokinase. Assuming a similar pattern of metabolism during pyruvate perfusions at $30°$ C, we may conclude that ATP produced in the mitochondria by the metabolism of pyruvate can be used for the maintenance of the action potential nearly as effectively as ATP produced by the metabolism of glucose.

Ischemic Hearts

Evidence for ischemia during the underperfusion period was: increased venous concentration of lactate and of ^{42}K, decreased high-energy phosphate compounds and glycogen, as the O_2 uptake fell from $100-120$ $\mu l/g$ wet wt/min to $18-24$ $\mu l/g/min$, and reactive hyperemia developed during the reperfusion period. As shown in Figure 2, the various substrates caused major differences in the reperfusion period. LDH release was higher in pyruvate than in glucose hearts, and even higher in acetate and in fatty acid hearts. Arrhythmias, measured as the peak incidence of abnormal beats per minute, were higher in acetate hearts but considerably higher in all nonglucose hearts than in glucose hearts.

The extent of LDH release was related to duration of ischemic arrest, which was much longer in acetate and in palmitate hearts (Bricknell and Opie, 1977), and only slightly longer in pyruvate than in glucose hearts. As ATP lack is held to be related to the severity of cardiac arrest during whole heart ischemia (Kübler and Spieckermann, 1970; Hearse, Stewart, and Braimbridge, 1975) we next measured ATP and CP at the end of the perfusion period. As expected, values in acetate and in palmitate hearts were very low, but, surprisingly, values for ATP in pyruvate hearts were similar to glucose values, and CP was actually 1 μmol/g higher in ischemic hearts perfused with pyruvate than in hearts perfused with glucose. The phosphate potential, here indirectly expressed as ATP + CP divided by Pi, was actually higher in ischemic pyruvate than in ischemic glucose hearts (Table 1, phosphate potential). Thus it was not the total ATP or CP that determined ischemic arrest and the reaction of the heart to reperfusion with the various substrates. We therefore turned our attention to the rate of production of glycolytic ATP, bearing in mind the theoretical arguments relating such ATP to membrane integrity.

Production rates of glycolytic ATP were calculated from the net glycogen change, the glucose uptake (if any), and a value of 2 ATP per unit glucose uptake and 3 ATP per C6 unit of net glycogen loss. That part of glycolytic flux not forming lactate was held to have undergone aerobic respiration, and ATP production was calculated from standard phosphorylation/oxidation (P/O) values (Opie, 1974). Because there were only small changes in the P/O ratio within 30 min of the onset of severe regional ischemia in the baboon (Lochner et al., 1975), P/O ratio changes were ignored for this calculation.

Glucose-perfused ischemic hearts had much higher rates of glycolytic ATP formation than pyruvate hearts in spite of total ATP and CP values, which were as high as or higher in pyruvate than in glucose hearts (Bricknell and Opie, 1977).

One possibility is that such increased glycolytic ATP actually contributed to the maintenance of membrane integrity and reduced reperfusion LDH release and arrhythmias. We cannot exclude, however, the possibility that increased glycolytic ATP is one of a constellation of changes with glucose hearts and that some other change could be more directly related to maintenance of membrane integrity. For example, Bricknell and Opie (1977) report that tissue

Table 1. Energy charge, here expressed by (ATP + PCr) ÷ (Pi), in hearts perfused with various substrates

Energy charge	$\dfrac{\text{ATP} + \text{PCR}}{\text{Pi}}$	
	Control	Ischemia
Glucose (11 mM)	1.48	0.55
Pyruvate (5 mM)	2.81*	1.10**
Acetate (4 mM)	1.47	0.20**
Palmitate (0.5 mM) (0.1 albumin)	0.92	0.11**

*$p < 0.005$ versus glucose.
**$p < 0.05$ versus glucose.

cyclic AMP is lower in glucose than in pyruvate- or acetate-perfused hearts, and cyclic AMP is widely held to influence membrane function. Podzuweit et al. (1976) have hypothetically suggested that cyclic AMP may act to provoke ventricular fibrillation in ischemic tissue. Recent information suggests that cyclic AMP may help regulate ion exchange across the cell membrane (Schneider and Sperelakis, 1974; Watanabe and Besch, 1974; Bittar, Chambers, and Schultz, 1976).

Electrophysiological Evidence for Role for Glycolytic ATP

First, Prasad and MacLeod (1969) used papillary muscle to show that the duration of the action potential was best maintained by glycolytically produced ATP when the tissue was subject either to anoxia or metabolic inhibitors. McDonald, Hunter, and MacLeod (1971) further showed that it was not the total ATP content but rather a particular pool of ATP, probably generated by glycolysis, that was involved in regulating the rate of repolarization. Second, Girardier and co-workers (Cheneval et al., 1972) showed that, in cultured fetal heart cells, glucose was more effective than pyruvate in maintaining total ATP and the duration of the action potential. Girardier and co-workers (Girardier, 1971; Hyde et al., 1972), therefore, formulated the hypothesis that glycolysis could be related to electrogenesis and that, more specifically, the ATP concentration in or near the plasma membrane may play a role in the promotion of the slow inward current associated with the plateau of the action potential. Recently Coraboeuf, Deroubaix, and Hoerter (1976) have discussed this hypothesis from the point of view of factors controlling the inward calcium current. The hypothesis also receives some support from the anatomical localization of enzymes of glycolysis; namely, in or near the sarcoplasmic reticulum and the cell membrane (Margreth, Muscatello, and Andersson-Cedergen, 1963).

However, Prasad and MacLeod (1969) were also able to show that pyruvate was able to maintain the action potential of well-oxygenated papillary muscle nearly as well as glucose. Girardier (1971) found evidence of a slower turnover between the proposed cytoplasmic pool of ATP and the ATP produced by oxidative phosphorylation. Glycolytic flux was, however, not measured, and the possibility remained that there was some residual glycolysis occurring from either exogenous glucose or endogenous glycogen. Our data on the pyruvate-perfused Langendorff heart show that mitochondrially produced ATP can maintain the action potential in the normoxic heart even though glycolysis is inhibited, but that the action potential duration is somewhat shortened.

Evaluation of Additional Evidence for Compartments of Cytoplasmic ATP

In 1969, Opie summarized the evidence favoring a small but rapidly turning over pool of "contractile ATP," which was chiefly the minor decrease of the content of ATP associated with decreased myocardial contractility, in contrast to a consistently larger decrease in CP. In 1970, Kübler and Spieckermann advanced kinetic data suggesting that ATP in the cytoplasm is contained in different compartments. Similarly, Gudbjarnason, Mathes, and Ravens (1970) formulated a functional compartmentation model to explain the observed lack of equilibrium of ATP and PCr during contraction and when the myocardium is ischemic. Further, Saks et al. (1974) put forward the hypothesis that PCr was the energy carrier from the mitochondria because its diffusion rate is significantly greater than that of ATP. Evidence from cardiac cell culture studies by Seraydarian (1974) also confirms that PCr is a unidirectional shuttle for $\sim$P between the source and the myofibrils and membranes.

Recently, however, Williamson et al. (1976) have stressed the importance of separating cytoplasmic ATP/ADP ratios from mitochondrial ratios. Using a number of assumptions, each of which needs critical evaluation, they have suggested that it is the cytoplasmic phosphate potential that changes dramatically during increased heart work, with lesser changes in the overall ATP. In spite of this, a "special activation" for mitochondrial respiratory regulation is also required. Heldt, Klingenberg, and Milovancev (1972) have provided direct evidence that the extramitochondrial ATP/ADP ratio in intact liver is considerably higher than the intramitochondrial ATP/ADP ratio. It may be argued that adenine nucleotide compartmentation could only take place in relation to cell membranes. However, enzyme complexes are thought to bind substrates or products, and, if the glycolytic enzyme complex is situated in relation to the sarcoplasmic reticulum or cell membrane, then there may yet be a physical explanation for presumed compartmentation of cytoplasmic adenine nucleotides.

Baba and Sharma (1971) studied the localization of LDH by histochemistry and have suggested that the sarcoplasmic reticulum is the site of glycolysis, especially in skeletal muscle. A preferential pathway for FFA uptake via the T-tubular system and with esterification in the sarcoplasmic reticulum has been shown by Stein and Stein (1968). Schwartz et al. (1976) have recently demonstrated that most of the glycogenolytic enzymes and glycogen are located within the sarcoplasmic reticulum. Forssmann and Girardier (1970), in a detailed study of the T system, have proposed that the Ca^{2+}-mediated excitation-contraction coupling occurs at the junction of the T system and the sarcoplasmic reticulum. Thus the control of the inward Ca^{2+} current could be modulated by the glycolytic ATP in the sarcoplasmic reticulum and the hypothesis of the electrophysiologists (Coraboeuf; Girardier and Hyde; McDonald, MacLeod, and Prasad) would have an anatomical basis.

The facts that: 1) creatine phosphokinase (CPK) has been shown to occur in the sarcoplasmic reticulum (Jacobus, 1975; Baba, Kim, and Farrell, 1976), and it would seem likely that CPK could participate in the PCr energy shuttle as proposed by Gudbjarnason et al. (1970); and 2) a Ca^{2+}-ATPase is vectorially oriented on the sarcoplasmic reticulum membrane and can both translocate Ca^{2+} inward and synthesize ATP by reverse action (de Meis, 1976) may be evidence that the sarcoplasmic reticulum is impermeable to ATP diffusion. On the other hand, evidence from studies on nerve membranes (Abood, 1969; Abood and Matsubara, 1968) has shown that ATP and not ADP is absorbed and firmly bound to membrane proteins. Although to a lesser degree than for brain tissue (64 nmol/g protein), ATP absorption and binding have been found in the heart (25 nmol ATP/g protein) and other excitatory tissue (Abood and Matsubara, 1968). Membrane-bound ATP would, therefore, constitute a nondiffusible pool. The strategically positioned glycolytic enzymes (Margreth *et al.,* 1963), especially membrane-bound phosphoglycerate kinase (Parker and Hoffman, 1967), could possibly explain a more generalized sub-membrane glycolytic ATP compartmentation.

Thus, while the anatomical and biochemical evidence for compartmentation of cytoplasmic ATP is by no means clear-cut, the available data are consonant with the concept.

Application to Promotion of Glucose Metabolism in Infarcting Tissue

In severely ischemic cells there are several lines of evidence suggesting that the severity of ischemia results in inhibition of glycolysis (Kübler and Spieckermann, 1970; Rivetto, Whitmer, and Neely, 1973; Opie, 1976), which in turn suggests that not much increase in anaerobic glycolysis is going to occur as a result of GIK (glucose-insulin-potassium) therapy. However, in the infarcting myocardium of the dog or the baboon, the existence of a collateral blood supply ensures that the predominant metabolism is still oxidative. Aerobic glycolysis would be increased if GIK increased glucose uptake by the peripheral infarct zone, as calculations suggest (Opie and Owen, 1976). Thus, it may be valuable to distinguish the effects of GIK on aerobic glycolysis (glycolytic flux with oxidative metabolism of pyruvate as its end product), and anaerobic glycolysis (with lactate and protons as ultimate end products, the protons being derived from splitting of ATP—see Gevers, 1977; Opie, 1976).

Based on arteriovenous differences across the heart, we conclude elsewhere that GIK increases aerobic glycolysis by the infarcting dog heart (Opie and Owen, 1976). Because there is preliminary evidence that glucose-fatty acid interaction in the ischemic zone is similar to that in the nonischemic zone (Opie, Owen, and Riemersma, 1973), it may be that glycolytic flux in the ischemic zone is also increased. The importance of such an increase in glycolytic ATP would lie in the data presented here and the hypothesis evolved from electrophysiological data.

Two points need emphasizing. First, GIK has many complex actions (Opie, 1975) and it is difficult to assess the role of changes of glycolytic flux in relation to all these changes. Secondly, changes in glucose metabolism are only one part of the complex changes occurring in developing human infarction. Provided the above reservations are clearly understood, a protective role for cytoplasmic glycolytic ATP may be suggested in minimizing the effects of ischemia in

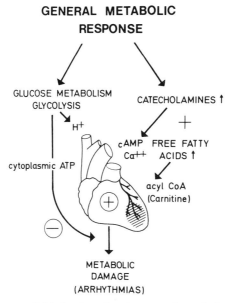

GENERAL METABOLIC RESPONSE

Figure 3. In acute myocardial infarction, there is a general metabolic response that includes glucose intolerance, increased catecholamines, and high blood free fatty acids (see Opie, 1975, for review). These changes can increase metabolic damage (indicated by + sign) and, possibly, help provoke arrhythmias. Catecholamines may exert an effect at a cellular level by cyclic AMP and/or calcium changes. Free fatty acids may act by intracellular accumulation of acyl CoA; carnitine may relieve such effects. Increased glycolysis can be induced therapeutically by administration of glucose and insulin; protons (H^+) are not expected to accumulate in moderately ischemic cells because the predominant pattern of metabolism is still oxidative (Opie, 1976) but increased provision of cytoplasmic ATP from glycolysis may be beneficial (see text).

developing infarction (Figure 3). It would be particularly informative to try to establish the links, if any, between glycolytic ATP and cytoplasmic cyclic AMP and membrane function during ischemia.

Acknowledgments The Chris Barnard Fund, the Harry Crossley Foundation, the Nelly Atkinson Fund, and the University of Cape Town are thanked for support. We thank Dr. T. Podzuweit for the measurements of cyclic AMP referred to, and for discussions.

REFERENCES

ABOOD, L. G. 1969. Calcium-adenosine triphosphate-lipid interactions and their significance in the excitatory membrane. Neurosci. Res. 2:41–70.
ABOOD, L. G., and MATSUBARA, A. 1968. Properties of an ATP-binding protein isolated from membranes of nerve endings. Biochim. Biophys. Acta 163:539–549.

BABA, N., S. KIM, and E. C. FARRELL. 1976. Histochemistry of creatine phosphokinase. J. Mol. Cell. Cardiol. 8:599–617.

BABA, N., and SHARMA, H. 1971. Histochemistry of lactic dehydrogenase in heart and pectoralis muscles of rat. J. Cell. Biol. 51:621–635.

BING, R. J. 1965. Cardiac metabolism. Physiol. Rev. 45:171–213.

BITTAR, E. E., CHAMBERS, G., and SCHULTZ, R. 1976. Mode of stimulation by adenosine 3':5'-cyclic monophosphate of the sodium efflux in barnacle muscle fibres. J. Physiol. (London) 257:561–579.

BRICKNELL, O. L., and OPIE, L. H. 1977. The effects of substrates on lactate dehydrogenase release and arrhythmias in the underperfused and in the reperfused isolated rat heart. Submitted for publication.

CHENEVAL, J-P., HYDE, A., BLONDEL, B., and GIRARDIER, L. 1972. Heart cells in culture: Metabolism, action potential and transmembrane ionic movements. J. Physiol. (Paris) 64:413–430.

CORABOEUF, E., DEROUBAIX, E., and HOERTER, J. 1976. Control of ionic permeabilities in normal and ischemic heart. Circ. Res. 38: (Suppl. 1)92–97.

De MEIS, L. 1976. Regulation of steady state level of phosphoenzyme and ATP synthesis in sarcoplasmic reticulum vesicles during reversal of the Ca^{2+}-pump. J. Biol. Chem. 251: 2055–2062.

FORSSMANN, W. G., and GIRARDIER, L. 1970. A study of the T system in rat heart. J. Cell. Biol. 44:1–19.

GEVERS, W. 1977. Generation of protons by metabolic processes in heart cells. J. Mol. Cell. Cardiol. In press.

GIRARDIER, L. 1971. Dynamic energy partition in cultured heart cells. Cardiology 56:1–6.

GUDBJARNASON, S., MATHES, P., and RAVENS, K. G. 1970. Functional compartmentation of ATP and creatine phosphate in heart muscle. J. Mol. Cell. Cardiol. 1:325–339.

HEARSE, D. J., STEWART, D. A., and BRAIMBRIDGE, M. V. 1975. Hypothermic arrest and potassium arrest. Metabolic and myocardial protection during elective cardiac arrest. Circ. Res. 36:481–489.

HELDT, H. W., KLINGENBERG, M., and MILOVANCEV, M. 1972. Differences between the ATP/ADP ratios in the mitochondrial matrix and in the extramitochondrial space. Eur. J. Biochem. 30:434–440.

HYDE, A., CHENEVAL, J-P., BLONDEL, B., and GIRARDIER, L. 1972. Electrophysiological correlates of energy metabolism in cultured rat heart cells. J. Physiol. (Paris) 64:269–292.

JACOBUS, W. E. 1975. Heart creatine kinase: Heterogeneous composition of the mammalian M-B isoenzyme. J. Mol. Cell. Cardiol. 7:783–791.

KLINGENBERG, M., and PFAFF, E. 1966. Structural and functional compartmentation in mitochondria. In J. M. Tager, S. Papa, E. Quagliariello, and E. C. Slater (eds.), Regulation of Metabolic Processes in Mitochondria, pp. 180–201. Elsevier Publishing Company, Amsterdam.

KREBS, H. A., and HENSELEIT, K. 1932. Untersuchungen über die Harnstoffbildung im Tierkörper. Hoppe Seylers Z. Physiol. Chem. 210:33–66.

KÜBLER, W., and SPIECKERMANN, P. G. 1970. Regulation of glycolysis in ischemic and anoxic myocardium. J. Mol. Cell. Cardiol. 1:351–377.

LANGENDORFF, O. 1895. Untersuchungen am überlebenden Säugethierherzen. Pfluegers Arch. 61:291–332.

LOCHNER, A., OPIE, L. H., OWEN, P., KOTZE, J. C. N., BRUYNEEL, K., and GEVERS, W. 1975. Oxidative phosphorylation in infarcting baboon and dog myocardium: Effects of mitochondrial isolation and incubation media. J. Mol. Cell. Cardiol. 7:203–217.

MARGRETH, A., MUSCATELLO, U., and ANDERSSON-CEDERGEN, E. 1963. A morphological and biochemical study on the regulation of carbohydrate metabolism in muscle cell. Exper. Cell Res. 32:484–509.

McDONALD, T. F., HUNTER, E. G., and MacLEOD, D. P. 1971. Adenosinetriphosphate partition in cardiac muscle with respect to transmembrane electrical activity. Pfluegers Arch. 322:95–108.

OPIE, L. H. 1969. Metabolism of the heart in health and disease. Part II. Amer. Heart J. 77:100–122.

OPIE, L. H. 1974. Myocardial energy metabolism. Adv. Cardiol. 12:70–83.

OPIE, L. H. 1975. Metabolism of free fatty acids, glucose and catecholamines in acute myocardial infarction: Relation to myocardial ischaemia and infarct size. Amer. J. Cardiol. 36:938–953.

OPIE, L. H. 1976. Effects of regional ischemia on metabolism of glucose and fatty acids: Relative rates of aerobic and anaerobic energy production during myocardial infarction and comparison with effects of anoxia. Circ. Res. 38: (Suppl. 1)52–68.

OPIE, L. H., and OWEN, P. 1976. Effect of glucose-insulin-potassium infusions on arterio-venous differences of glucose and of free fatty acids and on tissue metabolic changes in dogs with developing myocardial infarction. Amer. J. Cardiol. 38:310–321.

OPIE, L. H., OWEN, P., and RIEMERSMA, R. A. 1973. Relative rates of oxidation of glucose and free fatty acids by ischaemic and non-ischaemic myocardium after coronary artery ligation in the dog. Eur. J. Clin. Invest. 3:419–435.

PARKER, J. S., and HOFFMAN, J. F. 1967. The role of membrane phosphoglycerate kinase in the control of glycolytic rate by active cation transport in human red blood cells. J. Gen. Physiol. 50:893–916.

PODZUWEIT, T., LUBBE, W. F., and OPIE, L. H. 1976. Cyclic adenosine monophosphate, ventricular fibrillation, and antiarrhythmic drugs. Lancet 1:341–342.

PRASAD, K., and MacLEOD, D. P. 1969. Influence of glucose on the transmembrane action potential of guinea pig papillary muscle. Metabolic inhibitors, ouabain, $CaCl_2$, and their interaction with glucose, sympathomimetic amines, and aminophylline. Circ. Res. 24:939–950.

ROVETTO, M. J., WHITMER, J. T., and NEELY, J. R. 1973. Comparison of the effects of anoxia and whole heart ischaemia on carbohydrate utilization in isolated working rat hearts. Circ. Res. 32:699–711.

SAKS, V. A., CHERNOUSOVA, G. B., VORONKOV, I. I., SMIRNOV, V. N., and CHAZOV, E. I. 1974. Study of energy transport mechanism in myocardial cells. Circ. Res. 35:138–149.

SCHNEIDER, J. A., and SPERELAKIS, N. 1974. The demonstration of energy dependence of isoproterenol-induced transcellular Ca^{2+} current in isolated perfused guinea pig hearts; an explanation for the mechanical failure of ischemic myocardium. J. Surg. Res. 16:389–403.

SCHWARTZ, A., PITTS, B. J. R., LANE, L. K., ENTMAN, M. L., and WOOD, J. M. 1976. The Na^+,K^+-ATPase enzyme system and the sarcoplasmic reticulum: modulators of calcium in the heart. Presented at the 8th International Meeting of the International Study Group for Research in Cardiac Metabolism, 26–29 May, 1976, Tokyo, Japan.

SERAYDARIAN, M. W. 1974. Studies on the control of energy metabolism in mammalian cardiac muscle cells in culture. In P. E. Roy and P. Harris (eds.), Recent Advances in Studies on Cardiac Structure and Metabolism. Vol. 8. The Cardiac Sarcoplasm, pp. 181–190. University Park Press, Baltimore.

STEIN, O., and STEIN, Y. 1968. Lipid synthesis, intracellular transport and storage. III. Electron microscopic radioautographic study of the rat heart perfused with tritiated oleic acid. J. Cell. Biol. 36:63–77.

WATANABE, A. N., and BESCH, H. R., JR. 1974. Cyclic adenosine monophosphate modulation of slow calcium influx channels in guinea pig hearts. Circ. Res. 35:316–324.

WILLIAMSON, J. R. 1965. Glycolytic control mechanisms: I. Inhibition of glycolysis by acetate and pyruvate in the isolated, perfused rat heart. J. Biol. Chem. 240:2308–2321.

WILLIAMSON, J. R., FORD, C., ILLINGWORTH, J., and SAFER, B. 1976. Coordination of citric acid cycle activity with electron transport flux. Circ. Res. 38:(Suppl. 1)39–51.

Mailing address:
Dr. O. L. Bricknell
MRC Ischaemic Heart Disease Research Unit,
Department of Medicine, Groote Schuur Hospital,
Cape Town (South Africa).

Recent Advances in Studies on
Cardiac Structure and Metabolism, Volume 11
Heart Function and Metabolism
Edited by T. Kobayashi, T. Sano, and N. S. Dhalla
Copyright 1978 University Park Press Baltimore

CONTROL OF ENERGY PRODUCTION IN CARDIAC MUSCLE: EFFECTS OF ISCHEMIA IN ACIDOSIS

J. R. WILLIAMSON, C. STEENBERGEN, G. DELEEUW, and C. BARLOW

Department of Biochemistry and Biophysics,
University of Pennsylvania, Philadelphia, Pennsylvania, USA

SUMMARY

Evidence is summarized indicating that mitochondrial respiration and citric acid cycle activity in the intact heart are controlled by the cytosolic phosphate potential and mitochondrial NAD oxidation-reduction state. Data are presented showing that the effect of respiratory acidosis is greater than that of metabolic acidosis in inhibiting left ventricular pressure development in the perfused rat heart, because of a greater fall of intracellular pH under the former conditions. Respiratory acidosis is shown to be readily associated with tissue hypoxia as a result of an increased vascular resistance and diminished flow rate through the coronary circulation. In nonischemic respiratory acidosis, the rate of ATP production is well balanced by the rate of ATP utilization, and tissue ATP and creatine-P levels remain approximately normal. Partially ischemic respiratory acidosis was associated with low tissue levels of ATP and creatine-P and high tissue levels of lactate and NADH. Ischemic areas with sharp border zones were visualized during and after an abrupt decrease of perfusion fluid pH by directly photographing NADH fluorescence from the surface of perfused hearts. Reversal of the hypodynamic state with partially ischemic respiratory acidosis could not be achieved by augmenting the coronary flow by means of an external pump. The demonstration of the existence of sharp zones of high pyridine nucleotide fluorescence adjacent to normal zones indicates a great heterogeneity of coronary perfusion and the existence of steep oxygen gradients in the intact heart.

INTRODUCTION

Respiratory Control in the Intact Heart

The left ventricle of the heart is capable of responding to a wide range of work loads induced by an increase of preload atrial filling pressure or afterload of aortic pressure. As cardiac work increases, the demand for oxygen increases proportionately, and is met by autoregulatory increase of coronary blood flow and an increased oxygen extraction. In normal well-oxygenated myocardium the

Supported by contract NO1-HV-52995 under the Myocardial Infarction Program, National Heart and Lung Institute, and National Institutes of Health Grants HL-14461, HL-18708, and GM-07170.

rate of ATP generation by oxidative metabolism is strictly controlled by the rate of ATP utilization, and stores of high energy phosphate intermediates in the tissue are well maintained.

The isolated perfused rat heart cannulated at the left atrium and the aorta (Neely et al., 1967) has proved to be a very useful preparation for studying functional correlations between mechanical performance and energy metabolism (Neely and Morgan, 1974). Using a modification of this perfusion method that allowed the left atrial filling rate and ventricular output to be varied over a wide range, previous studies from this laboratory have shown, for instance, a linear relationship between left ventricular filling rate and total myocardial oxygen consumption or ATP production rate (Williamson et al., 1976a). In the presence of insulin to facilitate glucose entry, glucose oxidation increased in proportion to oxygen uptake and accounted for most of the respiratory fuel. With fatty acids also present, glucose oxidation was greatly inhibited at all ventricular filling rates (Williamson et al., 1976a) and fatty acids replaced glucose as the respiratory fuel (Oram, Bennetch, and Neely, 1973). In further studies, hearts were perfused with 1 mM pyruvate in order to oxidize cytosolic and reduce mitochondrial pyridine nucleotides, and subjected to a carefully controlled four-fold increase of work load by raising the left atrial filling pressure (Illingworth et al., 1975). Under these conditions, the pyridine nucleotide fluorescence, as measured from the surface of the heart, decreased rapidly as ventricular output and oxygen consumption increased, indicating a rapid oxidation of mitochondrial pyridine nucleotides as flux through the phosphorylating electron transport chain increased. Analyses of hearts frozen rapidly during the first minute after the work transition showed a small fall of the ATP/ADP ratio, but a larger decrease of the creatine-P/creatine ratio and increase of inorganic phosphate. Thus the phosphate potential (ATP/ADP $\times$ Pi), calculated from total tissue metabolite contents, decreased to half its initial value within the first 20 sec. By taking into account the fact that adenine nucleotides in the cell are compartmented between the cytosolic and mitochondrial spaces such that the cytosolic ATP/ADP ratio is much greater than that in the mitochondria, the observed four-fold increase of respiration after the work transition correlated well with a four-fold decrease of the cytosolic phosphate potential (Williamson et al., 1976a). Furthermore, the calculated cytosolic ADP concentration (50 μM) was commensurate with values found to give half-maximum stimulation of respiration in isolated mitochondria in the presence of ATP (Davis and Lumeng, 1975).

The conclusion reached from these studies is that mitochondrial respiration in the intact heart (as in isolated mitochondria) is controlled by the cytosolic phosphate potential, and that coordination between the rate of delivery of reducing equivalents from the citric acid cycle and their oxidation by the respiratory chain is achieved largely as a result of alterations of the mitochondrial pyridine nucleotide oxidation-reduction state (see LaNoue, Nicklas, and Williamson, 1970; Williamson and LaNoue, 1975). Similarly, negative inotropic agents that inhibit Ca^{2+} flux across the sarcolemma, such as La^{3+}, verapamil, or ruthenium red, produce a fall of oxygen consumption as left ventricular pressure declines and a reduction of pyridine nucleotide oxidation-reduction state (Williamson et al., 1974; unpublished observations). The ATP and creatine-P contents of the heart remained high, provided the coronary flow was maintained (Williamson et al., 1974), indicating that mitochondrial ATP generation is well coupled to the rate of ATP utilization at low as well as high rates of cardiac work.

METHOD AND RESULTS

Effects of Respiratory and
Metabolic Acidosis on Cardiac Contractility and Metabolism

It is well recognized that acidosis produces a negative inotropic effect on cardiac muscle, although the molecular mechanisms for this effect are not completely understood (Tsien, 1976; Williamson et al., 1976b). We have previously demonstrated (Williamson et al., 1975) that metabolic acidosis (low bicarbonate concentration) causes a much smaller and slower decrease of left ventricular pressure than respiratory acidosis in the perfused rat heart. Figure 1 demonstrates the effect on left ventricular pressure development of rapid transitions of the perfusion fluid from an artificial buffer to a bicarbonate-CO_2 buffer at three different pH values, 7.0, 6.8, and 6.6 (see figure legend for experimental details). It is seen from Figure 1 that perfusion with the bicarbonate-CO_2 buffer (respiratory acidosis) caused a rapid further fall of left ventricular pressure, even though the pH of the perfusion fluid remained unchanged.

Table 1 shows that with artifical buffer perfusion (25 mM MES) the intracellular pH fell to a smaller degree than with respiratory acidosis when the pH of the perfusion fluid was decreased to a similar extent. Furthermore, provided oxygen delivery to the myocardium was adequate, the tissue contents of high energy phosphate intermediates remained elevated with both high pCO_2 and artificial buffer acidosis, while lactate accumulated in the tissue to only a small extent. The conclusion reached from these studies is that the greater degree of inhibition of ventricular tension development observed with respiratory, rather than metabolic, acidosis at the same extracellular pH value is due to a greater fall of intracellular pH under the former conditions. This is presumably caused by the higher permeability of the cell membrane to CO_2 than to H^+. A possible two-site explanation for the effects of H^+ on cardiac muscle (see Williamson et al., 1975; Williamson et al., 1976b) is that extracellular $[H^+]$ affects the Ca^{2+} entry per beat during the slow phase of the action potential,

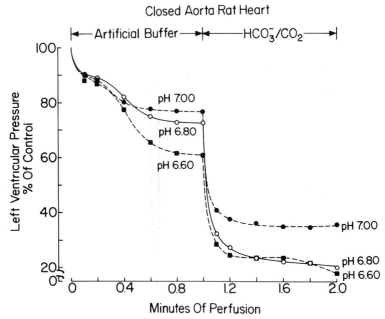

Figure 1. Effect of CO_2 versus H^+ on myocardial contractility. Rat hearts were perfused initially with Krebs bicarbonate medium equilibrated at pH 7.4 with 95% O_2 and 5% CO_2 containing 1.25 mM Ca^{2+}, 5 mM glucose, and 10^{-2} U/ml of insulin under conditions of closed aorta perfusion (Williamson *et al.*, 1976b). At time zero, perfusion was switched to artificial buffer equilibrated with 100% O_2 in which the bicarbonate of Krebs medium was replaced by 5 mM MES (2-*N*-morpholino ethane sulfonic acid; pK_a 6.15), 5 mM MOPS (2-*N*-morpholino propane sulfonic acid; pK_a 7.2), and 5 mM Tris [tris(hydroxymethyl)-aminomethane; pK_a 8.3]. After 1 min, perfusion was switched to 25 mM bicarbonate medium equilibrated with O_2 and CO_2 in order to provide the designated pH values.

while intracellular $[H^+]$ affects the availability of intracellular Ca^{2+} to troponin, or, more directly, Ca^{2+} binding to troponin in the actomyosin complex.

Ischemic and Nonischemic Respiratory Acidosis

Table 1 also shows the effect of oxygen deficiency developing during respiratory acidosis. This ischemic respiratory acidosis is to be distinguished from non-ischemic respiratory acidosis, in which an adequate oxygen supply was ensured by retrograde pumping through the aorta to maintain the coronary flow rate above 7 ml/min. Tissue hypoxia was evidenced by elevated tissue contents of lactate and NADH and decreased contents of ATP and creatine-P, accompanied by a further fall of intracellular pH. The cytosolic pyridine nucleotides also became more reduced, as evidenced by a rise of the lactate/pyruvate ratio. Ischemic respiratory acidosis may be distinguished from high flow anoxia by a greater accumulation of tissue lactate and a lower intracellular pH (Table 1).

Table 1. Effects of respiratory and metabolic acidosis in perfused rat hearts[a]

Perfusion condition	pH_e	pH_i	Lactate	ATP	Creatine-P	NADH	Lactate/Pyruvate	ATP/ADP
			μmol/g dry wt					
Bicarbonate control	7.33	7.05 ±0.02	2.24 ±0.4	22.4 ±0.7	29.7 ±0.9	0.27 ±0.06	16 ± 4	6.5
Nonischemic respiratory acidosis	6.75	6.76 ±0.03	4.5 ±0.5	21.6 ±0.7	26.0 ±1.3	0.28 ±0.06	70 ±6	5.7
Ischemic respiratory acidosis	6.79	6.69 ±0.04	16.5 ±1.9	16.1 ±1.2	10.9 ±1.2	1.28 ±0.03	131 ±9	2.4
High flow anoxia	7.21	6.93 ±0.03	12.9 ±0.8	16.8 ±0.8	3.5 ±0.6	1.85 ±0.12	167 ±36	2.8
MES buffer control	7.21	7.16 ±0.03	3.8 ±0.8	23.7 ±0.8	32.9 ±0.6			6.3
MES buffer acidosis	6.77	7.01 ±0.03	6.0 ±2.0	23.3 ±1.2	32.9 ±1.5			6.6

[a]Hearts paced at 300 beats/min were perfused for 15 min with Krebs bicarbonate medium containing 5 mM glucose and 10^{-2} U/ml of insulin at pH 7.4 followed by a further 3-min perfusion at the lowered pH. In nonischemic respiratory acidosis coronary flow was maintained by retrograde aortic pumping whenever the flow fell below 7 ml/min. [^{3}H]Sorbitol was used to measure the extracellular space and [^{14}C]DMO distribution between extracellular and intracellular spaces was used to calculate the intracellular pH. Respiratory acidosis was induced by an increase of pCO_2. Metabolic acidosis was induced by use of 25 mM MES (2-N-morpholino ethane sulfonic acid) to replace bicarbonate and by adjusting the pH with HCl. pH_e refers to the effluent pH, while pH_i refers to the intracellular pH.

The onset of ischemia with respiratory acidosis was associated with diminished contractile performance, as illustrated in Figure 2. The left side of Figure 2 shows a pH transition from 7.4 to 6.8 that was induced by increasing the CO_2 content of the gas mixture equilibrating the reservoir supplying the left atrium. This caused a gradual fall of the effluent pH, compared with an abrupt pH transition produced by switching to bicarbonate buffer pre-equilibrated at pH 6.8, as in the trace shown on the right side of Figure 2. Recordings of the effluent pH and percent effluent oxygen tension for this experiment are shown in Figure 3. Partial recovery of left ventricular performance, coronary flow rate, and effluent oxygen tension (see Figures 2 and 3) was achieved in the slow pH transition by a small decrease of the rate of electrical pacing, as indicated in the bottom trace of Figure 2. With the rapid pH transition, left ventricular pressure remained depressed, coronary flow fell to about 1 ml/min, and the effluent oxygen concentration fell to zero.

Whenever oxygen delivery to the myocardium falls below the oxygen requirements for the prevailing workload, oxygen deficiency in the tissue is revealed by an increased state of reduction of the pyridine nucleotides and

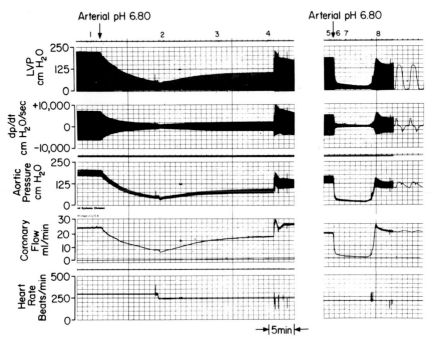

Figure 2. Comparison of nonischemic and ischemic respiratory acidosis transitions. Rat hearts were perfused with Krebs bicarbonate medium as in Figure 1. The numbers at the top of the figure refer to the times when photographs of the heart were taken (see Figures 4 and 5).

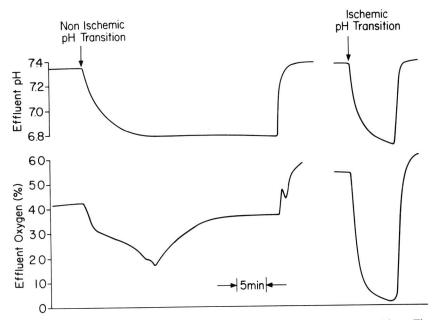

Figure 3. Comparison of nonischemic and ischemic respiratory acidosis transitions. The experiment was the same as shown in Figure 2.

respiratory chain components. Tissue pyridine nucleotide oxidation-reduction changes may be monitored on a continuous basis by surface fluorometry (cf. Figure 6), or by a new technique of flash photography, using xenon flash tubes fitted with Corning 5840 filters to provide 330–380 nm excitation, and Corning 9788 plus Wratten 45 filters over the camera lens to allow transmission of NADH fluorescence in the 430–510 nm region to the camera film (Barlow and Chance, 1976; Williamson *et al.*, 1977). In the experiment shown in Figure 2, such photographs of the heart were made at times denoted by the numbers at the top of the figure. Figure 4 shows four pictures taken during the slow pH transition. White areas in the photographs denote areas of high pyridine nucleotide fluorescence and therefore a high level of tissue NADH. Picture 1 shows a uniform texture of the heart surface in the control perfusion, except for a reflection artifact in the upper left side, indicating uniform oxygenation of the tissue and pyridine nucleotide oxidation-reduction state. In picture 2, taken at the time of the greatest fall of left ventricular pressure, many discrete areas of localized ischemia are visualized. These disappear as coronary perfusion is restored (pictures 3 and 4), even though the effluent pH remains constant at pH 6.8 (see Figure 3). On the other hand, with the rapid pH transition, Figure 5 shows that areas of ischemia develop rapidly and grow in size and density as perfusion continues. As

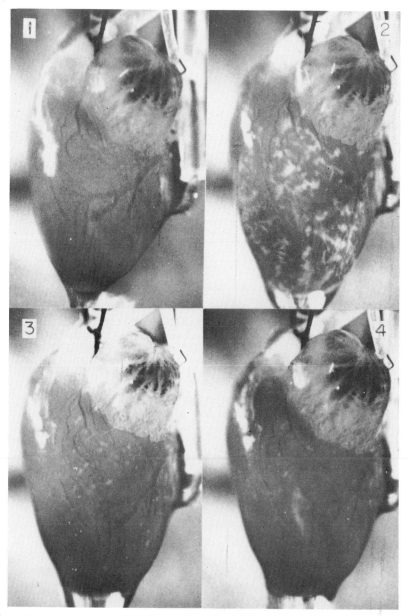

Figure 4. Photographs of NADH fluorescence from the perfused rat heart during a nonischemic (final state) pH transition (see Figures 2 and 3).

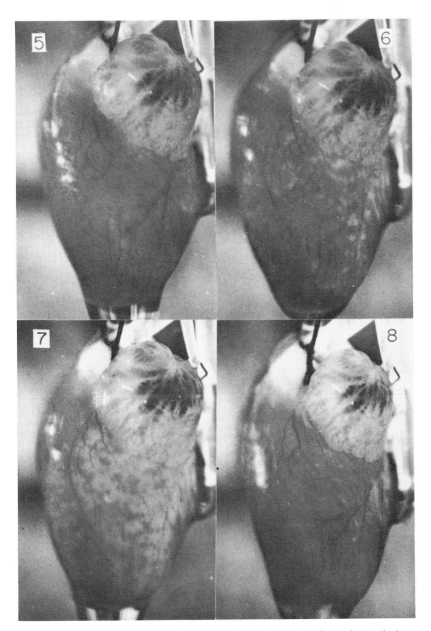

Figure 5. Photographs of NADH fluorescence from the perfused rat heart during an ischemic (final state) pH transition (see Figures 2 and 3).

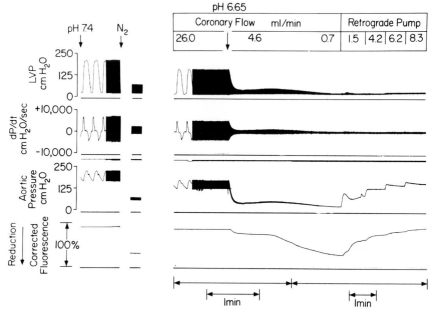

Figure 6. Respiratory acidosis pH transition followed by retrograde pumping. Rat hearts were perfused with Krebs bicarbonate medium, as in Figure 1. The left side of the figure shows anoxic calibrations, where N_2 replaced O_2 in the equilibrating gas mixture.

shown in picture 8 of Figure 5, these areas disappear when perfusion at pH 7.4 is restored.

Ischemia during respiratory acidosis can be prevented or reversed by augmentation of the coronary flow by means of a retrograde pump feeding fluid into the aorta and hence to the coronary circulation. This effect is depicted in Figure 6, which illustrates a rapid pH transition from pH 7.4 to 6.65. Left ventricular pressure, dP/dt, and aortic pressure fell rapidly, while pyridine fluorescence increased to almost the fully anaerobic value after a short delay. By this time the coronary flow had fallen to below 1 ml/min. Augmentation of the coronary flow in stages to above 8 ml/min produced reoxidation of the pyridine nucleotides but failed to restore contractile function. Thus, it is the increased intracellular [H⁺] *per se,* rather than tissue hypoxia or ATP deficiency, that accounts for the failure of ventricular pressure development in acidosis (see also Williamson *et al.,* 1975).

REFERENCES

BARLOW, C., and CHANCE, B. 1976. Ischemic areas in perfused rat hearts: Measurements by NADH fluorescence photography. Science 193:909–910.

DAVIS, E. J., and LUMENG, L. 1975. Relationships between the phosphorylation potentials generated by liver into mitochondria and respiratory state under conditions of adenosine diphosphate control. J. Biol. Chem. 250:2275–2282.

ILLINGWORTH, J. A., FORD, W. C. L., KOBAYASHI, K., and WILLIAMSON, J. R. 1975. Regulation of myocardial energy metabolism. In P. E. Roy and P. Harris (eds.), The Cardiac Sarcoplasm, pp. 271–290. University Park Press, Baltimore, Md.

LaNOUE, K. F., NICKLAS, W. J., and WILLIAMSON, J. R. 1970. Control of citric acid cycle activity in rat heart mitochondria. J. Biol. Chem. 245:102–111.

NEELY, J. R., LIEBERMEISTER, H., BATTERSBY, E. J., and MORGAN, H. E. 1967. Effect of pressure development on oxygen consumption by isolated rat heart. Amer. J. Physiol. 212:804–814.

NEELY, J. R., and MORGAN, H. E. 1974. Relationship between carbohydrate and lipid metabolism and the energy balance of the heart. Annu. Rev. Physiol. 36:413–459.

ORAM, J. R., BENNETCH, S. L., and NEELY, J. R. 1973. Regulation of fatty acid utilization in isolated perfused rat hearts. J. Biol. Chem. 248:5299–5309.

TSIEN, R. W. 1976. Possible effects of hydrogen ions in ischemic myocardium. Circ. 53 (Suppl. I):14–16.

WILLIAMSON, J. R., and LaNOUE, K. F. 1975. Feedback control of the citric acid cycle. 1976a. Coordination of citric acid cycle activity with electron transport flux. In H. Morgan and L. O. K. Wildenthal (eds.), Regulation of Cardiac Metabolism. Circ. Res. (Suppl. I) 38:39–51.

WILLIAMSON, J. R., and LANOUE, K. F. 1975. Feedback control of the citric acid cycle. Pan-American Association of Biochemical Societies Revista 4:53–62.

WILLIAMSON, J. R., SCHAFFER, S. W., FORD, C., and SAFER, B. 1976b. Contribution of tissue acidosis to ischemic injury in the perfused rat heart. Circ. 53 (Suppl. I):3–14.

WILLIAMSON, J. R., SAFER, B., RICH, T., SCHAFFER, S., and KOBAYASHI, K. 1975. Effects of acidosis on myocardial contractility and metabolism. Acta Med. Scand. (Suppl.) 587:95–111.

WILLIAMSON, J. R., SCHAFFER, S. W., SCARPA, A., and SAFER, B. 1974. Investigation of the calcium cycle in perfused rat and frog hearts. In N. S. Dhalla (ed.), Myocardial Biology, Vol. 4, pp. 375–392. University Park Press, Baltimore, Md.

WILLIAMSON, J. R., STEENBERGEN, C., RICH, T., DELEEUW, G., BARLOW, C., and CHANCE, B. 1977. The nature of ischemic injury in cardiac tissue. Spectrum Publications, Inc., Holliswood, N.Y. In press.

Mailing address:
Dr. J. R. Williamson,
Department of Biochemistry and Biophysics,
Medical School G3,
University of Pennsylvania,
Philadelphia, Pennsylvania 19174 (USA).

Recent Advances in Studies on
Cardiac Structure and Metabolism, Volume 11
Heart Function and Metabolism
Edited by T. Kobayashi, T. Sano, and N. S. Dhalla
Copyright 1978   University Park Press   Baltimore

ALTERATION IN CALCIUM METABOLISM IN MITOCHONDRIA ISOLATED FROM ISCHEMIC AND REPERFUSED MYOCARDIUM

C. F. PENG, M. L. MURPHY,
J. J. KANE, and K. D. STRAUB

Veterans Administration Hospital and
University of Arkansas for Medical Sciences,
Little Rock, Arkansas, USA

SUMMARY

This study determines the effect of ischemia and reperfusion on energy-linked Ca^{2+} uptake by myocardial mitochondria. The left anterior descending coronary artery was occluded in 14 mature pigs for 2 hr. In seven animals the ligature was released and the ischemic zone reperfused for 2 additional hours. After sacrifice, mitochondrial function was measured in normal and reperfused or ischemic areas of the left ventricle, using a polarographic method. Mitochondria were prepared without EDTA by standard procedures and Ca^{2+} uptake measured by $^{45}Ca^{2+}$ isotope tracer. Uptake of Ca^{2+} by mitochondria derived from ischemic myocardium is markedly impaired with or without phosphate. Reperfusion may accentuate this impairment. The presence of exogenous Ca^{2+} inhibits the ability of ischemic or reperfused mitochondria to phosphorylate ADP.

INTRODUCTION

A defect in electron flow in mitochondria isolated from ischemic pig myocardium has been previously demonstrated in this laboratory, and this impairment was not improved by 2 hr of reperfusion (Kane *et al.,* 1975). Furthermore, it has been noted that a significant change in calcium concentration did not occur in permanently ischemic myocardial cells, in contrast to the report that calcium is greatly increased in ischemic myocardium and mitochondria when reperfused (Shen and Jennings, 1972). The increase of mitochondrial calcium concentration as well as the defect in electron flow implies that all energetic functions of mitochondria could be impaired. The present studies were undertaken to examine the effect of acute ischemia and reperfusion on energy-linked calcium uptake by heart mitochondria. The effect of calcium on oxidative phosphorylation by mitochondria from ischemic and reperfused myocardium was also investigated.

METHODS

The pig was chosen as the experimental model because the coronary artery pattern is similar to the heart of man. Myocardial ischemia and reperfusion were performed by ligation and recirculation as described, and the tissue samples were minced and homogenized by methods similar to those previously outlined (Kane *et al.*, 1975). Mitochondria were isolated and suspended in a medium containing 0.25 M sucrose and 0.05 M Tris buffer at pH 7.4. Calcium uptake and oxidative phosphorylation were determined by the Millipore filter technique and polarographic method, respectively.

RESULTS

Calcium uptake by mitochondria isolated from normal, ischemic, and ischemic-reperfused myocardium is shown in Table 1. Calcium uptake by ischemic mitochondria was greatly reduced regardless of whether glutamate, malate plus pyruvate, or succinate plus rotenone was used as substrate. Mitochondria obtained from ischemic-reperfused myocardium accumulated even less Ca^{2+} than ischemic mitochondria. In the presence of Pi (inorganic phosphate), mitochondria from ischemic myocardium accumulated about 51 to 58 nmol Ca^{2+}/mg

Table 1. Effect of acute ischemia and reperfusion on respiratory-linked Ca^{2+} uptake by mitochondria*

Substrate used	Phosphate (mM)	Ca^{2+} accumulation by mitochondria (nmol/mg protein)		
		Normal mitochondria	Ischemic mitochondria	Ischemic-reperfused mitochondria
		(17)**	(10)**	(7)**
Glutamate	0	67 ± 11†	22 ± 9	18 ± 13
Malate and pyruvate	0	74 ± 12	37 ± 11	16 ± 6
Succinate plus rotenone	0	65 ± 18	23 ± 15	18 ± 4
Glutamate	3	172 ± 33	51 ± 15	22 ± 17
Malate and pyruvate	3	175 ± 22	53 ± 10	26 ± 6
Succinate plus rotenone	3	181 ± 26	58 ± 30	37 ± 14

*Experimental medium contained 10 mM Tris buffer, pH 7.4, 80 mM KCl, 100 mM sucrose, glutamate (10 mM), malate and pyruvate (10 mM), succinate (10 mM) plus rotenone (6 μg/ml), Pi (3 mM). Mitochondria (2.0–2.5 mg protein) and $^{45}Ca^{2+}$ (400 nmol) were added in the reaction mixture at 30°C. Ca^{2+} uptake was measured 2 min after Ca^{2+} was added.
**Number of animals used.
†Mean and standard deviation.

protein while normal mitochondria accumulated as much as 172–181 nmol Ca^{2+}/mg protein with the substrates used. The capacity of ischemic mitochondria to accumulate Ca^{2+} in the presence of Pi was further damaged by 2 hr reperfusion of ischemic myocardium (22, 26, and 37 nmol Ca^{2+}/mg protein with glutamate, malate plus pyruvate, and succinate, respectively). Hence, the impairment of Ca^{2+} uptake by ischemic and ischemic-reperfused mitochondria in the presence of Pi is more pronounced than in the absence of Pi. Calcium uptake results are probably more representative of the *in vivo* condition in the presence of Pi than in the absence of Pi.

Since ischemic myocardial mitochondria shows a defect in the ability to accumulate Ca^{2+}, it is thus interesting to see whether Ca^{2+} has any functional effect on ischemic myocardial mitochondria. The effect of Ca^{2+} on ADP-stimulated oxygen consumption by mitochondria is shown in Figure 1. It can be seen that addition of 400 nmol Ca^{2+} slows ADP-induced mitochondrial respiration in all mitochondrial preparations. Furthermore, the state 3–4 transition that occurs in normal mitochondria is completely eliminated in ischemic and ischemic-reperfused mitochondria. Thus, additional oxygen consumption related to ADP-phosphorylation cannot be identified in ischemic and ischemic-reperfused mitochondria after addition of Ca^{2+}.

The efficiency of oxidative phosphorylation in mitochondria as determined by ADP/0 ratios is summarized in Table 2. The ADP/0 ratio in normal mitochondria is not significantly altered by the addition of Ca^{2+}, but in ischemic and ischemic-reperfused mitochondria there is no stimulation of oxygen consumption by ADP. Therefore, calculation of ADP/0 ratio is not applicable. These results indicate that the ability of ischemic mitochondria to phosphorylate ADP is inhibited by exogenous Ca^{2+}.

DISCUSSION

This study demonstrates that the energy-linked Ca^{2+} accumulation by mitochondria from ischemic and ischemic-reperfused myocardium is markedly impaired, and that ADP phosphorylation by ischemic mitochondria is completely inhibited by ionic Ca^{2+}. The findings imply that the efficiency of energy production by myocardial mitochondria is closely related to the efficiency of mitochondria in accumulating Ca^{2+} from the cytosol. The marked decrease in the rate of Ca^{2+} uptake by ischemic mitochondria was demonstrated by Schwartz et al. (1973), while the reduction of the steady-state amount of Ca^{2+} accumulation by ischemic mitochondria with or without Pi was observed in this study. In the absence of permeable anions, such as inorganic phosphate or acetate, Ca^{2+} is thought to bind to the mitochondrial membrane instead of being transported to the internal matrix area (Schuster and Olson, 1974). A decrease in energy-linked Ca^{2+} uptake by ischemic mitochondria in the absence of Pi therefore implies that

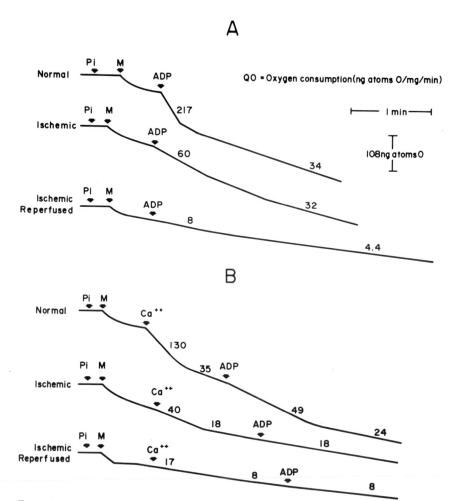

Figure 1. Effect of calcium on ADP induced mitochondrial respiration (glutamate substrate). Experimental conditions were the same as in Table 1. Inorganic phosphate (Pi), mitochondria (M), ADP and Ca²⁺ were added to incubation mixture as indicated. Numbers adjacent to each trace represent the rate of oxygen consumption.

either the alteration of membranous Ca^{2+} binding sites occurred in ischemic mitochondria or ischemic mitochondria contain higher endogenous Ca^{2+} than normal mitochondria. The release of Ca^{2+} from ischemic mitochondria during steady-state respiration has been demonstrated by Schwartz *et al.* (1973). This suggests that a marked reduction of Ca^{2+} accumulation is attributed to the leakage of Ca^{2+} from ischemic mitochondria. In addition, ischemic mitochondria have been shown to be deficient in cytochrome components (Schwartz *et al.*,

Table 2. Effect of calcium on oxidative phosphorylation in myocardial mitochondria (glutamate substrate)

Mitochondria	Addition of calcium (nmol)	No. of animals	Rate of respiration (ng atoms O/mg/min)	ADP/O ratio*	R.C.R.†
Normal	0	8	217 ± 30	2.9 ± 0.4	6.5 ± 1.0
	400	8	59 ± 16	2.5 ± 0.6	2.0 ± 0.4
Ischemic	0	4	72 ± 14	1.7 ± 0.1	1.8 ± 0.4
	400	4	20 ± 2	NA‡	NA‡
Ischemic-	0	4	12 ± 3	NA‡	NA‡
reperfused	400	4	10 ± 2	NA‡	NA‡

*The ratio of nmol ADP phosphorylated to ng atoms oxygen consumed.

†The ratio of oxygen consumed in the presence of ADP to oxygen consumed after
complete phosphorylation of ADP.

‡Not applicable.

1973), Krebs cycle intermediates, and adenine nucleotides (Calva *et al.,* 1966;
Jennings, Herdson, and Sommers, 1969), which may be important in stabilizing
mitochondrial Ca^{2+} (Lehninger and Carafoli, 1967).

The defect of electron flow in ischemic mitochondria has been found to be
further damaged by 2-hr reperfusion of ischemic myocardium (Kane *et al.,*
1975). A similar observation made in this study is that reperfusion accentuates
the impairment of mitochondrial Ca^{2+} accumulation. The deterioration of mitochondrial components and functions has been induced by massive Ca^{2+} loading
(Lehninger and Carafoli, 1967); thus the further impairment by reperfusion
could be attributed to an increase of Ca^{2+} content.

Ca^{2+} inhibits ADP phosphorylation in ischemic mitochondria. This is probably related to a decreased ability of ischemic mitochondria to accumulate Ca^{2+},
thus a great amount of external Ca^{2+} competes with ADP to utilize high energy
derived from substrate oxidation. However, the inhibition of ADP phosphorylation by added Ca^{2+} in ischemic-reperfused mitochondria is not significantly
different from that of ADP phosphorylation in the absence of added Ca^{2+}. This
is expected, since Shen and Jennings (1972) reported that no significant change
in Ca^{2+} concentration was noted in permanently ischemic myocardium, but
tissue Ca^{2+} was markedly increased in ischemic-reperfused myocardium. It is
thus possible that oxidative phosphorylation is already inhibited by increased
endogenous Ca^{2+} in ischemic-reperfused mitochondria. Therefore, the addition
of Ca^{2+} has no further effect on oxidative phosphorylation in ischemic-reperfused mitochondria.

Recently, the protection of ischemic myocardium by Nifedipine, a calcium
antagonist, has been demonstrated by Henry, Weiss, and Sobel (1975). It seems
likely that any intervention during the reperfusion of ischemic myocardium

should consider Ca^{2+} flow through ischemic myocardial cells. The preservation of ischemic mitochondrial ATP production following reperfusion thus might be accomplished by lowering the cellular ionic Ca^{2+} concentration.

REFERENCES

CALVA, E., MUJICA, A., NUNEZ, R., et al. 1966. Mitochondrial biochemical changes and glucose-KC1-insulin solution in cardiac infarct. Amer. J. Physiol. 211:71–76.

HENRY, P. D., WEISS, E. S., and SOBEL, B. E. 1975. Protection of ischemic myocardium with nifedipine, a calcium antagonist. Abstracts of the 48th Scientific Sessions. Circulation Supplement II: p. 23.

JENNINGS, R. B., HERDSON, P. B., and SOMMERS, H. M. 1969. Structural and functional abnormalities in mitochondria isolated from ischemic dog myocardium. Lab. Invest. 20:548–557.

KANE, J. J., MURPHY, M. L., BISSETT, J. K., DE SOYZA, N., DOHERTY, J. E., and STRAUB, K. D. 1975. Mitochondrial function, oxygen extraction, epicardial S-T segment changes and tritiated digoxin distribution after reperfusion of ischemic myocardium. Amer. J. Cardiol. 36:218–224.

LEHNINGER, A. O., and CARAFOLI, E. 1967. Energy-linked ion movements in mitochondrial system. *In* F. F. Nord (ed.), Advances in Enzymology, Vol. 29, p. 259. Interscience, New York.

SCHUSTER, S. M., and OLSON, M. S. 1974. Studies of the energy-dependent uptake of divalent metal ions by beef heart mitochondria. J. Biol. Chem. 249:7151–7158.

SCHWARTZ, A., WOOD, J. M., ALLEN, J. C., BORNET, E. P., ENTMAN, M. L., GOLDSTEIN, M. A., SORDAHL, L. A., and SUZUKI, M. 1973. Biochemical and morphological correlates of cardiac ischemia. I. Membrane systems. Amer. J. Cardiol. 32:46–61.

SHEN, A. C., and JENNINGS, R. B. 1972. Myocardial calcium and magnesium in acute ischemic injury. Amer. J. Pathol. 67:417–433.

Mailing address:
Dr. M. L. Murphy,
Veterans Administration Hospital,
300 E. Roosevelt Road,
Little Rock, Arkansas 72206 (USA).

Recent Advances in Studies on
Cardiac Structure and Metabolism, Volume 11
Heart Function and Metabolism
Edited by T. Kobayashi, T. Sano, and N. S. Dhalla
Copyright 1978   University Park Press   Baltimore

RELATIONSHIP BETWEEN ENERGY LIBERATION AND UTILIZATION IN ISCHEMIC CARDIAC MUSCLE

T. YAMAGAMI, N. SHIBATA, H. AKAGAMI, and S. TOYAMA

Department of Cardiology, The Center for Adult Diseases, Osaka,
Osaka, Japan

SUMMARY

Mitochondrial respiration, succinate dehydrogenase coenzyme Q reductase, and myosin B were investigated in ischemic myocardium from experimental myocardial infarction in dogs. Respiratory control ratio of mitochondria was impaired by ischemia at 60 min after coronary ligation, and oxygen consumption was inhibited 120 min later. Enzyme activity of succinate dehydrogenase coenzyme Q reductase was decreased at 6 hr after coronary ligation. Calcium ion sensitivity of myosin B declined 12 hr after coronary ligation. However, adenosine triphosphatase activity of myosin A from infarcted myocardium was not different from that of the intact one. These results suggest that interaction in the sequence of enzyme complexes was first impaired in ischemic myocardium and that deterioration of enzyme activity was then manifested.

INTRODUCTION

It is well known that the energy liberation system is impaired at the early stage of myocardial infarction in infarcted myocardium. On the other hand, the energy utilization system has not been clarified yet. The authors previously reported (1976) that loose coupling of the oxydative phosphorylation was revealed first in the mitochondria prepared from infarcted myocardium at the early stage. However, enzyme activity of the contractile protein was little involved at that stage of myocardial infarction, i.e., the grade of superprecipitation of myosin B from infarcted myocardium at 60 min after coronary ligation was similar to that of myosin B from intact myocardium. Moreover, it was suggested that the mitochondria from intact myocardium provided ATP well enough to achieve complete superprecipitation of myosin B, while the mitochondria from infarcted myocardium hardly provided ATP to the myosin B, resulting in incomplete superprecipitation.

Further investigation of mitochondrial oxydative phosphorylation and myosin B in myocardial infarction was studied, and the relation between energy

---

This study was supported by Research Grant for Adult Disease, Osaka, Japan.

liberation and the energy utilization system in ischemic cardiac muscle is discussed herein.

MATERIALS AND METHODS

Mongrel dogs were anesthetized by intravenous administration of sodium pentobarbital. The anterior descending branch of the left coronary artery was completely ligated at the origin under open chest surgery with artificial respiration with room air. Cardiac muscle of the left ventricular free wall was removed at 1, 3, 12, 24, and 48 hr after operation. The infarcted and noninfarcted myocardium were separately obtained. Mitochondrial fraction and myosin B were prepared from each specimen.

Mitochondrial fraction was prepared by Chance and Hagihara's method (Chance and Hagihara, 1963) and oxydative phosphorylation was studied polarographically according to the method of Hagihara (1961). The details have been described elsewhere (Yamagami, Morita, and Yamamura, 1967). Submitochondrial particles were prepared by differential centrifugation method in 0.1 M Tris chloride buffer (pH 7.4) containing 0.25 M sucrose, and succinate dehydrogenase coenzyme Q reductase (complex II) was measured by the reduction of dichlorophenol indophenol spectrophotometrically, according to the method of Ziegler and Rieske (1967).

Myosin B was extracted by Fanburg's method (Fanburg, Finekl, and Martonosi, 1964), and ATPase activity was measured by liberation of inorganic phosphate according to Martin and Doty (1949) at high ($\mu = 0.6$) and low ($\mu = 0.06$) ionic strength. Superprecipitation of myosin B was calculated according to Ebashi (1963). Five percent polyacrylamide gel disc electrophoresis (SDS electrophoresis) was carried out on myosin B dissolved in 8 M urea containing 1% sodium dodecyl sulfate, according to the method of Weber and Osborn (1969).

The details of each experimental condition are described in the legend of each figure.

RESULTS

Oxydative Phosphorylation of Mitochondria

In the mitochondria from intact cardiac muscle, oxygen consumption rate (QO_2) was 146 ± 8.7 natom O/mg/min, ADP/O ratio was 2.8 ± 0.05, and respiratory control ratio (RC) was 6.2 ± 0.52, as shown in Figure 1. At 30 min after myocardial infarction, QO_2 was 128 natom O/mg/min, ADP/O was 2.8, and RC was 3.8 ($p < 0.01$) in the mitochondria from infarcted myocardium. After 60 min, each figure turned to 132, 2.7, and 3.1, respectively. Consequently, no significant difference was found in oxydative phosphorylation between mitochondria from intact and mitochondria from infarcted cardiac muscle at 60 min

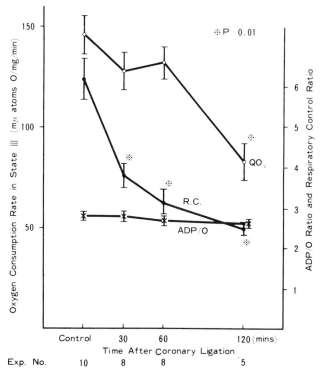

Figure 1. Mitochondrial respiration from infarcted myocardium. (Vertical bars = Mean ± S.E.) Reaction medium: 0.3 M mannitol, 0.1 M phosphate buffer (pH 7.4), 5 mM $MgCl_2$, 4 mM α-ketoglutarate. QO_2: Oxygen consumption rate. RC: Respiratory control ratio.

duration of ischemia except RC. However, in the mitochondria from infarcted myocardium removed 120 min after coronary ligation, QO_2 was 83 natom O/mg/min, ADP/O was 2.6, and RC was 2.5. Statistical differences were also found between mitochondria from intact myocardium and those from infarcted myocardium in both QO_2 ($p < 0.01$) and RC ($p < 0.005$).

Complex II

Enzyme activity of complex II of submitochondrial particles prepared from intact cardiac muscle was 15.05 ± 0.59 nmol/mg/min, as shown in Figure 2. The enzyme activity of submitochondrial particles from noninfarcted myocardium was almost the same as that from intact cardiac muscle, except for the submitochondrial particles prepared from noninfarcted area that was removed 3 hr after coronary ligation. In this exceptional specimen, enzyme activity was 24.11 ± 0.91 nmol/mg/min and significantly higher than that from intact cardiac muscle ($p < 0.001$). In the submitochondrial particles from infarcted myocardium

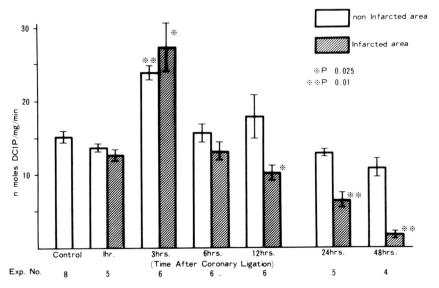

Figure 2. Specific activity of succinate dehydrogenase coenzyme Q reductase in submitochondrial particles from infarcted and noninfarcted myocardium. (Vertical bars = Mean ± S.E.) Reaction medium: 0.25 M sucrose, 0.1 M phosphate buffer (pH 7.0), 0.01 mM EDTA, 20 mM succinate, 0.035 mM dichloroindophenol.

removed at 1 hr after coronary ligation, the specific activity of complex II was 12.68 nmol/mg/min and not different from that of intact myocardium. AT 3 hr after coronary ligation, the specific activity of complex II of infarcted myocardium was increased as shown in noninfarcted myocardium. It was 27.67 ± 3.22 nmol/mg/min, and significantly higher than that of the intact one ($p <$ 0.025). Enzyme activity of complex II was quickly decreased thereafter; it was 13.36 at 6 hr, and 12.10 at 12 hr after coronary ligation. At 48 hr after coronary ligation, the specific activity of complex II of submitochondrial particles prepared from infarcted myocardium was 6.51 ± 1.01 nmol/mg/min and lower than that from intact myocardium ($p < 0.01$).

Percent change of the specific activity of complex II of submitochondrial particles prepared from infarcted cardiac muscle to that from noninfarcted cardiac muscle of the same animal is shown in Figure 3. The ratios at 1 hr and 3 hr after coronary ligation were 96% and 114%, respectively. Therefore, no significant differences were found between noninfarcted area and infarcted area. However, this ratio was 85.6% ($p < 0.05$) at 6 hr, 62.1% ($p < 0.025$) at 24 hr, and 50.5% ($p < 0.01$) at 48 hr after coronary ligation. Consequently, the specific activity of complex II decreased in the infarcted area compared with nonin-

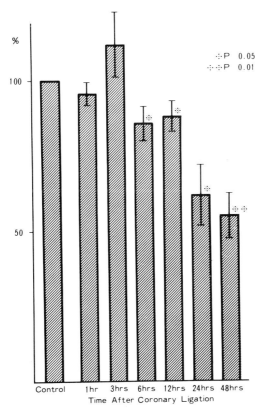

Figure 3. Percent change of specific activity of succinate dehydrogenase coenzyme Q reductase of submitochondrial particles from infarcted myocardium compared to that from noninfarcted myocardium obtained from same animal. (Vertical bars = Mean ± S.E.)

farcted area of the same animal, when the duration of ischemia was 6 hr or longer.

Myosin B

Superprecipitation of cardiac myosin B prepared from experimental myocardial infarction is shown in Figure 4. As seen in the figure, the grade of superprecipitation was almost equal in all materials, being irrelevant to the duration of ischemia (within 24 hr), when calcium ion was present in the reaction medium. The superprecipitation of myosin B extracted from intact myocardium was inhibited in the presence of EGTA with no addition of calcium ion, but that of myosin B from infarcted myocardium removed at 24 hr after coronary ligation was little inhibited under the same condition. In myosin B from infarcted

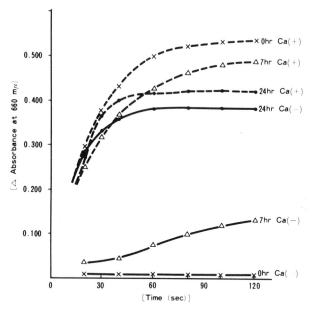

Figure 4. Superprecipitation of cardiac myosin B from infarcted myocardium. Reaction medium: 10 mM Tris maleate buffer (pH 7.0), 1 mM $MgCl_2$, 0.06 M KCl, 0.1 mM ATP, and 5 mM EGTA (Ca (–)) or 1 mM $CaCl_2$ (Ca (+)). Myosin B was extracted from intact myocardium (0 hr) or after 7 hr and 24 hr of ischemia.

myocardium removed at 7 hr after coronary ligation, EGTA partially inhibited superprecipitation.

These differences in superprecipitation may be due to ATPase activity of myosin B in each condition.

In myosin B from intact myocardium, magnesium-dependent ATPase in the medium containing EGTA at low ionic strength ($\mu = 0.06$) was 64.3 ± 5.9 nmol Pi/mg/min. The activity of myosin B from infarcted myocardium was lower; it was 29 in ischemia for 3 hr, 40 in ischemia for 6 hr, and 28 in ischemia for 15 hr. However, in myosin B for 24-hr coronary ligation, the magnesium-dependent ATPase activity was 98 nmol Pi/mg/min, considerably higher than the control level. The calcium-activated ATPase activity showed a tendency similar to that of magnesium-dependent ATPase. It was 125 nmol Pi/mg/min in myosin B from intact myocardium, and decreased to 68.9 nmol Pi/mg/min in myosin B from infarcted myocardium after the duration of ischemia for 3 hr, 72.4 nmol Pi/mg/min for 6 hr, and 45.5 nmol Pi/mg/min for 15 hr, but it was 117.1 nmol/mg/min for 24-hr duration of ischemia.

Calcium sensitivity in myosin B ATPase activity was calculated using the following formula at low ionic strength:

$$\text{Calcium sensitivity} = \frac{\text{calcium-activated ATPase activity}}{\text{magnesium-dependent ATPase activity}} \times 100$$

The sensitivity was 203% in myosin B from intact myocardium. It was increased to 274% in myosin B from infarcted myocardium for 3-hr duration of ischemia. However, the duration of ischemia became longer, and the sensitivity diminished; it was 194% in myosin B for infarcted myocardium for 6 hr, 168% for 15 hr, and 120% ($p < 0.01$) for 24 hr, as shown in Figure 5.

On the other hand, EDTA-activated ATPase activity of myosin B at high ionic strength, which represented myosin A ATPase, was 200–260 nmol Pi/mg/min in myosin B extracted from intact or infarcted myocardium.

These results indicate that some subcomponents of myosin B were denatured in myocardial infarction.

SDS electrophoretic pattern of myosin B is shown in Figure 6. A band of molecular weight of 34,000 was found in control myosin B, but it disappeared in myosin B extracted at 24 hr after coronary ligation. In the rest of two specimens, extracted at 3 hr and at 6 hr, the band was partially exhausted

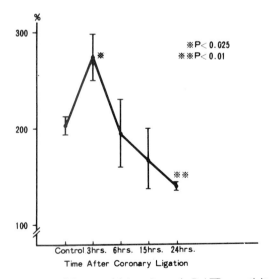

Figure 5. Percent change of calcium sensitivity of myosin B ATPase activity from infarcted myocardium. (Vertical bars = Mean ± S.E.) Experimental conditions were the same as in Figure 4.

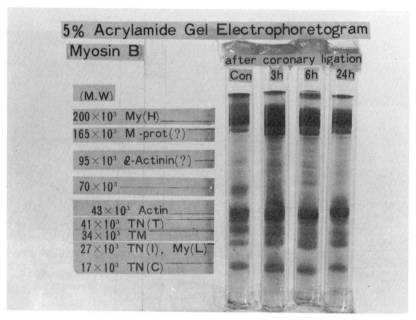

Figure 6. Five percent polyacrylamide gel electrophoretic pattern of cardiac myosin B from infarcted myocardium. Myosin B was dissolved in 8 M urea containing 1% sodium dodecyl sulfate. Electrophoresis: 5 mA/tube, stained with coomassie blue. M.W.: molecular weight; My (H): heavy meromyosin; M-prot: M-protein; TN (T): troponin-T; TM: tropomyosin; TN (I): troponin-I; My (L): light meromyosin; TN (C): troponin-C. Myosin B was extracted from intact myocardium (Con) or 3 hr (3h), 6 hr (6h), and 24 hr (24h) after coronary artery ligation.

compared to intact control. The other bands in myosin B were not different in all specimens.

DISCUSSION

Mitochondrial respiration was impaired in infarcted myocardium, which was characteristic of decrease of RC, and was followed by reduction of QO_2. Schwartz *et al.* (1973) reported that the mode of impairment of mitochondrial respiration in myocardial infarction was the inhibition of oxygen consumption, and disagreed with our previous results. From the facts described herein, it is supposed that the earliest impairment in infarcted mitochondria is the decrease of RC, which is followed by inhibition of oxygen consumption, since the decrease in RC was recognized at 60 min after coronary ligation and the inhibition of QO_2 was recognized at 120 min after coronary ligation. Enzyme activity of complex II was not inhibited in the early stage of infarction even when the oxygen consumption was inhibited after the duration of ischemia for 3 hr. Enzyme activity of complex II was inhibited after 6-hr or longer duration of ischemic state, compared with noninfarcted area.

Furthermore, enzyme activity of myosin B was not impaired at the early stage of myocardial infarction, as was mentioned previously. Myosin A ATPase activity did not change even in the ischemic condition for 24 hr. However, a component corresponding to tropomyosin, a band of 34,000 of molecular weight in SDS electrophoresis, may decline with the duration of ischemia in myocardium. This finding may explain the decrease of calcium sensitivity of myosin B in both ATPase activity and superprecipitation; nevertheless, an ATPase activity of myosin A is not affected by ischemia.

These biochemical changes of myocardium in myocardial infarction are summarized in Figure 7. As shown in the figure, enzyme activity of complex II and calcium sensitivity are both increased after 3 hr of ischemia. Biochemical reaction or protein synthesis may be accelerated in ischemic myocardium at the

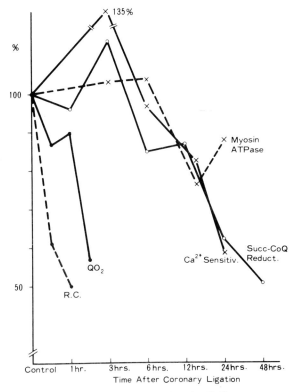

Figure 7. Percent change of respiratory control ratio (RC), oxygen consumption ratio (QO_2), succinate dehydrogenase coenzyme Q reductase (Succ-CoQ Reduct.), myosin ATPase, and calcium sensitivity of myosin B (Ca^{2+} sensitiv.) from infarcted myocardium to those from intact myocardium.

early stage. Hinterberger and Wollenberger (1976) mentioned previously that protein synthesis was not completely inhibited in the ischemic myocardium. Anyhow, biochemical change in the myocardium after myocardial infarction is suggested as enhancement of decrease in RC, inhibition of oxygen consumption in mitochondria, increase in some enzyme activity (complex II and calcium sensitivity of myosin B), and finally deterioration of enzyme activity.

It is supposed from these results that the first step of biochemical change in infarcted myocardium is the impairment of interaction in the sequence of enzyme complexes. Thereafter, compensatory activation of enzyme complex may be displayed, although interaction in the sequence of enzyme complexes was not improved by the compensatory activation. These enzyme activities in myocardium may finally be inhibited after 6 hr or more of ischemia.

REFERENCES

CHANCE, B., and HAGIHARA, B. 1963. Intracellular respiration. Phosphorylating and non-phosphorylating oxydation reactions. Fifth International Congress of Biochemistry, p. 3. Pergamon Press, New York.

EBASHI, S. 1963. Calcium binding activity of vesicular relaxing factor. J. Biochem. (Tokyo) 50:236–244.

FANBURG, B., FINEKL, R. M., and MARTONOSI, A. 1964. The role of calcium in the mechanism of relaxation of cardiac muscle. J. Biol. Chem. 239:2298–2306.

HAGIHARA, B. 1961. Techniques for the application of polarography to mitochondrial respiration. Biochim. Biophys. Acta 46:134–142.

HINTERBERGER, U., and WOLLENBERGER, A. 1976. Protein synthesis in cell-free systems from total ischemic rat myocardium. In P. Harris, J. Bing, and A. Fleckenstein (eds.), Recent Advances in Studies on Cardiac Structure and Metabolism, Vol. 7, pp. 341–347. University Park Press, Baltimore.

MARTIN, J. B., and DOTY, D. M. 1949. Determination of inorganic phosphate. Modification of isobutyl alcohol procedure. Anal. Chem. 21:965–967.

SCHWARTZ, A., WOOD, J. E., ALLEN, J. C., BORNET, E. P., ENTMAN, M. I., COLDSTEIN, M. A., SORDAHL, L. A., and SUZUKI, M. 1973. Biochemical and morphological correlation of cardiac ischemia. Amer. J. Cardiol. 32:46–61.

SHIBATA, N., YAMAGAMI, T., and TOYAMA, S. 1976. Energy metabolism in the infarcted cardiac muscle: The interaction of contractile protein and mitochondria. In P. Harris, J. Bing, and A. Fleckenstein (eds.), Recent Advances in Studies on Cardiac Structure and Metabolism, Vol. 7, pp. 145–152. University Park Press, Baltimore.

WEBER, K., and OSBORN, M. 1969. The reliability of molecular weight determinations by dodecyl sulfate-polyacrylamide gel electrophoresis. J. Biol. Chem. 244:4406–4412.

YAMAGAMI, T., MORITA, K., and YAMAMURA, Y. 1967. Mitochondrial respiration of experimentally produced ischemic heart muscle in dogs. Jpn. Heart J. 8:132–141.

ZIEGLER, D., and RIESKE, J. S. 1967. Preparation and properties of succinate dehydrogenase coenzyme Q reductase. Methods Enzymol. 10:231–235.

Mailing address:
Dr. T. Yamagami
Department of Cardiology,
The Center for Adult Diseases, Osaka,
1-3 Nakamichi, Higashinari-ku,
Osaka, 537 (Japan).

Recent Advances in Studies on
Cardiac Structure and Metabolism, Volume 11
Heart Function and Metabolism
Edited by T. Kobayashi, T. Sano, and N. S. Dhalla
Copyright 1978   University Park Press   Baltimore

AN EXPERIMENTAL STUDY OF THE EFFECT OF GLUCOSE-INSULIN-POTASSIUM SOLUTION ON ENERGY METABOLISM OF INFARCTED CARDIAC MUSCLE

T. UENO, T. ISHIYAMA, Y. MORITA,
Y. HATANAKA, J. AZUMA, T. TANIMOTO,
K. OGURA, H. HASEGAWA, K. S. SHIN,
N. TSUKAMOTO, and Y. YAMAMURA

The Third Department of Internal Medicine, Osaka University Hospital,
Fukushima 1-1-50, Fukushima-ku, Osaka 553, Japan

SUMMARY

The effect of GIK (glucose-insulin-potassium) infusion on the energy liberation of the infarcted heart muscle was studied experimentally in relation to epicardial electrocardiographic changes and cardiac dynamics. In the case of 30-min coronary ligation, the spread of the zone showing ST segment elevation was not depressed significantly, but the mean voltage values of ST elevations were suppressed in the peri-infarcted area, and the uncoupling of oxidative phosphorylation in the peri-infarcted area was also obscured by the GIK treatment. Cardiac dynamics did not change with GIK treatment. On the other hand, in the 60-min coronary ligation, the spread of the zone showing ST segment elevation was reduced significantly and the negative inotropism induced by coronary ligation was suppressed with GIK infusion. However, the uncoupling of oxidative phosphorylation in the infarcted area and in the peri-infarcted area did not show any significant improvement. Therefore, the disturbed energy metabolism of the peri-infarcted area of 30-min ligation might be improved by the effect of GIK infusion. These data suggested that the GIK infusion improved the energy liberation of the so-called twilight zone at 30 min after ligation, and then reduced the genuine infarcted zone after 60 min of ligation.

INTRODUCTION

Recently the effects of GIK (glucose-insulin-potassium solution) infusion on acute myocardial infarction have been re-evaluated, but the mode of action remains unknown. These authors reported previously that oxidative phosphorylation was uncoupled in the infarcted canine myocardium. Moreover, the authors observed thereafter that the occurrence of ventricular fibrillation was reduced and the deterioration of myocardial contractility was protected in experimental myocardial infarction when GIK was infused before and during experimental procedures. In the present study, the authors explored whether or not GIK infusion modifies the alteration of myocardial energy liberation as well as ST elevation in epicardial electrocardiogram of the infarcted and the peri-infarcted areas in relation to the change of chronotropic-inotropic state in experimental coronary occlusion.

MATERIAL AND METHODS

Mongrel dogs weighing from 8 to 14 kg were anesthetized with intravenous injection of 20 to 30 mg/kg of sodium pentobarbital. Left ventricular pressure, the first derivative of left ventricular pressure, and lead II electrocardiogram were recorded intermittently by a polygraph. Electrocardiographic epicardial mapping was performed serially.

Thirty or sixty minutes after coronary ligation, dogs were sacrificed and pieces of myocardia were removed from the infarcted area, the peri-infarcted area, and the noninfarcted area. Mitochondria were isolated by Chance and Hagihara's method from each area, and their respiration was measured polarographically; then oxygen consumption rate (QO_2) in state 3 and in state 4, respiratory control index, and ADP/O ratio were calculated. Glutamate was used as a substrate. Dogs were divided into four groups. In the first group, left anterior descending coronary artery (LAD) was ligated for 30 min without GIK treatment. In the second group, LAD was ligated for 30 min with GIK infusion. In the other two groups, LAD was ligated for 60 min with or without GIK infusion. Contents of this solution were 200 ml of 10% glucose, 4 U of regular insulin, and 8 meq of potassium. Infusion was started 30 min prior to ligation, and was continued throughout experimental procedures.

RESULTS AND DISCUSSION

Studies on Cardiac Dynamics

In dogs with 30-min ligation without GIK infusion, negative inotropism appeared with negative chronotropism in most cases. In dogs with 30-min ligation with GIK infusion, either positive or negative inotropism of a slight degree occurred. The chronotropic change was minimum. When LAD was ligated 60 min without GIK infusion, cardiac dynamics showed negative inotropism with positive chronotropism immediately after ligation, and then recovered gradually toward the control level. When LAD was ligated for 60 min with GIK infusion, cardiac dynamics showed negative inotropism with positive chronotropism immediately after coronary ligation, then recovered more rapidly, and eventually positive inotropism appeared.

Studies on Epicardial Electrocardiographic Mapping

Table 1 shows the results on ST segment elevation in the epicardial electrocardiograms. Compared with the groups without GIK treatment, the number of sites where the ST segment elevated severely was decreased significantly 60 min after ligation with GIK, although this effect was not apparent 30 min after ligation with GIK. Thereafter, the mean voltage values of ST elevation at the peri-infarcted area and the infarcted area were compared. Thirty minutes after the LAD ligation, GIK infusion suppressed the mean voltage values of ST elevations in the peri-infarcted areas significantly, but at 60 min after ligation, the suppressive effect disappeared. In the infarcted area, GIK infusion did not influence the mean voltage values of ST elevation significantly 30 min or 60 min after LAD ligation.

Studies on Mitochondrial Respiration

Figure 1 shows the effects on mitochondrial respiration of 30-min ligation. The upper half of the figure shows the data without GIK treatment. QO_2 state 4 increased and respiratory control (RC) decreased in both the peri-infarcted and the infarcted areas, compared with the noninfarcted area. The degrees of the impairment were similar in both areas. The lower half of the figure shows data for GIK infusion. In the peri-infarcted area, the increase in QO_2 state 4 and the decrease of RC were lesser than in those of the dogs without GIK. Figure 2 shows the effects on mitochondrial respiration of 60-min ligation. The upper

Table 1. Number of ST elevated sites of epicardial electrocardiographic mapping after experimental ligation of canine left anterior descending coronary artery

	ST elevation (mV)			
	$ST < 1$	$1 \leqslant ST \leqslant 2$	$2 < ST$	Total
30 min after ligation				
No treatment	14	4	39	57
GIK infusion	12	4	18	34
		(not significant)		
60 min after ligation				
No treatment	12	5	30	47
GIK infusion	18	12	17	47
		($p < 0.01$)		

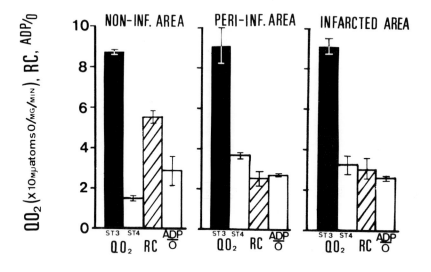

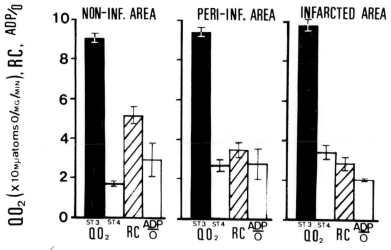

Figure 1. Effects of GIK infusion on the infarcted, the peri-infarcted, and the noninfarcted canine heart mitochondrial respiration. Dogs were sacrificed 30 min after ligation of left anterior descending coronary artery. The *upper half* shows the cases with GIK and the *lower half* shows the cases with GIK infusion. Glutamate was used as a substrate. (Abbreviations are: QO_2, oxygen consumption rate; ST 3, state 3; ST 4, state 4; RC, respiratory control index; ADP/O, ADP/O ratio.)

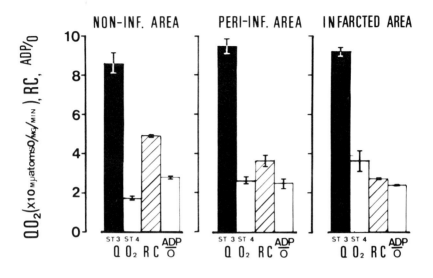

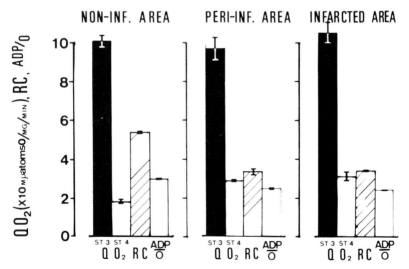

Figure 2. Effects of GIK infusion on the infarcted, the peri-infarcted, and the noninfarcted canine heart mitochondrial respiration. Dogs were sacrificed 60 min after ligation of left anterior descending coronary artery. The *upper half* shows the cases without GIK and the *lower half* shows the cases with GIK infusion. Glutamate was used as a substrate. (For abbreviations, see the legend to Figure 1.)

half of the figure shows the data without GIK treatment. QO_2 state 4 increased and RC decreased in both the peri-infarcted area and the infarcted area, compared with the noninfarcted area. These results indicated the uncoupling of oxidative phosphorylation in the peri-infarcted area as well as in the infarcted area.

Mailing address:
Teiichi Ueno, M.D.,
The Third Department of Internal Medicine,
Osaka University Hospital,
Fukushima 1-1-50, Fukushima-ku,
Osaka 553 (Japan).

Recent Advances in Studies on
Cardiac Structure and Metabolism, Volume 11
Heart Function and Metabolism
Edited by T. Kobayashi, T. Sano, and N. S. Dhalla
Copyright 1978   University Park Press   Baltimore

EFFECT OF XANTHINE OXIDASE INHIBITOR ON MYOCARDIAL ISCHEMIA

T. MINAGA, K. TAKEDA, T. NAKAMURA,
A. KIZU, and H. IJICHI

The Second Department of Internal Medicine,
Kyoto Prefectural University of Medicine, Kyoto, Japan

SUMMARY

The xanthine oxidase inhibitor, 4-hydroxypyrazolo(3,4-d) pyrimidine (HPP), Allopurinol, caused augmentation of myocardial uptake of [^{3}H]hypoxanthine, which was eventually completely incorporated into ATP. The decrease of [^{32}P]orthophosphate incorporation into ATP induced by isoproterenol was restored by HPP administration.

INTRODUCTION

DeWall *et al.* (1971) reported a protective action of HPP in acute myocardial ischemia. The breakdown of adenine nucleotides in ischemia has been well known. Catalysis by xanthine oxidase is irreversible. However, hypoxanthine can be salvaged by reversion to inosine monophosphate by hypoxanthine-guanine phosphoribosyl transferase. In this paper the protective action of HPP in ischemic myocardium was investigated with respect to adenine nucleotides.

MATERIALS AND METHODS

[^{3}H]hypoxanthine and $H_3{}^{32}PO_4$ were obtained from The Radiochemical Centre, Amersham, England, and Commissarian A L Energie Atomique, France, respectively. HPP was provided by Burroughs Wellcome Co., London. Mice (dd-strain), weighing about 20 g, were used. Isoproterenol was dissolved in physiological saline and injected subcutaneously on 2 consecutive days (50 mg per kg body weight). HPP was added into the basal diet (0.1%). [^{3}H]hypoxanthine and ^{32}P were injected intraperitoneally, but for the metabolic experiments in the liver [^{3}H]hypoxanthine was injected into portal vein. Tissues were immediately homogenized in 3% perchloric acid. The supernatant was neutralized and adenine nucleotides were fractionated by a slightly modified method of Potter *et al.* Phosphate was determined by the method of Takahashi. The reduction of nitro blue tetrazolium (NBT) by heart slices was determined by the method of Baehner and Hathan (1968).

RESULTS

Myocardial uptake of radioactivity, 1 hr after injection of [³H]hypoxanthine, was significantly increased by HPP administration ($p < 0.001$). As shown in Figure 1, the incorporation of [³H]hypoxanthine into myocardial ATP fraction was increased by HPP administration ($p < 0.01$). Because it was difficult to investigate the time course of the metabolic fate of [³H]hypoxanthine in the myocardium, mouse liver was used instead of myocardium. In this metabolic experiment, a small amount of radioactivity was detectable in the adenine nucleotides at even 15 sec after intraportal injection of [³H]hypoxanthine. Thirty seconds after injection, the increase of radioactivity in adenine nucleotide corresponded with the decrease of labeled hypoxanthine and inosine. This was also seen at 1 min after injection, while at 5, 15, and 30 min after injection all radioactivity was incorporated into adenine nucleotides. Hepatic uptake of radioactivity and the incorporation of [³H]hypoxanthine into ATP fraction, 1 hr after injection, was also significantly increased by HPP administration ($p < 0.001$). As shown in Figure 1, at 1 min after injection, there was a significant increase in radioactivity of hypoxanthine fraction by HPP administration ($p < 0.001$). ³²P uptake in mouse heart was decreased by isoproterenol administration, but this decrease was restored by HPP administration. There was no difference between the ³²P-specific activity of the inorganic phosphate fraction from the isoproterenol group and that from the group administered isoproterenol and HPP. On the other hand, as shown in Figure 2, the ³²P-specific activity of organic phosphate fraction, especially in ATP fraction, differed significantly between groups ($p < 0.01$). The decrease in the NBT reduction of

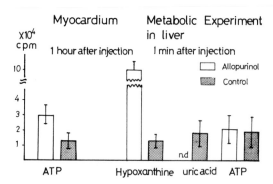

Figure 1. Incorporation of [³H]hypoxanthine. n.d. = not detectable. See text for explanation.

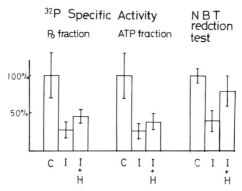

Figure 2. ^{32}P-specific activity. C = Control; I = isoproterenol administration; H = HPP administration. See text for explanation.

heart muscle induced by isoproterenol was restored by HPP administration ($p <$ 0.05).

DISCUSSION

HPP has been shown to have a protective effect against ischemic changes under certain conditions (Crowell, Jones, and Smith, 1969; DeWall *et al.,* 1971). The preservation of purine base and the increased resynthesis of ATP might be a cause of this effect. However, Cunningham, Keaueny, and Fitzgerald (1974) reported that significantly higher levels of ATP, ADP, and AMP were observed in HPP-treated animals during renal ischemia, and they speculated that the ac- cumulation of hypoxanthine might prevent the breakdown of ATP, ADP, and AMP. Our experiments were undertaken to examine re-utilization and synthesis of ATP, using [^{3}H]hypoxanthine and ^{32}P, but not the breakdown of ATP. As mentioned above, 1 min after injection of [^{3}H]hypoxanthine, there was a significant increase of radioactivity in hypoxanthine fraction by HPP administra- tion, and the radioactivity was rapidly and completely incorporated into the adenine nucleotides. It can be considered that accumulated hypoxanthine plays an important role as the substrate for the re-utilization, which induces an increase of incorporation of [^{3}H]hypoxanthine into adenine nucleotides. How- ever, hypoxanthine that accumulated through adenine nucleotide degradation in the ischemic state was rapidly and irreversibly converted by xanthine oxidase, and a significantly increased concentration of uric acid was consequently seen. Therefore, it is considered that accumulation of sufficient hypoxanthine for re-utilization does not occur without HPP administration.

As has been reported, HPP is taken up into the myocardium (Elion, Kovensky, and Hitchings, 1966) and xanthine oxidase activity is detectable in the myocardium; therefore, the site of action of HPP may be partially in the myocardium. In the last few years it has become apparent that HPP inhibits several enzymes in addition to xanthine oxidase. All of the actions of HPP are not yet well known.

It is well known that the decrease in ATP concentration induced by iso-proterenol is due to an increase in ATP degradation. However, in our experiments, an inhibition of ATP biosyntheses was also recognized and was restored by HPP administration. Calman and Bell (1973) postulated that tissue adenine nucleotide levels might be used as indicators of the viability of an organ following ischemic damage. It might thus be considered that the restoration of adenine nucleotides levels by HPP administration leads to increased cellular viability and consequently to a recovery of decreased NBT reduction. From these results and consideration, it is concluded that HPP has a protective action in myocardial ischemia with respect to adenine nucleotides.

REFERENCES

BAEHNER, R. L., and HATHAN, D. G. 1968. Quantivative nitroblue tetrazolium test in chronic granulomatous disease. New Engl. J. Med. 278:971–976.

CROWELL, J. W., JONES, C. E., and SMITH, E. E. 1969. Effect of allopurinol on hemorrhagic shock. Amer. J. Physiol. 216:744–748.

CUNNINGHAM, S. K., KEAUENY, T. V., and FITZGERALD, P. 1974. Effect of allopurinol on tissue ATP, ADP and AMP concentrations in renal ischaemia. Br. J. Surg. 61:562–565.

DeWALL, R. A., VASKO, K. A., STANLEY, E. L., and KEZDO, P. 1971. Responses of the ischemic myocardium to allopurinol. Amer. Heart J. 82:362–370.

ELION, G. B., KOVENSKY, A., and HITCHINGS, G. 1966. Metabolic studies of allopurinol, an inhibitor of xanthine oxidase. Biochem. Pharmacol. 15:863–880.

Mailing address:
Takeyoshi Minaga, M.D.,
The Second Department of Internal Medicine,
Kyoto Prefectural University of
Medicine,
Hirokoji Kawaramachi Kamikyo-ku,
Kyoto (Japan).

Recent Advances in Studies on
Cardiac Structure and Metabolism, Volume 11
Heart Function and Metabolism
Edited by T. Kobayashi, T. Sano, and N. S. Dhalla
Copyright 1978 University Park Press Baltimore

CALCIUM PARADOX: CHANGES IN HIGH-ENERGY PHOSPHATE COMPOUNDS OF ISOLATED PERFUSED RAT HEARTS

A. B. T. J. BOINK, T. J. C. RUIGROK,
A. H. J. MAAS, and A. N. E. ZIMMERMAN

Departments of Thoracic Surgery and Cardiology,
University Hospital, Utrecht, The Netherlands

SUMMARY

When isolated rat hearts are perfused with Ca^{2+}-containing medium, after a brief Ca^{2+}-free period, irreversible cell damage occurs (calcium paradox). This phenomenon is concomitant with a rapid consumption of myocardial high-energy phosphate stores, prior to the appearance of these compounds in the effluent perfusion medium. A possible mechanism for the origin of myocardial necrosis, caused by intracellular Ca^{2+} overload, is discussed.

INTRODUCTION

Reperfusion of isolated rat hearts with Ca^{2+}-containing medium, after a short Ca^{2+}-free perfusion period, causes irreversible loss of electrical and mechanical activity, and a considerable release of cell constituents. This phenomenon was named the "calcium paradox" (Zimmerman *et al.,* 1967). Ultrastructural changes, nearly identical to those observed in calcium paradox hearts, were found in hearts that were reoxygenated after a period of anoxic perfusion (Ganote *et al.,* 1975) or that were reperfused after a period of ischemia (Jennings and Ganote, 1974).

It has been suggested that intracellular calcium overload and subsequent "massive loading" of mitochondria with Ca^{2+} play an important role in the genesis of these injuries. It is well known that mitochondria are able to accumulate large amounts of Ca^{2+} at the expense of energy (Lehninger, Carafoli, and Rossi, 1967).

In the present study, high-energy phosphate compounds were assayed in rat hearts and perfusion medium during the calcium paradox procedure in order to test the current theory on the mechanism of Ca^{2+}-induced myocardial necrosis.

METHODS

Hearts from male Wistar rats of 200–250 g were used. The perfusion technique has been described elsewhere (Zimmerman *et al.*, 1967). After a 15-min stabilization period, the perfusion was changed to the Ca^{2+}-free medium. After 4 min of Ca^{2+}-free perfusion the hearts were reperfused with a Ca^{2+}-containing medium. The experiments were terminated by suddenly freezing the heart between aluminum blocks cooled to the temperature of liquid N_2 (Wollenberger, Ristau, and Schoffa, 1960). For the working up of the frozen tissue, and the determination of the high-energy phosphate compounds and creatine, commonly used techniques were followed (Bergmeyer, 1970).

RESULTS

Figure 1 shows the adenine nucleotides concentrations in isolated rat hearts during the periods of exposure to first Ca^{2+}-containing, then Ca^{2+}-free, and then Ca^{2+}-containing medium again. In Figure 2 the creatine phosphate (CP) and creatine content of the myocardium, and the total amount of creatine released during the various periods of reperfusion with Ca^{2+}, are given. The perfusion with Ca^{2+}-free medium induced an increase of the tissue CP and ATP levels by 20% and 10%, respectively, with regard to the control group. Reintroduction of Ca^{2+} in the perfusion medium resulted in a severe decline of CP and ATP levels within 0.5 min (65% and 45% decrease with respect to the content just prior to reperfusion with Ca^{2+}). In the same period there was an increase in myocardial creatine (15%), ADP (85%), and AMP (2800%). During continued reperfusion with Ca^{2+} the concentrations of all compounds decreased gradually. In the effluent perfusate, collected during reperfusion with Ca^{2+}, increasing amounts of creatine were found. The amounts of CP, ATP, and ADP in the effluent, collected during 2 min of reperfusion with Ca^{2+}, were small (CP, 1.4 ± 0.4; ATP, 0.7 ± 0.3; and ADP, 0.8 ± 0.2 μmol released/g dry tissue, ± S.D.). Relatively large amounts of AMP (3.5 ± 0.8 μmol/g dry weight) appeared in the effluent.

DISCUSSION

The finding that myocardial CP and ATP levels were decreased after 0.5 min of reperfusion with Ca^{2+}, whereas creatine, ADP, and AMP levels increased during this interval, points to a sudden consumption of high-energy stores, once Ca^{2+} was restored to the perfusion medium. When the sum totals of ATP + ADP + AMP are considered, it is clear that there is hardly any loss of these compounds from the hearts up to the first 30 sec of reperfusion. The decrease of this sum total after this period must be attributed mainly to further metabolism of the adenine nucleotides, as the effluent contained only very small amounts of ATP

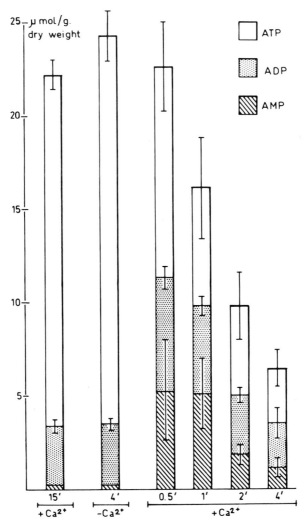

Figure 1. Concentration of the adenine nucleotides in isolated rat heart at the end of a 15-min perfusion period with standard medium, after 4 min of a subsequent perfusion with Ca^{2+}-free medium, and at different times of reperfusion with Ca^{2+}-containing medium. Each *bar* represents the average of 4 hearts ± S.D.

and ADP. The amount of AMP released is too small to compensate the difference in sum total between control perfusion and reperfusion with Ca^{2+}.

We suggest that this loss of energy stores during the calcium paradox is related to massive accumulation of calcium into the mitochondria, which is a highly energy-dependent process.

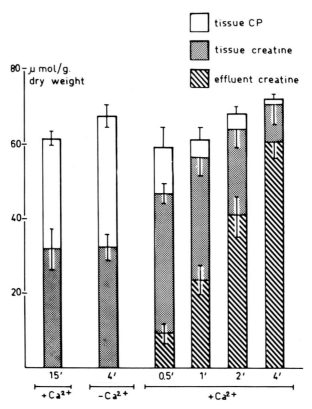

Figure 2. Concentration of creatine phosphate and creatine in the myocardium at the various stages of perfusion (see legend to Figure 1), and the amount of creatine released in the perfusion medium during the different periods of reperfusion with Ca^{2+}-containing medium. Each *bar* represents the average of 4 hearts ± S.D.

The normal intracellular ionized Ca^{2+} concentration in the myocardium ranges from 10^{-7} to 10^{-5} mol/liter. Scarpa (1974) has shown that at these concentrations mitochondrial Ca^{2+} uptake is markedly reduced. It has been suggested that during a Ca^{2+}-free perfusion period the selective permeability of the sarcolemma alters in such a way that, upon reintroduction of Ca^{2+} in the perfusion medium, this Ca^{2+} can enter the cell unrestrictedly. At a calcium concentration of 10^{-3} mol/liter the mitochondrial Ca^{2+} uptake mechanism reaches its maximal activity (Scarpa, 1974).

High-energy phosphate deficiency has been considered to be the crucial reaction in the origin of cardiac necrosis, caused by intracellular calcium overload (Fleckenstein, 1971). It is very unlikely, nevertheless, that the nearly complete exhaustion of CP and ATP we observed is directly responsible for the abrupt and massive cell damage during the calcium paradox. It should be considered that during an anoxic perfusion of 30 min, in the absence of glucose, myocardial CP and ATP concentrations fall to almost zero (Hearse and Chain, 1974), while these hearts exhibit only a slow release of enzymes (Hearse, Humphrey, and Chain, 1973; Ganote et al., 1975).

For the rest, it is beyond doubt that mitochondria, with their ability to accumulate massive quantities of calcium in preference to phosphorylating ADP, play an essential role in the origin of the calcium paradox phenomena. From the overall reaction for calcium phosphate deposition, displayed below, it is clear that "massive loading" of Ca^{2+} by mitochondria is coupled with an ejection of protons (Lehninger et al., 1967).

$$3\ Ca^{2+} + 2\ HPO_4^{2-} \rightarrow Ca_3(PO_4)_2 + 2\ H^+$$

The role of cytoplasmic acidification, as a result of intracellular calcium overload, in the origin of the calcium paradox should be considered.

Acknowledgments The authors are grateful to Mrs. Ineke Stolk-Mighorst and Miss Ria van Boesschoten for their skilled technical assistance.

REFERENCES

BERGMEYER, H. U. 1970. Methoden der enzymatischen Analyse, p. 2220. Verlag Chemie, Weinheim.

FLECKENSTEIN, A. 1971. Specific inhibitors and promoters of calcium action in the excitation-contraction coupling of heart muscle and their role in the prevention or production of myocardial lesions. In P. Harris and L. H. Opie (eds.), Calcium and the Heart, pp. 135–188. Academic Press, London.

GANOTE, C. E., SEABRA-GOMES, R., NAYLER, W. G., and JENNINGS, R. B. 1975. Irreversible myocardial injury in anoxic perfused rat hearts. Amer. J. Pathol. 80: 419–450.

HEARSE, D. J., and CHAIN, E. B. 1974. Effect of glucose on enzyme release from, and recovery of, the anoxic myocardium. In N. S. Dhalla (ed.), Recent Advances in Studies on Cardiac Structure and Metabolism, Vol. 3. Myocardial Metabolism, pp. 763–773. Urban & Schwarzenberg, München.

HEARSE, D. J., HUMPHREY, S. M., and CHAIN, E. B. 1973. Abrupt reoxygenation of the anoxic potassium-arrested perfused rat heart: a study of myocardial enzyme release. J. Mol. Cell. Cardiol. 5:395–407.

JENNINGS, R. B., and GANOTE, C. E. 1974. Structural changes in myocardium during acute ischemia. Circ. Res. 34 en 35 (Suppl. III):156–168.

LEHNINGER, A. L., CARAFOLI, E., and ROSSI, C. S. 1967. Energy-linked ion movements in mitochondrial systems. Adv. Enzymol. 29:259–320.

SCARPA, A. 1974. Kinetic studies of Ca^{2+} transport in mitochondria. In L. Ernster, R. W. Estabrook, and E. C. Slater (eds.), Dynamics of Energy-Transducing Membranes, pp. 473–482. Elsevier, Amsterdam.

WOLLENBERGER, A., RISTAU, O., and SCHOFFA, G. 1960. Eine einfache Technik der extrem schnellen Abkühlung grösserer Gewebestücke. Pfluegers Arch. 270:399–412.

ZIMMERMAN, A. N. E., DAEMS, W., HÜLSMANN, W. C., SNIJDER, J., WISSE, E., and DURRER, D. 1967. Morphological changes of heart muscle caused by successive perfusion with calcium-free and calcium-containing solutions (calcium paradox). Cardiovasc. Res. 1:201–209.

Mailing address:
A. B. T. J. Boink,
Department of Thoracic Surgery,
University Hospital,
Catharijnesingel 101,
Utrecht (The Netherlands).

Recent Advances in Studies on
Cardiac Structure and Metabolism, Volume 11
Heart Function and Metabolism
Edited by T. Kobayashi, T. Sano, and N. S. Dhalla
Copyright 1978   University Park Press   Baltimore

INFLUENCE OF ATP OR OXYGEN PLUS SUBSTRATE ON OCCURRENCE OF THE CALCIUM PARADOX

T. J. C. RUIGROK, A. B. T. J. BOINK, and A. N. E. ZIMMERMAN

Departments of Cardiology and Thoracic Surgery,
University Hospital, Utrecht, The Netherlands

SUMMARY

Reperfusion of Ca^{2+}-deprived rat hearts with Ca^{2+}-containing medium results in irreversible cell damage (calcium paradox). In this study this type of cell damage was studied in the anoxic rat heart, in the presence and absence of glucose. Creatine kinase (CK) release was used to define cell damage. Hearts were perfused successively with Ca^{2+}-containing medium (30 min), Ca^{2+}-free medium (5 min), and Ca^{2+}-containing medium (5 min).

In the presence of glucose, myocardial ATP was maintained at a fairly high concentration. Reperfusion with Ca^{2+} resulted in an immediate and massive release of CK.

In the absence of glucose, the ATP concentration was almost zero after 30 min. Reperfusion with Ca^{2+} did not result in release of CK. Massive release occurred as soon as these hearts were reoxygenated.

It is concluded that this type of calcium-induced cell damage only occurs in the presence of ATP, or oxygen plus substrate. Mitochondria most likely play a major role in the occurrence of the calcium paradox because of their ability to accumulate huge amounts of Ca^{2+} under these conditions.

INTRODUCTION

When isolated rat hearts are perfused with Ca^{2+}-containing medium, after a brief Ca^{2+}-free period, an irreversible loss of electrical and mechanical activity and a considerable release of cell constituents can be observed (calcium paradox; Zimmerman and Hülsmann, 1966). The intracellular calcium overload, occurring on reperfusion with Ca^{2+}, leads to extensive ultrastructural changes, among which are swelling of the mitochondria and formation of intramitochondrial electron-dense material (Zimmerman *et al.,* 1967). The role of calcium in a number of experimentally induced myocardial injuries has received ample attention (Jennings and Ganote, 1974; Ganote *et al.,* 1975). To test the theory that mitochondria, with their ability to accumulate huge amounts of Ca^{2+} in an energy-linked process, play an essential role in the origin of calcium-induced cardiac cell necrosis, the calcium paradox has been studied in the anoxic rat heart, in the presence and absence of substrate.

METHODS

Hearts obtained from male Wistar rats of 200–250 g were perfused at 37° C, according to Langendorff, at a constant pressure of 100 cm of water, with a modified Tyrode solution (Zimmerman and Hülsmann, 1966). After a 15-min stabilization period, the hearts were perfused for a period of 40 min with medium equilibrated with 95% N_2–5% CO_2:

a) in the presence of glucose. After 30 min of anoxic perfusion, the Ca^{2+} was omitted from this medium for 5 min.
b) in the absence of glucose. After 30 min of anoxic perfusion the Ca^{2+} was omitted from this medium for 5 min.
c) in the absence of glucose (merely anoxic, substrate-free perfusion).

Subsequently, the hearts were reoxygenated in the presence of glucose for a period of 40 min. Creatine kinase (CK) release from the myocardium was used to define cell damage and was expressed in international units per minute per gram dry weight.

RESULTS AND DISCUSSION

After 30 min of anoxic perfusion in the presence of glucose, the hearts still contained 80% of the amount of ATP that was present at the end of the 15-min control period of perfusion with normal oxygenated medium. The Ca^{2+} was then omitted from the medium for 5 min. Reperfusion with Ca^{2+} resulted in an immediate and massive release of CK from the anoxic hearts (Figure 1).

After 30 min of anoxic perfusion in the absence of glucose, the myocardial ATP content amounted to only 2% of the content at the end of the control perfusion period. Perfusion with Ca^{2+}-free medium and subsequent reperfusion with Ca^{2+} did not result in a marked increase of CK release from the anoxic hearts. Massive release of CK occurred as soon as these hearts were reoxygenated in the presence of glucose (Figure 2). This CK release was also seen when glucose was absent on reoxygenation. This can probably be explained by consumption of endogenous oxidizable substrate, other than glucose. It is well known that reoxygenation of anoxic hearts is accompanied with enzyme release (Hearse, Humphrey, and Chain, 1973; Ganote et al., 1975). Figure 3 shows that the CK release on reoxygenation after a merely anoxic substrate-free perfusion is much less pronounced than with a preceding Ca^{2+}-free period.

It is commonly accepted that during perfusion with Ca^{2+}-free medium the sarcolemma is affected in such a way that, on reperfusion with Ca^{2+}-containing medium, the Ca^{2+} can enter the cell freely. Our experiments show that the calcium paradox only occurs in the presence of ATP (Figure 1), or in the presence of oxygen plus substrate (Figure 2). The mitochondria most likely play

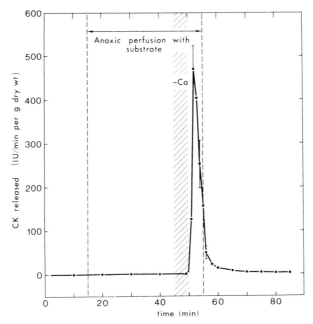

Figure 1. Effect of reperfusion with Ca^{2+} after a Ca^{2+}-free period (*shaded bar*), in the anoxic rat heart in the presence of glucose, on the release of CK (IU/min/g dry weight). Reperfusion with Ca^{2+} resulted in an immediate and massive release of CK. Values are given as mean ± S.E.M. (*n* = 4.)

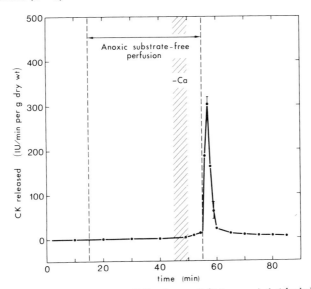

Figure 2. Effect of reperfusion with Ca^{2+} after a Ca^{2+}-free period (*shaded bar*), in the anoxic rat heart in the absence of glucose, on the release of CK (IU/min/g dry weight). Massive release of CK did not occur on reperfusion with Ca^{2+}, but only on reoxygenation of the heart. Values are given as mean ± S.E.M. (*n* = 4.)

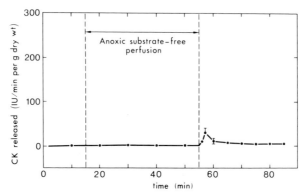

Figure 3. Effect of reoxygenation after an anoxic substrate-free perfusion on the release of CK (IU/min/g dry weight) from the isolated perfused rat heart. Reoxygenation resulted in a relatively slight release of CK. Values are given as mean ± S.E.M. ($n = 4$.)

a major role in the occurrence of the calcium paradox, because of their ability to accumulate massive quantities of Ca^{2+} under these conditions (Lehninger, Carafoli, and Rossi, 1967).

These findings might explain the massive loading of mitochondria with Ca^{2+} in myocardial tissue that occurs on reperfusion after a period of ischemia (Jennings and Ganote, 1974). During ischemia the mitochondria do not accumulate Ca^{2+}, because of the unavailability of ATP or oxygen and substrate. Arterial reperfusion, however, enables the mitochondria to accumulate Ca^{2+}, which can enter the cell freely in consequence of impaired membrane functions.

Acknowledgments The authors wish to thank Dr. A. H. J. Maas for his helpful advice, and Mrs. Ineke Stolk-Mighorst for excellent technical assistance.

REFERENCES

GANOTE, C. E., SEABRA-GOMES, R., NAYLER, W. G., and JENNINGS, R. B. 1975. Irreversible myocardial injury in anoxic perfused rat hearts. Amer. J. Pathol. 80: 419–450.

HEARSE, D. J., HUMPHREY, S. M., and CHAIN, E. B. 1973. Abrupt reoxygenation of the anoxic potassium-arrested perfused rat heart: a study of myocardial enzyme release. J. Mol. Cell. Cardiol. 5:395–407.

JENNINGS, R. B., and GANOTE, C. E. 1974. Structural changes in myocardium during acute ischemia. Circ. Res. 34/35 (suppl. III):156–168.

LEHNINGER, A. L., CARAFOLI, E., and ROSSI, C. S. 1967. Energy-linked ion movements in mitochondrial systems. Adv. Enzymol. 29:259–320.

ZIMMERMAN, A. N. E., DAEMS, W., HÜLSMANN, W. C., SNIJDER, J., WISSE, E., and DURRER, D. 1967. Morphological changes of heart muscle caused by successive perfusion with calcium-free and calcium-containing solutions (calcium paradox). Cardiovasc. Res. 1:201–209.

ZIMMERMAN, A. N. E., and HÜLSMANN, W. C. 1966. Paradoxical influence of calcium ions on the permeability of the cell membranes of the isolated rat heart. Nature 211: 646–647.

Mailing address:
Dr. T. J. C. Ruigrok,
Laboratory for Experimental Cardiology,
University Hospital,
Catharijnesingel 101,
Utrecht (The Netherlands).

Recent Advances in Studies on
Cardiac Structure and Metabolism, Volume 11
Heart Function and Metabolism
Edited by T. Kobayashi, T. Sano, and N. S. Dhalla
Copyright 1978   University Park Press   Baltimore

ROLE OF MYOCARDIAL LIPIDS
IN DEVELOPMENT OF CARDIAC NECROSIS

S. GUDBJARNASON, G. OSKARSDOTTIR,
J. HALLGRIMSSON, and B. DOELL

Science Institute and Department of Pathology,
University of Iceland, Dunhaga 3, Reykjavik, Iceland

SUMMARY

Significant alterations in fatty acyl composition of cardiac phospholipids and neutral lipids are induced by dietary cod liver oil in the rat. Increased dietary availability of docosahexaenoic acid (22:6ω3) leads to extensive replacement of linoleic acid (18:2ω6) and arachidonic acid (20:4ω6) in phospholipids. Dietary cod liver oil (10%) reduces isoproterenol stress tolerance and results in increased development of cardiac necrosis and mortality following isoproterenol treatment. It is suggested that diminished catecholamine stress tolerance may be related to altered synthesis of prostaglandins or related products.

INTRODUCTION

The purpose of this chapter is to examine the effects of myocardial lipid composition on development of cardiac necrosis. In this study we illustrate how dietary lipids may change the composition of cardiac lipids. We also suggest that polyunsaturated fatty acids in cardiac membrane lipids may have a role to play in regulation of myocardial metabolism and development of cardiac necrosis.

METHODS

The experiments were carried out on male Wistar rats, which were divided into several groups:

1. Control animals fed *ad libitum* a standard, commercial rat chow.
2. Animals fed a diet containing 10% cod liver oil. The animals were kept on this diet for at least 3 months before experimentation.
3. Animals fed a diet containing 10% cod liver oil, as in group 2. This group was injected intramuscularly with α-tocopherol, 20 mg once per week.
4. Animals on standard diet and injected intramuscularly with α-tocopherol, 20 mg once per week.

The various groups of animals were studied with or without isoproterenol treatment. Isoproterenol, 20–40 mg/kg, was injected twice according to the method of Rona (Rona *et al.,* 1959), the second injection 24 hr after the first injection. The surviving animals were then killed 48 hr after the first injection; the heart was removed and washed with ice-cold saline or water.

Myocardial lipids were extracted with chloroform-methanol (2:1) (Folch, Lees, and Sloane-Stanley, 1957). The extraction, separation, and saponification of lipids were carried out in the presence of the antioxidant BHT in order to prevent autoxidation of polyunsaturated fatty acids. The extracted lipids were separated into free fatty acids (FFA), neutral lipids (TG), and phospholipids (PL) by silicic acid chromatography and then analyzed by gas-liquid chromatography (Dittmer and Wells; Morrison and Smith, 1964).

The quality of separation was tested by TLC chromatography of lipid fractions. The separation and recovery of each sample were also estimated with the aid of an internal standard, i.e., a known amount of heptadecanoic methyl ester.

Calculations of the percentage distribution of methyl esters were performed by electronic integration with the Varian integrator and by triangulation of area peaks.

RESULTS

Dietary Fat and Cardiac Lipids

Figure 1 illustrates the relationship between the fatty acid composition of phospholipids and that of triglycerides in heart muscle. The fatty acid composition of cardiac lipids, both neutral lipids and phospholipids, is altered in animals on a diet containing cod liver oil. The most significant changes in neutral lipids are a decrease in linoleic acid and an increase in 20:1, 22:1, and 22:6. In phospholipids there is an increase in docosahexaenoic acid and decrease in linoleic acid.

Dietary availability of polyunsaturated fatty acids influences the composition of phospholipids to a much greater extent than it does that of triglycerides. Figure 1 illustrates the preferential incorporation of more unsaturated fatty acids into phospholipids. Increased dietary intake of docosahexaenoic acid, 22:6, results in a significant increase in the content of this fatty acid in phospholipids, but only a small increase in the content of 22:6 in glycerides. The linoleic acid is distributed almost equally between phospholipids and glycerides under normal conditions, whereas oleic acid seems to be preferentially incorporated into glycerides.

Figure 2 illustrates the relationship between linoleic acid, 18:2, and docosahexaenoic acid, 22:6, in phospholipids of normal rat heart muscle. This figure illustrates how the longer-chain and more unsaturated docosahexaenoic acid

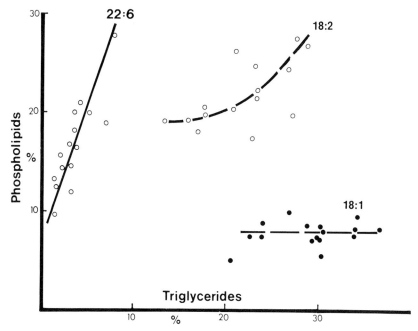

Figure 1. The relationship between the fatty acid composition of phospholipids and that of triglycerides in heart muscle.

replaces about one-third of linoleic acid in phospholipid. One-third of linoleic acid seems to be readily exchangeable for a more unsaturated fatty acid. Further increase in docosahexaenoic acid is possible, and leads to replacement of other fatty acids, such as stearic acid (Gudbjarnason and Oskarsdottir, 1975; Gudbjarnason and Hallgrimsson, 1976).

Table 1 illustrates the selectivity of phospholipid changes induced by cod liver oil. Phosphatidyl ethanolamine (PE) and phosphatidyl choline (PC) show extensive changes in fatty acid composition whereas cardiolipin does not show significant changes in composition. Cardiolipin contains mostly 18:2ω6 and this appears to be one of the main reasons why only one-third of 18:2 in total phospholipids can be replaced by 22:6ω3. These observations illustrate how dietary lipids modify both glycerides and phospholipids in heart muscle. The unsaturated fatty acids compete for incorporation into phospholipids and the more unsaturated fatty acids seem to be able to displace less unsaturated fatty acids.

Figure 3 illustrates a relationship between the ω-6 polyenoic fatty acids, i.e., linoleic and arachidonic acids, and the ω-3 polyenoic fatty acids (20:5ω3,

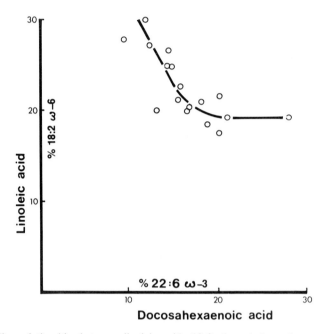

Figure 2. The relationship between linoleic acid, 18:2ω6, and docosahexaenoic acid, 22:6ω3, in phospholipids of heart muscle.

Table 1. Polyene fatty acyl composition of cardiac phospholipids

Phospholipids	Animal	18:2ω6 (%)	20:4ω6 (%)	22:6ω3 (%)
Phosphatidyl ethanolamine	Control	15.9	13.2	14.3
	CLO†	9.8*	5.7*	21.8*
Phosphatidyl choline	Control	26.3	10.8	1.7
	CLO	15.2*	10.6	7.5*
Cardiolipin	Control	71.5	0.4	3.6
	CLO	68.0	1.3	3.4
Phosph.-serine + Phosph.-inositol	Control	9.6	6.0	1.6
	CLO	7.4	5.1	2.6

*$n = 4$.
†CLO = animals fed a diet containing 10% cod liver oil.

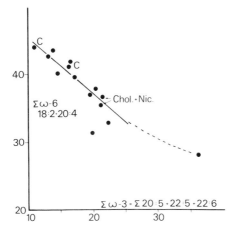

Figure 3. The relationship between the relative amount of ω-6 fatty acids (linoleic acid, 18:2ω6, and arachidonic acid, 20:4ω6) and ω-3 fatty acids (20:5ω3, 22:5ω3, 22:6ω3) in phospholipids of rat heart muscle.

22:5ω3, 22:6ω3). An inverse relationship exists between the ω-6 and ω-3 fatty acids, suggesting a competition between these fatty acids in heart muscle phospholipids.

Relation Between Cardiac Lipids
and Development of Catecholamine-Induced Myocardial Necrosis

The results in Table 2 show the fatty acid composition of heart muscle phospholipids before and after development of myocardial necrosis induced by isoproterenol stimulation, 40 mg/kg. Three groups of animals are represented, control animals, animals fed cod liver oil, and animals injected I.M. with α-tocopherol, 20 units per week for six weeks.

The relative amounts of palmitic, stearic, and oleic acids are the same in these groups of animals, whereas the phospholipids differ with respect to the relative content of polyenoic acids, i.e., 18:2, 20:4, and 22:6. Animals fed cod liver oil have considerably less of the ω-6 polyenoic acids, i.e., 18:2 and 20:4, and more of the ω-3 fatty acids, primarily 22:6 but also 20:5 and 22:5. Animals receiving α-tocopherol do show an increase in 20:4 and a decrease in 18:2.

After isoproterenol stimulation, the surviving animals were killed 48 hr after the first injection of isoproterenol. The animals fed cod liver oil usually died before or shortly after the second injection of isoproterenol, i.e., 20–30 hr after the first injection, and none of them survived 48 hr after the first injection. These animals had extensive myocardial necrosis.

Table 2. The fatty acid composition of heart muscle phospholipids before and after development of myocardial necrosis induced by isoproterenol (40 mg/kg)*

Percent fatty acid	Control		Animals fed CLO		α-Tocopherol	
	Before ($n = 4$)	After ($n = 3$)	Before ($n = 5$)	After ($n = 4$)	Before ($n = 5$)	After ($n = 4$)
16:0	12.9	13.5	12.1	10.9	12.7	13.7
	±0.1	±0.1	±0.4	±0.4	±0.3	±0.3
18:0	20.5	22.3	21.9	21.3	21.3	22.3
	±0.3	±0.6	±1.0	±0.5	±0.4	±0.1
18:1	8.2	9.1	8.5	10.1	7.9	9.4
	±0.8	±0.2	±0.4	±0.2	±0.3	±0.1
18:2	27.7	30.4	20.1	20.6	20.0	27.8
	±1.6	±1.0	±1.0	±1.1	±0.5	±0.9
20:4	16.6	13.1	11.1	9.4	20.3	11.6
	±0.9	±0.4	±0.5	±0.3	±1.0	±0.7
22:6	9.6	9.3	16.4	19.2	13.1	10.7
	±0.6	±0.9	±1.2	±0.7	±0.5	±0.9
Σ ω6	44.5	43.8	32.1	31.3	41.2	39.4
Σ ω3	11.0	11.0	19.9	25.2	14.4	12.6

*p values: 20:4–Control/CLO, before isoproterenol, $p < 0.005$; Control/α-Tocopherol, before isoproterenol, $p < 0.05$; α-Tocopherol, before/after isoproterenol, $p < 0.001$.

The increase in polyunsaturated fatty acids in phospholipids of cod liver oil–fed animals could make these lipids more susceptible to lipid peroxidation and membrane damage. In an attempt to retard such an effect, the animals were injected with α-tocopherol (vitamin E), 20 mg/week. When these vitamin E–treated animals were subjected to the isoproterenol stress they developed less necrosis and showed lower mortality than other groups. The fatty acid that seems to be of particular interest with respect to cardiac necrosis and mortality is arachidonic acid (Figure 4). The relative content of this fatty acid is lower in animals fed cod liver oil, and these animals have a 100% mortality at isoproterenol levels from 20–80 mg/kg. Control animals receiving vitamin E have an arachidonic acid level almost twice as high as the relative level of 20:4 in animals fed cod liver oil. Animals receiving vitamin E have lower mortality than the control group, i.e., 25% compared to 52% in the control group. When animals fed a diet containing 10% cod liver oil were injected with vitamin E, there was neither an increase in 20:4 levels of phospholipids, nor was there a decrease in mortality following stimulation.

The change in arachidonic acid level during isoproterenol stress may also be of significance (Figure 4, lower part). In the group with the lowest mortality the diminution or possibly the utilization of 20:4 is greatest, whereas the animals

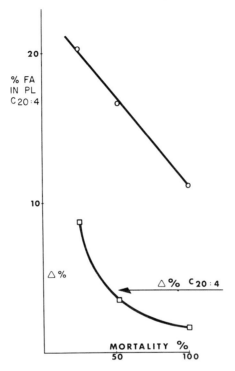

Figure 4. Upper part: The relationship between the relative content of arachidonic acid, 20:4ω6, in phospholipids of heart muscle and mortality following isoproterenol stimulation. *Lower part:* Diminution or change in the relative amount (Δ%) of arachidonic acid, 20:4ω6, in phospholipids of heart muscle during stimulation with isoproterenol.

with the highest mortality show little alteration in 20:4 of heart muscle phospholipids.

Metabolism of Polyene Fatty Acids in Heart Muscle

Figure 5 illustrates the oxygenation of 20:4ω6 and 22:6ω3 by cardiac microsomes. The cofactor in this assay is epinephrine, or adrenaline, and the product measured is adrenochrome (Takeguchi and Sih, 1972). These two substrates differ with respect to enzyme saturation, inhibitor sensitivity, and products formed. The products derived from 20:4ω6 are prostaglandins, endoperoxides, thromboxanes, and hydroxy fatty acids (Hamberg and Samuelsson, 1974; Hamberg, Svensson, and Samuelsson, 1976). The products derived from 22:6ω3 are unknown.

Figure 6 shows the effect of the PG-synthetase inhibitor indomethacin upon the oxygenation of 20:4ω6 and 22:6ω3. The oxygenation of the prostaglandin

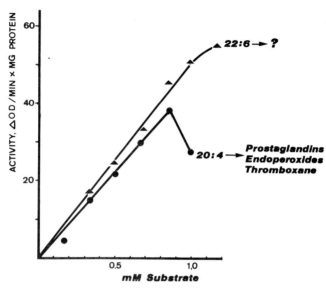

Figure 5. Oxygenation of arachidonic acid, 20:4ω6, and docosahexaenoic acid, 22:6ω3, by cardiac microsomes. Assay conditions: microsomal enzyme 10 μg protein; 1 mM L-epinephrine; 50 mM Tris-Cl; pH 8.3; 0–1.2 mM substrate; final volume, 3 ml. Rate of formation of adrenochrome is measured at λ_{480} nm.

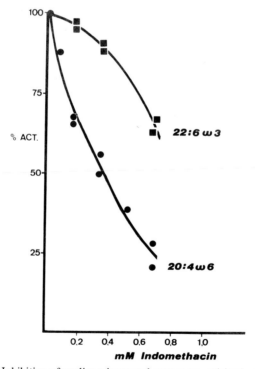

Figure 6. Inhibition of cardiac microsomal oxygenase activity by indomethacin.

precursor, 20:4ω6, is more sensitive to indomethacin than the oxygenation of 22:6ω3, suggesting different binding properties or different pathways for these substrates.

Membrane changes may also influence properties of membrane-bound enzymes. Figure 7 shows the inhibition of cardiac microsomal oxygenase and adrenochrome formation by Ca^{2+}. At normal Ca^{2+} levels there is no inhibition of oxygenase or PG-synthetase. At higher Ca^{2+} levels, above 4 mM, there are inhibition of PG synthesis and greater inhibition in older animals.

In animals fed cod liver oil, the Ca^{2+} sensitivity has increased considerably, suggesting that any increase in Ca^{2+} influx would diminish oxygenase activity.

DISCUSSION

The role of dietary fat in cardiovascular disease has thus far primarily been discussed with respect to the involvement of dietary lipids in atherosclerosis and

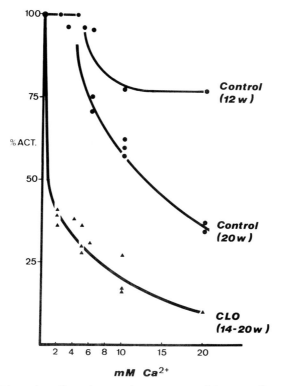

Figure 7. Inhibition of cardiac microsomal oxygenase activity by Ca^{2+}. Control animals were either 12 weeks or 20 weeks old. Animals fed CLO (cod liver oil, 10%) were 14–20 weeks old.

vascular occlusion. Dietary lipids may also cause extensive chemical modifications of various organs and change the composition of membrane lipids as well as the kinetic properties of membrane-bound enzymes. The polyunsaturated fatty acids of cardiac muscle seem to be more responsive to changes in the fatty acid composition of the diet than do those of other organs (Rieckehoff, Holman, and Burr, 1949; Widmer and Holman, 1950).

The polyene fatty acids of cardiac muscle are primarily located in membrane phospholipids. These polyene fatty acids contain 2–6 double bonds and arise from two different dietary sources, linoleic acid (18:2ω6) and α-linoleic acid (18:3ω3).

This study illustrates an extensive but selective alteration in fatty acyl composition of cardiac phospholipids induced by dietary cod liver oil. Cardiolipin, primarily located in mitochondria, does not change significantly, whereas PE and PC show significant changes in polyene composition: replacement of 18:2 and 20:4 by 22:6 in PE and replacement of 18:2 by 22:6 in PC.

An attempt was made to relate the alterations in polyene fatty acyl composition of membrane lipids to the diminution in isoproterenol stress tolerance in animals fed cod liver oil.

There are several ways in which changes in membrane lipid composition could influence stress tolerance: 1) Increase in polyene fatty acyl groups in phospholipids could increase membrane fluidity, permeability, lipid peroxidation, and instability. 2) Increase in polyene fatty acyl groups could alter properties of membrane-bound enzymes. 3) Alterations in polyene fatty acyl composition of phospholipids may affect those enzymatic processes that require specific membrane-bound polyene fatty acids as substrates, for example, prostaglandin synthetase.

It is possible that all three factors play a role in reduced catecholamine stress tolerance in cod liver oil–fed animals. In addition, vitamins D and A, contained in the cod liver oil, could also contribute to reduced isoproterenol tolerance. The cod liver oil–fed animals showed a normal growth rate, with an average body weight 7% above that of control animals. The daily dietary intake of vitamin D was 200 IU, and of vitamin A, 1,000 IU.

The reduced isoproterenol stress tolerance reflected in increased mortality of cod liver oil–fed animals following isoproterenol treatment may be related to the metabolism of membrane polyene fatty acids in heart muscle and possibly other organs. The extensive replacement of the ω-6 polyene fatty acids, 18:2 and 20:4, by the ω-3 polyene fatty acids, 20:5, 22:5, and 22:6, could affect myocardial prostaglandin synthesis and thereby influence the prostaglandin-mediated feed-back control of catecholamine action, such as control of intracellular lipolytic activity and norepinephrine release from nerve terminals in heart muscle (Steinberg *et al.,* 1970; Ramwell and Shaw, 1970).

Arachidonic acid, 20:4, is synthesized from linoleic acid, 18:2, and serves as a substrate for prostaglandin synthesis (Bergström, Carlson, and Weeks, 1968). A variety of polyenoic acids, mostly ω-6 fatty acids, can serve as substrates for PG synthesis, whereas some of the ω-3 fatty acids, such as 22:6, do not serve as substrates (Lands *et al.*, 1973). Figure 5 illustrates that both 20:4 and 22:6 serve as substrates for cardiac microsomal oxygenases. The products derived from 20:4 are prostaglandins and other products (Hamberg *et al.*, 1976), whereas the products of 22:6 are unknown, but they are not prostaglandins.

The extensive alteration in fatty acyl composition of membrane lipids in cod liver oil–fed animals may also influence the properties of membrane-bound enzymes, and alter K_m and inhibitor sensitivity. Figure 7 illustrates an increase in Ca^{2+} sensitivity of myocardial PG-synthetase with age or cod liver oil diet. Administration of isoproterenol has been shown to increase Ca^{2+} influx (Fleckenstein, 1971) and could thus diminish PG-synthetase or oxygenase activity *in vivo*.

The hypothesis is proposed that reduced isoproterenol stress tolerance in animals fed cod liver oil may in part be related to altered synthesis of prostaglandins or related products, possibly by way of altered substrate availability and by alterations in properties of the PG-synthetase complex.

REFERENCES

BERGSTRÖM, S., CARLSON, L. A., and WEEKS, J. R. 1968. The prostaglandins: A family of biologically active lipids. Pharmacol. Rev. 20:1–48.

DITTMER, J. C., and WELLS, M. A. Quantitative and qualitative analysis of lipids and lipid components. *In* J. M. Lowenstein (ed.), Methods of Enzymology, Vol. 14, Lipids. Academic Press, New York.

FLECKENSTEIN, A. 1971. Specific inhibitor and promoters of calcium action in the excitation-contraction coupling of heart muscle and their role in the prevention or production of myocardial lesions. *In* P. Harris and L. Opie (eds.), Calcium and the Heart, Proceedings of the Meeting of the European Section of the International Study Group for Research in Cardiac Metabolism. Academic Press, New York.

FOLCH, J., LEES, M., and SLOANE-STANLEY, G. H. 1957. A simple method for the isolation and purification of total lipids from animal tissues. J. Biol. Chem. 226: 497–509.

GUDBJARNASON, S., and HALLGRIMSSON, J. 1976. The role of myocardial membrane lipids in the development of cardiac necrosis. Acta Med. Scand. (Suppl.) 587:17–26.

GUDBJARNASON, S., and ÓSKARSDÓTTIR, 1975. Changes in fatty acid composition of cardiac lipids accompanying myocardial necrosis. *In* A. Fleckenstein and G. Rona (eds.), Recent Advances in Studies on Cardiac Structure and Metabolism, Vol. 6, Pathophysiology and Morphology of Myocardial Cell Alterations, pp. 193–203. University Park Press, Baltimore.

HAMBERG, M., and SAMUELSSON, B. 1974. Prostaglandin endoperoxides. Novel transformation of arachidonic acid in human platelets. Proc. Natl. Acad. Sci. USA 71: 3400–3404.

HAMBERG, M., SVENSSON, J., and SAMUELSSON, B. 1976. Novel transformation of prostaglandin endoperoxides: Formation of thromboxanes. *In* B. Samuelsson and R. Paoletti (eds.), Advances in Prostaglandin and Thromboxane Research, Vol. I, pp. 19–28.

LANDS, W. E. M., LE TELLIER, P. R., ROME, L. H., and VANDERHOEK, I. Y. 1973. Inhibition of prostaglandin biosynthesis. *In* S. Bergström (ed.), Advances in Biosciences, Vol. 9, pp. 15–28. Pergamon Press Ltd., Oxford.

MORRISON, W. R., and SMITH, L. M. 1964. Preparation of fatty acid methylesters and dimethylacetals from lipids with boron-fluoride-methanol. J. Lipid Res. 5:600–608.

RAMWELL, P. W., and SHAW, J. E. 1970. Biological significance of the prostaglandins. Rec. Progr. Horm. Res. 26:139–187.

RIECKEHOFF, J. G., HOLMAN, R. T., and BURR, C. O. 1949. Polyethenoid fatty acid metabolism. Effect of dietary fat on polyethenoid fatty acids of rat tissues. Arch. Biochem. 20:331–340.

RONA, G., CHAPPEL, C. I., BALAZS, T., and GAUDRY, R. 1959. An infarct-like myocardial lesion and other toxic manifestations produced by isoproterenol in the rat. A. M. A. Arch. Pathol. 67:443–455.

STEINBERG, D., VAUGHAN, M., NESTEL, P., and BERGSTRÖM, S. 1970. Effects of prostaglandin E opposing those of catecholamines on blood pressure and on triglyceride breakdown in adipose tissue. Biochem. Pharmacol. 12:764–766.

TAKEGUCHI, C., and SIH, C. J. 1972. A rapid spectrophotometric assay for prostaglandin synthetase: Application to the study of non-steroidal antiinflammatory agents. Prostaglandins 2:169–184.

WIDMER, C., and HOLMAN, R. T. 1950. Polyethenoid fatty acid metabolism II. Deposition of polyunsaturated fatty acids in fat deficient rats upon single fatty acid supplementation. Arch. Biochem. 25:1–12.

Mailing address:
Dr. S. Gudbjarnason,
Science Institute, University of Iceland,
Dunhaga 3, Reykjavik (Iceland).

Recent Advances in Studies on
Cardiac Structure and Metabolism, Volume 11
Heart Function and Metabolism
Edited by T. Kobayashi, T. Sano, and N. S. Dhalla
Copyright 1978   University Park Press   Baltimore

ENERGY LIBERATION IN ABNORMAL CARDIAC MUSCLE

T. ISHIYAMA and Y. MORITA

The Third Department of Internal Medicine, Osaka University Hospital,
Fukushima 1-1-50, Fukushima-ku, Osaka 553, Japan

SUMMARY

Uncoupling of oxidative phosphorylation was suggested in experiments using the infarcted myocardium, even in dogs with 15-min ligation. The same type of disturbance in mitochondrial respiration was observed in dogs with reperfusion after 45-min ligation, whereas the disturbance was recovered in dogs with reperfusion after 15-min ligation.

INTRODUCTION

The heart is beating continuously, and therefore performs tremendous work. Thus, energy liberation is essential in consideration of cardiac metabolism. In energy liberation, subcellular oxidation, coupled with phosphorylation, is the essential process, and it is performed in mitochondria. The authors have studied mitochondrial respiration of canine heart muscle using the polarographic method developed by Hagihara (1961), in order to clarify disturbances of the subcellular mechanism of energy liberation.

METHOD AND RESULTS

For the first time, the authors studied an experimental ischemic heart that was produced by ligation of the stem of a coronary artery (Yamagami, Morita, and Yamamura, 1967). The effects on mitochondrial respiration are summarized in Table 1. With the intact heart muscle, the authors found that the oxygen consumption rate (QO_2) in state 3 was 83.0 ± 18.0 natoms O/mg protein/min, and QO_2 state 4 was 16.7 ± 5.08 natoms O/mg protein/min. Therefore, the respiratory control index (RCI), which was calculated by division of QO_2 state 3 by QO_2 state 4, was 5.65 ± 1.17, and the ADP/O ratio was 2.77 ± 0.19. Heart mitochondria isolated from the noninfarcted area of the left ventricle revealed deteriorated respiration. When the dogs were sacrificed 60 min after ligation at the stem of left circumflex coronary artery, mitochondria isolated from the

Table 1. Respiration of canine heart mitochondria in experimental myocardial infarction*

Condition of heart muscle	Oxygen consumption rate		Respiratory control index	ADP/O ratio
	State 3	State 4		
	(natoms O/mg protein/min)			
Intact	83.0 ± 13.0	16.7 ± 5.08	5.65 ± 1.17	2.77 ± 0.19
Noninfarcted	91.0 ± 18.8	18.4 ± 5.60	5.16 ± 1.07	2.81 ± 0.18
Infarcted				
15 min	105.1 ± 21.6	36.1 ± 10.8	3.10 ± 1.09	2.68 ± 0.08
30 min	87.2 ± 19.0	28.8 ± 9.15	3.20 ± 0.90	2.65 ± 0.30
60 min	87.8 ± 9.03	45.9 ± 11.3	2.03 ± 0.49	2.71 ± 0.29

*Glutamate was used as a substrate. Numerical values are mean ± S.D.

infarcted area showed remarkable acceleration of the QO_2 state 4. This state is an experimentally prepared condition of mitochondrial suspension *in vitro,* where the phosphate acceptor, ADP, is absent. Therefore, in this state, oxidation is proceeding but phosphorylation is not concurrent. QO_2 state 3 was within normal range. Therefore, RCI was deteriorated but ADP/O ratio was unchanged. These results suggested the occurrence of uncoupling of oxidative phosphorylation in the mitochondria isolated from the infarcted heart muscle. These changes were observed in the mitochondria isolated from the infarcted myocardium of the dogs that were sacrificed 15 or 30 min after coronary ligation. This fact suggested that the change of mitochondrial respiration revealed a relatively early stage of myocardial ischemia.

These changes of mitochondrial respiration in the ischemic heart were analyzed experimentally. Table 2 shows the experimental results on mitochondrial respiration in hypoxic hearts induced by various methods. Hypoxic myocardium produced by blood-letting for 60 min from the femoral artery revealed deteriorated RCI due to the accelerated QO_2 state 4. Then, the intact canine hearts were extirpated and immersed in saline ($38°$ C) for 60 min without coronary perfusion, and the mitochondria were isolated. These mitochondria did not show any deterioration of RCI. In the same condition, however, when the extirpated hearts were forced to pulsate in the saline by electrical stimulation, QO_2 state 4 was accelerated and RCI was deteriorated. These experimental results suggested that hypoxic hearts without beating did not reveal any disturbance of energy liberation, but hearts in states of hypoxia with beating revealed the disturbance of energy liberation, as shown in the blood-let hearts *in vivo* or in the ischemic hearts due to coronary ligation. Therefore, it is suggested that

Table 2. Respiration of canine heart mitochondria in experimental hypoxic myocardium*

Condition of heart muscle	Oxygen consumption rate		Respiratory control index	ADP/O ratio
	State 3	State 4		
	(natoms O/mg protein/min)			
Intact	83.0 ± 18.0	16.7 ± 5.08	5.65 ± 1.67	2.77 ± 0.19
Blood-letting	90.4 ± 8.20	33.8 ± 7.95	2.76 ± 0.54	2.82 ± 0.38
Extirpated				
Without beating	97.6 ± 22.3	20.4 ± 9.10	5.26 ± 1.69	2.70 ± 0.41
With beating	82.8 ± 11.0	29.2 ± 8.18	3.04 ± 1.04	2.76 ± 0.16

*Glutamate was used as a substrate. Numerical values are mean ± S.D.

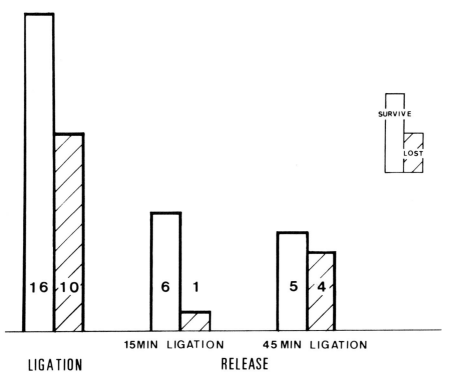

Figure 1. Fatality of dogs in experimental groups. (Survive: survived for 60 min, then sacrificed; lost: died due to ventricular fibrillation.)

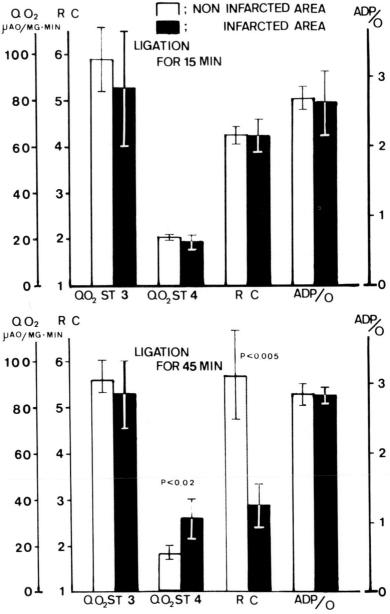

Figure 2. Respiration of canine heart mitochondria in experimental coronary reperfusion. The *upper figure* is that of the 15-min ligation followed by 60-min reperfusion; the *lower figure* is that of 45-min ligation followed by 60-min reperfusion. (QO_2: oxygen consumption rate; ST 3: state 3; ST 4: state 4; RC: respiratory control index; ADP/O: ADP/O ratio; numerical values are mean ± S. E.)

the mechanism of the disturbance of energy liberation of myocardium is beating under hypoxic states.

Further experiments were performed in order to ascertain whether or not changes of beating frequency and/or force of beating of the infarcted myocardium modified mitochondrial respiration (Morita *et al.,* 1974). Positive chronotropism and/or positive inotropism tended to accelerate the uncoupling of oxidative phosphorylation. On the other hand, negative chronotropism and/or negative inotropism mitigated the RCI.

The next problem that the authors studied as a related experiment was the effect of reperfusion of the ligated coronary artery. Many reports have been published on the effects of coronary reperfusion in surgical cases of ischemic heart diseases or experimental coronary occlusion. The authors found that the coronary reperfusion did not always bring on favorable effects, but caused sudden death in some dogs in the early stage of coronary reperfusion. As shown in Figure 1, coronary ligation caused sudden death due to ventricular fibrillation in 10 out of 26 dogs (38%). Dogs whose coronary ligations were released after 15 min revealed ventricular fibrillation only in 1 dog out of 7 dogs (14%). On the contrary, dogs whose coronary ligations were released after 45 min revealed an apparently high incidence of ventricular fibrillation: 4 dogs out of 9 dogs (44%). These effects of reperfusion were studied from the standpoint of electrocardiography, cardiac dynamics, and myocardial energy liberation.

Here, the authors present the results of myocardial energy liberation. Figure 2 shows the changes of mitochondrial respiration. The upper figure is the 15-min ligation followed by coronary release for 60 min. QO_2 state 3, QO_2 state 4, RCI, and ADP/O ratio did not show any significant differences between the infarcted and the noninfarcted areas. As shown in Table 1, QO_2 state 4 was accelerated and RCI was deteriorated in the dogs with 15-min coronary ligation. Therefore, these results suggested that the 15-min ligation followed by coronary release for 60 min recovered the disturbed mitochondrial respiration due to coronary ligation. On the other hand, as shown in the lower figure, the 45-min ligation followed by coronary release for 60 min showed significant differences in QO_2 state 4 and RCI between the infarcted and the noninfarcted areas. These changes of mitochondrial respiration were just the same as those of coronary ligation without release, suggesting uncoupling of oxidative phosphorylation.

In summary, it is suggested that the disturbed mitochondrial respiration due to coronary ligation occurs even in the early stage, and if the ligation is sustained for 45 min it might be irreversible even by coronary perfusion.

REFERENCES

HAGIHARA, B. 1961. Techniques for the application of polarography to mitochondrial respiration. Biochim. Biophys. Acta 46:134–142.

MORITA, Y., ISHIYAMA, T., TSUKAMOTO, N., and YAMAMURA, Y. 1974. Effects of isoproterenol, propranolol and artificial pacing on hemodynamics and energy liberation of the infarcted heart in dogs. Jpn. Heart J. 15:579–592.
YAMAGAMI, T., MORITA, Y., and YAMAMURA, Y. 1967. Mitochondrial respiration of experimentally produced ischemic heart muscle in dogs. Jpn. Heart J. 8:132–141.

Mailing address:
Taro Ishiyama, M.D.,
The Third Department of Internal Medicine,
Osaka University Hospital,
Fukushima 1-1-50, Fukushima-ku,
Osaka 553 (Japan).

Recent Advances in Studies on
Cardiac Structure and Metabolism, Volume 11
Heart Function and Metabolism
Edited by T. Kobayashi, T. Sano, and N. S. Dhalla
Copyright 1978 University Park Press Baltimore

MYOCARDIAL ENERGY
AND ELECTROLYTE METABOLISM DURING
EXERCISE IN PATIENTS WITH CIRCULATORY DISEASE

I. SEKI, H. AKIOKA, N. GOTO,
H. KAMIDE, Y. HIGASHIHARA, K. MORI,
K. FUJIWARA, H. HIGUCHI, A. TERAUCHI,
I. SANO, A. IMAOKA, N. KISHIMA,
K. KONDO, and T. MIYAGI

The First Department of Internal Medicine,
Osaka Medical College, Takatsuki, Japan

SUMMARY

In 43 patients with various circulatory diseases, the coronary blood flow and myocardial metabolism of oxygen, carbohydrates, fats, inorganic phosphate (Pi), creatine (Cr), and potassium (K) were measured before and during bicycle ergometry (50 w, 15 min), along with ECG changes and cardiac performance. The energy expenditure was 4.4 kcal per min and 64 kcal in 15 min. The ECT changes were quite similar to that of Master's double two-step test. The limitation of coronary vascular response was seen in cases with normotensive coronary disease as a main cause of cardiac ischemic changes during exercise. In cases with idiopathic cardiomyopathy or rheumatic mitral stenosis, similar disorders of ECG changes and myocardial metabolism were seen, in spite of no remarkable disturbance of coronary vascular response. The simultaneous output or decrease of uptake of Pi and Cr during exercise, in cases with cardiac ischemia, indicates the mobilization of stored energy from myocardial creatine phosphate, and it appeared a more physiological response, compared with anaerobic carbohydrate metabolism. Potassium output from ischemic heart was seen during exercise. In the K myocardial uptake there was a significant difference between patients with and patients without ischemic ECG changes, regardless of the dominant influence of its arterial concentration. As to the reduction of S-T changes during exercise, there was no evidence suggesting unfavorable signs of ischemic heart, as far as the present study is concerned.

INTRODUCTION

Since Lombardo *et al.* (1953), many studies on human myocardial metabolism and coronary circulation during exercise were reported. The close relationship of ECG patterns or angina pectoris to myocardial metabolism was clearly demonstrated by Parker *et al.* (1969a, 1969b). However, the effect of coronary circulation upon them in clinical cases is still obscure (Rowe *et al.*, 1965; Cohen *et al.*, 1966). In a previous study, the relation between ECG changes and myocardial oxygen demand-and-supply during Levy's hypoxemia test with coronary venous catheterization was shown (Seki, 1960). This chapter is a comprehensive study of myocardial energy and potassium (K) metabolism and coronary circulation, relating them with cardiac mechanical performance and ECG changes during exercise, in which the selection of cases and the severity of exercise loading were scheduled to induce coronary insufficiency in most ischemic hearts, without confusion. The simultaneous measurement of inorganic phosphate (Pi) and creatine (Cr) was made in order to estimate the mobilization of stored energy from myocardial creatine phosphate, as previously reported (Mori, 1972; Seki and Akioka, 1973).

MATERIAL AND METHODS

In 43 patients, consisting of 5 with neurocirculatory asthenia (NCA), 8 with hypertension without coronary insufficiency (HT), 8 with hypertensive coronary failure (HTC), 8 with normotensive coronary heart disease (CHD), excluding severe coronary occlusion, and 14 with other heart diseases (HD), such as mitral stenosis or idiopathic cardiomyopathy, coronary catheterization was performed and coronary blood flow (CBF) (N_2O method) and myocardial metabolism of oxygen (O_2), glucose, lactate, pyruvate, non-esterified fatty acid (NEFA), ketone bodies, Pi [modification of Folin Wu method (Taussky and Shorr, 1953)], Cr [modification of Fiske Subbarow method (Bosnes and Taussky, 1945) and enzyme method], and K were measured, before and 15 min after starting bicycle ergometry at a rate of 50 W. The details of the method are already given (Higuchi, 1972; Mori, 1972; Higashihara, 1973; Fujiwara, 1975).

RESULTS

Energy Expenditure and Cardiac Function (Table 1)

General oxygen consumption increased to about 4 times that of pretest value and the energy expenditure for the exercise test was nearly the same in each group: 4.4 kcal per minute and 64 kcal in 15 minutes. The cardiac output also increased similarly in all groups. However, blood pressure, left ventricular work (LVW), and myocardial tension (MT) were the highest in the HT group, both at rest and during exercise. In the CHD group, heart work was the lowest at rest, but the increase was the largest among the groups.

Coronary Circulation and Myocardial Oxygen Metabolism (Table 1)

Myocardial oxygen consumption (MOC) had high positive correlation with CBF before and during exercise, regardless of coronary or heart disease (r = 0.92, r = 0.98), but it was not so linear with cardiac work, especially not in coronary and heart diseases. CBF and MOC did not significantly differ among the groups at rest, but during exercise they increased significantly in cases without coronary disorder, namely, in NCA, HT, and HD groups. They did not significantly increase in cases of coronary disease, HTC and CHD. The CBF during exercise in CHD was the lowest of all groups. The ratio of MOC to LVW or MT was maintained only in NCA, and in other groups it decreased significantly.

Myocardial Metabolism of Carbohydrates and Fats

The arterial concentration of lactate and pyruvate increased significantly during exercise in all groups. The myocardial usage of carbohydrates increased significantly in NCA and HT, chiefly due to increases in CBF and arterial concentration, but in HTC and CHD the myocardial usage of carbohydrates did not increase significantly due to poor response of CBF. In CHD and HD, there were many patients in which the myocardial extraction ratio of lactate and pyruvate inverted to negative, indicating anaerobic carbohydrate metabolism. The arterial concentration of NEFA generally decreased; 10 or 15 min after starting exercise, myocardial extraction tended to decrease, but the myocardial usage was maintained in many groups. Between the myocardial extraction and arterial level of NEFA, there was a significant positive correlation at rest, but it disappeared during exercise.

Myocardial Metabolism of Creatine Phosphate (Figure 1)

Cr was extracted by the myocardium in correlation with its arterial concentration at rest, but the correlation disappeared during exercise. In most cases without ECG changes, or NCA and HT groups, the myocardial uptake of Cr and Pi was maintained, but in CHD, HTC, and HD groups, the uptake of both metabolites was reduced or turned to negative. The myocardial extractions of Cr and Pi did not correlate with each other at rest but they did correlate during exercise. These findings indicate the mobilization of stored energy in myocardial creatine phosphate in cases of coronary and heart disease.

Myocardial Uptake of Potassium (Figure 2)

The mean value of the arterial concentration of K was increased significantly during exercise, as well as the coronary venous concentration. However, the myocardial uptake of K was maintained in the cases without ECG changes. In many cases with changes, the uptake turned to negative. The change of myocardial uptake of K was significantly different between the two groups. The myocardial uptake of K correlated with its arterial concentration even during exercise or at rest. The K output from the cardiac muscle in patients with ECG changes was observed, with no exception, when the arterial serum level of K was below 4.0 mEq/liter during the exercise.

Table 1. Myocardial energy metabolism and hemodynamics during bicycle ergometry†

		NCA (n = 5)	H T (n = 8)	HTC (n = 8)	CHD (n = 8)	H D (n = 14)
CBF	R	59.7 ± 9.8 **	66.7 ± 5.3 *	1.8 ± 0.2	58.8 ± 3.1	71.8 ± 4.8 *
ml/100g/min	E	132.5 ± 41.7	98.3 ± 7.6	88.0 ± 12.4	84.7 ± 10.9	119.4 ± 11.1
MOC	R	6.4 ± 0.9	7.0 ± 0.7	6.8 ± 0.8	6.4 ± 0.5 *	7.2 ± 0.5 ***
ml/100g/min	E	14.4 ± 4.4	10.7 ± 0.4	9.3 ± 1.4	9.2 ± 1.3	12.6 ± 1.2
Glucose	R	18.2 ± 4.7	15.6 ± 2.8	14.6 ± 3.7	10.9 ± 2.3	7.4 ± 2.4
extr. ratio %	E	13.3 ± 4.1	16.1 ± 2.8	13.4 ± 5.2	4.8 ± 3.8	7.3 ± 2.9
Lactate	R	25.4 ± 5.8	30.9 ± 7.8 **	30.1 ± 9.6	21.0 ± 10.4	37.2 ± 6.3 **
extr. ratio %	E	33.6 ± 6.3	27.0 ± 4.2	26.0 ± 2.3	10.3 ± 5.9	14.6 ± 5.4
Pyruvate	R	35.2 ± 4.7	41.7 ± 3.6	31.9 ± 12.6	28.4 ± 6.1	33.4 ± 5.2
extr. ratio %	E	37.0 ± 1.3	34.1 ± 6.2	33.4 ± 5.2	24.2 ± 11.7	25.0 ± 8.1
NEFA	R	13.6 ± 3.3	12.7 ± 2.0	10.9 ± 3.0	10.5 ± 0.7	10.4 ± 1.2
extr. ratio %	E	12.2 ± 4.0	6.2 ± 1.4	6.6 ± 1.9	9.8 ± 2.0	9.1 ± 1.3
Keton	R	22.4 ± 10.7	0.6 ± 19.5	20.8 ± 8.4 *	14.9 ± 6.3	−13.9 ± 12.9
extr. ratio %	E	31.7 ± 12.1	6.5 ± 11.6	−5.4 ± 11.4	−10.5 ± 18.3 *	−25.5 ± 18.4 *
Pi	R	3.8 ± 1.0	2.3 ± 1.3	1.2 ± 1.2	2.7 ± 0.9	1.2 ± 0.6

extr. ratio %	E	5.4 ± 1.9	2.7 ± 0.9	−0.7 ± 2.0	−1.8 ± 1.8	−1.8 ± 0.8
Creatine	R	−5.8 ± 3.3 **	−9.3 ± 3.8 *	7.7 ± 15.2	6.6 ± 7.1	0.2 ± 4.5
extr. ratio %	E	26.3 ± 17.3	12.0 ± 3.7 *	−25.7 ± 11.8	−4.9 ± 8.5	−6.3 ± 7.6
K	R	−5.7		5.2 ± 4.2	8.2 ± 5.8	−2.4 ± 2.4
extr. ratio %	E	0.4		0.1 ± 6.5	2.9 ± 3.0	−0.3 ± 3.5
HR	R	86.5 ± 8.4 **	83.3 ± 6.3 **	72.6 ± 4.4 ***	76.6 ± 5.0 ***	86.3 ± 4.3 ***
beats/min	E	113.2 ± 5.4	121.6 ± 9.4	103.3 ± 4.7	117.3 ± 10.1	139.5 ± 6.9
mBP	R	92.1 ± 4.6 *	110.8 ± 6.2 ***	101.3 ± 4.2 ***	96.1 ± 4.2 *	88.7 ± 3.7 ***
mmHg	E	96.2 ± 8.5	131.0 ± 5.7	121.3 ± 4.5	104.7 ± 4.2	103.6 ± 4.7
LVW index	R	4.6 ± 0.9 *	7.2 ± 0.9 *	4.4 ± 0.3 ***	3.7 ± 0.4 ***	5.6 ± 0.9 ***
MT	E	9.6 ± 2.0	22.6 ± 3.5	13.6 ± 1.1	16.5 ± 3.3	20.5 ± 3.1
	R	13.8 ± 1.9 **	17.3 ± 1.5 ***	12.5 ± 0.5 ***	11.6 ± 0.6 ***	13.3 ± 0.6 ***
dyne/cm 10^{-6}	E	21.4 ± 2.7	36.4 ± 3.0	26.1 ± 1.8	26.4 ± 2.4	32.6 ± 2.5

† Abbreviations are: NCA = neurocirculatory asthenia; HT = hypertension without coronary insufficiency; HTC = hypertensive coronary failure; CHD = normotensive coronary heart disease; HD = other heart diseases; CBF = coronary blood flow; MOC = myocardial oxygen consumption; R = rest; E = exercise; NEFA = non-esterified fatty acid; HR = heart rate; BP = blood pressure; LVW = left ventricular work; MT = myocardial tension; *$p < 0.05$; **$p < 0.01$; ***$p < 0.001$. Values are expressed as mean ± S.E.

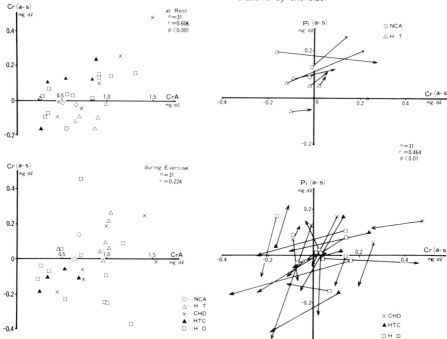

Relationship between myocardial extraction of creatine and the arterial concentration.

Relationship between changes of myocardial extraction of inorganic phosphate and creatine by exercise.

Figure 1. Arterial creatine (CrA) and myocardial uptake of creatine (Cr(a–s)) and inorganic phosphate (Pi(a–s)) at rest, during exercise, and the change by exercise.

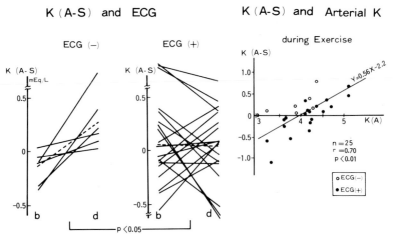

K (A-S) and ECG

K (A-S) and Arterial K

Figure 2. Significant difference between the change of myocardial uptake of potassium (K(A–S)) in cases without ECG change (ECG(–)) and with changes (ECG(+)) before (b) and during (d) exercise, and correlation of K(A–S) with arterial potassium (K(A)) during exercise.

594

ECG Change and Myocardial Energy Metabolism

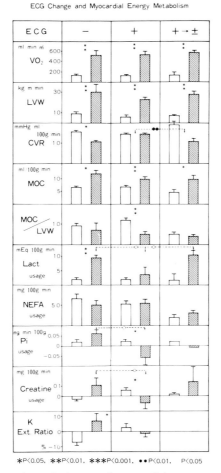

Figure 3. Mean value and standard error of myocardial energy metabolism at rest (white column) and during exercise (black column) in 3 groups; without (−), with (+), and improved (+ → ±) ischemic ECG changes during exercise.

ECG Changes and Myocardial Metabolism (Figure 3)

The ECG changes during bicycle ergometry were quite similar to those of Master's double two-step test in all cases except for two. In 17 cases, there was no ischemic change, in 22 cases there were changes, before and/or after exercise test, and in 4 patients, the ischemic ECG changes were diminished during exercise. Among the 3 ECG change groups, there was no significant difference in the myocardial energy metabolism at rest. During exercise, in the normal ECG group, coronary vascular resistance decreased significantly and MOC per LVW was maintained. In the ischemic ECG change group, there was no significant decrease in coronary vascular resistance, and the ratio of MOC to LVW decreased significantly. The myocardial use of lactate and pyruvate during exercise in this group was the lowest among the groups. In the improved ECG group, the coronary circulatory response and myocardial use of lactate were as good as in the normal ECG group. Considering the present data, we could not find any evidence indicating that this ECG change was an unfavorable sign.

**Feature of Myocardial Energy Balance
During Exercise in Circulatory Diseases (Figure 4)**

To illustrate the special feature of coronary response and myocardial energy metabolism of each disease group during exercise, a schematic drawing was made. The mean value and standard error of LVW (W), CBF (F), MOC (O), myocardial extraction ratio of lactate (L), Pi (P), and Cr (C), and the summation of S–T depression in leads I, II, III, and V4 (E) during exercise were compared, and the scales of the parameters were so determined that the mean value of NCA falls on the same line, except for ECG change, which is marked, based on zero line. In Figure 4 one can clearly see the remarkable increase in LVW with the good response of CBF and the early mobilization of stored energy from creatine phosphate without anaerobic carbohydrate metabolism or ischemic ECG change in the HT group. In the HD group, anaerobic carbohydrate metabolism and ischemic ECG changes were similarly seen, in spite of good response of CBF.

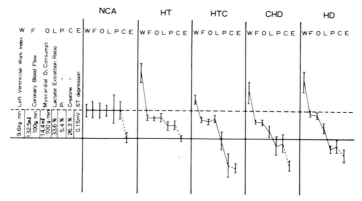

Feature of Myocardial Energy Balance
during Exercise in various circulatory Disease

Figure 4. Mean value and standard error of left ventricular work (W), coronary blood flow (F), myocardial oxygen consumption (O), myocardial extraction ratio of lactate (L), inorganic phosphate (P), and creatine (C), and S–T deviation during exercise in circulatory diseases. The scale of parameters is so determined that the mean value of NCA falls on the same line, except for the ECG change, which is on the zero line.

DISCUSSION

To elucidate the special feature of coronary vascular response in coronary disease, the following were considerations of this study. First, the intensity of exercise loading was determined in reference to ECG changes during exercise, in order to induce coronary insufficiency in most of the ischemic heart. This fact was verified when results quite similar to Master's double two-step test were obtained. Second, the selection of controls and patients and the classification of disease were carefully done to avoid confusion. Finally, the severe cases of coronary occlusion were excluded in order to avoid misleading deviations from apparently normal findings in myocardial oxygen extraction or in production of lactate through pathological bypass across the fibrous tissue. The limitation of coronary vascular response in coronary disease was suggested in this study, and the fact was confirmed in our previous study of 146 patients with the use of various coronary dilating agents (Seki, Kamide, and Miyazawa, 1974). From these observations, it is certain that in coronary disease the relative myocardial oxygen want, anaerobic carbohydrate metabolism, and ischemic ECG changes were caused chiefly by a disorder in the regulation of coronary circulation. However, the ECG changes did not indicate any change of coronary circulation essentially, but a chemical one, due to myocardial metabolic disorders. Therefore, it is no wonder that the same changes of ECG and myocardial metabolism during exercise appear in patients with idiopathic cardiomyopathy (Brink and Lewis, 1967), or rheumatic mitral stenosis, in spite of nearly normal coronary response (as shown in Figure 4). Chiong and Parker (1975) observed the release of lactate, K, Pi, and CPK by arterial pacing and proposed a myocardial ischemic syndrome. We have found the simultaneous output or decrease of uptake of Pi and Cr in ischemic heart during exercise. These changes indicate more directly the mobilization of stored energy from the myocardial creatine phosphate. The comparison of myocardial energy balance in various circulatory diseases shows the fact that it is more a physiological response than an anaerobic carbohydrate metabolism, and it would be based on a small compartment and a high turnover rate of ATP used for contraction (Opie, 1969). In spite of the dominant influence of the arterial concentration of K upon myocardial uptake, among many other factors, and of the significant increase of the arterial concentration, K was released from the ischemic heart during exercise. It may be due to cardiac hypoxia (Gerligs, Miller, and Gilmore, 1969), as far as the relative myocardial oxygen want was proven in CHD and HD groups. It is of clinical importance that the K was released from the heart muscle without exception when the arterial concentration during exercise was below 4.0 mEq/liter. The oxygen expenditure of the test is equal with that of cycling on plain ground. In relation with the diminution of S–T depression or normalization of inverted T wave during exercise, we, contrary to many investigators, could find neither circulatory nor metabolic evidence that it is an unfavorable sign.

REFERENCES

BONSNES, R. W., and TAUSSKY, H. H. 1945. On the colorimetric determination of creatine by the Jaffe reaction. J. Biol. Chem. 158:581–591.

BRINK, A. J., and LEWIS, C. M. 1967. Coronary blood flow, energetics, and myocardial metabolism in idiopathic mural endomyocardiopathy (14 patients). Amer. Heart J. 73:339–348.

CHIONG, M. A., and PARKER, J. O. 1975. Metabolic indicators of myocardial ischemia in man. *In* G. Rona (ed.), Recent Advances in Studies on Cardiac Structure and Metabolism, Vol. 10, pp. 141–157. University Park Press, Baltimore.

COHEN, L. S., ELLIOT, W. C., KLEIN, M. D., and GORLIN, R. 1966. Coronary heart disease, clinical cineangiographic and metabolic correlations. Amer. J. Cardiol. 17:153–168.

FUJIWARA, K. 1975. Study on myocardial carbohydrate and energy metabolism during exercise in patients with circulatory diseases. Jpn. Cir. J. 39:623–646.

GERLIGS, E. D., MILLER, D. T., and GILMORE, J. P. 1969. Oxygen availability: A determinant of myocardial potassium balance. Amer. J. Physiol. 216:559–562.

HIGASHIHARA, Y. 1973. Myocardial lipid metabolism during exercise in clinical cases. Jpn. Circ. J. 37:657–658 (672–681).

HIGUCHI, H. 1972. Coronary circulation, myocardial oxygen metabolism and general hemodynamics during exercise and relation to electrocardiographic changes in patients with circulatory diseases. Jpn. Circ. J. 36:847–850 (875–904).

LOMBARDO, T. A., ROSE, L., TAESCHLER, M., TULUY, S., and BING, R. J. 1953. The effect of exercise on coronary blood flow, myocardial oxygen consumption and cardiac efficiency in man. Circulation 7:71–78.

MORI, K. 1972. The effect of exercise on myocardial metabolism of inorganic phosphorus and creatine in patients with circulatory disease. Jpn. Circ. J. 36:1119–1120 (1123–1135).

OPIE, L. H. 1969. Metabolism of the heart in health and disease. Part II. Amer. Heart J. 77:100–122.

PARKER, J. O., CHIONG, M. A., WEST, R. O., and CASE, R. B. 1969a. Sequential alterations in myocardial lactate metabolism, S–T-segments and left ventricular function during angina induced by atrial pacing. Circulation 40:113–131.

PARKER, J. O., WEST, R. O., CASE, R. B., and CHIONG, M. A. 1969b. Temporal relationships of myocardial lactate metabolism, left ventricular function and S–T segment depression during angina precipitated by exercise. Circulation 40:97–112.

ROWE, G. G., AFONSO, S., LUGO, J. E., CASTILLO, C. A., BOAKE, W. C., and CRUMPTON, C. W. 1965. Coronary blood flow and myocardial oxidative metabolism at rest and during exercise in subjects with severe aortic valve disease. Circulation 32:251–257.

SEKI, I. 1960. Clinical pathophysiological studies between myocardial oxygen demand-and-supply and electrocardiographic changes in induced anoxemia. Jpn. Circ. J. 24:695–735.

SEKI, I., and AKIOKA, H. 1973. On myocardial energy metabolism during exercise in patients with circulatory disease. Symposium, Cardiac Metabolism, on the Vth APCC in Singapore. Singapore Med. J. 14:347–348.

SEKI, I., KAMIDE, H., and MIYAZAWA, K. 1974. Über die Einschränkung der koronaren Krieslaufreaktion unter vershiedenen Belastungen bei Koronarerkrankungen und die Genese der Herzmuskelschädigung. Folia Angiol. 22:448–454.

TAUSSKY, H. H., and SHORR, E. 1953. A microcolorimetric method for the determination of inorganic phosphorus. J. Biol. Chem. 202:675–685.

Mailing address:
Ichiro Seki, M.D.,
First Department of Internal Medicine, Osaka Medical College,
Daigaku-cho, Takatsuki, Osaka (Japan).

Recent Advances in Studies on
Cardiac Structure and Metabolism, Volume 11
Heart Function and Metabolism
Edited by T. Kobayashi, T. Sano, and N. S. Dhalla
Copyright 1978   University Park Press   Baltimore

STUDIES ON MYOCARDIAL MITOCHONDRIA IN FAILING DOG HEARTS: STUDIES BY ELECTRON SPIN RESONANCE (ESR) SPECTROMETRY

Y. SUZUKI, N. YAMAZAKI, K. OGAWA,
K. MIZUTANI, N. KAKIZAWA, M. YAMAMOTO,
M. OKUBO, and M. YOSHIDA

Second Department of Internal Medicine, Nagoya University,
School of Medicine, Nagoya, Japan

SUMMARY

The formation of free radicals, which was represented by the concentration of free radicals in state 4 respiration, and the respiratory control ratio were studied in the myocardial mitochondria isolated from dog hearts that were failing due to aortic constriction.

Both formation and respiratory control ratio were lowered, compared to each control value, in acute and chronic heart failure. A positive correlation was recognized between free radicals in state 4 respiration and respiratory control ratio.

From these results it was concluded that there was uncoupling of oxidative phosphorylation in the mitochondria isolated from failing dog hearts. Measurement of free radicals in state 4 respiration, as well as respiratory control ratio, is a useful method for evaluation of the function of oxidative phosphorylation.

INTRODUCTION

Free radicals are chemical compounds that have one or more unpaired electrons and that can be detected by electron spin resonance (ESR) spectrometry. Biological application of this method was carried out by Commoner in 1954 (Commoner, Townsend, and Pake, 1954). He suggested that free radicals observed in surviving mammalian tissues were due to the free radicals produced as a result of the enzymatic oxidation-reduction activity in mitochondria, and that their concentrations were related to the biological origin of the tissue and varied with certain physiological and pathological conditions.

We have reported that free radicals were increased by the addition of succinate to mitochondrial preparation and that the concentration, as well as respiratory control ratio, might be a useful index for the evaluation of the function of oxidative phosphorylation in mitochondria (Suzuki *et al.*, 1974).

In order to investigate the energy production system of myocardial mitochondria in failing hearts, we report, in this chapter, on the free radical formation of myocardial mitochondria isolated from failing dog hearts by use of ESR spectrometry, and the results are compared with those of respiratory control ratio measured at the same time.

MATERIALS AND METHODS

Twenty-one adult mongrel dogs were used as experimental animals. They were divided into four groups: 1) acute heart failure; 2) acute sham-operation; 3) chronic heart failure; and 4) chronic sham-operation.

Heart failure was induced by the constriction of the proximal portion of the ascending aorta to about 25% of normal size for 3 hr in acute heart failure and to about 40% of normal size for two weeks in chronic heart failure. Heart failure was confirmed hemodynamically by elevation of left ventricular end-diastolic pressure and histologically by congestion of pulmonary capillaries.

Myocardial mitochondria were prepared by Chance and Hagihara's method (Chance and Hagihara, 1963) and the respiration was measured polarographically, using succinate as substrate.

Free radicals in each respiratory state were measured in liquid nitrogen by use of a JES-ME-3X ESR spectrometer. In this chapter free radical concentration is represented by ESR intensity, which was calculated from the ratio of maximum deflection of the ESR signals of the samples to that of the standard signals of manganase chloride inserted in the same resonance cavity of the ESR spectrometer. The details of the method have been described in a previous report (Suzuki, 1975).

RESULTS

ESR signals in each respiratory state are shown in Figure 1. ESR intensity is significantly increased by the addition of succinate to mitochondrial preparation (state 4 respiration) compared with mitochondrial preparation alone (state 1 respiration), and is decreased by the addition of ADP (state 3 respiration). ESR intensity in state 4 respiration was used as a parameter for the evaluation of the function of oxidative phosphorylation.

In acute heart failure, ESR intensity in state 4 respiration was lower than in the control, 0.135 ± 0.024 (S.D.) compared with 0.160 ± 0.013, although this difference was not statistically significant ($p < 0.1$). Respiratory control ratio was significantly lower than in the control, i.e., 2.80 ± 0.83 compared with 4.11 ± 0.57 ($p < 0.05$).

In chronic heart failure, ESR intensity in state 4 respiration was significantly lower than in the control, i.e., 0.101 ± 0.037 compared with 0.163 ± 0.022 ($p <$

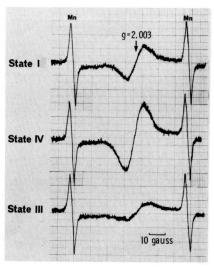

Figure 1. ESR signals in each respiratory state are seen in the center ($g = 2.003$). Mn represents the signals of manganase chloride as a magnetic field marker. The magnetic field increases to the right along the abscissa. The signal in state 4 respiration is the largest in size and the signal in state 3 is the smallest. ESR intensity was calculated from the ratio of maximum deflection of the signals of the samples to that of the standard signals of manganase chloride.

0.01). Respiratory control ratio was also significantly lower than in the control, i.e., 2.36 ± 0.49 compared with 4.03 ± 0.47 ($p < 0.01$) (Table 1).

A positive correlation was recognized between ESR intensity in state 4 respiration and the logarithm of respiratory control ratio ($p < 0.001$) (Figure 2).

Table 1. ESR intensity in state 4 respiration and respiratory control ratio of the myocardial mitochondria*

Group	n	ESR intensity in state 4 respiration (mg protein)	Respiratory control ratio
Acute heart failure	5	0.135 ± 0.024	2.80 ± 0.83
Acute sham	5	0.160 ± 0.013	4.11 ± 0.57
		($p < 0.1$)	($p < 0.05$)
Chronic heart failure	6	0.101 ± 0.037	2.36 ± 0.49
Chronic sham	5	0.163 ± 0.022	4.03 ± 0.47
		($p < 0.01$)	($p < 0.01$)

*Each value represents the mean ± S.D., and n is the number of dogs used for the experiment.

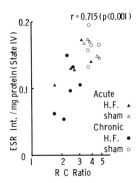

Figure 2. Relationship between ESR intensity in state 4 respiration and respiratory control ratio.

DISCUSSION

A great number of investigations have been carried out both in humans and experimental animals, concerning the impairment of energy production system in failing hearts. However, the results have been conflicting.

These studies have been carried out by the measurement of oxygen and substrate uptake by the method of coronary sinus catheterization (Blain *et al.,* 1956; Gudbjarnason *et al.,* 1962), by measurement of energy-rich compounds such as ATP and phosphocreatinine in tissue (Feinstein, 1962; Olson, 1964), and by polarographic measurement of oxygen consumption, P/O ratio, ADP/O ratio, and respiratory control ratio of mitochondria (Schwarz and Lee, 1962; Lindenmayer, Sordahl, and Schwartz, 1968).

In this study we tried to estimate the function of oxidative phosphorylation of mitochondria, using a new technique of ESR spectrometry, by measurement of free radicals in state 4 respiration that represent free radicals produced by the addition of succinate to mitochondrial preparation.

We have already reported that, in the studies on dogs with experimental infarction, reduction in ESR intensity in state 4 respiration suggested uncoupling of oxidative phosphorylation of mitochondria, because the same phenomena could be seen in the mitochondria treated by dinitrophenol as an uncoupler.

CONCLUSIONS

From the results in this study, it is concluded that:

1. Lowered ESR intensity in state 4 respiration and respiratory control ratio suggest that there is uncoupling of oxidative phosphorylation of myocardial mitochondria isolated from failing dog hearts induced by aortic constriction, and

the degree of uncoupling is more severe in chronic heart failure than in acute heart failure.

2. A good correlation between these two parameters suggests that the measurement of free radicals in state 4 respiration, as well as of respiratory control ratio, is also a useful method for the evaluation of the function of oxidative phosphorylation; nevertheless, the theoretical implication of these two parameters has not yet been made clear.

REFERENCES

BLAIN, J. M., SCHAFER, H., SIEGEL, A. L., and BING, R. J. 1956. Studies on myocardial metabolism. VI. Myocardial metabolism in congestive failure. Amer. J. Med. 20:820–833.

CHANCE, B., and HAGIHARA, B. 1963. Intracellular respiration. Phosphorylating and non-phosphorylating oxidation reactions. The fifth international congress of biochemistry, p. 3. Macmillan Co., New York.

COMMONER, B., TOWNSEND, J., and PAKE, G. E. 1954. Free radicals in biological materials. Nature 174:689–691.

FEINSTEIN, M. B. 1962. Effects of experimental congestive heart failure, ouabain, and asphyxia on the high-energy phosphate and creatine content of the guinea pig heart. Circ. Res. 10:333–346.

GUDBJARNASON, S., HAYDEN, R. O., WENDT, V. E., STOCK, T. B., and BING, R. J. 1962. Oxidation reduction in heart muscle. Theoretical and clinical considerations. Circulation 26:937–945.

LINDENMAYER, G. E., SORDAHL, L. A., and SCHWARTZ, A. 1968. Reevaluation of oxidative phosphorylation in cardiac mitochondria from normal animals and animals in heart failure. Circ. Res. 23:439–450.

OLSON, R. E. 1964. Abnormalities of myocardial metabolism. Circ. Res. 15 (Suppl. II):109.

SCHWARTZ, A., and LEE, K. S. 1962. Study of heart mitochondria and glycolytic metabolism in experimentally induced cardiac failure. Circ. Res. 10:321–332.

SUZUKI, Y. 1975. Studies on the free radicals in myocardial mitochondria by electron spin resonance (ESR) spectrometry: Studies on experimental infarction dogs. Jpn. Circ. J. 39:683–691.

SUZUKI, Y., YAMAZAKI, N., OGAWA, K., MIZUTANI, K., KAKIZAWA, N., YAMAMOTO, M., MIYAGISHIMA, Y., MORI, K., SUGIURA, M., OKUBO, M., and YOSHIDA, M. 1974. Studies on myocardial metabolism by electron spin resonance (ESR) spectrometry (Report 14): Relationship of respiration and free radical formation of myocardial mitochondria in experimental infarction dogs. Jpn. Circ. J. 38:584.

Mailing address:
Dr. Yoshikasu Suzuki,
Second Department of Internal Medicine,
Nagoya University, School of Medicine,
65 Tsurumacho, Showaku, Nagoya (Japan).

Recent Advances in Studies on
Cardiac Structure and Metabolism, Volume 11
Heart Function and Metabolism
Edited by T. Kobayashi, T. Sano, and N. S. Dhalla
Copyright 1978   University Park Press   Baltimore

DISTURBANCE OF MYOCARDIAL ENERGY LIBERATION IN EXPERIMENTAL CHARCOAL EMBOLISM OF CANINE PULMONARY ARTERY

T. TANIMOTO, T. ISHIYAMA, Y. MORITA,
Y. HATANAKA, T. UENO, J. AZUMA,
K. OGURA, H. HASEGAWA,
N. TSUKAMOTO, and Y. YAMAMURA

The Third Department of Internal Medicine, Osaka University Medical School,
Fukushima 1-1-50, Fukushima-ku, Osaka, Japan

SUMMARY

Experimental charcoal embolism of the pulmonary artery was produced in dogs. Changes in hemodynamics, electrophysiology, and cardiac energy liberation were observed. The effects of histaminic and antihistaminic drugs on these changes were also studied. After two infusions of charcoal suspension, acute right ventricular overloading was recognized hemodynamically and electrophysiologically. Mitochondria isolated from both ventricles exhibited uncoupling of oxidative phosphorylation polarographically. These changes were enhanced with histamine injection and reduced with diphenhydramine injection. Histamine was seen to have some uncoupling effects on the heart mitochondria and a slight effect on cardiac dynamics. It is concluded that oxidative phosphorylation of the heart mitochondria was uncoupled in the acute stage of experimental pulmonary embolism, and that histamine might emphasize this change directly or indirectly or both, that is, directly affecting the myocardial cell metabolism, and indirectly aggravating myocardial hypoxia through pulmonary vasoconstrictive action.

INTRODUCTION

Many investigations of cor pulmonale have been published, including aspects of clinical, electrocardiographic, hemodynamic, and respiratory function changes. However, changes of myocardial metabolism, especially of the energy metabolism, have not been clear, because it is interesting but difficult to evaluate myocardial energy metabolism directly in clinical cases. The states of myocardial energy metabolism may vary with the causes and severity of cor pulmonale, because the factors influencing the metabolic disturbances in cor pulmonale are thought to be numerous and complicated. There are few techniques available *in vivo* for detection of these factors. Therefore, the present study was intended to prove the alteration of the energy liberation in isolated heart mitochondria in consideration with the changes of cardiac dynamics and electrocardiographic findings. As the first step, the authors intended to study an acute phase of cor pulmonale produced experimentally by charcoal embolism of the pulmonary artery in dogs. Subsequently, the effects of histamine were studied in the acute phase of cor pulmonale. Histamine is known to be released from the lung tissue and is considered to modify myocardial metabolism.

MATERIAL AND METHODS

Mongrel dogs weighing 10–12 kg were anesthetized by intravenous injection of pentobarbital sodium. Two catheters were inserted into the outflow tract of the right ventricle. Right ventricular pressure was obtained through the catheter via the right jugular vein, and charcoal powder suspension was infused through the catheter via the femoral vein. Electrocardiogram, vectorcardiogram, and right ventricular pressure were monitored and recorded intermittently. After 60 min, the animals were sacrificed and the hearts were extirpated. Heart mitochondria were isolated from both ventricular myocardia. Mitochondrial oxygen consumption rate was measured polarographically with an oxygen consumption recorder. Oxygen consumption rates in state 3 and state 4, respiratory control index, and ADP/O ratio were calculated.

Dogs were divided into four groups. In Group 1, were the cases of the pulmonary charcoal embolism. In this group, charcoal suspension was infused through the catheter, repeating twice at an interval of 20 min. Group 2 were the cases of pulmonary charcoal embolism with histamine injection. Charcoal embolism was produced the same as in Group 1. Moreover, in this group histamine was injected four times, at intervals of 15 min before and after embolization. Group 3 were the cases of pulmonary charcoal embolism with diphenhydramine injection. This drug was injected 30 min before charcoal infusion. Group 4 were the cases of histamine injections without charcoal infusion. In this group, histamine was injected four times, at intervals of 15 min, but charcoal was not infused.

RESULTS

Hemodynamic Studies

In Group 1, as shown in Figure 1, heart rate (HR) did not change significantly, but right ventricular systolic pressure (RVSP) increased immediately after the charcoal infusion. The abrupt rise of RVSP was transient, and RVSP remained at a high level for more than 40 min. In Group 2, HR tended to decrease by repeated histamine injections. The change of RVSP due to embolization was similar to Group 1, and seemed to be slightly influenced by histamine. In Group 3, dogs were treated with diphenhydramine prior to charcoal infusion. Although

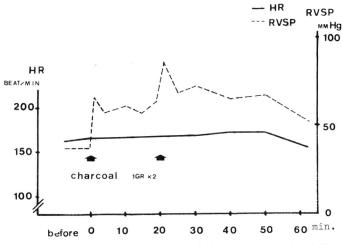

Figure 1. Hemodynamic changes of an example of Group 1 (charcoal embolism group). Changes of heart rate (HR) and right ventricular systolic pressure (RVSP) are illustrated.

HR did not change significantly, the rise of RVSP due to embolization subsided within 30 min. In Group 4, HR tended to decrease slightly. RVSP increased transiently by histamine injection.

Electrocardiographic and Vectorcardiographic Studies

Electrocardiographic and vectorcardiographic QRS changes suggesting acute right ventricular overloading were classified into four categories, i.e., severe, moderate, mild, and unchanged. The results are shown in Table 1. In Group 1, severe and moderate changes were proved in one out of eight dogs. In Group 2, no dog revealed any severe changes but moderate changes were found in three

Table 1. Incidence of electrocardiographic (ECG) and vectorcardiographic (VCG) QRS changes suggesting acute right ventricular overloading

Experimental group	ECG and VCG QRS changes				
	Severe	Moderate	Mild	Unchanged	Total
1. Charcoal embolism	1	1	3	3	8
2. Charcoal embolism with histamine injection		3		1	4
3. Charcoal embolism with antihistaminic drug injection			4	1	5
4. Histamine injection without charcoal embolism				5	5
Total	1	4	7	10	22

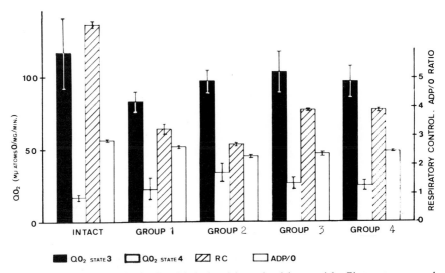

Figure 2. Respiration of mitochondria isolated from the right ventricle. Glutamate was used as a substrate. (QO_2: oxygen consumption rate; RC: respiratory control; ADP/O: ADP/O ratio.)

out of four dogs. On the contrary, the changes of the diphenhydramine treatment group ranged in mild degree or less. Histamine revealed no effect on QRS in electrocardiographic and vectorcardiographic findings in Group 4.

Studies on Respiration of Heart Mitochondria

Respiration of mitochondria isolated from the right ventricle is shown in Figure 2. In Group 1, oxygen consumption rate of mitochondria decreased in state 3 and increased in state 4; thus respiratory control index was deteriorated, but ADP/O ratio remained within normal range. These changes were thought to be the uncoupling of oxidative phosphorylation. Respiratory control index was markedly deteriorated in Group 2, but the deterioration of the respiratory control index was mitigated considerably in Group 3. Histamine had a slight uncoupling effect on the heart mitochondria. Similar changes were also recognized in the left ventricular mitochondria.

Mailing address:
Takuji Tanimoto, M.D.,
The Third Department of Internal Medicine,
Osaka University Hospital,
Fukushima 1−1−50, Fukushima-ku,
Osaka 553 (Japan).

Recent Advances in Studies on
Cardiac Structure and Metabolism, Volume 11
Heart Function and Metabolism
Edited by T. Kobayashi, T. Sano, and N. S. Dhalla
Copyright 1978   University Park Press   Baltimore

A BACTERIAL CARDIOTOXIN:
THERMOSTABLE DIRECT HEMOLYSIN
PRODUCED BY *VIBRIO PARAHAEMOLYTICUS*

T. HONDA, K. GOSHIMA, Y. TAKEDA, and T. MIWATANI

Department of Bacteriology and Serology, Research Institute for Microbial Diseases,
Osaka University, Yamada-kami, Suita, Osaka, Japan;
and Biological Research Laboratories, Central Research Division,
Takeda Chemical Industries, Ltd., Yodogawa, Osaka, Japan

SUMMARY

Thermostable direct hemolysin was purified extensively from the culture filtrates of *Vibrio parahaemolyticus*. The purified hemolysin was a protein and its homogeneity was demonstrated by sodium dodecyl sulfate-polyacrylamide gel disc electrophoresis and analytical ultracentrifugation. The purified hemolysin had a lethal effect when injected into mice and rats either intravenously or intraperitoneally. Its lethal effect was rapid, a dose of 10 μg of the hemolysin per rat killing the animals after about 2 min.

Studies by electroencephalography and electrocardiography showed that following intravenous injection of the hemolysin the electroencephalogram remained normal for quite a long time after the heart of the animals had stopped beating. Depression of intra-atrial and intraventricular conduction of electrical activation, including atrioventricular block, was observed in electrocardiograms of animals injected with the hemolysin.

From these results it is concluded that the thermostable direct hemolysin of *V. parahaemolyticus* is a cardiotoxin.

According to the statistics reported by the Ministry of Health and Welfare of Japan, cases of food poisoning due to *Vibrio parahaemolyticus* in Japan constitute about 20 to 30% of all cases of food poisoning and about 50 to 70% of the cases of bacterial food poisoning recorded during the past 12 years (Miwatani and Takeda, 1976).

Thermostable direct hemolysin produced by *V. parahaemolyticus* has been studied by several workers (Zen-Yoji *et al.*, 1971; Nikkawa *et al.*, 1972; Sakurai, Matsuzaki, and Miwatani, 1973) and it has been reported that the thermostable direct hemolysin is a pathogenic factor of *V. parahaemolyticus* infection (Miyamoto *et al.*, 1969).

This chapter reports purification and cardiotoxicity of the purified thermostable direct hemolysin produced by *V. parahaemolyticus*.

MATERIALS AND METHODS

Isolation and Purification of the Thermostable Direct Hemolysin

Thermostable direct hemolysin was isolated from culture filtrates of *V. para-haemolyticus* as described previously (Honda *et al.*, 1976a) and purified by

609

successive column chromatographies on DEAE-cellulose, hydroxylapatite, and Sephadex G-200, as described previously (Honda *et al.*, 1976a).

Assay of Lethal Toxicity

The lethal toxicity of the purified hemolysin was assayed by injecting the hemolysin intravenously into either 4- to 6-week-old mice (ddO strain) or 12- to 15-week-old rats (Sprague-Dawley strain) and measuring the survival time of the animals.

Electroencephalography

Electroencephalograms of rats after injection of the purified hemolysin under anesthesia with 800 mg of urethane per kg of body weight were recorded with a Nihon-Koden polygraph. The two leads were placed in the hippocampus and the motor area, respectively. Electrocardiogram obtained with a unipolar chest lead around the apex of the heart was recorded simultaneously.

Electrocardiography

Electrocardiograms of rats after injection of the purified hemolysin under anesthesia with 800 mg of urethane per kg of body weight were recorded with a Nihon-Koden polygraph. Three leads were used: one from electrodes in the right and left forelegs, one from electrodes in the right foreleg and left hind leg, and one from electrodes in the left foreleg and left hind leg.

RESULTS

Purification of the Thermostable Direct Hemolysin and Demonstration of the Identity of the Hemolysin with the Lethal Toxin Produced by *V. parahaemolyticus*

The culture filtrate of *V. parahaemolyticus* was fractionated with ammonium sulfate, and the hemolytic activity and lethal toxicity of each fraction were examined. It was found that both hemolytic activity and lethal toxicity were isolated by adding 35.1 g of solid ammonium sulfate per 100 ml of culture filtrate (55% saturation of ammonium sulfate). The crude toxic fraction was purified by successive column chromatographies on DEAE-cellulose, hydroxyl-apatite, and Sephadex G-200. On DEAE-cellulose column chromatography the lethal toxin was eluted with about 0.4 M NaCl and coincided with the hemolytic activity. On further chromatographies on hydroxylapatite and Sephadex G-200, the lethal toxin was consistently eluted with the hemolytic activity.

Physicochemical Properties of Purified Thermostable Direct Hemolysin

Homogeneity of the purified thermostable direct hemolysin was examined by SDS-polyacrylamide disc gel electrophoresis and ultracentrifugation. The purified hemolysin gave a single band on SDS-polyacrylamide disc gel electrophoresis and also formed a single symmetric peak on sedimentation analysis.

The purified hemolysin was found to be a pure protein. Five hundred micrograms of the purified hemolysin did not contain detectable amounts of carbohydrate and phospholipid. The sedimentation coefficient was calculated to be 6.9S. The molecular weight of the purified hemolysin was determined to be about 42,000 by Sephadex G-100 gel filtration. The isoelectric point of the purified hemolysin was around pH 4.2.

Lethal Toxicity of the Toxin to Mice and Rats

The lethal toxicity of the purified hemolysin to mice and rats was studied. Intravenous injection of the hemolysin killed mice very rapidly, and 5 μg of the hemolysin per mouse killed the animals within 1 min. An amount of 10 to 25 μg of the hemolysin killed rats in about 2 min (Table 1). When injected with the hemolysin, the animals became motionless and sometimes showed signs of cramp.

Electroencephalography of Rats Injected with Hemolysin

Changes in the electroencephalograms of rats injected with the hemolysin were studied. In this experiment a rat weighing 445 g was injected intravenously with 15 μg of the hemolysin and its electroencephalogram and electrocardiogram were recorded simultaneously. The electroencephalograms showed no significant change after intravenous injection of the hemolysin. On the other hand, the electrocardiogram showed that the voltage increased about 13 sec after the

Table 1. Lethal activity of the purified thermostable direct hemolysin after intravenous injection into mice and rats

Amount of hemolysin injected (μg of protein/animal)	Survival time after injection
Mice	(sec)
10.0	35.5 ± 4.8
5.0	49.0 ± 8.4
2.5	561.2 ± 368.8
1.0	1,121.5 ± 291.0
0.5	No death
Rats	(min)
25.0	1.87 ± 0.22
10.0	2.15 ± 0.36
7.5	7.00 ± 1.53
5.0	180.00 ± 174.00
2.5	No death

injection and that the heart stopped beating 33.5 sec after the injection. The electroencephalogram remained normal for more than 50 sec. This indicates that the effect of the toxin was primarily on the heart and that the heart stopped beating before the activity of the brain was affected.

Electrocardiography of Rats Injected with Hemolysin

For further studies on changes in the electrocardiogram of rats injected with the hemolysin, three leads were used for electrocardiography. A typical example is shown in Figure 1, in which a rat weighing 448 g was injected intravenously with 7.5 μg of the hemolysin. The hemolysin was administered at 0 sec. At about 15 sec after the injection, the P wave became wider and higher

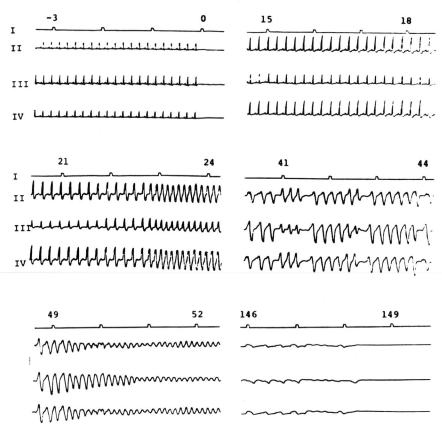

Figure 1. Electrocardiogram of a rat injected with the purified thermostable direct hemolysin. 7.5 μg of the hemolysin was injected into a rat weighing 448 g at zero time. Line I, time in seconds; line II, lead from a combination of electrodes in the right and left forelegs; line III, lead from a combination of electrodes in the right foreleg and left hind leg; line IV, lead from a combination of electrodes in the left foreleg and left hind leg.

than normal. This suggests changes in intra-atrial impulse conduction. At about this time the voltage of QRS became higher and ST-T changed, suggesting changes in intraventricular impulse conduction. At about 17 to 18 sec after the injection, prolongation of the PQ interval was observed, suggesting inhibition of atrioventricular conduction. Then at about 41 sec after the injection the patterns showed change of exciting foci of the ventricle and the heart rate decreased due to reduced excitation of the heart muscle. Ventricular flutter developed about 50 sec after the injection and the heart stopped beating after 148 sec.

DISCUSSION

This chapter reports that the thermostable direct hemolysin produced by *V. parahaemolyticus* has lethal toxicity and that the lethal toxicity is due to the cardiotoxic activity of the toxin. Intravenous injection of the purified hemolysin killed mice and rats within a few minutes. Electrocardiographic changes were observed shortly after administration of the hemolysin, whereas no significant electroencephalographic changes were observed even after the heart has stopped beating. The various changes in the electrocardiogram were observed, among which depression of intra-atrial and intraventricular excitation was the most marked effect. From these observations we conclude that intravenous injection of the lethal toxin (hemolysin) primarily affects the heart, so that animals died a few minutes after its administration. Intraperitoneal injection of the hemolysin also killed the animals, although this route was less effective than the intravenous route (Honda *et al.,* 1976a). When injected intraperitoneally, the hemolysin probably entered the bloodstream and so affected the heart. The cardiotoxicity of the thermostable direct hemolysin of *V. parahaemolyticus* is described more in detail elsewhere (Honda *et al.,* 1976a and 1976b; Miwatani and Takeda, 1976).

REFERENCES

HONDA, T., TAGA, S., TAKEDA, T., HASIBUAN, M. A., TAKEDA, Y., and MIWATANI, T. 1976a. Identification of lethal toxin with thermostable direct hemolysin produced by *Vibrio parahaemolyticus* and some physicochemical properties of the purified toxin. Infect. Immun. 13:133–139.

HONDA, T., GOSHIMA, K., TAKEDA, Y., SUGINO, Y., and MIWATANI, T. 1976b. Demonstration of the cardiotoxicity of thermostable direct hemolysin (lethal toxin) produced by *Vibrio parahaemolyticus*. Infect. Immun. 13:163–171.

MIWATANI, T., and TAKEDA, Y. 1976. *Vibrio parahaemolyticus*–A causative bacterium of food poisoning. Saikon Publishing Co., Tokyo.

MIYAMOTO, Y., KATO, T., OBARA, Y., AKIYAMA, S., TAKIZAWA, K., and YAMAI, S. 1969. In vitro hemolytic characteristic of *Vibrio parahaemolyticus:* Its close correlation with human pathogenicity. J. Bacteriol. 100:1147–1149.

NIKKAWA, T., OBARA, Y., YAMAI, S., and MIYAMOTO, Y. 1972. Purification of a hemolysin from *Vibrio parahaemolyticus*. Jap. J. Med. Sci. Biol. 25:197–200.

SAKURAI, J., MATSUZAKI, A., and MIWATANI, T. 1973. Purification and characterization of thermostable direct hemolysin of *Vibrio parahaemolyticus*. Infect. Immun. 8:755–780.

ZEN-YOJI, H., HITOKOTO, H., MOROZUMI, S., and LECLAIR, R. A. 1971. Purification and characterization of a hemolysin produced by *Vibrio parahaemolyticus*. J. Infect. Dis. 123:665–667.

Mailing address:
Takeshi Honda,
Department of Bacteriology and Serology,
Research Institute for Microbial Diseases,
Osaka University, Yamada-Kami, Suita, Osaka 565 (Japan)

Recent Advances in Studies on
Cardiac Structure and Metabolism, Volume 11
Heart Function and Metabolism
Edited by T. Kobayashi, T. Sano, and N. S. Dhalla
Copyright 1978   University Park Press   Baltimore

STOPPING OF SPONTANEOUS BEATING OF CULTURED MOUSE AND RAT MYOCARDIAL CELLS BY A TOXIN (THERMOSTABLE DIRECT HEMOLYSIN) FROM *VIBRIO PARAHAEMOLYTICUS*

K. GOSHIMA[1], T. HONDA, Y. TAKEDA, and T. MIWATANI

Biological Research Laboratories, Central Research Division,
Takeda Chemical Industries, Ltd., Yodogawa, Osaka 532, Japan;
and Department of Bacteriology and Serology,
Research Institute for Microbial Diseases,
Osaka University, Suita, Osaka 565, Japan

SUMMARY

Low concentrations of thermostable direct hemolysin from *Vibrio parahaemolyticus* stopped the spontaneous beating of cultured mouse and rat myocardial cells. These low concentrations depolarized the maximal diastolic potential and inhibited the generation of action potential of cultured myocardial cells. The toxin lost its activity when preincubated with ganglioside, G_{T1} or G_{M1}. G_{T1} was more effective than G_{M1}. High concentrations of the toxin caused morphological damage of cultured mouse and rat myocardial cells, but did not stop the beating, or cause morphological damage of cultured chick myocardial cells.

INTRODUCTION

Vibrio parahaemolyticus is a causative bacterium of food poisoning. Recently, a highly purified toxin (thermostable direct hemolysin) was obtained from the culture filtrates of *V. parahaemolyticus* (Honda *et al.*, 1976a). The toxin is a simple protein with a molecular weight of about 42,000. The toxin has a hemolytic activity on human, rat, and mouse erythrocytes (Takeda *et al.*, 1975), and has a strong lethal activity on rats and mice. Electrocardiographic abnormalities developed immediately after intravenous injection of small amounts of the toxin into rats (Honda *et al.*, 1976b, Miwatani and Takeda, 1976).

It is well known that when the component cells of fetal mouse, fetal rat, and embryonic chick heart are separated with the aid of trypsin and cultured *in vitro*, both single isolated myocardial cells and cell clusters beat spontaneously. The cultured myocardial cells function in a manner essentially similar to the

---

[1] Present address: Institute of Molecular Biology, Faculty of Science, Nagoya University, Chikusa-ku, Nagoya 464 (Japan).

adult heart *in situ* (Goshima, 1969, 1975, and 1976). The cultured cells, and especially single isolated cells are separated anatomically and functionally from nerves, connective tissue, and blood vessels, and so they can be used to see whether a toxin exerts its cardiotoxic effect directly, or indirectly, on myocardial cells.

In the work described in this chapter the effects of the toxin on the spontaneous beating of cultured mouse, rat, and chick myocardial cells were studied (Honda *et al.*, 1976b; Goshima *et al.*, 1977).

RESULTS AND DISCUSSION

As shown in Table 1, on addition of more than 0.05 μg/ml of the toxin from *V. parahaemolyticus,* mouse myocardial cell clusters stopped spontaneous beating within 0.5 to 3 min. There were no detectable differences in the potassium, sodium, and calcium concentrations or the pH values of the culture medium before and 5 min after addition of 0.2 μg/ml of the toxin to the cells.

As shown in Figure 1, on addition of 0.25 μg/ml of the toxin the maximal diastolic potentials gradually became depolarized, and the amplitude of action potentials gradually decreased and finally disappeared. This suggests that the

Table 1. Effects of toxin from *Vibrio parahaemolyticus* on the spontaneous beating of mouse, rat, and chick myocardial cell clusters cultured *in vitro*

Toxin (μg/ml)[¶]	Beat stopped*	Beat restarted[†]	Time (min)[‡]
Fetal mouse myocardial cells[§]			
0.03	0/5	—	—
0.05	3/14	3/3	7 ± 3
0.10	11/14	11/11	9 ± 4
0.20	14/14	14/14	17 ± 8
Fetal rat myocardial cells[§]			
0.10	5/5	5/5	7 ± 4
0.20	5/5	5/5	13 ± 6
Embryonic chick myocardial cells[§]			
50	0/6	—	—

*Ratio of number of cell clusters that stopped beating on addition of the toxin to total number of cell clusters examined.

†Ratio of number of cell clusters regaining beat on further incubation in the presence of the toxin to number of cell clusters that stopped beating after addition of the toxin.

‡Mean time (±S.D.) between stopping and restarting beating.

§Mouse, rat, and chick myocardial cells were cultured as described previously (Goshima, 1977). after cultivation for 1 day, microscopic observations were performed at 36°C in the following medium: 116 mM NaCl, 5.4 mM or 1.0 mM KCl, 1.8 mM CaCl$_2$, 0.8 mM MgSO$_4$, 0.9 mM NaH$_2$PO$_4$, 5.5 mM glucose, amino acids, vitamins, 5% fetal bovine serum, and 10 mM BES (one of Good's buffers), at pH 7.3.

¶0.1 μg toxin/ml: 2.4 × 10^{-9} M.

0.25 µg Toxin/ml

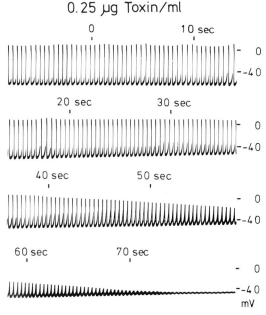

Figure 1. Transmembrane potential recorded from a mouse myocardial cell cluster. Electrical recording was made by the method described previously (Goshima, 1976). 0.25 µg/ml of the toxin from *Vibrio parahaemolyticus* was added at time 0. No beating was observed microscopically after 80 sec.

toxin increased the ionic permeability of the cell membrane. Detailed electrophysiological studies on this problem will be reported by Seyama *et al.* (1977).

As shown in Table 1, on further incubation of the cells in the presence of 0.05 to 0.2 µg/ml of the toxin the beating started again spontaneously. The interval between the times when the beating stopped and started again was longer on addition of higher concentrations of the toxin. The restoration is mainly due to denaturation of the toxin during incubation at low concentrations at 36°C.

The activity of the toxin to stop the beating of mouse myocardial cells was inhibited by preincubation of the toxin with ganglioside G_{T1} or G_{M1}. G_{T1} was more effective than G_{M1}.

The toxin from *V. parahaemolyticus* also inhibited the normal beating of single isolated mouse myocardial cells (Table 2). Two to 5 min after addition of 0.05 to 0.5 µg/ml of the toxin, the number of cells beating rhythmically decreased and the numbers of quiescent cells and of cells showing irregular, faint fibrillatory movements increased. On further incubation in the presence of the toxin, however, most of the quiescent cells (morphologically normal) and those

Table 2. Effects of toxin from *Vibrio parahaemolyticus* on the spontaneous beating of single isolated mouse myocardial cells cultured *in vitro*

Toxin (μg/ml)	Time after addition (min)	Quiescent cells among total cells	Beating cells among total cells†	Rhythmic and arrhythmic‡ beating cells among total beating cells	
				Rhythmic	Arrhythmic
0	–	20 ± 4*%	80 ± 4*%	92 ± 3*%	8 ± 3*%
0.05	2–5	23 ± 5	77 ± 5	67 ± 18	33 ± 18
	15–20	17 ± 2	83 ± 2	89 ± 6	11 ± 6
0.20	2–5	32 ± 4	68 ± 4	23 ± 14	77 ± 14
	60–65	19 ± 4	81 ± 4	86 ± 7	14 ± 7
0.50§	2–5	77 ± 10	23 ± 10	5 ± 8	95 ± 8
	60–65	66 ± 5	34 ± 5	64 ± 19	36 ± 19

*Mean ±S.D. of values in 3 independent experiments. Total of 100 to 200 cells were examined with each concentration of the toxin.

†Both rhythmic and arrhythmic beating cells among total single isolated myocardial cells.

‡Cells showing irregular, faint fibrillatory movements of high frequency (100 to 300 oscillations/min).

§Morphologically damaged cells appeared.

Table 3. Effects of bacterial toxins* and tetrodotoxin on the spontaneous beating of mouse
myocardial cell clusters cultured *in vitro*

Toxin (μg/ml)	Effect on beating
Vibrio parahaemolyticus toxin (0.1, 0.2)	Stopped
Cholera enterotoxin (0.1, 2.5)	No effect
Tetanus toxin (1.6, 16)	No effect
Diphtheria toxin (26, 130)	No effect
Staphylococcus enterotoxin (300, 600)	No effect
Tetrodotoxin (1, 10, 100)	No effect

*Highly purified toxins from *V. cholerae, C. tetani, Coryne. diphtheriae*, and *S. aureus* were kindly supplied by Dr. N. Ohtomo (Chemo-Sero-Therapeutic Research Institute, Kumamoto), Dr. M. Matsuda (Osaka University), Dr. T. Uchida (Osaka University), and Dr. S. Katsuno (Hyogo Medical College), respectively.

showing irregular beating regained their normal, rhythmic beating. On addition of less than 0.2 μg/ml of the toxin, mouse myocardial cells did not degenerate. However, on addition of more than 0.5 μg/ml of the toxin, morphologically damaged cells appeared.

We tested several other bacterial toxins and tetrodotoxin on the spontaneous beating of mouse myocardial cell clusters cultured *in vitro.* As shown in Table 3, highly purified toxins from *Vibrio cholerae, Clostridium tetani, Corynebacterium diphtheriae* and *Staphylococcus aureus* had no significant effects on the beating. Tetrodotoxin also had no effect.

The spontaneous beating of cultured rat myocardial cells also stopped and degenerated on addition of the toxin from *V. parahaemolyticus* in the same way as it did in the cultured mouse myocardial cells (Table 1). In contrast, cultured chick myocardial cells showed normal beating and normal morphology even on addition of 50 μg/ml of the toxin (Table 1).

The toxin from *V. parahaemolyticus* also stopped the spontaneous beating of isolated adult rat atrial preparations. From these observations we concluded that thermostable direct hemolysin produced by *Vibrio parahaemolyticus* has a direct cardiotoxic activity on mice and rats (Goshima *et al.,* 1977).

REFERENCES

GOSHIMA, K. 1969. Synchronized beating of and electrotonic transmission between myocardial cells mediated by heterotypic strain cells in monolayer culture. Exp. Cell Res. 58:420–426.

GOSHIMA, K. 1975. Further studies on preservation of the beating rhythm of myocardial cells in culture. Exp. Cell Res. 92:339–349.

GOSHIMA, K. 1976. Arrhythmic movements of myocardial cells in culture and their improvement with antiarrhythmic drugs. J. Mol. Cell. Cardiol. 8:217–238.

GOSHIMA, K., HONDA, T., HIRATA, M., KIKUCHI, K., TAKEDA, Y., and MIWATANI, T. 1977. Stopping of the spontaneous beating of mouse and rat myocardial cells *in vitro* by a toxin from *Vibrio parahaemolyticus.* J. Mol. Cell. Cardiol. 9:191–213.

HONDA, T., TAGA, S., TAKEDA, T., HASIBAN, M. A., TAKEDA, Y., and MIWATANI, T. 1976a. Identification of lethal toxin with thermostable direct hemolysin produced by *Vibrio parahaemolyticus* and some physicochemical properties of the purified toxin. Infect. Immun. 13:133–139.

HONDA, T., GOSHIMA, K., TAKEDA, Y., SUGINO, Y., and MIWATANI, T. 1976b. Demonstration of the cardiotoxicity of thermostable direct hemolysin (lethal toxin) produced by *Vibrio parahaemolyticus.* Infect. Immun. 13:163–171.

MIWATANI, T., and TAKEDA, Y. 1976. *Vibrio parahaemolyticus*–A causative bacterium of food poisoning. Saikon Publishing Co., Tokyo.

SEYAMA, I., IRISAWA, H., HONDA, T., TAKEDA, Y., and MIWATANI, T. 1977. Effect of hemolysin produced by *Vibrio parahaemolyticus* on membrane conductance and mechanical tension of rabbit myocardium. Jap. J. Physiol. 27:43–56.

TAKEDA, Y., TAKEDA, T., HONDA, T., SAKURAI, J., OHTOMO, N., and MIWATANI, T. 1975. Inhibition of hemolytic activity of thermostable direct hemolysin of *Vibrio parahaemolyticus* by ganglioside. Infect. Immun. 12:931–933.

Mailing address:
Kiyota Goshima, Ph.D.,
Institute of Molecular Biology,
Faculty of Science,
Nagoya University,
Chikusa-ku, Nagoya 464 (Japan).

Recent Advances in Studies on
Cardiac Structure and Metabolism, Volume 11
Heart Function and Metabolism
Edited by T. Kobayashi, T. Sano, and N. S. Dhalla
Copyright 1978   University Park Press   Baltimore

INCREASE IN MEMBRANE CONDUCTANCE AND POSITIVE INOTROPIC ACTION OF HEMOLYSIN PRODUCED BY *VIBRIO PARAHAEMOLYTICUS* ON RABBIT MYOCARDIUM

I. SEYAMA, H. IRISAWA, T. HONDA, T. TAKEDA, and T. MIWATANI

Department of Physiology, School of Medicine,
Hiroshima University, Hiroshima;
and Department of Bacteriology and Serology,
Research Institute for Microbial Disease,
Osaka University, Suita, Osaka, Japan

SUMMARY

The effects of purified thermostable direct hemolysin from the cultured filtrate of *Vibrio parahaemolyticus* on both S—A node cells and atrial cells were studied electrophysiologically. Hemolysin caused the membrane conductance to increase, thereby causing membrane depolarization. The major ion responsible for this depolarization was Na^+, but other ions, such as K^+ and Ca^{2+}, also participated. Positive inotropic action of hemolysin was observed, and the Na—Ca exchange mechanism was enhanced after hemolysin treatment.

INTRODUCTION

Purified, thermostable direct hemolysin from the cultured filtrate of *Vibrio parahaemolyticus* is a protein (molecular weight, about 42,000). The purified hemolysin shows a lethal effect, presumably by its distinguished cardiotoxicity (Honda *et al.*, 1976a and 1976b). The mechanisms of the action of hemolysin in S—A node and right atrial cells have been studied by means of a single sucrose-gap method (Noma and Irisawa, 1974; Seyama, 1976).

RESULTS

Effect of Hemolysin on Membrane Potential

Figure 1 gives a typical example of the effect of hemolysin of 2.5 μg/ml on the action potential of the rabbit S—A node. During the application of hemolysin, reduction of the overshoot and the maximum diastolic potential were observed. After the cessation of the spontaneous activity, the resting potential continued to depolarize. The electrical stimulation after the cessation of the spontaneous activity elicited an action potential of a low rising rate, small amplitude, and

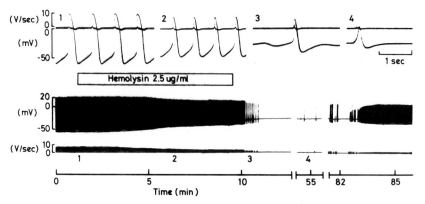

Figure 1. Effect of hemolysin (2.5 μg/ml) on the action potential of S—A node. *Upper row,* fast speed, and *lower row,* slow record.

small after-hyperpolarization (Figure 1). Since the excitability remained even after the pacemaker activity had ceased, cessation of the spontaneous activity might mainly be produced by both the disturbance of the pacemaker mechanism and the partial cathodal block due to the depolarization of the membrane.

The reduction of the after-hyperpolarization of the S—A node action potential in response to hemolysin suggests the reduction of the intracellular K^+ concentration, due to an increased membrane conductance to Na^+. In order to confirm this possibility, changes of the membrane resistance were measured in a quiescent S—A node preparation by applying constant anodal current pulses (Figure 2). Accompanying the depolarization of the resting membrane, the membrane resistance reduced by 20%, indicating the increase of the permeability of the membrane to Na^+. The action potential elicited as the anodal break excitation (bottom graph in Figure 2) showed a similar trend, as has been shown in Figure 1. Also, similar findings were obtained in the isolated atrial muscles. In order to explain the effect of hemolysin on the action potential—generating mechanism, the action potentials before and after the application of hemolysin were compared, keeping the resting potential constant at −100 mV by application of anodal pulses. There was essentially no change in the pattern of action potential primed before and after hemolysin treatment. Therefore, it is considered that hemolysin at this concentration depolarized the membrane without affecting the action potential generating mechanisms. The depolarization of the membrane and also the increased slope conductance of the membrane are the direct cause of the hemolysin in both the S—A node cells and the atrial fibers. Such a finding indicates that one of the major mechanisms of the action of hemolysin on these muscles is the increase of the membrane conductance to Na^+.

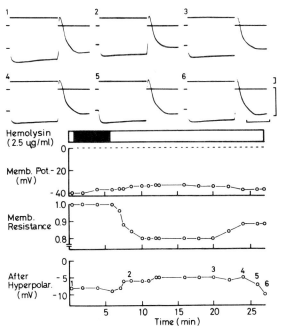

Figure 2. Changes in the membrane resistance of a quiescent S–A node cell. *Upper vertical bar,* 5 × 10⁻⁵ A, *lower vertical bar,* 50 mV, and *horizontal bar,* 500 msec.

Changes in Membrane Conductance in Low Na⁺ Tyrode Solution

From the above results it is suggested that the action of hemolysin might be caused by an increase in the membrane conductance to Na^+. Further supportive evidence was obtained by applying constant pulses of 1×10^{-5} A across the single sucrose-gap in an atrial fiber. When 30% Na Tyrode was perfused, membrane was hyperpolarized by 8.6 mV within 4 min. Addition of 10 μg/ml of hemolysin to this specimen caused a gradual depolarization of the membrane by 8.6 mV; the membrane depolarized to the original resting potential. The depolarization of the membrane in response to 10 μg/ml hemolysin was obviously small within 30% Na Tyrode, because, within control Tyrode, 8 μg/ml hemolysin depolarized the resting membrane by 17.7 mV. Following 8.1-min perfusion of the hemolysin within 30% Tyrode, the normal Tyrode (143 mM $[Na]_o$) without hemolysin was perfused. Membrane again depolarized by 8.6 mV, and the slope conductance increased extremely under this condition. This experiment shows that the depolarization of the membrane in response to hemolysin was caused mainly by an increased Na^+ permeability of the membrane in response to hemolysin in normal Tyrode. However, after the depolarizing action of the membrane by hemolysin, tetrodotoxin, TTX, apparently failed to hyperpolarize the membrane, indicating that the increased conductance is not solely due to Na^+ permeability. Because the depolarization of the membrane caused by Grayanotoxin 1 (GTX 1) reversibly hyperpolarized the membrane by TTX in rabbit atrium (Seyama, unpublished observation), the depolarizing action of hemolysin is nonspecific to Na^+, compared to GTX.

Effect of Hemolysin on Mechanical Tension

Hemolysin caused a positive inotropic action of the right atrial trabecula. Transient potentiation of the phasic tension was followed by a progressive increase in the diastolic tension. Accompanying the elevation of diastolic tension, the phasic tension gradually decreased. The diastolic tension continued to elevate as long as 10–15 min, even after washing with normal Tyrode. As the phasic tension was increased, the rate of rise of tension increased. Tonic tension returned to the control level after 30- to 60-min perfusion in normal Tyrode.

Contracture of Atrial Fibers in Na^+-Depleted Tyrode

When the concentration of extracellular Na^+ was lowered to less than 30% of the normal Tyrode, contracture of the muscle was observed (Lüttgau and Niedergerke, 1958; Vassort, 1973; Irisawa and Noma, 1976). This contracture was explained by an increase of intracellular Ca concentration, due to Na-Ca exchange mechanism (Reuter and Seitz, 1968). After an application of hemolysin, concentration of Na^+ within the cell was increased as a result of the increased membrane conductance; therefore, the contracture due to Na-Ca exchange became more pronounced. Since these inotropic effects of hemolysin were not affected by the presence of propranolol, it is unlikely that the positive inotropic effect would be due to the action of discharged norepinephrine. These experimental results indicate that the unique cardiotoxic action of hemolysin is caused by an increased membrane conductance to several ions, especially to extracellular Na^+ in normal Tyrode.

REFERENCES

HONDA, T., GOSHIMA, K., TAKEDA, Y., SUGINO, Y., and MIWATANI, T. (1976a). Demonstration of the cardiotoxicity of the thermostable direct hemolysin (lethal toxin) produced by *Vibrio parahaemolyticus*. Infect. Immun. 13:163–171.

HONDA, T., TAGA, S., TAKEDA, T., HASIBAN, M. A., TAKEDA, Y., and MIWATANI, T. 1976b. Identification of lethal toxin with the thermostable direct hemolysin produced by *Vibrio parahaemolyticus* and some physicochemical properties of the purified toxin. Infect. Immun. 13:133–139.

IRISAWA, H., and NOMA, A. 1976. Contracture and hyperpolarization of the rabbit sinoatrial node cells in Na-depleted solution. Jpn. J. Physiol. 25:133–144.

LÜTTGAU, H. C., and NIEDERGERKE, R. 1958. The antagonism between Ca and Na ions on the frog's heart. J.Physiol.143:486–505.

NOMA, A., and IRISAWA, H. 1974. The effect of sodium ion on the initial phase of the sinoatrial pacemaker action potentials in rabbits. Jpn.J.Physiol. 24:617–632.

REUTER, H., and SEITZ, N. 1968. The dependence of calcium efflux from cardiac muscle on temperature and external ion composition. J.Physiol. 195:451–470.

SEYAMA, I. 1976. Characteristics of the rectifying properties of the sino-atrial node cell of the rabbit. J. Physiol. 255:379–397.

VASSORT, G. 1973. Influence of sodium ions on the regulation of frog myocardial contractility. Pfluegers Arch. 339:225–240.

Mailing address:
Dr. I. Seyama,
Department of Physiology,
School of Medicine, Hiroshima University,
Kasumi 1-2-3, Hiroshima 734 (Japan).

Author Index

Abe, H., 279
Abe, Y., 73
Aizawa, K., 313
Aizawa, Y., 313
Akagami, H., 539
Akera, T., 401
Aki, K., 343
Akioka, H., 589
Anazawa, S., 325
Aomine, M., 73
Aoyagi, R., 313
Arita, M., 45, 85
Azuma, J., 549, 605

Barlow, C., 521
Bauman, Kl., 175
Besch, H. R., Jr., 219, 227, 423, 431
Blanck, J., 199
Bleeker, W. K., 51
Boink, A. B. T. J., 559, 565
Bor, P., 495
Bornet, E. P., 195
Bouman, L. N., 51
Brandt, R., 501
Bricknell, O. L., 509
Brody, T. M., 401

Carlson, L. A., 355
Chance, B., 307
Clapier-Ventura, R., 143
Cole, H. A., 111
Coraboeuf, E., 11
Csete, K., 495

Dagenais, G. R., 385
de Bruijne, J., 19
Deleeuw, G., 521
Dhalla, N. S., 457
Dimino, M. J., 349
Dirschinger, J., 501
Doell, B., 571
Dunnett, J., 213

Ebashi, S., 93, 185
Eitenmüller, J., 319

Elfont, E. A., 349
Entman, M. L., 195
Ezrailson, E. G., 195

Farmer, B. B., 431
Fassold, E., 489
Fleck, E., 501
Fozzard, H. A., 3
Frearson, N., 111
Fricke, U., 393
Fujiwara, K., 589

Gailis, L., 385
Gibbons, W. R., 3
Goshima, K., 609, 615
Goto, M., 37, 57, 73
Goto, N., 589
Gudbjarnason, S., 571

Hall, D., 301
Hallgrimsson, J., 571
Harris, R. A., 431
Harrow, J. A. C., 457
Hasegawa, H., 549, 605
Hashimoto, K., 451
Hasselbach, W., 205
Hatanaka, Y., 549, 605
Hatano, R., 481
Hathaway, D. R., 423, 431
Higashihara, Y., 589
Higuchi, H., 589
Hiraoka, M., 31, 79
Honda, T., 609, 615, 621
Horackova, M., 137
Hughes, G. W., 349

Ijichi, H., 555
Ikemoto, Y., 57
Ikeo, T., 437
Ikezono, E., 481
Imai, S., 335
Imanaga, I., 441
Imaoka, A., 589
Irisawa, H., 25, 621
Ishiyama, T., 549, 583, 605

Isselhard, W., 319
Ito, Y., 293
Ito, Y., 185

Jones, L. R., 219, 227
Jongsma, H. J., 19
Julien, P., 385

Kaijser, L., 355
Kakizawa, N., 599
Kako, K. J., 369
Kaku, T., 273
Kamide, H., 589
Kamiyama, A., 131
Kane, J. J., 533
Katano, Y., 335
Katz, A. M., 205
Khatter, J. C., 121
Kinoshita, N., 279
Kirchberger, M. A., 265, 285
Kishima, N., 589
Kitazawa, T., 93
Kiyomoto, A., 437
Kizu, A., 555
Klaus, W., 393
Kohama, K., 93
Koizumi, T., 185
Kondo, K., 589
Krasnow, N., 297
Kumazawa, T., 481
Kumazawa, T., 473
Kuramoto, K., 273
Kurihara, S., 181

Leung, L.-K., 249
Levey, G. S., 195
Lieberman, M., 19
Loracher, C., 501
Löw, H., 355
Luka, N. L., 473

Ma, S. K., 249
Maas, A. H. J., 559
Mackaay, A. J. C., 51
Mashima, H., 149
Mason, D. T., 103
Matsuda, H., 451

Matsumura, K., 343
Matsuo, H., 279
Matsuoka, M., 313
Matsushita, S., 273
Matsuura, H., 293
Mäurer, W., 319
McNeill, J. H., 413
Merin, R. G., 473
Mikawa, K., 343
Minaga, T., 555
Miwatani, T., 609, 615, 621
Miyagi, T., 589
Mizutani, K., 599
Moir, A. J. G., 111
Mongo, K., 143
Mori, H., 343
Mori, K., 589
Morita, Y., 549, 583, 605
Murakami, M., 273
Murooka, H., 313
Murphy, M. L., 533

Nagamoto, Y., 45, 85
Nagano, M., 325
Nagao, T., 437
Nakagawa, M., 481
Nakagawa, Y., 335
Nakajima, H., 437
Nakamura, T., 555
Nakano, T., 273
Nawrath, H., 419
Nayler, W. G., 213, 489
Niki, T., 343
Nimura, Y., 279
Nishi, K., 63
Noma, A., 25

Ogawa, K., 599
Ogura, K., 549, 605
Ohmori, F., 279
Ohta, N., 467
Okazaki, K., 467
Okubo, M., 599
Olgaard, M. K., 401
Opie, L. H., 509
Oshino, N., 307
Oskarsdottir, G., 571
Otorii, T., 335

Peak, H. J., 355
Peng, C. F., 533

Perry, S. V., 111
Pitts, B. J. R., 195
Platt, M. R., 169
Ponce Zumino, A., 69
Prasad, K., 121

Raffo, A., 285
Redl, A., 501
Reichel, H., 175
Reinecke, H., 319
Repeck, M. W., 349
Repke, D. I., 205
Roulet, M. J., 143
Roy, P.-E., 385
Rudolph, W., 501
Ruigrok, T. J. C., 559, 565
Ruiz-Ceretti, E., 69

Saeki, Y., 131
Saikawa, T., 45, 85
Saito, N., 325
Saito, T., 467
Sakai, M., 273
Sakai, T., 181
Sakakibara, H., 279
Sakata, S., 467
Sano, I., 589
Sano, T., 31, 79
Sato, M., 437
Sawanobori, T., 79
Schanne, O. F., 69
Schraven, E., 363
Schwartz, A., 195
Seki, I., 589
Seyama, I., 621
Shapiro, W., 407
Shibata, N., 539
Shigekawa, M., 205
Shin, K. S., 549
Singal, P. K., 121
Smettan, G., 199
Solaro, R. J., 111
Steenbergen, C., 521
St. Louis, P. J., 235, 241
Straub, K. D., 533
Sulakhe, P. V., 235, 241, 249, 257
Sulakhe, S. J., 257
Sunamori, M., 481
Suzuki, T., 481

Suzuki, Y., 599
Szekeres, L., 495

Tada, M., 265, 279
Takeda, K., 555
Takeda, K., 335
Takeda, T., 621
Takeda, Y., 609, 615
Takenaka, F., 63, 379
Takeo, S., 379
Tamura, K., 313
Tamura, M., 307
Tanaka, Y., 467
Tanimoto, T., 549, 605
Taubent, K., 407
Templeton, G. H., 169, 407
Terauchi, A., 589
Toll, M. O., 159
Tomino, T., 467
Tomino, Y., 467
Tonogai, R., 467
Toyama, S., 539
Tsuda, Y., 37
Tsukada, T., 451
Tsukamoto, N., 549, 605
Tsuyuguchi, N., 343

Ueba, Y., 293
Ueno, T., 549, 605

Vághy, P., 495
Van Eerd, P.-C., 93
Van Ginneken, A. C. G., 19
Van Winkle, W. B., 195
Vasdev, S. C., 369
Vassort, G., 137, 143

Wahlqvist, M. L., 355
Watanabe, A. M., 219, 227, 423, 431
Weisfeldt, M., 169
Welter, H., 319
Whitty, A. J., 349
Wide, L., 355
Wikman-Coffelt, J., 103
Will, H., 199
Willerson, J. T., 169, 407
Williamson, J. R., 521

Wilmshurst, E. G., 355
Wollenberger, A., 199

Yamagami, T., 539
Yamamoto, M., 599
Yamamoto, N., 481
Yamamura, Y., 549, 605

Yamazaki, N., 599
Yatani, A., 37
Yoshida, M., 599
Yoshikawa, Y., 63

Zaror-Behrens, G., 369
Zimmerman, A. N. E., 559, 565

Subject Index

Acetaldehyde, effect on functioning of cardiac muscle at ultrastructural level, 489–494

Acetylcholine
  effects on atrial muscle, 57–61
  response of sinoatrial node cells to, 63–68

Acidosis, energy production in cardiac muscle, 521–531

Action potential
  in atrial muscle, fluoride effects on, 73–78
  from AV node, effects of TTX and verapamil on upstroke components, 69–72

Adenine nucleotides, myocardial, after adenosine infusion, 319–323

Adenosine, myocardial adenine nucleotides after infusion of, 319–323

Adenosine monophosphate
  cyclic
    α-adrenergic reduction of, 431–436
    calcium transport regulation mediated by, 265–272
    effect on extracellular calcium distribution and contractility in heart, 293–296
    protein kinase dependent on, 273–278

Adenosine triphosphatase, myofibrillar activity, 490

Adenosine triphosphatase inhibitors, effect on cardiac electromechanics, 121–130

Adenosine triphosphate
  effects on atrium, 37–44
  glycolytic, production of, during ischemia, 509–519
  influence of, on occurrence of calcium paradox, 565–569
  quinidine influence on calcium binding in presence of, 457–465

Adenylate cyclase, cardiac, subcellular localization of, 227–234

Adrenergic amines, thyroid hormone-induced supersensitivity to cardiac phosphorylase-activating effect of, 413–418

α-Adrenergic reduction of cAMP in ventricular myocardial cells, 431–436

Aging, ventricular contraction duration and diastolic stiffness, 169–173

Anesthesia
  halothane, effects on hemodynamics and myocardium, 467–471
  inhalation, dose-dependent depression of cardiac function and metabolism by, 473–480

Anoxia, effects on reaction of fast sodium system, 79–83

Antiarrhythmic agents, inotropic and chrontropic effects of, on ventricular tissue, 451–455

Aorta, effect of diltiazem on calcium- and noradrenaline-induced contractions of, 437–440

Artery, regulation of contraction, 185–191

Atrial muscle
  effects of ACh and cyclic nucleotides on, 57–61
  fluoride effects on action potential, contraction, and membrane currents, 73–78

Atrium
  effects of ATP and sodium pump on, 37–44
  restitution of full myocardial contractility in, 175–179

[3H] Atropine binding by cardiac plasma membrane-enriched fractions, 249–256

Automaticity, electrically induced, in ventricular myocardium, 45–49

Biochemical aspects, 193–304
Biophysical aspects, 91–192

631

Blood flow, regional myocardial,
    alterations induced by nitrates
    in coronary artery disease,
    501–505

Calcium
    accumulation and release of, by
        cardiac microsomal fractions,
        213–218
    accumulation by microsomes and
        mitochondria, 490
    cAMP effect on extracellular
        distribution of, in heart,
        293–296
    and contraction dynamics, 149–157
    effect of diltiazem on aortic
        contractions induced by,
        437–440
    initial accumulation rates by cardiac
        sarcoplasmic reticulum, 199–204
    metabolism in mitochondria in
        ischemia and after reperfusion,
        533–538
    modulation of, in heart, 195–198
    movement of, and ventricular
        contraction, 131–135
    release of, in excitation-contraction
        coupling, 8
    transport and release by
        sarcoplasmic reticulum,
        205–212
Calcium binding by mitochondria and
    microsomes, influence of
    quinidine on, 457–465
Calcium binding sites of troponin in
    contractile processes, 97–100
Calcium concentration in medium,
    dynamic responses of heart to
    changes in, 159–167
Calcium current
    in cardiac muscle, 13–16
    in excitation-contraction coupling,
        5–8
    membrane, in cardiac excitation,
        37–44
Calcium ions
    in cardiac contractility, 93–101

chronotropic effects of, at different
    temperatures, 51–55
Calcium paradox
    changes in high energy phosphate
        compounds of heart during,
        559–564
    influence of ATP or oxygen plus
        substrate on occurrence of,
        565–569
Calcium transport
    cardiac sarcolemmal, 241–247
    effect of protein kinase on, in
        sarcoplasmic reticulum, 279–284
    by sarcoplasmic reticulum,
        phospholamban in, 265–272
Carbocromene, influence on heart
    FFA metabolism, 363–367
Carbohydrates, myocardial
    metabolism of, 591
Cardiac muscle
    abnormal, energy liberation in,
        583–588
    effect of acetaldehyde on
        functioning of, 489–494
    effect of rapid cooling, 181–184
    effects of insulin on, 441–450
    energy liberation and utilization in
        ischemia, 539–548
    energy production in ischemia and
        acidosis, 521–531
    frequency-dependent changes in
        electromechanical and (Na^+,K^+)-
        ATPase activity, 121–130
    infarcted, effect of glucose-insulin-
        potassium solution on energy
        metabolism of, 549–554
    ionic basis of excitation mechanism
        in, 11–18
    isometric dynamic response to
        $[Ca^{2+}]$ changes of medium,
        159–167
    mechanochemical model, 155
    metabolism of individual fatty
        acids in, 369–377
    tetanic contraction of, 150–151
Cardiopulmonary bypass, effects of
    morphine and halothane on
    cardiac function before and
    after, 481–487

Cardiotoxin, bacterial, 609–614, 615–620, 621–625

Catecholamines
    effects on myocardial energy metabolism, 335–341
    myocardial necrosis induced by, 575–577
    role of phospholamban in action of, on muscle, 270

Cations, divalent, binding by cardiac myosin, 103–109

Chlorpromazine, intraventricular conduction disturbance after, 85–90

Chronotropic effects of calcium and magnesium ions, 51–55

Circulation, coronary, uptake and release of insulin in, 355–361

Circulatory disease, myocardial energy and electrolyte metabolism, 589–598

Contractility
    cardiac
        calcium ion in, 93–101
        effects of acidosis on, 523–524
        effect of cAMP, 293–296
    myocardial
        and cyclic nucleotides, 419–422
        delay in diastolic restitution of full, 175–179
        effects of halothane, 467–471

Contraction
    arterial smooth muscle, regulatory mechanism in, 185–191
    of atrial muscle, fluoride effects on, 73–78
    cardiac, sodium-calcium exchange in regulation of, 137–141
    dynamics of, and calcium, 149–157
    ventricular
        aging, and duration of, 169–173
        rate-dependent change of, and calcium movements, 131–135

Contracture, rapid cooling, 182–184

Cooling, rapid, effect on cardiac muscles, 181–184

Coronary artery disease, changes induced by nitrates, 501–505

Creatine phosphate, myocardial metabolism of, 591

Cyclic nucleotides, effects on atrial muscle, 57–61

Cytochrome aa$_3$, absorption during a heartbeat, 310–311

Dephosphorylation of sarcoplasmic reticulum phosphoprotein, 285–291

Digitalis glycosides, effects on myocardial stiffness, 407–411

Diltiazem, effect on calcium- and noradrenaline-induced aortic contractions, 437–440

Electrical aspects of excitation-contraction coupling, 3–10

Electrocardiogram
    and a cardiotoxin, 610, 612–613
    changes in, and myocardial metabolism, 595–596
    in pulmonary embolism, 607–608

Electroencephalogram and a cardiotoxin, 610, 611–612

Electrogenic transport mechanisms in cardiac muscle, 11–13

Electrolytes
    dependence of cardiac glycoside actions on, at cellular and subcellular levels, 393–399
    myocardial metabolism of, during exercise, 589–598

Electromechanics of cardiac muscle, 121–130

Electron spin resonance spectrometry, studies on myocardial mitochondria by, 599–603

Electrophysiological aspects, 1–90

Electrophysiology of heart cells, 19–24

Embolism, pulmonary, disturbance of myocardial energy metabolism in, 605–608

Energetics of left ventricle, heat loss in, 313–317

Energy, liberation and utilization in
     ischemic cardiac muscle,
     539–548
Energy liberation
  in abnormal cardiac muscle,
     538–588
  myocardial, disturbance of, in
     pulmonary embolism, 605–608
Energy metabolism
  cardiac, spectroscopic approach to,
     307–312
  of infarcted cardiac muscle, effect
     of glucose-insulin-potassium
     solution, 549–554
  myocardial
     catecholamine effects, 335–341
     during exercise, 589–598
  in specialized muscle of heart,
     343–347
Energy production in cardiac muscle
     in ischemia and acidosis,
     521–531
Enflurane, depression of cardiac
     function and metabolism by,
     473–480
Epicardial electrocardiographic
     mapping, 551
Epinephrine, effect on frequency-force
     relationship, 126
Excitation
  cardiac, membrane calcium current
     in, 37–44
  premature in ventricular muscle,
     31–36
Excitation-contraction coupling,
     electrical aspects of, 3–10
Excitation mechanism in cardiac
     muscle, ionic basis of,
     11–18
Exercise
  insulin uptake and release during,
     355–361
  myocardial energy and electrolyte
     metabolism during, 589–598

Fatty acids
  free
     content in myocardial interstitial
        spaces, 385–389
     heart metabolism of, 363–367

metabolism of individual in heart
     muscle, 369–377
  myocardial, and cardiac
     performance, 379–384
  polyene, metabolism in heart
     muscle, 577–579
Fluoride, effects on action potential,
     contraction, and membrane
     currents of atrial muscle, 73–78
Frequency-force relationship
  effect of ATPase inhibitors,
     124–125
  effect of epinephrine, 126
  effect of quinidine, 126–127
  effect of rubidium, 125–126

Glucose
  insulin uptake and release during
     infusion of, 355–361
  metabolism in infarcting tissue,
     516–517
Glucose-insulin-potassium solution,
     effect on energy metabolism of
     infarcted cardiac muscle,
     549–554
Glycosides, cardiac, electrolyte
     dependence at cellular and
     subcellular levels, 393–399
Guanylate cyclase, membrane-bound
     and soluble, of cardiac and
     skeletal muscle, 257–263

Halothane
  depression of cardiac function and
     metabolism by, 473–480
  effects on cardiac function before
     and after cardiopulmonary
     bypass, 481–487
  effects on hemodynamics and
     myocardium, 467–471
Heart
  AMP-dependent protein kinase from
     heart, 273–278
  carbocromene influence on FFA
     metabolism, 363–367
  changes in high energy phosphate
     compounds during calcium
     paradox, 559–564

depression of function and
    metabolism of, by inhalation
    anesthetics, 473–480
energy metabolism in specialized
    muscle of, 343–347
modulation of calcium in, 195–198
myocardial fatty acid and
    performance of, 379–384
production of glycolytic ATP during
    ischemia, 509–519
respiratory control in, 521–523
Heartbeat, stopping of, by
    cardiotoxin, 615–620
Heart cells, electrophysiology of,
    19–24
Heart failure, myocardial
    mitochondria in, 599–603
Heart-lung preparation, pH effect on
    myocardium of, 325–333
Heat loss in energetics of left ventricle,
    313–317
Hemodynamics
    effects of anesthetics on, after
        cardiopulmonary bypass,
        482–484
    effects of halothane on, 467–471
    in pulmonary embolism, 606–607
Hemolysin, thermostable direct,
    produced by *Vibrio
    parahaemolyticus,* 609–614,
    615–620, 621–625
Hyperthyroidism, cholinergic
    antagonism of effects of
    isoproterenol, 423–429
Hypoxia, effects on myocardial
    stiffness, 407–411

Insulin
    effects on mammalian cardiac
        muscle, 441–450
    immunoreactive, uptake and release
        in coronary circulation, 355–361
Intraventricular conduction
    disturbance after chlorpromazine
    treatment, 85–90
Ischemia
    calcium metabolism in
        mitochondria, 533–538
    energy liberation and utilization in
        cardiac muscle, 539–548

energy production in cardiac muscle,
    521–531
myocardial, effect of xanthine
    oxidase inhibitor, 555–558
production of glycolytic ATP
    during, 509–519
Isoproterenol
    effects in hyperthyroidism, 423–429
    effects of
        in absence of glucose, 380–383
        in presence of glucose, 380

Lanthanides, interaction with muscle
    microsomes, 297–304
Lipids, myocardial, role in
    development of cardiac necrosis,
    571–582

Magnesium ions, chronotropic effects
    of, at different temperatures,
    51–55
Membrane conductance, increase in,
    by hemolysin, 621–625
Membrane currents in atrial muscle,
    fluoride effects on, 73–78
Metabolic aspects, 305–389
Metabolic inhibitors, effects on
    reaction of fast sodium
    system, 79–83
Methoxyflurane, depression of cardiac
    function and metabolism by,
    473–480
Microsomal fractions, cardiac, calcium
    accumulation and release by,
    213–218
Microsomes
    cardiac, intact vesicles of membranes
        of, 219–225
    muscle, interaction of lanthanides
        with, 297–304
    quinidine influence on calcium
        binding, 457–465
Mitochondria
    action of nitroglycerin on, 495–500
    myocardial
        studies by ESR spectrometry,
            599–603
        transmural differences in, 349–354

Mitochondria (*continued*)
  oxidative phosphorylation of,
    540–541
  quinidine influence on calcium
    binding, 457–465
  respiration of, 551–554, 608
  role in regulating intracellular
    calcium ion concentration,
    93–97
Morphine, effects on cardiac function
  before and after
  cardiopulmonary bypass,
  481–487
Muscle
  arterial smooth, regulatory
    mechanism in contraction of,
    185–191
  cardiac, *see* Cardiac muscle
  cardiac and skeletal, membrane-
    bound and soluble guanylate
    cyclase, 257–263
  interaction of lanthanides with
    microsomes of, 297–304
  role of phospholamban in
    catecholamine action on, 270
  specialized, of heart, energy
    metabolism in, 343–347
  see also specific organ
Myocardium
  adenine nucleotides in, after
    adenosine infusion, 319–323
  alpha receptors and cAMP in,
    431–436
  calcium metabolism in ischemia,
    533–538
  catecholamine effects on energy
    metabolism in, 335–341
  cyclic nucleotides and
    contractility of, 419–422
  effect of xanthine oxidase inhibitor
    on ischemia, 555–558
  effects of halothane, 467–471
  effects of hypoxia and digitalis
    glycosides on stiffness of,
    407–411
  energy and electrolyte metabolism
    during exercise in patients with
    circulatory disease, 589–598
  energy liberation disturbance in
    pulmonary embolism, 605–608

  fatty acids and cardiac performance,
    379–384
  free fatty acid content in
    interstitial spaces, 385–389
  metabolic effect of pH on, 325–333
  relaxation of, 143–147
  role of lipids in development of
    cardiac necrosis, 571–582
  transmural mitochondrial differences
    in, 349–354
  ventricular, electrically induced
    automaticity in, 45–49
Myofibril, protein phosphorylation,
  111–120
Myosin
  cardiac, divalent cation binding by,
    103–109
  phosphorylation of, 111–114
Myosin B in ischemic myocardium,
  543–546

(Na^+, K^+)-ATPase activity, frequency-
  dependent changes in cardiac
  muscle, 121–130
Necrosis, cardiac, role of myocardial
  lipids in development of,
  571–582
Nitrates, changes induced by, in
  coronary artery disease,
  501–505
Nitroglycerin, action on heart
  mitochondria, 495–500
Noradrenaline, effect of diltiazem on
  aortic contractions induced by,
  437–440
Nucleotides, cyclic, and myocardial
  contractility, 419–422

Ouabain, effect on sodium movement
  in cardiac cells, 401–405
Oxygen concentration during
  contraction-relaxation of heart,
  308–310

Pathophysiological aspects, 507–625
pH, metabolic effect on myocardium
  of heart-lung preparation,
  325–333

Pharmacological aspects, 391—505
Phosphate
    changes in high energy compounds
        during calcium paradox,
        559—564
    in study of calcium accumulation
        and release by cardiac
        microsomal fractions, 213—218
Phospholamban
    in cAMP-mediated regulation of
        calcium transport by
        sarcoplasmic reticulum,
        265—272
    distribution in different types of
        muscle, 268—269
    effect of protein kinase on
        phosphorylation of, 279—284
Phosphoprotein phosphatase,
    dephosphorylation of
    sarcoplasmic reticulum
    catalyzed by, 285—291
Phosphorylase, cardiac, activation by
    adrenergic amines, 413—418
Phosphorylation of cardiac
    myofibrillar proteins, 111—120
Potassium, myocardial uptake of, 591
Protein kinase
    AMP-dependent, from heart,
        273—278
    effect on sarcolemmal calcium
        accumulation, 241—247
    effects in sarcoplasmic reticulum,
        279—284
Proteins, cardiac myofibrillar,
    phosphorylation of, 111—120
Pulmonary artery, myocardial energy
    liberation during embolism of,
    605—608

Quench-flow measurements of Ca²⁺
    accumulation, 199—204
Quinidine
    effect on frequency-force, 126—127
    influence on ATP-linked calcium
        binding by mitochondria and
        microsomes, 457—465

Redoximeter, effects of
    catecholamines on myocardial

energy metabolism studied by,
    335—341
Rubidium, effect on frequency-force
    relationship, 125—126

Sarcolemma
    cardiac
        calcium transport and
            accumulation, 241—247
        isolation and enzymatic
            characterization of, 235—240
        subcellular localization of cardiac
            adenylate cyclase, 227—234
Sarcoplasmic reticulum
    cardiac
        Ca²⁺ transport and release by,
            205—212
        dephosphorylation of 22,000-
            dalton phosphoprotein of,
            285—291
        initial rates of Ca²⁺ accumulation
            by, 199—204
        slow calcium uptake by, 206—208
        effects of protein kinase, 279—284
        phospholamban in calcium transport
            by, 265—272
        subcellular localization of cardiac
            adenylate cyclase, 227—234
Sinoatrial node cells
    response to acetylcholine, 63—68
    voltage-clamp experiments by
        double microelectrode
        technique, 25—29
Sodium-calcium exchange in
    regulation of cardiac
    contraction, 137—141
Sodium current in cardiac muscle,
    13—16
Sodium movement in cardiac cells,
    effect of ouabain on, 401—405
Sodium pump
    effects on atrium, 37—44
    electrogenic, contribution to
        response of node cell to ACh,
        63—68
Sodium system, fast, effects of anoxia
    and metabolic inhibitors on
    reaction of, 79—83

Spectrometry, electron spin resonance, studies on myocardial mitochondria by, 599—603

Spectroscopy, cardiac energy metabolism, 307—312

Thyroid hormone, supersensitivity to cardiac phosphorylase-activating effect of adrenergic amines, 413—418

Troponin
  phosphorylation of, 114—119
  role of calcium binding sites of, in contractile processes, 97—100

TTX, effects on upstroke components of action potential from AV node, 69—72

Tyrode, low sodium solution, and membrane conductance, 623—624

Vectorcardiogram in pulmonary embolism, 607—608

Ventricle
  conduction disturbance after chlorpromazine, 85—90
  divalent cation binding by myosin, 103—109
  inotropic and chronotropic effects of antiarrhythmic agents on, 451—455

left
  aging and diastolic stiffness, 169—173
  alterations induced by nitrates in coronary artery disease, 501—505
  heat loss in energetics of, 313—317
  rate-dependent contraction change in, and calcium movements, 131—135
  role of slow inward current on premature excitation in, 31—36

Verapamil, effects on upstroke components of action potential from AV node, 69—72

Vesicles, cardiac microsomal, and vectorial properties of integral enzymes, 219—225

Vibrio parahaemolyticus, thermostable direct hemolysin produced by, 609—614, 615—620, 621—625

Voltage-clamp studies
  by double microelectrode technique, in sinoatrial node cell, 25—29
  of excitation-contraction coupling, 4—8
  of heart cells, 26—27

Xanthine oxidase inhibitor, effect on myocardial ischemia, 555—558